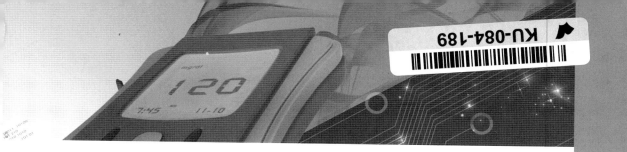

Diabetes Management in Primary Care

SECOND EDITION

Jeff Unger, MD

Founder, Unger Primary Care Center
Director of Metabolic Studies
Catalina Research Institute
Chino, California
Assistant Professor of Family Medicine
Loma Linda University School of Medicine
Loma Linda, California

Edited by Zachary Schwartz

Wolters Kluwer | Lippincott Williams & Wilkins
Health
Philadelphia • Baltimore • New York • London
Buenos Aires • Hong Kong • Sydney • Tokyo

Senior Acquisitions Editor: Sonya Seigafuse
Senior Product Manager: Kerry Barrett
Vendor Manager: Alicia Jackson
Senior Manufacturing Manager: Benjamin Rivera
Senior Marketing Manager: Kimberly Schonberger
Senior Designer: Joan Wendt
Production Service: SPi Global

Printed in China

Library of Congress Cataloging-in-Publication Data
Unger, Jeff, M.D.
  Diabetes management in primary care / Jeff Unger; edited by Zac Schwartz. — 2nd ed.
      p. ; cm.
  Includes bibliographical references and index.
  ISBN 978-1-4511-4295-2
  I. Schwartz, Zac. II. Title.
  [DNLM: 1. Diabetes Mellitus—therapy. 2. Primary Health Care. WK 815]
  616.4'62—dc23

                                                          2012016534

To purchase additional copies of this book, call our customer service department at (800) 638-3030 or fax orders to (301) 223-2320. International customers should call (301) 223-2300.

Visit Lippincott Williams & Wilkins on the Internet: at LWW.com. Lippincott Williams & Wilkins customer service representatives are available from 8:30 am to 6 pm, EST.

10 9 8 7 6 5 4 3 2 1

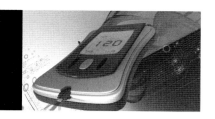

Dedication

*This remarkable project is dedicated to my talented and extraordinary family.
To my wife and soul-mate, Lisa, who once said she "looked forward to growing old
with me"—it's time to go to Jamaica! To Sarah (AKA Bear), who guards
the front desk of my office as if it were a national treasure.
I am so proud of you! To Brett—a son and big brother famous for carrying his
sister up and down a waterfall three times—Don't worry; we'll find your hat as
soon as I finish writing this book! To Muffin, who loves to read me "bedtime stories"
consisting of journal articles I've written using words she can't pronounce—
you are writing songs that will make the whole world sing! To Gracie, who has lost
out on spending so many weekends with her "Daddu" while he worked on this book.
Daddy loves you for always having your finger on my continuous glucose sensor.
Thanks for always asking, "Are you OK, Daddy?" Finally, I would like to thank
my guardian angels who gave me the inner strength to bring
this project to a safe and healthy conclusion:
Papa, Nanalea, Mom, and Bubby and Granny.*

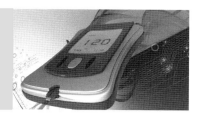

Foreword

I remember asking to be the speaker at a dinner program in Costa Mesa, California for a newly released diabetes medication a few years ago. As an endocrinologist I really enjoy introducing new drugs, technologies, and concepts to primary care physicians (PCPs), or for that matter, anyone who wants to listen to me preach about the importance of intensifying glycemic control. That night there must have been at least 20 practitioners in the restaurant who were very interested in what I had to say as well as picking my brain about my diabetes experience.

With over 5,000 Americans each day being diagnosed with diabetes, there is a sense of urgency in screening high-risk patients for prediabetes and instituting prevention strategies early as well as aggressive clinical management of diabetes. The basic concept of diabetes management remains to minimize "glycemic burden." When patients are diagnosed as having prediabetes, simply introducing them to healthy lifestyle interventions such as reducing their dietary intake of saturated fat and walking 30 to 45 minutes each day will prevent many of them from progressing to T2DM or even help them to revert back to normal glucose tolerance. Do you think I'm going to see these high-risk patients in my clinic? No way…I am too busy taking care of complicated patients with diabetes with complicated regimens and unfortunately with advanced complications due to years and years of poor control. (More on this later) This is why it is so important that PCPs feel comfortable incorporating proven strategies related to prevention, early detection, and aggressive management of diabetes into their daily interaction with all patients.

Managing a patient with prediabetes, or even newly diagnosed diabetes, is a lot easier than trying to fix all the complex, interrelated complications I see in patients with advanced disease. Who would you guys rather take care of on a busy Friday afternoon? A high-risk patient whom you've just identified as having prediabetes with an A1C of 6.3% and no apparent complications, or "Aunt Sally" who is brought in on a gurney by paramedics for chest pain and found to have a blood glucose value of 481 mg/dL?

I'm in no way suggesting the PCPs should handle only the "easy" cases of diabetes. In fact, anything I do primary care doctors can do as well. As a teacher, I am delighted to see that more clinicians are not only interested in initiating insulin earlier, but adding on meal time insulin and GLP-1 analogues and encouraging their patients to become more adept at self-management. Patients are also getting smarter and more active with their own care by carrying in articles to their PCPs describing everything from insulin pump therapy and continuous glucose sensing to websites helping them become volunteers for clinical trials. Consumer programs such as Taking Control of Your Diabetes have taught hundreds of thousands of patients since 1995 how their lives might be enhanced through a variety of education portals including national conferences, TV, books, newsletters, and an active website. The word has spread to health-care providers, consumers, government officials, and the pharmaceutical industry that we, as members of the diabetes community, are a powerful and united voice. *Our ultimate goal is to STOP diabetes after which we may focus our efforts on other disease states that also require our attention.*

My relationship with Jeff Unger started many years ago. As Jeff explains it, I was the one who actually got him interested in the field, diabetes…although this may not be exactly factual. (Jeff still claims that before we met, he really wanted to be a forensic pathologist!) We have shared the podium at many conferences over the years and even presented national diabetes programs on live TV. Jeff's energy, passion, and desire to teach diabetes is unmatched amongst his primary care peers. *The second edition of Diabetes Management in Primary Care covers every topic one needs to care for patients in the outpatient setting. Some of the concepts discussed in the book, such as cultural diversity, the relationship between cancer and diabetes, the slow death of an injured beta-cell, and the effect of sleep deprivation and insulin resistance are worthy of a guest appearance on "The Edelman Report" (www.tcoyd. org). Any clinician who reads this book should develop a heightened level of confidence in assisting patients with diabetes to live life to their fullest potential.*

That dinner in Costa Mesa many years ago was very special for me because Dr. Unger was also in attendance. Although the drug which was being promoted had just been approved by the FDA, Jeff had already been working with the medication within his primary care–based clinical trials program. I was able to sit down, relax, eat my steak, and advance the slide deck while Dr. Unger pretty much convinced everyone in attendance, including me, that the drug in question was safe, was effective, and had multiple advantages over other antihyperglycemic medications. By the end of the evening, all of us in attendance had become better clinicians and students in the disease state of diabetes.

Some may suggest that the secrets of successfully stopping diabetes rest within the pages of this textbook. For those who doubt my words, read on…

Steven V. Edelman, MD
Professor of Medicine in the Division of Endocrinology, Diabetes, and Metabolism
University of California at San Diego (UCSD)
Founder and Director of Taking Control of Your Diabetes (TCOYD)

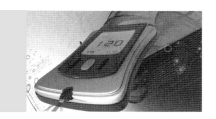

Preface

Let the reader of the second edition of *Diabetes Management in Primary Care* be forewarned… I will be looking for you!

One of my favorite lecture tactics when speaking to large groups of clinicians is to ask the audience this very simple question, "Who amongst you has cared for a patient with diabetes in the past 2 weeks whom you consider to have been 'noncompliant'?" Immediately 90% of the people in the crowd not only raise their hands but also relate a story on noncompliance with another attendee (whom they have never met) about their most problematic patient. (By the way, the remaining 10% of audience members who did not raise their hands are each living with diabetes.) The lecture hall briefly becomes filled with laughter and tales about patients who are totally inept at diabetes self-management.

Soon, those attendees who are so pleased to have finally determined that the true barrier to successful diabetes management is patient incompetence stop smiling as I challenge them with the following barrage of questions: "OK, so your patients are noncompliant with their diabetes management? Let's turn the mirror on ourselves for just a few minutes. How many of you in the audience are willing to check your blood glucose levels four times each day? How many of you know how to count carbohydrates? How many of you know how to inject insulin? How many of you can appropriately dose insulin based on the pre-meal glucose value *and* add in a correction factor if the sugar is over 200 mg/dL? How many of you exercise 5 days a week for 30 minutes each session? How many of you know how to monitor for and predict impending hypoglycemia? If you were on glucocorticoids, how would you adjust your insulin doses to minimize those nasty postprandial excursions? How many of you would remember to take your blood pressure medications, your statin, your aspirin, and three of your oral antidiabetic agents every day and remember to get them refilled monthly? How many of you have seen an eye doctor in the past year? A dentist? A nephrologist? How many of you with sexual dysfunction feel comfortable discussing this complication with your primary care physician? Do you snore? Do you get least 7 to 8 hours of sleep each night? If you are on metformin and have stage 3 kidney disease, do you know how to modify the dose of that drug? While we're at it, what drug doses should be monitored and adjusted for patients with renal insufficiency? If you have a patient with mental illness and diabetes, which of these two chronic illnesses should be managed preferentially? If you have a body mass index over 40 kg/m^2, would you consider undergoing metabolic surgery to minimize your cardiovascular risk? If you personally had diabetes, could you do everything you are asking your patients to do each and every day and maintain an A1C of less than 7%? Now, let me ask the question once again, "How many of you in the audience have seen a patient in the past 2 weeks whom you consider as being noncompliant?" This time, no one raises their hand.

Perhaps out of respect for the disease state or the speaker, the audience now begins to focus on what they can do as a group as well as individually to assist those patients who can make up 40% of their primary care population. They understand that diabetes is a complicated, progressive, and mysterious chronic disease that requires self-dedication and perseverance. Treatment decisions must be made multiple times each day by patients based on what information they are provided by their physician and educator. Patients also realize that each therapeutic option they consider at any time may ultimately be vetoed by their "significant other" who may be either a guardian angel or a member of the dreaded "diabetes police corp."

When I began writing this second edition of *Diabetes Management in Primary Care*, I wanted to address the complex and, perhaps, controversial issues facing PCPs in today's office setting. As a group, PCPs manage patients with infertility, sleep apnea, cancer, severe clinical obesity, Parkinson's disease, asthma, peripheral vascular disease, and coronary artery disease. We are trained to screen high-risk patients for chronic diseases and evaluate others for mental illness. Our offices are havens for obese adolescents who are rapidly becoming the flag bearers of type 2 diabetes in the United States. Pharmaceutical companies continue to provide us with new oral and injectable agents to manage our hyperglycemic patients. More novel agents are likely to be introduced in the near future. The federal government appears to be more concerned with monitoring meaningful use data than incentivizing practitioners who dare to accept the challenges related to screening, prevention, and reversal of those afflicted with impaired glucose intolerance.

Diabetes Management in Primary Care provides enough resources, rational thought, and even some controversial political analysis for readers of all levels. Although written by a family physician who himself has type 1 diabetes, the content covers topics related to everything from cultural diversity to adjusting insulin doses for patients during chemotherapy. The aim of every chapter is simply to provide clinicians with the most appropriate means of patient-centered intensification of care. I will provide you with the tools you need for successful diabetes management. All the reader has to do is explore the options presented and choose what appears to be the most rational, safe, and evidence-based route toward achieving one's targeted metabolic goals.

The second edition of *Diabetes Management in Primary Care* was written to enlighten PCPs on what they may be overlooking while treating their patients with diabetes. Patients rely on their physicians for guidance, insight, coaching, and confidence in their struggle to minimize their glycemic burden. Although the disease may appear overwhelming at times, one should remember the "top five" rules required for successful diabetes self-management: (1) Know your metabolic treatment targets. (2) Understand how to achieve those treatment targets. (3) Stop smoking. (4) Become adherent to the prescribed behavioral and pharmacologic treatment regimen. (5) Make certain that your provider is dedicated to teaching patients successful diabetes self-management.

Some of my peer reviewers have suggested that the book is the most comprehensive review of diabetes they have ever read. Still, these words mean little unless the reader understands the concepts upon which they were written. My undertaking in writing this book was to slow the epidemic of diabetes in the United States by improving the care provided to this population by primary care physicians. By the year 2050, one-third of all adults in the United States will be diagnosed with diabetes. May I suggest that your dedication to studying the content of this textbook might be our best opportunity to slow the explosive progression of this extraordinary disease?

Jeff Unger, MD
Founder, Unger Primary Care Center
Director of Metabolic Studies
Catalina Research Institute
Chino, California

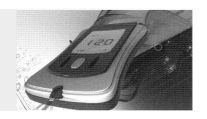

Acknowledgments

As I am a physician trained in family medicine, some may question the scientific validity of some or all of the content contained within this comprehensive book about diabetes management. While writing the manuscripts for each chapter, I wanted to make certain that the scientific statements implied by myself and my publisher were accurate, evidence-based, clinically relevant, and practical. Each chapter was evaluated by an "expert reviewer" whose suggestions were incorporated into the final manuscript. Several of my "mentors" volunteered their expertise and valuable time to tutoring me about complex concepts, which I have hopefully been able to translate into meaningful, practical, and clinical terms for our primary care audience. A special thanks to Drs. Stanley Schwartz (*do you ever sleep?*), Bob Chilton (*the National Geographic Photographer of Cardiology*), Jason Brett, Alan Moses, Todd Hobbs (*Yes, "you guys" are going to cure diabetes some day*), Tim Heise (*who now loves country music*), Ted Okerson (*my metabolic surgery mentor*), Bryan Gallagher (*a guy who dreams about PCOS every night—I think*), Titus Gylvin (*Dallas Cowboys? Who are they?*), Javier "Firecracker" Morales, Joe Tibaldi (*The Lord of Flatbush Diabetes*), Jeff Freeman (*GLP-1 is in his blood—fortunately*), Anshul Varshney (*Injecting the eye is fun. Giving an insulin shot—are you crazy?*), Richard Bruck (*my next book will be on cardiology*), Robert Henry (*just greeting him should qualify you for CME credit*), Jeff Koch (*the greatest lipid teacher of all time*), Alan Dietzek (*he wants everyone to know he is a surgeon*), Doug Muchmore (*yes, Doug, you are FAST*), Juan Frias (*Chino, NOT Chico*), Michael Cobble (*Grandma told you about the sugar. You should have listened*), and Rabbi Dovid Weiss (*baruch ha-shem*)!

Without hesitation, my highest level of gratitude goes to my Dad, Dr. Donald Unger, and my Grandpa, Dr. Leon Unger. Both are past Presidents of the American College of Allergy and instrumental at creating and evolving this essential medical specialty. As a senior med student I remember seeing the disappointment on both their faces when I announced that I had opted to pursue a career in family medicine rather than apply for the expected allergy fellowship. In retrospect, both are to blame for my defection to primary care. As a child, I used to accompany my Dad on house calls and watch him administer aminophylline to severely asthmatic patients. After the patients began to breathe comfortably, they would always say, "Thank you, Dr. Unger!" I also spent time with my Grandfather at his office in Chicago. I always noticed a special bond that Grandpa had with his patients. Grandpa would smile, hold their hands, and reassure them that all would be well. Quite comforting knowing that treatment options historically for asthma in the 1950s consisted of prednisone, Benadryl, and epinephrine. Yet, patients DID get better, and were very appreciative of the doctor's efforts. I guess I wanted to be just like them, and Uncle Charlie, Cousin Maj, Uncle Jerry, Cousin Randy, and everyone else in my family who was, or is, a physician. You are **ALL** my heroes!

I would like to dedicate Chapter 8 (diabetes and cancer) to my father-in-law, Les Davis, who succumbed to pancreatic cancer last year. The challenges of managing both his diabetes and the pancreatic cancer came to light while Papa was being chastised by a hospital nurse and a dietitian for eating ice cream and "being a terrible diabetic!" Hanging my head in shame as if I had been convicted of violating my Hippocratic Oath, I nevertheless saw my scheming cousin, Stevie, spoon feeding Papa the forbidden snack. When the "food police" left the room, we high-fived each other after which I simply adjusted the dose of his insulin to match his carbohydrate intake. Two hours later his blood glucose level was 125 mg/dL. A team approach is often needed when dealing with complex diabetes conditions, and it sure helps when Stevie is on your side!

Finally, I appreciate the time and dedication that each of the following clinicians has spent helping me teach others how to manage such a challenging and fascinating disease state. These mentors provided me with ideas, manuscript reviews, photographs, and other documents that assisted me in the authorship of this comprehensive primary care–oriented textbook.

Lippincott "Hall of Fame Expert Reviewers" for *Diabetes Management in Primary Care,* **2nd edition.**

- Andy Ajello
- Navin Amin, MD
- Tim Bailey, MD
- Reinhard Beel
- Lotte Bjerre Knudsen, MD
- Larry Blonde, MD
- Bruce Bode, MD
- Susan Bonner-Weir, PhD
- Jason Brett, MD
- Richard Bruck, MD
- Stephen Brunton, MD
- Joe Calleros
- Jack Carlson, MD
- Robert Chilton, DO
- Michael Cobble, MD
- Nechama Cohen
- Barry Cole, MD
- Phil Cryer, MD
- David D'Alessio, MD
- Ralph DeFronzo, MD
- Alan Dietzek, MD
- Rabbi Dovid Weiss
- Steve Edelman, MD
- Danny Farber, MD
- Jerry Farber, MD
- Juan Frias, MD
- Jeff Freeman, DO
- Bryan Gallagher, MD
- Alan Garber, MD, PhD
- Satish Garg, MD
- Carlos Gonzalez, MD
- Titus Gylvin, MD
- Tim Heise, MD
- Robert Henry, MD
- Don Hilty, MD
- Irl Hirsch, MD
- Todd Hobbs, MD
- Todd Houtman
- Jeff Jackson, MD
- Klaus Jensen, MD
- Lotte Bjerre Knudsen
- Jeff Koch, MD
- Jack Leahy, MD
- David Maggs, MD
- Wayne Martin, MD
- Juris Meier, MD
- Luigi Meneghini, MD
- Javier Morales, MD
- Stephen Mouhapt, MD
- Doug Muchmore, MD
- Ted Okerson, MD
- Jesper Ostegaard Jensen
- Jerzy Paprocki, MD
- Chris Parkin, MS
- Joan Perez, CDE
- Athena Phyllis-Tsmikas, MD
- Dan Pollom, MD
- Bill Polonsky, PhD
- Richard Pratley, MD
- David Price, MD
- Michael Robinson, MD
- Julio Rosenstock, MD
- Stanley Schwartz, MD
- Leo Seaman, MD
- Fannie Smith, MD, PhD
- Bill Tamborlane, MD
- Joe Tibaldi, MD
- Donald L. Unger, MD
- Anshul Varshney, MD
- Gordon Weir, MD
- John West, MD
- Yizhen Xu, MD

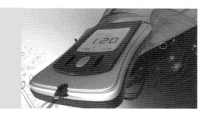

Contents

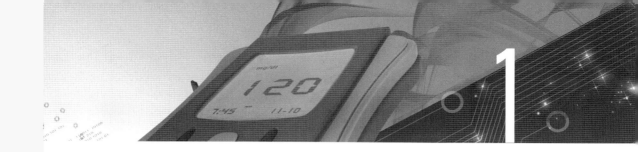

Introduction to Diabetes

Everybody gets so much information all day long that they lose their common sense.
—Gertrude Stein, American writer (1874–1946)

Primary Care Physicians Are the Cornerstone for Diabetes Care in the United States

Management of the patient with diabetes mellitus—a chronic, progressive, and potentially disabling illness—epitomizes the spirit of primary care medicine. Although specialists are often asked to evaluate and treat patients who have advanced complications or require complex treatment regimens, 90% of patients with diabetes can successfully be managed in a primary care setting.[1,2] Primary care physicians (PCPs) can screen high-risk patients for diabetes, initiate treatment to reduce hyperglycemia, monitor and fine-tune pharmacologic therapies, as well as detect and manage microvascular and macrovascular complications. Family physicians also provide a portal for important life-altering information to their patients, such as access to certified diabetes educators (CDEs) and registered dietitians (RDs).

We are our patients' first line of defense for ensuring that their pregnancies have favorable outcomes, when we begin to discuss preconception planning with adolescents with diabetes. Armed with the knowledge that eating disorders are frequently encountered in adolescent patients with type 1 diabetes mellitus (T1DM), we are able to elicit a history of the "danger signs" that are suggestive of this dangerous behavior pattern. Athletes seek our advice on how to manage their medication therapy when they are training for a marathon or seeking to join the high school football team. We are on the front lines for patients complaining of sleep disorders.

As specialists in the management of chronic disease states, we understand the frustrations that our patients express in wanting to "eliminate" medications on each visit because their metabolic targets may actually be improving. Unfortunately, modifying a disease state does not translate into a cure. Diabetes is a chronic progressive disease often coexisting with hypertension, hyperlipidemia, atherosclerosis, major depression, sleep disorders, obesity, painful neuropathy, and sexual dysfunction. Some fortunate individuals actually manage to navigate through the "mine fields of glycemic burden" unscathed and develop no long-term microvascular or macrovascular complications. Others may start as role models for other patients by maintaining near normal metabolic control for years, only to develop neuropathy, cancer, Parkinson disease, or hearing loss later in life.

Because PCPs monitor every aspect of their patient's metabolic history, we should not hesitate to share this information openly with other specialists. Imagine the appreciation an ophthalmologist would likely show if a patient arrived at his or her office complete with an updated medical history, A1C level, and lipid panel. Most specialists are forced to provide patient care without having access to this information, which may delay the integration of certain therapies into the patient's treatment regimen. For example, how could a nephrologist offer any advice to a patient who says only, "My doctor sent me to you because he thinks my kidneys are failing. But honestly, I feel just fine!" Where is the patient's estimated glomerular filtration rate (eGFR), hemoglobin, A1C level, serum calcium, intact parathyroid hormone level, or test for urinary albumin excretion? What medications is the patient taking? Is there a family history of chronic kidney disease? Does the patient have hypertension or hyperlipidemia? Is the patient smoking? Timely and comprehensive communication with specialists not only enhances coordination of care, but minimizes the liklihood of subjecting patients to redundant or costly testing procedures..

PCPs have a unique opportunity to evaluate, predict, and prevent many of the devastating long-term complications associated with diabetes. Simply identifying patients at high risk for diabetes developing based on their family history, ethnicity, history of gestational diabetes, or body-fat distribution should warrant the introduction of lifestyle and behavioral interventions that could delay or prevent the onset of diabetes. Intensive and customized management designed to normalize hyperglycemia and other metabolic anomalies early in the course of the disease can improve outcomes.[3–5]

• The Diabetes Pandemic

Twenty-six million Americans have diabetes and an additional 79 million Americans are estimated to have prediabetes. Approximately 5% to 10% have T1DM, 90% to 95% have type 2 diabetes mellitus (T2DM), and 1% to 5% are diagnosed with disorders such as gestational diabetes, monogenetic diabetes (MODY), or secondary causes of diabetes such as cystic fibrosis. With increasing numbers of the obese, the elderly, and members of higher-risk minority groups in the population, prevalence is increasing.[6] Twenty-seven percent of all patients with diabetes, and 7 million Americans with prediabetes are unaware that they are afflicted with the disorder.[6] Projections from the CDC indicate that the prevalence of diabetes is likely to increase fourfold within the next 40 years. By 2030, 55.5 million adults aged 18 to 79 years will have diabetes with the prevalence rising to 86.6 million adults by 2050. Assuming an adult population of 306 million and an undiagnosed diabetic population of 13.7 million in 2050, as many as one in three adults in the United States will have diabetes by midcentury (Fig. 1-1).[7]

A study conducted by the Institute for Alternative Futures (IAF) identified California, Texas, Florida, New York, Ohio, Illinois, Georgia, Pennsylvania, North Carolina, and Michigan as "diabetes hot spots," where the burden of diabetes will be greatest within the next 15 years.[8] The IAF diabetes model estimates that the overall number of people in the United States living with diabetes will increase 64% by 2025 to 53.1 million. This equates to one in seven Americans. The resulting medical and societal cost of diabetes will be almost $514 billion—a 72% increase from 2010 and comparable to the total budget for Medicare in 2010.[9]

Currently, the 10 states identified as diabetes hot spots shoulder nearly 60% of the cost from diabetes or approximately $176 billion of the total $299 billion. In 15 years, the aggregate direct cost of diabetes care to these 10 states is projected to jump to $297 billion, nearly exceeding the entire cost of diabetes care within the entire United States today.[8] (The prevalence and cost of diabetes for each of the 50 states plus 13 major metropolitan areas for the years 2000, 2010, 2015, and 2025 may be found at www.altfutures.org/diabetes2025.)

These projections provide further insight into the growing threat of diabetes toward public health. The burden for preventing, screening, and managing diabetes will lie within the primary care domain. Cost may best be mitigated by preventing costly long-term complications. This will require cost-effective disease prevention programs targeting high-risk populations. High-risk patients will require customized programs designed to encourage the adaptation of healthy lifestyle changes into

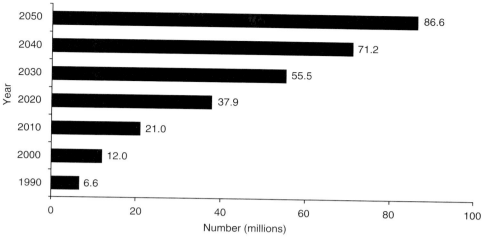

Figure 1-1 • Estimated Prevalence of Diagnosed Type 2 Diabetes in the United States from 1990 to 2050
From 2010 through 2050 the prevalence of T2DM in the United States will increase fourfold with one in every three adults becoming diagnosed with the disorder. (An increase in diabetes prevalence rates of 165%.) Reference: Boyle JP, Thompson TJ, Gregg EW, et al. Projection of the year 2050 burden of diabetes in the U.S. adult population: dynamic modeling of incidence, mortality, and prediabetes prevalence. *Popul Health Metr.* 2010;8:29; National Diabetes Information Clearinghouse: http://diabetes.niddk.nih.gov/dm/pubs/overview/#scope. Accessed October 20, 2011.

one's daily routine. Lifestyle intervention is the least expensive of all diabetes intervention programs, yet the most difficult to initiate and maintain over time. For clinicians who believe changing behaviors should be second nature, try brushing your teeth with your opposite hand. Not so easy to do. Right?

Rates of diabetes are increasing worldwide. At least 171 million people currently have diabetes, and this figure is likely to more than double to 366 million by 2030. The top ten countries, in numbers of people with diabetes, are currently India, China, the United States, Indonesia, Japan, Pakistan, Russia, Brazil, Italy, and Bangladesh. The greatest percentage increase in rates of diabetes will occur in Africa over the next 20 years. At least 80% of people in Africa with diabetes are undiagnosed, and many in their 30s to 60s will die from diabetes in that continent.[10]

The prevalence of T2DM varies widely among various racial and ethnic groups. T2DM is more prevalent among Hispanics, Native Americans, African Americans, and Asians/Pacific Islanders than in non-Hispanic whites. Indeed, the disease is becoming virtually pandemic in some groups of Native Americans and Hispanic people. T2DM is less common in non-Western countries where the diet contains fewer calories and daily caloric expenditure is higher. However, as people in these countries adopt Western lifestyles, weight gain and T2DM are becoming virtually epidemic.

Diabetes Prevalence is Increasing in Children and Adolescents

PCPs are observing an increase in the incidence of T2DM within their adolescent patient population, particularly in high-risk racial and ethnic groups. New onset T2DM now accounts for 8% to 45% of all pediatric diabetes cases.[11] In the years 2002 to 2005, among children and adolescents aged 10 to 19 years, the estimated rate of new cases of T1DM was 18.6 per 100,000 per year, compared with the estimated rate of new cases of T2DM of 8.5 per 100,000 per year.[12]

Not infrequently, adolescents who are diagnosed with T2DM have evidence of islet autoimmunity (see Table 1-1). Obese adolescents with T2DM who are autoantibody positive have severe insulin deficiency and pancreatic β-cell failure as opposed to those who test antibody negative.[13] The presence or absence of autoantibodies in children or adolescents will distinguish whether the patient has T1DM or T2DM. Any patient with clinical evidence of diabetes who tests autoantibody negative should be diagnosed as having T2DM (Table 1-1).[14]

Obesity in adolescents is the environmental trigger that ignites the fuse of the overworked and overstressed pancreatic β-cells. The body may respond in one of two ways to this growth-induced physiologic stress. As in adults, individuals with "super β-cell" are able to produce enough insulin to maintain euglycemia for a prolonged period of time. Those patients who progress to clinical diabetes fall victim to the "accelerator hypothesis," which contends that β-cell function and mass are genetically programmed to fail over time. Patients who develop diabetes are simply unable to maintain normal β-cell function over time. Those individuals who elicit an autoimmune response within their islets will progress more rapidly toward chronic hyperglycemia and become ketosis prone against a

 TABLE 1-1. Differentiating T1DM and T2DM in Young Patients

Diagnostic Characteristic	T1DM	T2DM
Weight	20% may be overweight.	Virtually all BMI > 85th percentile for age
Typical clinical course	Usually rapid onset 35%–40% present with diabetic ketoacidosis.	Slow onset Ketonuria at diagnosis = 33% Mild DKA at diagnosis = 5%–25% Other presenting symptoms include blurry vision, monilial vaginitis, polyuria, and polydipsia. Hyperglycemic, hyperosmolar, nonketotic state may be life threatening.
Genetic predisposition	5% with T1DM Up to 30% may have with T2DM. A family history of T2DM increases risk of T1DM two- to threefold.	74%–100%: first to second degree with T2DM
Comorbidities	Thyroid, adrenal, vitiligo, celiac	Polycystic ovary syndrome, acanthosis nigricans, coronary artery disease, obstructive sleep apnea, dyslipidemia
C-peptide level	C-peptide can be preserved at diagnosis.	Normal or increased
Antibodies	85% have islet autoimmunity: 8.1% have ICA 30% have GAD 35% have IAA	Negative autoantibodies
Interpretation of antibody status	Positive autoimmunity suggests the major pathogenesis is defective insulin secretion.	Negative autoimmunity suggests the major pathogenesis is impairment of endogenous insulin action for both glucose and fat metabolism.
Recommended therapies	Insulin Lifestyle modification	Lifestyle modification Metformin is the only oral agent that is FDA approved in children and adolescents Insulin

ICA, Islet cell antibody; GAD, glutamic acid decarboxylase; IAA, Insulin autoantibodies.
Adapted from Tfayli H, Bacha F, Gungor N, et al. Phenotypic type 2 diabetes in obese youth: insulin sensitivity and secretion in islet cell antibody-negative versus -positive patients. *Diabetes*. 2009;58:738–744.

background of obesity and insulin resistance. Exogenous physiologic insulin replacement therapy will be needed in these patients[15]

Lifestyle modification remains the treatment of choice for adolescents with T2DM. Long-term outcome studies evaluating the safety and efficacy of intensive dietary and exercise therapies versus pharmacotherapies have not been performed in the adolescent population. However, few could argue that some weight reduction with guidance provided by a certified diabetic educator or a registered dietitian is undesirable. PCPs should insist that patients eliminate sugary drinks and high-caloric foods from their daily diets. Meal skipping may become a precursor to disordered eating behaviors. Daily exercise should be encouraged. Determining the true benefits of adapting healthy lifestyle changes is problematic as approximately 65% of adolescent patients with T2DM treated with lifestyle intervention alone are lost to follow-up.[16]

Currently, metformin is the only FDA-approved oral agent for the management of T2DM in children and adolescents.[17] In a randomized placebo-controlled trial of metformin in adolescents with new-onset T2DM, metformin treatment resulted in a significantly lower A1C after 16 weeks compared with placebo (7.5% vs. 8.6%).[18] Metabolic surgery may be considered for patients with T2DM having a BMI greater than 35 kg per m^2 in association with serious comorbidities (sleep apnea, heart disease, and hypertension, which is discussed in detail in Chapter 10).

Comorbid hyperlipidemia in adolescent patients with T2DM must also be managed aggressively. The accepted targeted goals include an LDL-C of less than 100 mg/dL, triglycerides less than 150 mg/dL, and HDL-C greater than 35 mg/dL. Pharmacotherapy for LDL with a statin should be considered when the LDL-C is greater than 160 mg/dL. Statin therapy has been shown to be safe and effective in adolescent patients. Triglyceride levels greater than 1,000 mg/dL should be treated with a fibric acid to reduce the risk of pancreatitis.[19]

The differences in response to treatment and prevention of long-term complications between obese adolescent patients with either T1DM or T2DM have yet to be clearly determined.

Can Primary Care Providers Make a Positive Impact on National Trends Related to Diabetes Care?

The National Health Survey Act of 1956 established an effective means by which the continued assessment of the health and welfare of U.S. citizens could be evaluated.[20] Since 1959, eight separate surveys, evaluating over 130,000 individuals have been completed under the supervision of the Department of Health and Human Services. Originally, two separate surveys on nutrition and health issues were conducted. In 1970, the National Nutrition Surveillance System and the National Health Examination were combined to form the National Health and Nutrition Examination Survey (NHANES).

NHANES data are collected by "probability sampling." The country is divided into geographic areas, known as "primary sampling units" (PSUs). The PSUs are then combined to form strata that are divided into a series of neighborhoods. Inhabitants living within these neighborhoods are chosen randomly to determine their eligibility for NHANES participation. In theory, each selected participant represents approximately 50,000 comparable U.S. residents. Eligible participants are referred to local mobile examination centers where they undergo comprehensive historical interviews, physical examinations, and laboratory studies. (The diabetes questionnaire for NHANES 2008 may be accessed at http://www.cdc.gov/nchs/nhanes/nhanes2007-2008/DIQ_E.htm#DIQ190C.)

NHANES provides important insight into many chronic disease states including obesity, diabetes, arthritis, cardiovascular disorders, COPD, cholelithiasis, kidney disorders, osteoporosis, and cancer. Data obtained from NHANES are used by researchers, health care professionals, and public health officials to design a variety of public health initiatives directed at improving the health outcomes of U.S. citizens.

NHANES data have demonstrated that glycemic control in the United States has actually improved substantially from 1999 through 2004. In 1999, only 37% of patients achieved the ADA desired A1C target of less than 7%, whereas in 2004, 55.7% of individuals were successful at attaining an A1C below 7% (Fig. 1-2). This important achievement also proposes that a 0.5%

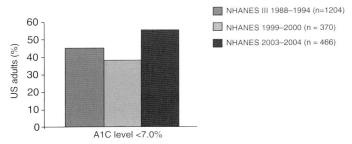

Figure 1-2 • **Adults with Previously Diagnosed Diabetes Achieving ADA-recommended A1C Goal**
ADA, American Diabetes Association; NHANES, National Health and Nutrition Examination Survey.
Reference: National Institutes of Health. The National Diabetes Education Program: 10 years of progress
1997–2007. August 2007. Available at: www.ndep.nih.gov/media/ndep_progressrpt07.pdf. Accessed
December 22, 2011.

reduction in A1C when maintained over 10 years would produce a 10.7% reduction in diabetes complications while improving all-cause mortality and direct costs attributed to glycemic burden.[21]

Much of the efforts for improving the outcomes of patients with diabetes are attributed to the efforts of primary care providers who supervise and deliver care to over 90% of all patients with diabetes in the United States. Just as the NHANES data have demonstrated a nearly 19% improvement in the number of patients achieving their ADA recommended A1C target of less than 7%, the U.S. health care system is experiencing critical shortages of primary care clinicians. Those PCPs who remain on the front lines of diabetes care are the target of incessant political debates as to the most cost-effective and rational means by which health care may be delivered equally to all people living in the United States. Physicians have had to invest in electronic medical records, e-prescribing, and software to achieve 25 Meaningful Use objectives. More importantly, what health care delivery systems might prove the most beneficial for society as a whole? Should the responsibility for cost-effective health care delivery be placed in the hands of the private sector or the government? With 60% of the adult population expected to have diabetes by year 2050, implementation of novel health care systems is imperative. PCPs should carefully evaluate the risks and benefits of any fundamental change suggested to their existing practice prior to enrolling in an alternative and untested program. Let us take a look at some of the controversial aspects of health care delivery in the United States today as it relates to diabetes management and primary care.

Patient-centered Medical Homes: Offering Privatization of Medical Care

An estimated 65 million Americans live in officially designated primary care shortage areas. The number of medical students entering adult primary care careers in internal and family medicine is on the decline. The United States spends more on specialist care per capita than any other industrialized country.[22] Coordination of patient care between PCPs, specialists, and hospitals is also deficient in many communities. Patients lack the sophistication to optimize their own pharmacologic treatment plans when prescribed medications by multiple providers.

In today's economic environment, one is hard pressed to provide cost-effective and efficient care to every patient with diabetes who becomes integrated into one's practice. Still, several patient-centered primary care-based groups have developed innovative health-care delivery models which have proven to be cost-effective while improving outcomes.

Patient-centered medical homes (PCMHs) provide a health care setting that facilitates partnerships between individual patients, their personal PCP, and a team of medical professionals. Medical homes assure that patients acquire the care that is most appropriate in a timely manner while taking into account one's individual cultural and linguistic orientation.

TABLE 1-2. Services Provided by Medical Family Homes

- Primary care advocacy for patients who are members of the medical home
- Appropriate, timely, and evidence-based interventions for both acute and chronic illnesses
- Initiation and integration of psychological counseling as well as behavioral interventions for patients with mental illness and chronic diseases, which, in theory, will improve long-term outcomes and adherence to treatment regimens
- Reproductive care that may be directed by qualified PCPs
- Integrated care in conjunction with specialists and adjunctive therapists if required
- Supportive care provided within hospitals, home, community, or nursing homes by PCPs and ancillary staff members
- Emphasis toward education and support for self-care and preventive care
- End-of-life support for terminally ill patients and their families
- Service coordination and referral, the goals of which are to allow patients to attain timely and appropriate consultation
- No co-pays, co-insurance, or deductibles
- Unhurried 30- to 60-min office visits
- Phone consultations and e-mail access to primary care providers
- Onsite pharmacy

Adapted from Rossner WW, Colwill JM, Kasperski J, et al. Progress of Ontario's family health team model: a patient-centered medical home. *Ann Fam Med.* 2011;9:165–171.

The services to patients with diabetes provided by a PCMH are summarized in Table 1-2. The primary corporate objectives of PCMH include the following:

1. Access to a personal *trusting* physician who directs a medical team responsible for the patient's care.
2. Patient care should maintain "whole-person orientation." Patients with diabetes would be comanaged with a certified diabetic educator, a pharmacist to make certain the patient is adherent to their pharmacologic regimen, a behavioral interventionist when necessary, and timely specialist referral.
3. Preventive care is the core benefit provided by PCMH.
4. Equally important is the desire of the medical home to assure that the patient is satisfied with the care and consultations that are being provided to him or her.
5. Corporate philosophy of medical homes recognize the value that PCPs add to their patient's well-being, especially if patients are afflicted with a chronic progressive disease such as diabetes. As such, physicians are compensated based on productivity. Patients within a medical home will pay monthly "membership fees" allowing them 24/7 access to their PCP. The membership fee allows physicians to see fewer patients per day while providing more comprehensive care to each person. Satisfaction for this practice model among patients and staff members is passionate within the medical homes.

Medical homes were initially established in 1967 as a means of caring for chronically ill children. Over the past 7 to 10 years, the medical home movement in association with a flourishing primary care environment has validated a means by which more Americans can access care for both acute and chronic illnesses while reducing overhead medical costs.[23]

Prior to achieving a designation as an official medical home, a primary care practice must achieve standards at three different levels including 30 separate elements of certification by the National Committee for Quality Assurance (NCQA) (Table 1-3).

TABLE 1-3. NCQA Standards Used to Designate Medical Homes in the United States

Access and communication	Has written standards for patient access and patient communication. Uses data to show standards for patient access and communication are being met.
Patient tracking and registry	Uses paper or electronic-based charting tools to organize clinical information. Uses data to identify important diagnoses and conditions in practice.
Care management	Adopts and implements evidence-based guidelines for three conditions.
Patient self-management support	Actively supports patient self-management.
Test tracking	Tracks tests and identifies abnormal results systematically.
Referral tracking	Tracks referrals using a paper-based or electronic system.
Performance reporting and improvement	Measures clinical and service performance by physician or across the practice. Reports performance across the practice or by physician.

More than 100 demonstration projects have already confirmed the effectiveness of the PCMH concept with a variety of approaches and populations. A study comparing claims data from 2010 of noted declines of 35% to 82% in ER visits, hospitalizations, hospitalization days, specialty visits, and surgeries of patients enrolled in a Washington-based medical home (Qliance Medical Group) with that of traditionally managed patients.[24]

Group Health—a Seattle-based nonprofit health insurance venture—encompasses a clinic of 8 physicians and 9,200 patients. After becoming designated as a medical home, standard visit times were increased from 20 to 30 minutes and staffing levels were expanded for other member services. Within 1 year, clinician work experience and clinical quality of care improved.[25] Substantial upfront investments were recouped due to a decline in ER visits, urgent care visit, and acute hospitalizations.[25] Group Health estimates a return of investment of $1.50 for every $1 invested in its medical home.[22]

Pay for performance within medical homes are based on a number of biomatrix standards including the number of patients screened for lipids, A1C levels, albuminuria, colon cancer, diabetic retinopathy, chronic kidney disease, peripheral neuropathy, pap smears, mammograms, osteoporosis, smoking history, and family history of diabetes-related complications. Additional financial incentives are provided to cover the cost of "high-risk patients" including those with mental illness or those who have a history of frequent hospitalizations or nonadherence to pharmacotherapy. Some medical homes are reimbursed for sending reminder cards to patients related to preventive services or appointments.[26]

Critics might argue that members might be confused about the "philosophy" of being a member of a medical home. This confusion might limit the cost-effectiveness of these ventures. However, unlike Accountable Care Organizations (ACOs), patients of medical homes are fully aware that they are members of that specific medical care service provider. ACO patients may not be informed of their membership and are free to seek medical care through a provider without affiliation to their assigned ACO.

Medical homes that are operated by privately funded PCPs have a tremendous potential for improving access to care and long-term outcomes for patients with all chronic illnesses including diabetes. Successful implementation of the medical home model in the United States will require PCPs to integrate both acute and preventive care for their chronically ill patients who have diabetes.

An interdisciplinary team with behavioral medicine, pharmacists, midlevel care providers, and specialists must rely upon an integrated electronic medical record system to track data from point of care visits and long-term outcomes. Finally, providers will need to become "high-level customer service representatives." Customized, cohesive, and targeted care for patients with diabetes will be supervised by the PCP, some of whom have been trained as thought leaders in the field of diabetes. Patients must accept their providers as their teachers, advocates, and disease coaches rather than just prescription writers for insulin, metformin, and test strips.

The United States faces major shortages of PCPs for care of adults. If the current U.S. primary care practice model continues as it is today, 44,000 additional family physicians and general internists would be needed in 2025 to maintain the current number of visits for each adult as the population increases and ages.[27] An additional 3,000 PCPs would be required to begin practicing annually in order to achieve this goal. Adoption of PCMHs could become part of the solution to reduced primary care availability and services. With fewer PCPs to manage the burgeoning diabetes population, one could anticipate that patients will not initiate treatment until their disease state is further advanced and complications less amenable to reversal.

• Accountable Care Organizations: The Government's Solution to Diabetes Health-Care Delivery

One fundamental flaw of the U.S. health care system is failing to reward health-care providers who work proactively to prevent chronic diseases from occurring or progressing. Instead, compensation favors clinicians who see patients more frequently, request more ancillary services, and perform more costly procedures on patients who have expensive chronic disorders. There is little doubt that the best health-care delivery system in the world is facing major financial hurdles in the next decade. Under current law, Medicare spending, the largest health-care purchaser and largest driver of federal entitlement costs and federal debt, is expected to rise from $523 billion in 2010 to $932 billion in 2020.[28] Medicare's long-term unfunded liabilities—the total cost of benefits promised but not paid for—amount to an incredible $36.8 trillion![29] Facing this unimaginable deficit, Congress decided to come up with a program for managing Medicare health-care delivery that could not lose a dime... at least for the Medicare Trust Fund! Let us now take a look at the Government mandated Accountable Care Organizations. As we do, ask yourselves if ACOs will likely add to the successful management of patients with chronic diseases such as diabetes. Also, if you were a senior patient on Medicare, who would you rather have as your health-care provider: a primary care medical home or an ACO?

ACOs take up only seven pages of the massive 1990-page proposed affordable health act, but has become one of the most befuddling of all provisions. Hospital and provider groups are preparing to form ACOs despite outwardly complaining that this program has created more risks than rewards while imposing onerous reporting requirements.

The ACOs are being promoted, at least in theory, as a means by which health-care costs may be contained while improving overall quality of care for millions of Americans. From a philosophical, or mythologic, perspective (if you prefer), ACOs will be developed to realign payment incentives by shifting the focus from high patient care to one of value and performance.[30] Similar to medical homes, the ACOs want doctors to "voluntarily" see fewer fee-for-service patients, while documenting various quality measures of high performance with each individual.

The Centers for Medicare and Medicaid Services (CMS) define an ACO as "an organization of health-care providers that agrees to be accountable for quality, cost, and overall care of Medicare beneficiaries who are enrolled in the traditional fee-for-service program who are assigned to it."[31] ACOs that succeed in delivering high quality care and reducing health care costs will receive a share of the money the government saves on patients registered to that ACO. The Department of Health and Human Services predicts that ACOs could save Medicare up to $940 million during the first 4 years of its implementation, which is far less than 1% of Medicare's anticipated spending during that same period!

ACOs will include physicians working in group practices or networks of practices and hospitals. ACOs must have at least 5,000 patient "beneficiaries" as well as the technologic ability to report data on cost and quality for Medicare fee-for-service patients. As in the classic movie "The Dirty Dozen," every ACO will attempt to unify a large group of providers with a hospital or several hospitals, some of whom are fierce local or regional competitors, for the benefit of all. With so many political adversaries and self-interests involved in local and regional medical politics, many insiders believe that the ACO concept will be doomed to failure.

In Medicare's traditional fee-for-service payment system, doctors and hospitals are compensated based upon the number of tests and procedures they perform. This incentivizes physicians to order more ancillary services and procedures that will increase their income. Remember, ACOs want doctors to spend MORE quality time with patients, but doctors know that in a fee-for-service enterprise, the winners are those that schedule the most appointments. Perhaps if doctors schedule fewer patients, hospitalizations, and surgery numbers will also decrease and money will be saved.

ACOs would continue the *same* traditional fee-for-service program, while creating savings incentives that they hope would pay bonuses to frugal doctors over the long term. Savings in health care costs would be derived from groups of physicians who see fewer patients, order fewer tests, keep their patients out of the hospital, and reduce the number of invasive procedures individuals may require.

But wait! Congress was smart when they legislated the ACO program. There could be only one loser in this game and two winners. If costs could NOT be contained, or if performance and savings benchmarks were not met, the ACO would be responsible for *all* penalties... not the government! After all, Medicare has $36.8 trillion in unfunded liabilities. Why should this entitlement program take on any additional debt when liability can be passed on to a third party? If, by chance, the ACO was profitable, incentive bonuses would be provided to the members. Some rural ACOs may be eligible to receive government start-up costs in advance to help them build the infrastructure necessary for coordinated care. Before any ACO members get excited about these bonuses, the government intends to withhold distribution of any funds for up to 2 years, making certain that all of the patient costs have been appropriated.

The government will begin receiving its initial round of applications for the ACO Shared Savings Program in January 2012, and the first ACOs are expected to launch in April. CMS created a second strategy, called the Pioneer Program, allowing high-performing health systems to potentially recover more of the expected health care savings in exchange for accepting greater financial risk.

Table 1-4 lists the variables and reservations related to ACO development and strategic planning. Prior to contracting with an ACO, providers are strongly encouraged to consider the risks and benefits of working within the confines of these organizations.

Has the ACO concept undergone performance field testing? The "Physicians Group Practice Demonstration" was a directive originally decreed by Congress in 2000 designed to field test a system by which physicians who accepted traditional fee-for-service patients could be rewarded for their high-quality and cost-effective medicine.[32] The project was eventually launched after 5 years of bureaucratic delays. Ten of the most respected large multispecialty groups in the country were selected as test sites including the Marshfield Clinic, St. John's, Geisinger, Park Nicollet, and Billings. Two pilot sites were associated with academic medical centers—the University of Michigan and Dartmouth.

Physician groups in the demo continued to receive their regular Medicare compensation while sharing in any savings generated. Each group had to attain 32 predetermined quality metrics and exceed a savings threshold of 2%. By the 4th year of the demo, all 10 groups met at least 29/32 quality goals and by the 5th year, 7 groups achieved benchmark-level performance on all 32 measures. All PGPs increased their quality scores on diabetes management by at least 9% over 5 years.

Now, let us take a look at the cost savings incurred by the groups who had done so well with patient metrics. Despite their reputation as being some of the most highly regarded medical groups in the United States, only two of the PGP participants (St. John's and Forsyth) were able to exceed a 2% savings threshold during the 1st year of the demo and five surpassed the threshold of 2% after 3 years. St. John's earned 15% of the total savings earning $13.9 million. At the end of the pilot

TABLE 1-4. Variables and Uncertainties Regarding Accountable Care Organizations

Variable	ACO Concept	Reservations Associated with ACO Concept
Patient membership	Patients ("attributed beneficiaries") who are members of the ACOs are assigned to specific PCPs for medical services.	Attributed beneficiaries WILL NOT be aware of their ACO affiliation and may continue to seek services from PCPs of their choice even outside of their designated ACO. This will limit the ability of the ACO to contain cost. The ACO cannot force a patient to receive care by their physician members. How will costs be contained?
Physician compensation	ACOs are based on fee-for-service compensation.	ACOs will work ONLY if the providers get paid LESS for the same patient services. Few believe that providers will voluntarily lower their fees and see fewer patients to support their ACOs.
Hospital and physician competition	ACOs will require collaboration between hospitals, independent physicians, large medical groups, and other service organizations.	The track record for managed care efforts between hospitals and providers has been poor. Contracts between third-party payers and hospitals have failed in the past due to inadequate resources, weak hospital boards, and the inability of hospitals and medical groups to control costs of services and contain expenses. In some cases, local hospitals and physician groups will have to work together in a single ACO. Prior to forming an ACO, these entities were likely in competition. The local medical politics in some communities may limit the cohesiveness and ultimate success of the ACOs. Success will be dependent upon how well hospitals and providers can work together to coordinate a multitude of services such as outpatient clinics, urgent care facilities, home health, and palliative care. A hospital with a dysfunctional staff or administration cannot succeed. Effective leadership is a necessity for ACO implementation.
Stakeholders	CMS is concerned about cost-effective health-care delivery. Little emphasis is placed on engaging the "attributed beneficiaries" in ways by which they too may be able to help reduce their own medical costs.	ACOs place little to no emphasis on preventive medicine care and health-care educational services. Attributed beneficiaries will not be aware that they are members of a given ACO! How can costs be contained in such a large cohort of patients?
Capital expense planning	Hospital budgets will need to be reworked to include start-up costs for ACOs and coordinated care.	ACO incentive payments may not be realized for 2–3 y. Money for other capital expenses will be reduced. In California, this may impact retrofitting of hospitals to comply with seismic safety standards by 2013.[a]

(Continued)

TABLE 1-4. Variables and Uncertainties Regarding Accountable Care Organizations *(Continued)*

Rush to judgment	ACOs are a serious public policy issue requiring a great deal of thought and perspective. Entities are rushing to become the first established ACOs in a community.	Economists fear that ACOs will have a significant downside resulting in hospital mergers, closures, primary care practice purchases, and provider consolidation. This will leave fewer independent hospitals and physicians. Greater market share gives the ACOs more leverage in negotiations with insurers driving up health care costs and lowering the ultimate health care savings of everyone, including the tax payers!
Legal concerns	Each ACO must have legal counsel.	ACOs could violate antitrust and antifraud laws, which limit market power, increase prices, and stifles competition. In rural communities, the ACOs could grow so large that they would employ all of the providers in a region.
Start-up costs	CMS estimates start-up costs will be $1.76 million. Upfront money will need to come from the ACO providers in the form of a cash investment.	ACOs will not recover any costs for at least 1–2 y. CMS will withhold a percentage of the profit made by each ACO.
Risks	ACO regulations require the consortium to establish adequate financial security allowing CMS to collect any money owed if the ACO fails to attain its performance targets.	ACOs will need to place cash into an escrow account, which the government can "steal" if the group fails to save the government money. Members of an ACO MUST understand that this is NOT a two-way street. ONLY the ACO is at risk for losses. The government cannot lose!
Profits and losses	After each contract year, CMS will pay the ACO "a portion" of earned Medicare savings or determine how much the ACO must pay CMS.	Note here that the ACO will not be paid its entire savings fee. A percentage will be withheld by the government. The ACO will distribute profits based on a formula that incentivizes providers to meet the ACO's overall objectives. The specifics of these formulas are open for individual negotiation among ACO provider members. A provider who has a stellar performance may still be at financial risk for the entire ACO. Therefore, providers must carefully assess their binding ACO contracts prior to signing.
Disciplinary action	A disciplinary process will be used by individual ACOs to manage providers who do not help the consortium achieve its financial or clinical goals.	Each provider will be carefully monitored for performance. Doctors who manage high risk, nonadherent patients, or those patients whose special needs may find the corrective action plan intrusive.

[a]California's hospital seismic safety law, its implementation, history, and progress. http://www.google.com/#hl=en&cp=51&gs_id=6n&xhr=t&q=Retrofitting±hospital±for±earthquakes±in±California&pf=p&sclient=psy-ab&pbx=1&oq=Retrofitting±hospital±for±earthquakes±in±California&aq=f&aqi=&aql=&gs_sm=&gs_upl=&bav=on.2,or.r_gc.r_pw.,cf.osb&fp=96ce8927a7c42694&biw=1360&bih=712. Accessed December 23, 2011.
From Becker's Hospital Review. 5 problems with ACOs. November 19, 2010. http://www.beckershospitalreview.com/hospital-physician-relationships/5-problems-with-acos.html. Accessed December 23, 2011.

program (year 5), only four of the groups received bonus money totaling $29 million as their share of saving $36 million for the Medicare Trust Fund.[33] Two groups achieved their quality performance targets by year 5 (Billings and Middlesex) yet received no shared savings incentive payments as these groups were unable to minimize costs for their patients. Another group, Everett, received a payment of only $129,268 in year 2, but no other cash payments for their participation. In summary, only 2 of the 10 groups were able to generate savings in all 5 years. One major health system required 3 years before exceeding the savings threshold. One group with 30 years of managed care experience qualified for bonus compensation in just a single year.

This is very sobering news for physicians, hospitals, and other providers who are planning to invest their time, money, and efforts into forming an ACO. The minimum savings threshold that CMS has proposed for ACOs is 2% (or 3.9% for plans with fewer patients). Yet ACOs will have to share losses as well as gains by the 3rd year. Based on the data derived from the government's own pilot project, which recruited some of the most highly regarded medical groups in this country, successful implementation of the ACO concept will be very difficult and lead to higher overall health-care costs.

Group Diabetes Visits

Group diabetes visits provide an innovative and efficient approach for managing patients with chronic diseases, such as diabetes, pain, asthma, hypertension, hyperlipidemia, coronary artery disease, and obesity within a private office or large medical group.[34] Group visits are typically supervised by a nurse, CDE, RD, pharmacist, psychologist, and physician, although not all health-care providers need be present at each group encounter. Group visits augment the traditional face-to-face primary care office visit by offering patients more lengthy visits, peer interaction, and subject intensive education. Unlike group education classes, group visits must include documentation of each patient's vital signs, medication list, a degree of individualized care, and the reasons for the encounter.

If properly managed, group visits can lower A1Cs and improve lipids and medication adherence over a 3-year period.[35] Trento et al. demonstrated that providing health care in groups of patients with T2DM resulted in improved metabolic control compared with usual care.[36] Group patients demonstrated significantly increased knowledge of T2DM and expressed improved quality of life versus those patients managed with usual care. Another study targeting patients with T2DM aged 16 to 75 having an A1C greater than 8.5% or no recorded A1C within 1 year were offered monthly 2-hour group visits in 6-month cycles. The group visits were led by a CDE, a behaviorist, a pharmacist, and two diabetologists. Patients continued to receive their routine care from their PCPs within the HMO to which they were assigned. Patients who participated in the group visits demonstrated improvement in diabetes control, satisfaction with health-care services, and reduced health-care utilization.[37] Group visits may also be used effectively to improve adherence to the ADA standards of care for uninsured or inadequately insured patients with T2DM.[38] The diabetes focused group visit may also reduce health-care costs while improving patient and clinician satisfaction.[39]

Incorporating group diabetes visits into a primary care practice requires strategic planning on behalf of all professional staff members. A staff meeting should be held during which the roles of each facilitator are clearly defined. Newsletters, patient handouts, and e-blasts can be used to encourage patients to enroll in a group visit.

The group visit encounter should be efficient, enlightening, and appropriately coded (see Table 1-5). Visits last approximately 2 hours and include six to ten patients. Participating patients should sign a statement of confidentiality protecting the HIPA rights of all members of a group (Fig. 1-3). Upon entering the group, patients will have their vital signs recorded by the medical assistant and should be provided with any written educational material that will be discussed at the session. Patients may also be provided with notepads and pens to record notes or questions for the facilitators.

The meeting opens with the lead facilitator providing an introduction of the topic at hand. For example, if the theme is foot care, one may discuss the risk factors for diabetic neuropathy (duration

TABLE 1-5. Group Visit Questions and Answers

Question	Answer
How many patients per group visit?	3–10 would be the most efficient number.
How often would you schedule a group visit?	Every 1–3 mo depending on physician, CDE, and patient availability
When is the best time for a group visit?	During office hours or even after hours, which would accommodate your patients who would not have to miss work to attend the group
What is the length of the group visit?	2 h total 30 min for vital signs 30 min spent with CDE 30 min spent with facilitator 30 min for chart notations
Suggested topics of discussion for group classes	• Preventing diabetes complications • Preconception planning • Smoking cessation • Healthy lifestyle intervention • Diabetes for the disinterested. Getting back into the game • Carbohydrate counting • Insulin pump group meeting • Insulin pen demonstrations • Diabetes and depression • Managing diabetic neuropathy • Foot care • Managing diabetic retinopathy • Cancer risk and diabetes • Prediabetes • Monogenetic diabetes (MODY) • Diabetes and mental illness • Diabetes management based upon diverse cultural values
How are eligible patients notified of the group availability?	Posters, postcards, and phone calls from office staff inviting them to the class on behalf of the clinician Explain to all patients that the group visit will be charged as an office visit. Patients may be required to provide a co-pay at the time of the visit.
What are the staff responsibilities on group visit day?	Bring all charts to the visit room. Set up the room for maximum efficiency of communication. Circle or horseshoe is best for discussion. Prepare any handouts and document them in patient chart. Prepare informed consent for group visit and place in medical record when signed. Have flip chart available. Name tags for all staff members.
What group guidelines should be provided at the start of the group session?	Explain that group visits are provided as an alternative means to attain medical care that works. Some patients may not like the format, and others will. No one is required to say anything they feel uncomfortable about. However, by participating actively, everyone should learn more about managing their own diabetes. Suggestions on diabetes self-management will be greatly appreciated by all.

(Continued)

TABLE 1-5. Group Visit Questions and Answers *(Continued)*

Question	Answer		
Responsibilities during the group visit	Medical assistant collects vitals.	CDE/pharmacist/ psychologist can provide predetermined medical education on specific topics of interest.	Physician goes over care plan with each patient and documents group visit in medical record. Care plan can be based on the topic discussed by CDE, pharmacist, or psychologist.
What else does clinician do during the group session?	Serve as a facilitator during questions and answers. Encourage full participation of all patients. If someone asks a question, get other patient's feedback rather than providing your own opinion.		
What are the codes for a group visit?	For group visits you do not need to do any exam other than vital signs to code a 99213 or 99214 for established patients as long as you have satisfied the history and level of complexity requirements as indicated in Figure 1-4. Be certain your ICD 9 code reflects the level of control, type of diabetes, and any comorbidities.		

of diabetes, age, obesity, smoking, high cholesterol), the symptoms of diabetic sensory neuropathy, how to differentiate DSN from arthritic pain, and pathogenesis. Patients can be asked about their experience with symptoms such as "feet that tingle, burn and hurt while you are at rest." The facilitator can demonstrate a brief foot exam for the group and explain that each patient will subsequently undergo a similar exam prior to the conclusion of the visit. Patients at high risk for peripheral vascular disease may be referred for ankle brachial index (ABI) testing. The facilitator should encourage group participation by everyone in attendance.

At the conclusion of the visit, patients are provided with appointments to their PCPs and the next group visit. The facilitator is responsible for properly documenting and coding the encounter on each patient's medical record.

Many patients prefer group to individual visits as they have more quality time with the clinician, CDE, pharmacist, and even visiting specialists. They also enjoy meeting with other team members with whom they share a chronic disease state.

Medicare does not reimburse the group education component of group visits unless it is provided by a CDE. E & M codes may be billed using the extent of history, physical exam, decision-making, and complexity model (see Fig. 1-4). Documentation is vital for reimbursement. Figure 1-4 may be used as a template for documentation and coding.

• Keys to Efficient Diabetes Management: A Primary Care Perspective

Within busy primary care practices, successful diabetes management requires an organized, calculated, and predetermined strategic approach toward the initial assessment and subsequent follow-up visit for each patient. This can be a daunting task during an 8- to 12-minute visit. Therefore, being familiar with the diabetes standards of care allows the physician to focus on customized care at the time of each visit. Table 1-6 provides an extensive summary of the most recently published evidence-based standards of care for patients with diabetes as published professional societies such as the American Diabetes Association, American Heart Association, American Cancer Society, and the U.S. Preventive Services Task Force (USPSTF).

Sample Group Visit Consent Form

Date:
Dear Patient

You are voluntarily consenting to participate in a Diabetes Group Medical Visit. During this visit you, and other patients, may share personal health related information. This information will be used to help instruct other members of the group to become more active and efficient participants in their own diabetes care. You do not have to provide any information to the group that you feel is uncomfortable or private. We also ask that any medical issues that are addressed in this room not be disseminated to any of your friends, relatives or associates. Your privacy, as well as the privacy of others in the group is vitally important to all.

The group will consist of educational discussions related to exercise, diet, medications, and devices used to manage diabetes. Your vital signs will be taken and additional exams will be performed as indicated. These exams (such as a foot examination) may be performed in private if you would prefer.

The group visit is billed as a regular office visit, and, as such you will be responsible for paying for the co-pay or for the entire visit based upon your 3rd party payor requirements.

The group visit may replace some of your routine visits for diabetes but you will still have some privately scheduled appointments with your regular primary care physician.

You of course have the option to not come to the group visits. If you have questions about this process please discuss them with your physician or the office administrator.

Name:

Patient signature:

Your signature indicates that you have read the above, understand what it says and agree to attend group visits

CONSENT TO ATTEND A GROUP VISIT

I, hereby voluntarily consent to participate in a "Diabetes Group Medical Visit" in which I and other patients may share personal health information, if they wish on a purely voluntary basis. This information will be used to help educate the group about various health topics and which may help improve my care.

The group meeting will consist of discussions of current medical conditions, pertinent educational information, and open discussions with other patients on diabetes and subjects of interest to the group.

To the extent needed I may be examined in the group for a blood pressure reading, foot exam or other areas. If you wish to have these parts of the exam done in a private examining room just let us know.

The group visit may replace some of your routine visits for diabetes but you will still have some privately scheduled appointments needed with your doctor in the future. You of course have the option to not come to the group visits.

I have read the above, understand what it says and agree to attend group visits.

Name (Printed) _____

Signature _____

Today's Date _____

Figure 1-3 • Sample Group Visit Consent Form

Clinical Group Visit Chart

Comments:

Assessment: (ICD -9 or ICD-10 code for diabetes controlled with or without complications)
(For ICD-10 coding, see on-line chapter on coding).
> (Include codes for co-existing disorders such as hypertension, chronic kidney disease, neuropathy, depression, etc.)

Management Plan (Mark all that apply):
- Discussed targets and management of A1C
- Discussed targets and management of lipids
- Discussed targets and management of blood pressure
- Recommended ASA daily.
- Discussed and encouraged activity.
- Discussed and encouraged diet
- Discussed smoking cessation
- Discussed preconception planning
- Discussed insulin pump therapy
- Discussed home blood glucose monitoring, paired glucose testing
- Discussed continuous glucose sensors
- Discussed depression
- Discussed sick day management
- Discussed insulin/GLP-1 delivery devices
- Discussed medication adherence
- Discussed carb counting
- Discussed prevention of complications
- Reviewed medication options; risks, benefits and side effects
- Changed medication
- Reviewed foot care
- Met with CDE
- Met with pharmacist
- Met with psychologist
- Met with specialist
- Spent more than 50% of visit counseling re: therapy options and management of diabetes.

ICD-9 Charge code: 99213   99214   99215

ICD-9 Code	Chief complaint history	History: HPI	Patient family/ social history	Review of systems	Medical decision making
99213	Required	1–3 elements	Pertinent	Not required	Low complexity
99214	Required	4+ elements (or 3+ chronic diseases)	2-9 systems	1 element	Moderate complexity

Adapted from Coding "Routine" Office Visits: 99213 or 99214? Family Practice Management, September 2005

Figure 1-4 • Clinical Group Visit Chart

TABLE 1-6. Evidence-based Diabetes Standards of Care Summary

Patient name:
Diabetes type: T1DM, T2DM, GDM, MODY, Type 1B, Other
Age when initially diagnosed with diabetes:
Metabolic measures:

	Standards of Care Recommendations (Based on Published Guidelines from the American Diabetes Association, American Cancer Society, and American College of Cardiology)	Evidence-based Grading System	Comment
Lifestyle Interventions			
Exercise	Patients with diabetes should perform exercise of moderate intensity (targeting 50–70% of maximum heart rate) for at least 150 minutes per week. Activity should be spread over a minimum of 3 days with no more than 2 consecutive days of inactivity.	A	Patients with autonomic neuropathy should undergo a thorough cardiovascular evaluation before initiating any intense training program.
	If not contraindicated, patients with T2DM should be encouraged to incorporate resistance training into their regimen.	A	
Smoking cessation	Should be evaluated at each visit	A	Include smoking cessation counseling as needed at each visit (B).
Diabetes self-management education (DSME)	Patients should receive DSME at the time of diagnosis and as needed thereafter.	B	DSME can result in cost-savings and improve outcomes. Therefore, DSME should be fully reimbursed by third party payors.
Hypoglycemia	For conscious patients, take 15–20 g of carbohydrate. Repeat blood glucose testing after 15 min. If level remains low, repeat dose of 15–20 g of carbs.	E	
	Glucagon emergency kit should be prescribed to all patients at risk for developing severe hypoglycemia. Family members or caregivers must be instructed on the use of glucagon.	E	
	Patients with hypoglycemia awareness autonomic failure (HAAF) should be encouraged to raise their glycemic targets for several weeks to minimize their risk of hypoglycemia and reverse hypoglycemia unawareness.	B	

Bariatric surgery	May be considered for adults with BMI >35 kg/m² especially with difficult to control diabetes associated with multiple comorbidities	B	78% of patients with diabetes undergoing bariatric surgery undergo remission of diabetes (normalization of blood glucose levels in the absence of medications) sustained for over 2 y. Remission rates are higher with gastric bypass than lap banding procedures.
Medical nutrition therapy (MNT)	Treatment plans should be individualized to achieve treatment goals and provided by an RD.	A	
	Weight loss is recommended for all obese and overweight patients using low-fat, calorie-restricted, or Mediterranean diets for up to 2 y.	A	
	Saturated fat intake should be <7% of total calories.	B	
	Intake of trans fat should be minimized to reduce LDL-C.	E	
	Adults should limit alcohol intake to ≤1 drink per day for women and ≤2 drinks per day for men.	E	
	Routine supplements are not advised.	A	
Metabolic Targets			
A1C (Adults)	• <7% (For most nonpregnant adults)	B	Perform the A1C test quarterly in patients whose therapy has changed or not at their glycemic target.
	• <6.5% for patients with short duration of diabetes, long life expectancy, and no significant heart disease	C	
	• <8% for patients with a history of severe hypoglycemia, limited life expectancy, advanced complications, and extensive comorbid complications	B	Perform the A1C test at least biannually in patients who are meeting treatment goals and who have stable glycemic goals.
A1C (children and adolescents)	• <8.5% (ages 0–6 y)		Due to vulnerability of hypoglycemia, unpredictable dietary intake, and physical activity. Can target <8% if patient does not have excessive hypoglycemia
	• <8% (ages 6–12 y)		A lower goal of <7.5% is reasonable if this can be achieved without excessive hypoglycemia.
	• <7.5%		A lower goal of <7% is reasonable if this can be achieved without excessive hypoglycemia.

(Continued)

TABLE 1-6. Evidence-based Diabetes Standards of Care Summary (Continued)

	Standards of Care Recommendations (Based on Published Guidelines from the American Diabetes Association, American Cancer Society, and American College of Cardiology)	Evidence-based Grading System	Comment
Lipids		E	Measure annually. Patients with low risk lipid profile (LDL < 100 mg/dL, HDL > 50 mg/dL, and TG < 150 mg/dL) may be tested every 2 yrs.
		A	Statins should be added to lifestyle intervention regardless of baseline lipid levels for diabetic patients with (a) overt CAD and (b) anyone over age 40 who has one or more risk factors for CAD.
		B	Statins are contraindicated in pregnancy.
	LDL-cholesterol Target <100 mg/dL or <70 mg/dL in high-risk patients	A	
	HDL-cholesterol Target >40 mg/dL in men and >50 mg/dL in women	C	
	Triglycerides Target <150 mg/dL	C	
	Apo B (measure in statin-treated patients in whom the LDL cholesterol goal is <70 mg/dL and the non-HDL cholesterol target is <100 mg/dL)	E	
Blood Pressure	Measure at each visit (see chapter on microvascular complications for individualized targets).	C	
	Systolic target is <130 mm Hg.	B	
	Diastolic target is <80 mm Hg.	B	
	Based on patient characteristics, treatment should be individualized.	E	Attempt lifestyle intervention for SBP of 130–139 mm Hg and DBP of 80–89 mm Hg for 3 months. If treatment goals not achieved, initiate pharmacotherapy.
		A	Patients with SBP ≥ 140 or DBP ≥ 90 mm Hg should receive pharmacotherapy and lifestyle intervention.
		B	Lifestyle intervention for hypertension consists of weight loss, exercise, and DASH (Dietary Approaches to Stop Hypertension Diet).

	If pharmacologic therapy is needed, initiate with an ACE inhibitor or an ARB.	C
	Add a thiazide diuretic to those with persistent hypertension and an estimated GFR ≥ 30 mL/min/1.73 m².	C
	Use a loop diuretic in those with persistent hypertension and an estimated GFR ≤ 30 mL/min/1.73 m².	C
	ACE inhibitors and ARBs are contraindicated in pregnancy.	E
Antiplatelet therapy	Used in primary prevention in most men aging >50 or women aging >60 with T1DM or T2DM and at least one additional major risk factor (family history of coronary heart disease, hypertension, smoking, dyslipidemia, or albuminuria).	C
	Patients with CAD and aspirin allergy may use clopidogrel 75 mg/d.	B
	Combination therapy with ASA (75–162) mg/d + clopidogrel (75 mg/d) is reasonable for up to 1 yr after an acute coronary syndrome event.	B

Vaccinations

Influenza	Influenza vaccine given to all patients with diabetes ≥6 months of age	C
Pneumococcal	Vaccinate all patients with diabetes age ≥2 yrs. A one-time revaccination is recommended for patients aging >64 previously immunized when they were younger than age 65 and if the vaccine was administered more than 5 yrs previously.	C
	Administer hepatitis B vaccination to adults with diabetes for disease control and prevention.	C
	Hepatitis B vaccination is recommended for persons with diabetes younger than 60 years as soon as feasible after diagnosis; persons with diabetes who are 60 years or older at the discretion of the treating clinician based on increased need for assisted blood glucose monitoring in long-term care facilities, likelihood of acquiring hepatitis B infection, its complications or chronic sequelae, and likelihood of immune response to vaccination. (CDC recommended adult immunization schedule: http://www.cdc.gov/mmwr/preview/mmwrhtml/mm6104a9.htm. Accessed 6/1/12)	C

(Continued)

TABLE 1-6. Evidence-based Diabetes Standards of Care Summary (Continued)

	Standards of Care Recommendations (Based on Published Guidelines from the American Diabetes Association, American Cancer Society, and American College of Cardiology)	Evidence-based Grading System	Comment
Screening for Comorbid Complications			
Coronary artery disease screening and treatment	Routine screening in asymptomatic patients does not improve outcomes and is not warranted.	A	Candidates for cardiac testing include those with typical or atypical cardiac symptoms and an abnormal resting EKG.
	Patients with known CAD should be placed on aspirin, ACE inhibitors, and a statin unless contraindicated.	C,A	
	Patients with a history of acute myocardial infarction should be maintained on a β-blocker for at least 2 years post event.	B	
	Thiazolidinediones (TZDs) should be avoided in patients with symptomatic heart failure.	C	
	Metformin may be used in patients with stable CHF and renal function but avoided in unstable or hospitalized patients with CHF.	C	
	Candidates for cardiac testing include those with typical or atypical cardiac symptoms and an abnormal resting EKG.	A	
Nephropathy	Annual test to assess urine albumin excretion in type 1 patients with diabetes duration of 5 yrs and in all type 2 patients at the time of diagnosis	B	
Microalbuminuria = 30–299 µg/mg creatinine (spot collection)	Measure serum creatinine and estimated GFR annually in all patients in order to stage chronic kidney disease.	E	
Macro (clinical) albuminuria ≥300 µg/mg creatinine (spot collection)	To reduce risk or slow the progression of nephropathy, optimize glucose control and blood pressure.	A	
	In patients with T2DM, hypertension, and microalbuminuria, both ACE inhibitors and ARBs delay progression of macroalbuminuria.	A	
	For patients with T1DM, hypertension and any degree of albuminuria, ACE inhibitors delay the progression of nephropathy.	A	

		If one class is not tolerated, the other should be substituted.	E	Renin-angiotensin system (RAS) inhibition delays onset of microalbuminuria but has demonstrated an unexpected higher rate of fatal cardiovascular events with olmesartan among patients with preexisting CAD. Patients using a RAS inhibitor should avoid using these drugs in combination with an ACE or an ARB, especially in patients with kidney disease. These drugs used in combination have been found to increase the risk of hyperkalemia, hypotension, stroke, and renal events (ALTITUDE Trial).
Retinopathy screening	B	Adults and children aged 10 yrs or older with T1DM should have an initial dilated and comprehensive eye examination by an ophthalmologist or optometrist within 5 yrs after the onset of diabetes.	
	B	Patients with T2DM should have an initial dilated and comprehensive eye examination by an ophthalmologist or optometrist shortly after the diagnosis of diabetes.	
	B	Subsequent examinations for T1DM and T2DM patients should be repeated annually by an ophthalmologist or optometrist. More frequent examinations will be needed if retinopathy is progressive.	
	B	Women with preexisting diabetes who are planning a pregnancy or who have become pregnant should have a comprehensive eye examination and should be counseled on the risk of development and/or progression of diabetic retinopathy. Eye examination should occur in the first trimester with close follow-up throughout pregnancy and for 1 yr postpartum.	Retinal photography with remote reading by experts has a great potential where ophthalmology consultation may not be readily available but are not a substitute for a comprehensive eye examination.

(Continued)

TABLE 1-6. Evidence-based Diabetes Standards of Care Summary *(Continued)*

	Standards of Care Recommendations (Based on Published Guidelines from the American Diabetes Association, American Cancer Society, and American College of Cardiology)	Evidence-based Grading System	Comment
Neuropathy	Screen at time of diagnosis for T2DM and annually using "simple tests" for sensory neuropathy. Patients with T1DM may be initially screened 5 yrs after the diagnosis followed by annual exams.	B	
	Annual comprehensive foot exam (include inspection, assessment of foot pulses, and testing for loss of protective sensation, vibration sense, pinprick, ankle reflexes, or vibration perception threshold).	B	
	Screen for autonomic neuropathy at time of diagnosis for T2DM and 5 y after diagnosis of T1DM. Specialized testing may not affect management or outcomes and is rarely needed.	E	
Cervical cancer	Every 2 yrs from age 21 to 29	A	Gardasil (human papilloma virus) vaccine provided as a series of three doses is recommended by the Advisory Committee on Immunization Practices for females beginning as young as 9 through age 26 who have not been exposed to the virus through prior sexual contact. The vaccine is also licensed for males aged 9–26 for prevention of genital warts caused by human papilloma virus types 6 and 11.
	Every 3 yrs for women age ≥30 yrs with a history of three negative cytology tests	A	
	Stop screening between age 65 and 70 with three consecutive normal cytology tests and no abnormal tests in the past 10 yrs (any older woman who is sexually active and has multiple partners should continue screening.).	B	
	Pap smears do not have to be performed if hysterectomy was performed for benign disease and patient has no history of high-grade CIN pathology.	B	

		Grade
	Gardasil protects against HPV types 6, 11, 16, and 18. Another vaccine, Cervarix (used primarily in England), protects against HPV types 16 and 18, which is responsible for 70% of cervical cancers and is associated with squamous cell carcinoma of the throat	
	HPV vaccination is recommended for preteen girls and boys at age 11 or 12 years. Preteens and teens should receive all 3 doses of HPV vaccine prior to the time of their initial sexual exposure. Only Gardasil, which is the only HPV vaccine approved for use in girls and boys, is protective against most genital warts, as well as cervical, anal, vaginal, and vulvar cancers. Vaccines are given at baseline, 1 or 2 months thereafter, and 6 months after baseline.	
Breast cancer (^^^)	Consider mammography every 1–2 yrs for women 40 yrs and older.	B
	Digital mammography is an option for younger women and those with denser breasts, although studies have not proven a reduction in mortality.	C
	Magnetic resonance imaging is recommended as an adjunct to screening mammography in women 30 yrs and older who are at high risk for breast cancer.	C
	BRCA genetic testing for high risk patients with a history of breast and or ovarian cancer (see [a] below for guidance and website).	
Osteoporosis Screening	The Cochrane collaboration found screening mammography to be unjustified.	
	Screen women age ≥65 without previous known fractures or secondary causes of osteoporosis.	B
	Screen women age ≤65 whose 10-year fracture risk is equal to or greater than that of a 65-year-old white woman without additional risk factors.	B

(Continued)

TABLE 1-6. Evidence-based Diabetes Standards of Care Summary *(Continued)*

	Standards of Care Recommendations (Based on Published Guidelines from the American Diabetes Association, American Cancer Society, and American College of Cardiology)	Evidence-based Grading System	Comment
	FRAX fracture risk assessment tool is available at: http://www.shef.ac.uk/FRAX/.		Age-matched hip fracture risk is significantly increased in both T1DM and T2DM for both men and women.
			T1DM is associated with osteoporosis.
			T2DM is associated with an increased risk of hip fracture despite higher bone mineral density.
			Educate patients regarding fall risk, supplemental vitamin D and calcium intake, avoidance of glucocorticoids and avoidance of TZDs.
			Consider pharmacotherapy for high-risk patients.
Colon cancer screening (^^^)	All adults 50 yrs and older should be screened for colorectal cancer.	A	Most colorectal cancers arise from adenomatous polyps.
	Routine screening for colorectal cancer should continue until age 75.	A	
	Options for colorectal cancer screening include:		
	(a) Annual fecal occult blood testing (FOBT)	A	
	(b) Flexible sigmoidoscopy every 5 yrs (with and without FOBT)	A	
	(c) Colonoscopy every 10 yrs	B	
Peripheral arterial disease	The USPSTF recommends against routine screening for PAD and carotid artery stenosis. Although the screening tests are non-invasive and accurate, the treatment of asymptomatic PAD beyond standard cardiovascular risk assessment and treatment, does not improve major health outcomes.	D	

	Due to the high prevalence of symptomatic PAD in patients with diabetes an ADA consensus statement on PAD published in 2003 suggested screening patients 50 yrs and older with ABI and those younger than age 50 with risk factors for PAD (smoking, hypertension, hyperlipidemia, and duration of diabetes >10 yrs). Patients with a positive ABI or symptomatic PAD should be referred for vascular assessment and surgical options.		
Psychological and social situation assessment	Psychological screening tests for depression, diabetes-related distress, anxiety, eating disorders, and cognitive impairment when diabetes self-management skills are deficient.	E	Attitudes about illness, expectations for medical management and outcomes, affect/mood, general and diabetes-related quality of life, resources (financial, social, and emotional), and psychiatric assessment. Psychosocial impairment will compromise health status. Lifetime prevalence of major depression in patients with diabetes is 28.5%. Simple patient screening test (Prime-MD = Primary Care Evaluation of Mental Disorders) is available online at http://www.psy-world.com/prime-md_print1.htm.

Optional Screening Tests
(Note: No formal recommendations have been published for these comorbidities)

Routine pure tone audiometry for hearing loss	The Hearing Handicap Inventory for the Elderly-Screening Version is available online: http://teachhealthk-12.uthscsa.edu/curriculum/vision-hearing/pa06pdf/0608E-eng.pdf.	Hearing loss affects two-thirds of adults with diabetes over age 50. Screening for hearing loss has not been demonstrated to slow the progression of the sensorineural hearing loss.
Autoimmune Hashimoto thyroiditis and celiac disease in children and adolescents with T1DM	*Thyroid* Thyroid peroxidase antibody (TPO) Thyroglobulin antibody *Celiac disease* IgA antiendomysial antibody	Prevalence of Hashimoto thyroiditis in patients with T1DM varies between 8% and 50%. Celiac disease coexists in 3%–8% of T1DM patients.

(Continued)

TABLE 1-6. Evidence-based Diabetes Standards of Care Summary *(Continued)*

	Standards of Care Recommendations (Based on Published Guidelines from the American Diabetes Association, American Cancer Society, and American College of Cardiology)	Evidence-based Grading System	Comment
Erectile and female sexual dysfunction	Questionnaire (IIEF) may be used as a screening tool for ED and is available online at www.dcurology.net/forms/ief.pdf. Female sexual dysfunction may be screened using the Female Sexual Distress Scale-Revised (FSDS-R) available online at www.obgynalliance.com/files/fsd/FSDS-R_Pocketcard.pdf.		Prevalence of ED is 35%–90%. The International Index of Erectile Function. In women with diabetes, the prevalence of sexual dysfunction is 47% (32% report vaginal dryness, 21% decreased libido, 15% have anorgasmia).
Androgen deficiency	Morning free and total testosterone, sex hormone–binding globulin. Optional tests: prolactin, FSH, LH, bone densitometry, and semen analysis if infertility is of concern Transferrin saturation if hereditary hemochromatosis is in the differential diagnosis		Patients with T2DM are twice as likely to have testosterone deficiency as age-matched controls. Hereditary hemochromatosis is associated with hypogonadotrophic hypogonadism and diabetes. Patients may present with fatigue, sexual dysfunction, myalgias, arthralgias, weight loss, and bronzing of the skin. If suspected, obtain transferrin saturation, which is >50% in patients having the disorder.
Obstructive sleep apnea	The Berlin Sleep Questionnaire may be used to screen obstructive sleep apnea and is available online: www.firstcoastcardio.com/files/Sleep.Questionnare.pdf If questionnaire is positive suggesting sleep apnea, consider performing an ApneaLink home study as described in Chapter 8. Definitive diagnosis requires a comprehensive sleep study.		Up to 70% of patients with diabetes have sleep apnea, which is associated with insulin resistance and obesity.
	American Diabetes Association Evidence-grading System		
Level A	Clear evidence from well-conducted, generalizable randomized controlled trials that are adequately powered, including: • Evidence from a well-conducted multicenter trial • Evidence from a meta-analysis that incorporated quality ratings in the analysis • Evidence from a well-conducted trial at one or more institutions		

Level B	Supportive evidence from well-conducted cohort studies, including:
	• Evidence from a well-conducted prospective cohort study or registry
	• Evidence from a well-conducted meta-analysis of cohort studies
Level C	Supportive evidence from poorly controlled or uncontrolled studies, including:
	• Evidence from randomized clinical trials with one or more major or three or more minor methodologic flaws that could invalidate the results
	• Evidence from observational studies with high potential for bias (such as case series with comparison to historical controls)
	• Evidence from case series or case reports
	Conflicting evidence with the weight of evidence favoring the recommendation
Level D	At least fair scientific evidence suggests that the risks of the clinical service outweigh potential benefits. Clinicians should not routinely offer the service to asymptomatic patients (*Note that this recommendation relates only to the USPSTF prostate cancer screening recommendations for 2011 and the task force recommendations against routine screening for peripheral arterial disease*).
Level E	Expert consensus or clinical experience[b]

(^^^) American Academy of Family Practice Strength of Recommendation Taxonomy (SORT)

Strength of Recommendation Grades	Basis for Recommendation
A	Consistent, good-quality patient-oriented evidence
B	Inconsistent or limited-quality patient-oriented evidence
C	Consensus, disease-oriented evidence, usual practice, expert opinion, or case series for studies of diagnosis, treatment, prevention, or screening

[a]BRCA genetic testing is available to screen for BRCA1 and BRCA2 mutations. Mutations in these genes have been linked to hereditary breast and ovarian cancers in women and breast and pancreatic cancers in men. Federal and state laws help ensure the privacy of a patient's genetic information and provide protection against discrimination in health insurance and employment practices. The likelihood of a harmful BRCA mutation being present is increased with certain familial patterns of cancer including: (A) Women who are not of Ashkenazi Jewish descent, but have two first-degree relatives (mother, daughter, or sister) diagnosed with breast cancer, one of whom was diagnosed at age 50 or younger; three or more first- or second-degree relatives (grandmother or aunt) diagnosed with breast cancer regardless of their age at diagnosis; a combination of first- and second-degree relatives diagnosed with breast and ovarian cancers (1 cancer type per person); a first-degree relative with bilateral breast cancer; a combination of two or more first- or second-degree relatives diagnosed with ovarian cancer regardless of age at diagnosis; a first- or second-degree relative diagnosed with both breast and ovarian cancers regardless of age at diagnosis and; breast cancer in a male relative. (B) For women of Ashkenazi Jewish descent, any first-degree relative diagnosed with breast or ovarian cancer; two second-degree relatives on the same side of the family diagnosed with breast or ovarian cancer. Approximately 2% of adult women in the general population will be BRCA positive. (http://www.cancer.gov/cancertopics/factsheet/Risk/BRCA).

[b]PSA screening should be performed on an individual basis after the patient is provided with informed consent related to the risks and benefits of prostate cancer screening. The United States Preventive Service Task Force (USPSTF) has concluded that screening for prostate cancer results in detection of more prostate cancers; small to no reduction in prostate cancer mortality after 10 years, and complications from false-positive PSA test results (including overdiagnosis and overtreatment). (Chou R, Croswell JM, Dana T, et al. Screening for prostate cancer: a review of the evidence for the U.S. Preventive Services Task Force. *Ann Intern Med.* 2011;155(11):762–771).

(Continued)

TABLE 1-6. Evidence-based Diabetes Standards of Care Summary (Continued)

http://www.aafp.org/online/en/home/publications/journals/afp/afpsort.html. Accessed December 29, 2011.

Rooke TW, Hirsch AT, Misra S, et al. 2011 ACCF/AHA focused update of the guideline for the management of patients with peripheral artery disease (Updating the 2005 Guideline). A report of the American College of Cardiology Foundation/American Heart Association Task Force on Practice Guidelines. *Circulation.*

American Diabetes Association. Standards of medical care in diabetes 2011. *Diabetes Care.* 2012;35(1):S2–S63.

American Diabetes Association. Peripheral arterial disease in people with diabetes (Consensus Statement). *Diabetes Care.* 2003;26:3333–3341.

U.S. Preventive Services Task Force. Screening for peripheral arterial disease. http://www.uspreventiveservicestaskforce.org/uspstf05/pad/padrs.htm. Accessed December 29, 2011

Adapted from: American Cancer Society American Cancer Society Guidelines for the Early Detection of Cancer http://www.cancer.org/Healthy/FindCancerEarly/CancerScreeningGuide-lines/american-cancer-society-guidelines-for-the-early-detection-of-cancer. Accessed September 16, 2011.

Enzlin P, Mathieu C, Demytteanere K. Diabetes and female sexual functioning: a state-of-the-art. Diabetes Spectrum. 2003;16:256–259.

Hirose K. Hearing loss and diabetes: you might not know what your're missing. *Ann Intern Med.* 2008;149(1):54–55.

Anderson RJ, Freedland KE, Clouse RE, et al. The prevalence of comorbid depression in adults with diabetes: a meta-analysis. *Diabetes Care.* 2001;24(6):1069–1078.

Malavige LS, Levy JC. Erectile dysfunction in diabetes mellitus. *J Sex Med.* 2009;6(5):1232–1247.

Hanukoglu A, Mizrachi A, Dalí I, et al. Extrapancreatic autoimmune manifestations in type 1 diabetes patients and their first-degree relatives. *Diabetes Care.* 2003;26:1235–1240.

Jackman RP, Judkins DZ. What screening tests should you use to evaluate a man with low testosterone? *J Fam Pract.* 2008;57(11):756–758.

American Association of Clinical Endocrinologists. Hypogonadism guidelines: https://www.aace.com/sites/default/files/hypogonadism.pdf.

Brissot P, Troadec MB, Bardou-Jacquet E, et al. Current approach to hemochromatosis. *Blood Rev.* 2008;224):195–210.

Wilkins T, Reynolds PL. Colorectal cancer: A summary of the evidence for screening and prevention. *Am Fam Physician.* 2008;78(12):1385–1392.

Screening for osteoporosis. Clinical summary of U.S. Preventive Services Task Force recommendation. http://www.uspreventiveservicestaskforce.org/uspstf10/osteoporosis/osteosum.htm. Accessed December 29, 2011.

Altitude Trial of Aliskiren added to ACE or ARB in patients with diabetes and concurrent kidney disease. http://www.clinicaltrials.gov/ct2/show/record/NCT00549757?term=ALTITUDE&rank=2

Quadrivalent human papillomavirus vaccine. Recommendations of the Advisory Committee on Immunization Practices (ACIP). MMWR recommendations and Reports. March 23, 2007/56(RR02); 1-24) http://www.cdc.gov/mmwr/preview/mmwrhtml/rr5602a1.htm Accessed December 28, 2011.

FDA licensure of quadrivalent human papillomavirus vaccine (HPV4, Gardasil) for use in males and guidance from the Advisor Committee on Immunization Practices (ACIP). *MMWR Morb Mortal.* May 28. 2010;59(20):630–632. http://www.cdc.gov/mmwr/preview/mmwrhtml/mm5920a5.htm. Accessed December 28, 2011.

Knutson D, Steiner E. Screening for breast cancer: Current recommendations and future directions. Am Fam Wkly Rep Physician. 2007;75(11):1660–1666.

Saslow D, Boetes C, Burke W, et al., for the American Cancer Society. American Cancer Society guidelines for breast screening with MRI as an adjunct to mammography. *CA Cancer J Clin.* 2007;57:76.

Silverstein MJ, Lagios MD, Recht A, et al. Image-detected breast cancer: state of the art diagnosis and treatment. *J Am Coll Surg.* 2005;201:587.

Clinical practice recommendations are published annually by the ADA. These recommendations consist of position statements that are produced under the auspices of the ADA by invited experts and approved by the Professional Practice and Executive Committee of the ADA Board of Directors. The recommendations are based on scientific evidence derived from scientific and medical peer-reviewed journals. Clinicians are encouraged to interpret the needs of each individual patient and consider comorbid and coexisting diseases such as age, education, and disability when prescribing or intensifying therapy. Most importantly, the ADA encourages clinicians to always consider patient values and preferences when prescribing the most appropriate treatment for each individual.[40]

The Art of Communication

Many patients compare their attempts at effectively communicating with their PCP as if they were contestants on the "Gong Show For Diabetics!" They look forward to their doctor's appointment with anxious anticipation. They are prepared to ask questions, discuss concerns about adverse drug effects, hypoglycemia, weight gain, or lack of drug efficacy. They may be experiencing a progression of one of their previously diagnosed complications or concerned as to why their A1C levels continue to rise despite being on an insulin pump for 2 years. Some patients may actually be thrilled to show their doctor their improved glucose logs or have the staff comment on their 3-lb weight loss. These patients and their families have little or no interest in the latest EMR tools or meaningful use requirements of an individual practice. They are asking for the clinician's undivided attention to their concerns, achievements, and perhaps failures. Providers all too often appear to be insensitive to the concerns of the patient and his family members. With one hand on the computer and the other on the escape hatch of the exam room, one could easily understand why patients become disinterested in their own diabetes self-management.

When I give lectures to large groups of physicians I often ask the question, "How many of you in the audience have seen a patient with diabetes in the past 4 weeks who you consider as being 'non-compliant' with their treatment regimen?" Immediately 90% of the hands in the audience are raised while many turn to their seated neighbors and quickly attempt to relate their favorite tale of dysfunctional self-care by one of their patients. The group is quickly silenced when they are reminded that diabetes is a complex, progressive, and often frustrating chronic disorder that challenges the most astute clinicians and patients. When people who do not have diabetes eat, their pancreas secretion of insulin maintains the plasma glucose in the consistent range of 85 to 140 mg per dL. Those with diabetes are not so lucky. Those who are using insulin, for example, have to check their blood glucose before they eat, calculate a correction factor, count the grams of carbohydrates they will be eating for that meal, and consider if they intend to increase their activity level within 4 hours of giving their meal time insulin. After eating, they can perform a 2-hour postprandial glucose check to making certain that they have not exceeded the ADA recommend level of 180 mg per dL. If they have, they have the option of providing a correction bolus based on the "rule of 1,800." Of course, when they correct, they will have to monitor once again 2 to 3 hours later to make certain they have not driven themselves into hypoglycemia. These same patients will need to take their ACE or ARB blood pressure medications, an aspirin, and a statin, as well as any additional drugs that are needed to control or prevent microvascular or macrovascular complications. Patients with diabetes will need to have lab testing performed at least twice a year and see the eye doctor annually. Those with long-term complications will require specialty referrals and comprehensive care. As the patient is attempting to monitor his glucose levels and bolus insulin, he is being observed by a neighbor, a friend, or a spouse eager to tell him "you are doing it all wrong." Despite the odds of failure, many patients actually do very well attaining their specified glycemic targets, admitting that each day is a challenge.

Returning my attention to the audience I again ask the question, "OK, how many of you have seen a patient in the past 4 weeks who has been non-compliant?" This time, they are silenced by the rhetorical query. Patients are not noncompliant. Physicians need to become better educators, coaches, and motivators for patients with diabetes. Only by understanding this disease state and confirming their willingness to learn will patients be successfully managed rather than treated toward failure. Why must a 21-year-old patient with an A1C of 12% complaining of weight loss, thirst, and blurred vision who begs to be placed on insulin have to be treated for another 3 months on an oral agent when clearly the need for intensive therapy exists? Is this patient noncompliant as well?

Because diabetes management is so complex from both a professional and patient perspective, choosing our battles appropriately will likely influence the success of our prescribed treatments. Patients with diabetes tend to worry endlessly about become a "diabetic invalid," a burden to their family who will invariably lose an eye, kidney, or foot to this miserable disease. Intensification of therapy to such individuals is interpreted not as a proactive approach designed to physiologically control glucose levels, but as a personal failure to achieve ideal glycemic control through one's personal dedication to lifestyle change. Some patients may eventually become disengaged with their diabetes self-management altogether. Others become obsessive about self-glucose monitoring and avoidance of hyperglycemia to the point that they become chronically hypoglycemic. Beware of the patient who presents proudly with an A1C of 5.3% and declares that he is "going to be complication free." In fact, these patients probably have hypoglycemia awareness autonomic failure and are unable to recognize the symptoms or effectively counterregulate the physiologic pathways associated with severe hypoglycemia.

Managing diabetes is actually quite simple if focus can be directed to five basic goals. Once a patient realizes that they may be responsible for only five interventions for successful diabetes management, their self-confidence will rise.

The "Top 5" Strategies for Successful Diabetes Management

Successful management of diabetes is based upon five fundamental strategies. Implementation of the five points listed in Table 1-7 will provide a road map for effective self-management of diabetes.

Elevating Your Knowledge Base about Diabetes

Those physicians who are serious about providing quality care and services to patients with diabetes should become the "the local expert" for the disorder. One could begin the process by joining professional organizations such as the American Diabetes Association (http://www.diabetes.org/about-us/become-a-member.html) and the American Association of Clinical Endocrinologists (www.aace.com). Membership in these organizations will allow access to online CME, medical journals, and newsletters, as well as regional and national meetings.

Physicians interested in integrating basic science, pharmacology, clinical medicine, and advanced patient care into their practices should consider becoming a clinical investigator for novel drug therapies. Clinical research is necessary to establish the safety and efficacy of medical products and practices. Expert opinions and consensus guidelines are based upon information attained from data derived from randomized controlled clinical trials. Patients who enroll in clinical trials do so with the hope that their participation will provide the sponsor with important valuable information regarding a drug, medical device, or a disease state. Most clinical trial volunteers are not charged for any professional medical services rendered during the course of the study. Therefore, physicians

 TABLE 1-7. Five Simple Interventions to Improve One's Likelihood of Becoming a Successful Diabetes Self-manager

1. Know your metabolic targets (A1C, blood pressure, lipids).

2. Understand how to best achieve these targets (behavioral and pharmacologic intervention).

3. Stop smoking. If the patient does not smoke, don't start!

4. Be adherent with the prescribed treatment regimen (pharmacologic and lifestyle).

5. Make certain that the care received is directed and supervised by providers who are dedicated to the successful management of patients with diabetes.

Top 5 courtesy of Bill Polonsky, PhD, CDE.

may offer study participation to all patients within a practice including those with no access to health insurance. Owing to the importance of gathering and reporting all data from patients enrolled in clinical trials, the protocols for managing such individuals are unique and require additional training by the "primary investigator" and the research staff. The FDA sponsors an annual clinical investigator training course for physicians who are interested in becoming expert trialists.[41] Various online, web-based, and live commercial courses are also available.

Pharmaceutical representatives may also provide guidance to physicians who truly wish to provide a high level of care to their patients with diabetes. Beside offering the typical patient education resources, some companies will provide certified diabetic educators to help train patients on everything from medical nutrition therapy to use of injection devices. Pharma rules are in place, which may restrict the location of training to an off-site venue. Physicians may also speak with company medical liaisons about specific questions or concerns they have related to an individual drug or product. The medical liaison is not a market representative and has at their disposal a more detailed database of scientific information from which they can answer most disease state and drug-specific medical inquiries.

Physicians who become thought leaders within their specialty are often sought out by various device and pharmaceutical companies as advisory board members. Advisory boards provide a forum of discussion on future clinical trial design, publication planning, research and development updates, safety and efficacy data, and integration of novel drugs into the current marketplace. Most importantly, the Ad Boards allow members the opportunity to interact professionally with some of the best minds in the industry.

The American Academy of Family Practice sponsors many continuing medical education courses on diabetes, which are available on their Web site: www.aafp.org. Additional CME is available for members of the American Association of Clinical Endocrinologists (https://www.aace.com/education/cme/asap).

Putting Primary Skill Training to Work for Patients with Diabetes

Diabetes provides PCPs with a unique opportunity to enhance the lives of patients by providing behavioral modification, preventive treatments, urgent therapies, and psychological support. In a patient with a history of gestational diabetes mellitus (GDM), in all likelihood, T2DM eventually will develop. The PCP would suggest that these high-risk patients begin a daily exercise regimen, coupled with strategies to reduce their weight, in an attempt to delay their progression toward diabetes. Children born to mothers with GDM whose birth weight exceeded 9 lb have a higher incidence of T2DM that develops during adolescence, which, in turn, would increase their risk of coronary artery disease during the second decade of life. Early intervention with patient education regarding lifestyle modification may be helpful in reducing the prevalence of obesity, diabetes, and heart disease in at-risk populations.

Preconception counseling can prevent microvascular complications and improve maternal/fetal outcomes. By initiating the discussion on preconception planning for all adolescent patients in the primary care setting, physicians are able to emphasize the benefits of attaining and maintaining targeted glycemic levels as soon as possible after the diagnosis of diabetes is made.

PCPs are trained in **behavioral intervention strategies.** By providing the proper guidance, therapeutic options, and encouragement to enhance successful outcomes, we can become a motivational force for our patients to replace harmful behaviors—such as smoking and inactivity—with healthy lifestyle interventions. Prescribing a basic exercise program, asking a patient to eat sensibly by using the ADA food pyramid (see Chapter 3), and providing patients with the tools necessary to perform home blood glucose monitoring (see Chapter 3) are neither time consuming nor counterproductive.

Our patients look to their PCP for **guidance** related to all aspects of their medical care from managing influenza to diagnosing the cause of their chronic headaches. Patients realize that diabetes is a complicated disorder that lacks a cure. However, by guiding patients toward the lowest and safest attainable A1C level, we will allow them to live longer, more productive lives in the comfort of their own homes and away from the unfriendly confines of the intensive care unit (ICU).

PCPs should always be alert for patients at risk not only for having prediabetes but those who might benefit substantially from **early diagnosis and intervention** of their abnormal metabolic profiles. PCPs are often consulted by patients who are concerned about acne, obesity, hirsutism, abnormal periods, and infertility. These patients may have polycystic ovary syndrome (PCOS), an endocrine disorder that predisposes the individual to diabetes and heart disease. Treating these patients with metformin or a thiazolidinedione (TZD) may allow them to become pregnant and improve their metabolic status.

Primary **prevention of diabetes-related complications** should be our first priority. Unfortunately, many of our patients are seen in our practices for the first time with poorly controlled diabetes of long duration. Our management must focus on secondary intervention strategies, as exemplified most often in patients with microvascular disease. Although we are unable to reverse the structural damage to neurons, nephrons, or the retina, we can certainly provide patients with the tools necessary to slow the rate of disease progression and limit their physical disabilities. Our approach should always be focused on complication surveillance.

Encourage patients to remove their shoes at each visit so that their feet can be inspected. Patients who are **insensate** should be given a monofilament to use on their own feet on a daily basis. Instead of telling a patient "I want you to inspect your feet each night and let me know if you see anything suspicious," ask the patient to use a monofilament on his or her feet each night before bedtime. In the case of patients who are insensate, you have my permission to tell them a "little white fib." "John, I'd like you to take this monofilament home with you. Beginning each night at bedtime, go ahead and touch your feet with the filament. Let me know when the feeling comes back into your feet (this is the white fib, by the way). As soon as you feel anything, let me know immediately. Oh, and if you happen to see any blisters, red spots, ulcers, or anything else that might concern you, I want to know about it right away! Go ahead and call my office. Thanks for helping us out here, John."

In reality, the feeling in John's feet will never return. However, this patient is at high risk for a plantar ulcer or a Charcot foot syndrome. The use of the monofilament essentially forces John to inspect his feet each night. If he sees a suspicious area on the foot, he knows he has permission to contact his doctor. This proactive approach might save a limb. Having done this with my own patients, I have found even more success when I contact these individuals by phone 1 week after providing them with their monofilament. I ask them the following question: "Hey John, this is your doctor. I'm just checking to see if you have felt any sensation in your feet since you started using that monofilament I gave you. Well, keep trying, because you never know when that tingling may return to your feet. Let me know if you see any funny stuff on your feet that concerns you. We'll see you next time around, and thanks for helping me keep you in such good shape!"

Patients with **chronic kidney disease** should be advised to stop smoking. They should be given statins to lower their low-density lipoprotein cholesterol (LDL-C) levels to less than 100 mg per dL, take aspirin, limit their dietary intake of red meat, begin using an ACE or an ARB, reduce their blood pressure to less than 120/75, and be screened for anemia. Although appearing complicated, if not a bit overwhelming, these tasks are mandated by the ADA practice management guidelines[42] and should be followed by all physicians caring for patients with diabetes.

PCPs may see one to two patients with **major depressive disorder** (MDD) each day, most of whom are at high risk for developing T2DM. Patients with T2DM and MDD share some common phenotypic characteristics: obesity, inactivity, cigarette smoking, and elevations in C-reactive protein. Not only do 80% of patients with T2DM have a history of MDD within 8 years of their initial diagnosis,[43] but depressed diabetes patients also have a higher risk of coronary artery disease than do diabetic patients without mood disorders.[44] Perhaps screening depressed patients for diabetes and patients with diabetes for depression should be considered.

Patients at risk for developing T2DM should be screened according to the ADA guidelines.[42] Lifestyle intervention should begin immediately for all high-risk individuals. Patients newly diagnosed with diabetes should be given combination drug therapy in addition to behavioral interventions. Failure to attain an A1C level of less than 7% should initiate a rapid progression to intensification of treatment based on recommended treatment guidelines published by the American Diabetes Association or The American Association of Clinical Endocrinologists.[45,46]

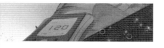

SUMMARY

As a chronic disease, diabetes offers an opportunity for PCPs to have a central role in managing and coordinating patient care. Diabetes has a broad spectrum of severity, with the majority of patients having a less severe and "less intimidating" form of the disease. Most patients with diabetes require pharmacologic regimens that are well established, widely used, and safe, allowing PCPs to provide care for many of their own patients and referring more complex cases to specialists. The coexisting disorders that accompany diabetes must be addressed by the PCP. Patients with chronic, poorly controlled hyperglycemia may have multiple complications that require the coordination and management skills of a shrewd practitioner. Finally, expertise in behavioral change and disease self-management is central to successful care of any chronic disease, especially diabetes. No one is better trained to promote patient adherence and self-management in chronic disease states than PCPs. Whereas specialty training focuses on managing a single disease state or organ, PCPs understand the connection between the mind and the body. We know our patients better than anyone else. If we can make our patients feel good about themselves and their efforts in diabetes self-management, we should be able to help patients expand their lifetimes and live complication-free lives.

Appropriate and timely physician compensation is certainly warranted for all physicians managing highly complex patients with chronic diseases. PCPs are highly trained specialists capable of screening, preventing, treating, and coordinating care of all patients with diabetes. Our practices are unique in that our patient population includes people of all ages, ethnicities, sexual orientations, literacy capabilities, psychological profiles, and medical comorbidities. Our relationships with patients are long and enduring. We are innovators of care yet often compensated as midlevel providers by third-party payers. We are lifelong students of medicine because we truly love to make our patients safe, healthy, and strong.

This book provides PCPs with the tools necessary to manage successfully the many medical challenges related to diabetes. Patients need our guidance to achieve their targeted metabolic goals through a variety of lifestyle interventions, prescribed pharmacologic therapies, and behavioral modifications. Simply admonishing a patient to "lose weight, exercise, eat right, and check your sugars" will most often result in a failed attempt at pleasing the medical provider. Patients will often incorporate a healthy lifestyle into their daily lives if they become partners in their own care and "students of diabetes pathophysiology."

What an exciting era we have entered as we attempt to lead our patients with diabetes down a road less littered with weakened bodies riddled by complications. Before the discovery of insulin in 1922, patients died as a direct result of diabetes. In modern times, patients with diabetes are living on average 45 years longer than they did before insulin was available. The long-term consequences of chronic hyperglycemia exposure result in morbidity and mortality from eye, kidney, neurologic, and cardiovascular diseases. Our landmark studies have taught us the importance of providing our patients with safe and effective "customized care." We know that overprescribing care to susceptible patients can be dangerous. Therefore, everyone has their own A1C target, which is dependent upon their age, existing comorbidities, duration of diabetes, and expected length of life.

Managing diabetes is certainly not an easy undertaking, yet we can always turn to our patients for guidance. One of my patients with end-stage renal failure who was on fluid restriction while on dialysis explained how he managed to control his thirst during the hot summer days in Southern California. "It's real easy, Doctor. If you drink from a straw, the liquid goes down real slow and that tends to quench your thirst better than when you down 12 ounce bottles of cold water as fast as you can!"

On behalf of all patients with diabetes and their families, thank you for taking the time to learn how to manage this complex disorder. I applaud your dedication to their cause.

REFERENCES

1. Unger J. Diabetes management in the new millennium (Editorial, Primary Care Edition). *Female Patient.* 2001;6:10–11.
2. Hiss RG. Barriers to care in non-insulin dependent diabetes mellitus: the Michigan experience. *Ann Intern Med.* 1996;124:146–148.
3. The Diabetes Control and Complications Trial/Epidemiology of Diabetes Interventions and Complications Research Group. Retinopathy and nephropathy in patients with type 1 diabetes four years after a trial of intensive therapy. *N Engl J Med.* 2000;342:381–389.
4. The Diabetes Control and Complications Trial/Epidemiology of Diabetes Interventions and Complications (DCCT/EDIC) Study Group. Intensive diabetes treatment and cardiovascular disease in patients with type 1 diabetes. *N Engl J Med.* 2005;353:2643–2653.
5. Diabetes Control and Complications Trial/Epidemiology of Diabetes Interventions and Complications Research Group. Intensive diabetes therapy and carotid intima-media thickness in type 1 diabetes mellitus. *N Engl J Med.* 2003;348:2294–2903.
6. U.S. Department of Health and Human Services, Centers for Disease Control and Prevention, 2011. National diabetes fact sheet: national estimates and general information on diabetes and prediabetes in the United States, 2011. Available at: http://www.cdc.gov/diabetes/pubs/pdf/ndfs_2011.pdf. Accessed October 20, 2011.
7. Boyle JP, Thompson TJ, Gregg EW, et al. Projection of the year 2050 burden of diabetes in the U.S. adult population: dynamic modeling of incidence, mortality, and prediabetes prevalence. *Popul Health Metr.* 2010;8:29.
8. Diabetes Data & Forecasts. 2025 Diabetes Forecasts for State and Metropolitan Areas Study by the Institute for Alternative Futures. This study utilizes a national model from Narayan. Impact of Recent Increase in Incidence on Future Diabetes Burden. *Diabetes Care.* 2006;9:2114–2116; the latest CDC projections by Boyle; U.S. Census Bureau population estimates; and latest CDC national diabetes statistics and state prevalence rates. www.altfutures.org/diabetes2025.
9. U.S. Department of Health and Human Services, Fiscal Year Budget in Brief. Available at: http://dhhs.gov/asfr/ob/docbudget/2010budgetinbriefl.html. Accessed December 18, 2011.
10. Wild S, Roglic G, Green A, et al. Global Prevalence of Diabetes. Estimates for the year 2000 and projections for 2030. *Diabetes Care.* 2004;27:1047–1053.
11. Fagot-Campagna A, Petitt DJ, Engelgau MM, et al. Type 2 diabetes among North American children and adolescents: an epidemiologic review and a public health perspective. *J Pediatr.* 2000;136:664–672.
12. Centers for Disease Control and Prevention: National Diabetes Fact Sheet: General Information and National Estimates on Diabetes in the United States 2011. Available at: http://www.cdc.gov/diabetes/pubs/figuretext11.htm!fig4. Accessed October 22, 2011.
13. Gilliam LK, Brooks-Worrell BM, Palmer JP, et al. Autoimmunity and clinical course in children with type 1, type 2, and type 1.5 diabetes. *J Autoimmunol.* 2005;25:244–250.
14. Tfayli H, Bacha F, Gungor N, et al. Phenotypic type 2 diabetes in obese youth: insulin sensitivity and secretion in islet cell antibody-negative versus-positive patients. *Diabetes.* 2009;58:738–744.
15. Dabelea D, D'Agostino RB Jr, Mayer-Davis EJ, et al. SEARCH for Diabetes in Youth Study Group: Testing the accelerator hypothesis: body size, beta cell function, and age at onset of type 1 (autoimmune) diabetes. *Diabetes Care.* 2006;29:1462–1463.
16. Reinehr T, Schober E, Roth CL, et al. DPV-Wiss Study Group. Type 2 diabetes in children and adolescents in a 2-year follow-up: insufficient adherence to diabetes centers. *Horm Res.* 2008;69:107–113.
17. Weigensberg MJ, Goran MI. Type 2 diabetes in children and adolescents. *Lancet.* 2009;373:1743–1744.
18. Jones KL, Arslanian S, Peterokova VA, et al. Effect of metformin in pediatric patients with type 2 diabetes: a randomized controlled trial. *Diabetes Care.* 2002;25:89–94.
19. Flint A, Arslanian S. Treatment of type 2 diabetes in youth. *Diabetes Care.* 2011;34(Suppl 2):S177–S183.
20. National Center for Health Statistics. Cycle I of the Health and Examination Survey: Sample and Response. United States: 1960–1962. *Vital Health Stat.* 1965;1(4):1–43.

21. Hoerger TJ, Segel JE, Gregg EW, et al. Is glycemic control improving in U.S. adults? *Diabetes Care*. 2008;31(1):81–86.

22. Health Affairs. Vol. 30 No. 10. Available at: http://www.healthaffairs.org/healthpolicybriefs/brief.php?brief_id=25. Accessed October 22, 2011.

23. Larson EB, Reid R. The patient-centered medical home movement why now? *JAMA* 2010;303(16):1644–1645.

24. Qliance Primary Care Specialist Brochure. Available at: http://www.qliance.com/pdf/Qliance+Current+Brochure.pdf. Accessed December 23, 2011.

25. Reid RJ, Fishman PA, Yu O, et al. Patient-centered medical home demonstration: a prospective, quasi-experimental, before and after evaluation. *Am J Manag Care*. 2009;15(9):e71–e87.

26. Rossner WW, Colwill JM, Kasperski J, et al. Progress of Ontario's family health team model: a patient-centered medical home. *Ann Fam Med*. 2011;9:165–171.

27. Valderas JM, Starfield B, Forrest CB, et al. Ambulatory care provided by office-based specialists in the United States. *Ann Fam Med*. 2009;7(2):104–111.

28. Centers for Medicare and Medicaid Services. 2011 Annual Report of the Boards of Trustees of the Federal Hospital Insurance and Federal Supplemental Medical Insurance Trust Funds. May 13, 2011, p. 55. Available at: https://www.cms.gov/ReportsTrustFunds/downloads/tr2011.pdf (September 19, 2011). Accessed December 27, 2011.

29. Moffit, R. The first stage of Medicare reform: Fixing the current program. The Heritage Foundation: Available at: http://www.heritage.org/research/reports/2011/10/the-first-stage-of-medicare-reform-fixing-the-current-program#_ftn6. Accessed June 1, 12.

30. Fisher ES, McClellan MB, Bertko J, et al. Fostering accountable health care: moving forward in Medicare. *Health Aff (Millwood)*. 2009;28:w219–w231.

31. Rice D, Roberts WL, Collinsworth A, et al. Diabetes and accountable care organizations: an accountable care approach to diabetes management. *ClinDiabetes*. 2011;29(2):70–72.

32. Physician Group Practice Demonstration succeeds in improving quality and reducing costs. Press release of the Centers for Medicare and Medicaid Services, August 8, 2011. Available at: https://www.cms.gov/apps/media/press/release.asp?Counter=4047.

33. Centers for Medicare and Medicaid Services. Physician group practice demonstration. Available at: https://www.cms.gov/DemoProjectsEvalRpts/downloads/PGP_Summary_Results.pdf. Accessed June 1, 2012.

34. Wellington M: Stanford Health Partners: Rationale and early experiences in establishing physician group visits and chronic disease self management workshops. *J Ambul Care Manag*. 2001;24:10–16.

35. Langford AT, Sawyer DR, Gioimo S, et al. Patient-centered goal setting as a tool to improve diabetes self-management. *Diabetes Educ*. 2007;33:139S–144S.

36. Trento M, Passera P, Tomalino M, et al. Group visits improve metabolic control in type 2 diabetes. *Diabetes Care*. 2001;24:995–1000.

37. Sadur CN, Moline N, Costa M, et al. Diabetes management in a health maintenance organization. *Diabetes Care*. 1991;12:2011–2017.

38. Clancy DE, Cope DW, Magruder KM, et al. Evaluating concordance to American Diabetes Association standards of care for type 2 diabetes through group visits in an uninsured or inadequately insured patient population. *Diabetes Care*. 2003;26:2032–2036.

39. Riley SB, Marshall ES. Group visits in diabetes care: a systematic review. *Diabetes Educ*. 2010;36(6):936–944.

40. American Diabetes Association. Standards of Medical Care in Diabetes. *Diabetes Care*. 2012;35(Suppl 1):S1–S2.

41. http://pharma.about.com/gi/o.htm?zi=1/XJ&zTi=1&sdn=pharma&cdn=b2b&tm=71&f=00&tt=2&bt=0&bts=0&st=10&zu=http%3A//www.fda.gov/ScienceResearch/SpecialTopics/CriticalPathInitiative/SpotlightonCPIProjects/ucm201459.htm

42. American Diabetes Association. Position Statement: Standards of Medical Care in Diabetes—2006. *Diabetes Care*. 2006;29:S4–S42.

43. Lustman PJ, Griffith LS, Clouse RE. Depression in adults with diabetes: results of 5-yr follow-up study. *Diabetes Care*. 1988;11:605–612.

44. Katon WJ, Lin EH, Russo J, et al. Cardiac risk factors in patients with diabetes mellitus and major depression. *J Gen Intern Med*. 2004;19:1192–1199.

45. Nathan DM, Buse JB, Davidson MB, et al. Medical management of hyperglycemia in type 2 diabetes: a consensus algorithm for the initiation and adjustment of therapy: a consensus statement of the American Diabetes Association and the European Association for the Study of Diabetes. *Diabetes Care*. 2009;32 (1):193–203.

46. Rodbard HW, Jellinger PS, Davidson JA, et al. Statement by an American Association of Clinical Endocrinologists/American College of Endocrinology consensus panel on type 2 diabetes mellitus: an algorithm for glycemic control. *Endocr Pract*. 2009;15:540–559.

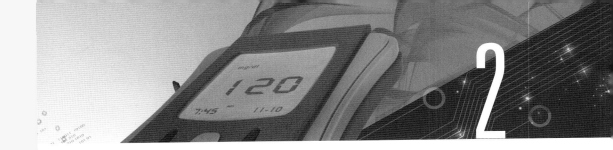

Prediabetes

The more you prepare, the luckier you appear.
—Terry Josephson, 20th/21st-century
   motivational author

Introduction One of the most common questions posed to thought leaders at continuous medical education meetings relates to the appropriate and timely management options for patients diagnosed with prediabetes. Patients frequently request information from their primary care physicians on ways that they may "cure diabetes." Other patients proudly declare that they were once diagnosed with diabetes. However, with the use of lifestyle intervention, prescribed or herbal medications, they appear to be symptom and diagnosis free. Chiropractors are now advertising in local newspapers ways by which their homeopathic services may reverse diabetic peripheral neuropathy and type 2 diabetes (T2DM). With over 1.8 million Google hits for "prediabetes" versus only 434,000 for "prehypertension," one could clearly understand the importance of early detection and prevention of diabetes. How one tests for, diagnoses, and treats prediabetes may have an enormous impact on a patient's life quality and longevity.

Prediabetes is strongly correlated with increased insulin resistance, which is a mediator for an adverse cardiometabolic profile.[1] Prediabetes is characterized by decreasing sensitivity of target tissues to the action of insulin, elevated blood glucose, and insulin concentrations in association with elevations of hepatic glucose production and atherogenic lipids. Clinical markers of prediabetes include elevated plasma glucose concentrations under fasting and/or postprandial conditions, increased serum triglycerides, and below normal levels of high-density lipoprotein cholesterol (HDL-C). A decrease in antiatherogenic HDL-C is indicative of impaired reverse cholesterol transport that, over time, accelerates atherosclerosis.

Abnormal visceral adipose tissue secretions influence multiple metabolic pathways that modulate glycemia and blood pressure control. Ultimately, the anti-inflammatory and proinflammatory balance becomes disjointed favoring inflammation, impaired glucose tolerance (IGT), circadian abnormalities in blood pressure control, endothelial cell dysfunction, and abnormal platelet adhesion.

The estimated relative risk (RR) for cardiovascular disease associated with IGT ranges from 0.97 to 1.30 and that associated with IFG ranges from 1.12 to 1.37. The risk is higher for patients having fasting glucose levels in the range of 110 to 126 mg per dL (Fig. 2-1).[2] Some reviews suggest that IGT doubles the risk for macrovascular disease.[3] The increased cardiovascular risk observed in patients with prediabetes is due to the endothelial changes that occur as one progresses toward clinical conversion to T2DM.[4]

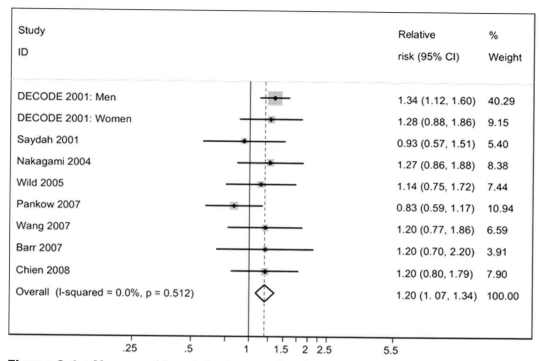

Figure 2-1 • Measures of Association between Impaired Glucose Tolerance and Cardiovascular Outcomes. The RR of cardiovascular disease in patients with prediabetes has been evaluated in several publications noted on the left side of the chart. The estimate of the RR (*represented by the diamond shape*) and confidence interval (*square box*—portrayed graphically as the weight estimate provided to each study) is shown at each data point. The overall summary of the estimated RR is shown on the last row of the graph. (Adapted from Ford ES, Zhao G, Li C. Pre-diabetes and the risk of cardiovascular disease. A systemic review of the evidence. J Am Coll Cardiol. 2010; 55: 1310–1131).

Because patients with prediabetes convert to clinical diabetes at the rate of approximately 6% to 29% over 4 years, targeting such high-risk patients for early therapeutic interventions would be key to the primary prevention of coronary artery disease.[5]

Although one could argue about when and how to treat patients diagnosed with prediabetes, the truth of the matter is that in virtually all cases therapeutic interventions are safer, less expensive, and more durable when initiated earlier rather than later after one is diagnosed with IGT. As a physician, wouldn't you rather treat an asymptomatic patient who presents for a routine physical exam and is found on screening to have a random blood glucose of 179 mg/dL and an A1C of 5.9%. The patient is overweight and has a family history of T2DM. Or, perhaps you would prefer evaluating a 65-year-old man, new to your practice with a 20-year history of poorly controlled diabetes and coronary artery disease?

Patients with prediabetes are often motivated to do whatever is necessary to avoid exposure to prolonged hyperglycemia and risking long-term complications. They know that early interventions, which normalize glucose levels will allow them to live lives comparable to those individuals who are euglycemic. Thus, these patients are eager to listen, learn, and adhere to any and all prescribed interventions including the adaptation of healthier lifestyles and pharmacologic therapies.

Prediabetes Definition and Prevalence

By definition, patients with prediabetes have evidence of impaired fasting glucose (IFG) (fasting glucose levels of 100 to 125 mg per dL), IGT [2-hour plasma glucose in a 75-g oral glucose

TABLE 2-1. Diagnostic Criteria for Prediabetes and Diabetes

	Fasting Plasma Glucose (mg/dL)	Two-hour Oral Glucose Challenge[a] (mg/dL)	A1C (%)
Normal	<100	<140	<5.6
Prediabetes	100–125	140–199	5.7–6.4
Diabetes	>126	>200[b]	≥6.5[c]

[a]Two-hour glucose challenge test should be performed using a glucose load containing 75 g of anhydrous glucose dissolved in water.
[b]In a patient with classic symptoms of hyperglycemia or hyperglycemic crisis, a random plasma glucose ≥ 200 mg/dL is also diagnostic of diabetes.
[c]A1C should be performed via a standardized laboratory test rather than a point of service screening test.

tolerance test (OGTT) of 140 to 199 mg per dL], or both IFG and IGT (Table 2-1).[6] Normal fasting glucose levels are <100 mg per dL, while 2-hour postprandial glucose values do not exceed 140 mg per dL in euglycemic individuals. Any random blood glucose level >200 mg per dL is considered diagnostic for diabetes. Patients with prediabetes have a glycemic burden favoring the development of microvascular and macrovascular complications.[7,8]

Six to ten percent of patients with IGT progress to clinical diabetes each year, whereas up to sixty-five percent of individuals with both IFG and IGT progress to clinical diabetes annually when compared to euglycemic subjects.[9] Therefore, aggressive screening and ambitious treatment of high-risk individuals targeting β-cell preservation may slow disease progression and theoretically improve outcomes. Table 2-2 lists the risk factors for patients at risk for developing prediabetes as well as those individuals who warrant screening for the disorder. Progression rates of IFG or IGT to diabetes vary according to degrees of initial hyperglycemia, racial and ethnic backgrounds, and environmental influences. The higher the glucose values, the greater the risk of progression to diabetes and diabetic complications.[10]

Fifty-seven million Americans have prediabetes (IFG, IGT or both),[11] whereas the worldwide incidence of prediabetes is projected to be 418 million in 2025.[12]

As the prevalence of and progression to diabetes have increased, diabetes-related complications and disease state mortality have emerged as an expensive major health care issue. The

TABLE 2-2. Screening Patients at High Risk for Developing Prediabetes

Patients at Risk for Developing Prediabetes	Whom to Target for Prediabetes Screening
• History of polycystic ovary syndrome • History of gestational diabetes • Children of parents with T2DM • Patients with abdominal obesity	• + Family history of diabetes • History of cardiovascular disease • Obesity • Sedentary lifestyle • Nonwhite ancestry • Previous history if IGT or IFG • History of hypertension • History of elevated triglycerides and low HDL-C or both • History of gestational diabetes • History of polycystic ovary syndrome • Delivery of a baby weighing >9 lbs • Patients with schizophrenia or bipolar disorder

Adopted from Garber AJ, Handelsman Y, Einhorn D, et al. Diagnosis and management of prediabetes in the continuum of hyperglycemia—when do the risk of diabetes begin? A consensus statement from the American College of Endocrinology and the American Association of Clinical Endocrinologists. *Endocr Pract.* 2008;14(7):933–945.

annual cost of diabetes is over $174 billion. Direct costs related to diabetes and diabetes-related complications are $116 billion.[13] More importantly, diabetes robs individuals of productive days, months, and years that they could spend with family members and within the community as valuable contributors to society.

As primary care physicians, we are most adept at screening for, diagnosing, and managing chronic diseases. When physicians focus on identifying patients who are at high risk for developing diabetes and actually make the diagnosis of prediabetes, lives can be changed forever.

Ironically, the diagnosis of "prediabetes" may have some negative connotations. For example, once a patient is diagnosed as having IGT, his or her health insurance coverage may change because the patient now has a "preexisting condition" consistent with diabetes. Additionally, life insurance policies may become more expensive as underwriters adjust costs based on projected life expectancy rates that are influenced by a high prevalence of cardiovascular disease in patients with diabetes.[14]

Nevertheless, physicians should provide patients with a positive outlook after one is diagnosed with prediabetes. Patients with prediabetes have an opportunity to intensively manage their glucose intolerance at the earliest stages of the disorder while inducing either metabolic memory or a legacy effect. In the long run, patients will be less likely to develop the microvascular and macrovascular complications associated with prolonged exposure to hyperglycemia.

Despite the clear origins of diabetes-related complications early in the prediabetic state, no medications are approved by the U.S. Food and Drug Administration (FDA) for treating either IFG or IGT. Third-party payers may reject claims for lifestyle treatments or educational programs targeting diabetes prevention. Confusion exists among health-care providers as to the appropriate therapeutic and metabolic targets that should be achieved in patients with prediabetes. What is certain is that the risks of developing microvascular and macrovascular complications occur at levels of hyperglycemia much lower than those that are currently defined as indicative of clinical diabetes.

Screening for Prediabetes

Patients suspected of having prediabetes may be screened with a glucose level obtained following an 8-hour overnight fast or after a 75-g oral glucose challenge given in the morning after an 8-hour fast. Testing for IGT rather than IFG appears to increase the sensitivity of diagnosing prediabetes.[15]

In 2010, the American Diabetes Association (ADA) adapted the A1C as a screening tool for diabetes and prediabetes. Point-of-care A1C assays are not sufficiently accurate for diagnostic purposes. Therefore, testing should be performed using methods that are certified by the National Glycohemoglobin Standardization Program.[16] A1C assays are also more sensitive for diagnosing prediabetes than simply screening patients with fasting glucose. One study suggested that A1C screening of high-risk patients would successfully identify nearly 38 million Americans, initially labeled as having normal glucose tolerance (NGT) based upon fasting glucose values, as actually having prediabetes![17]

A1C testing does have limitations as a screening tool. Compared with IFG and 2-hour postchallenge testing, A1C costs are approximately 50% higher. A1C levels can vary with patient's ethnicity as well as with certain anemias and hemoglobinopathies.[18] Any condition affecting red blood cell turnover such as pregnancy, recent blood loss, transfusion, anemias, or sickle cell trait will cause A1C reporting to be inappropriately lower as shown in Table 2-3.

Disease states such as renal insufficiency may directly affect A1C levels by interfering with the direct glycation of glucose to the hemoglobin structure. Alcohol ingestion may interfere with certain A1C assays, whereas elevated triglycerides artifactually decrease A1C levels.[19]

A1C has also been shown in prospective studies to predict progression toward clinical diabetes. In a systematic review following 44,000 individuals from 16 studies for up to 12 years, those with

TABLE 2-3. Conditions That Can Alter the Reliability of Glycosylated A1C Testing

Conditions That Elevate A1C Levels	Conditions That Lower A1C Levels
• Iron deficiency anemia • Any process that slows erythropoiesis (aplastic anemia), will increase A1C by maintaining an older erythrocyte cohort in the plasma • Alcoholism • Splenectomy • Hyperbilirubinemia • Medications (high dose salicylates, chronic opioid use)	• Any process that shortens the lifespan of erythrocytes (i.e., chronic kidney disease, liver disease, hemolytic anemia, hemoglobinopathies, recovery from blood loss) • Vitamins C and E by inhibiting glycation of the glucose to the hemoglobin • Pregnancy • Splenomegaly • Rheumatoid arthritis • Medications (antiretrovirals, ribavirin, dapsone) • Hypertriglyceridemia

Note: Patients with hemoglobinopathies, such as common sickle cell trait HgAS (found in 8% of African Americans) and the hemoglobin C trait (HgAC) (found in 2.3% of African Americans), may have abnormally high or low A1Cs depending on the testing method used. Patients with homozygous variant HgSS and HgCC also cannot be reliably tested for A1C levels. Instead, the diagnosis of diabetes must employ glucose criteria exclusively. A hemoglobin electrophoresis should be performed if the A1C is ≥ 15 or when the mean plasma glucose values do not correlate to the patient's A1C.
From Unger J. Fine-Tuning glycemic control using computerized downloading software: a case-based approach. In: Hirsch I, ed. *Insulin Therapy: Evolution and Practice.* Vol. 26; Supplement 2. Endocrinology and Metabolism Clinics of North America; Philadelphia, PA: Elsevier; 2007:46–68.

A1C levels between 5.5% and 6% had a 5-year progression rate of 9% to 25%. A1Cs ranging from 6% to 6.5% at baseline progressed to clinical diabetes over 5 years at the rate of 25% to 50%, a rate 20 times higher than those having A1C levels <5.0%.[20] An A1C level >5.7% is associated with a risk of diabetes progression equal to that of the high-risk participants in the Diabetes Prevention Program (DPP). Thus, the ADA has defined any A1C in the range of 5.7% to 6.4% as having pre-diabetes, those most likely to progress clinically to diabetes. As with serum glucose measurements, cardiovascular risk increases in direct proportion to A1C. Interventions should be most intensive and follow-up particularly vigilant for patients with A1C levels >6%.[21]

Diagnostic tests for prediabetes and diabetes should be repeated to rule out laboratory error unless the diagnosis is unequivocal. A screened symptomatic patient with an A1C of 7.9% and a random blood glucose of 265 mg per dL can simply be treated for diabetes. However, a patient with a screening A1C of 6.2 % and a normal 2-hour 75 gram post-glucose challenge value below 140 mg/dL should be re-screened. Preferably, the same test should be repeated for confirmation. If the initial A1C is 6.4% with the secondary screen performed 2 months later being 6.3%, the diagnosis of prediabetes is confirmed. One can also make the diagnosis of prediabetes if two different tests such as the A1C and the 2-hour post–glucose challenge are above the diagnostic thresholds.

Laboratory testing for plasma glucose values is far from perfect. The College of American Pathologists surveyed 6,000 commercial labs by retesting glucose values previously run on 32 different types of instruments. Using a comparable standardized glucose concentration specimen, 12% of the commercial labs would have reported values with a potential for misclassifying the patient's level of glucose tolerance.[22] Thus, a patient who is noted to have a fasting plasma glucose value of 122 mg per dL should always be retested to make certain the patient is not classified inappropriately as having prediabetes.

Additionally A1C may be useful as a screening tool for patients who present to the emergency department for management of an acute illness. An A1C > 5.7% performed in the acute care setting has a sensitivity of 54.8% and a specificity of 71.3% for detecting prediabetes. An A1C of 6% has a sensitivity of 76.9% and a specificity of 87.3% for diagnosing diabetes in the acute care setting.[23]

Individuals with an A1C of 5.7% to 6.4% have a risk of developing clinical diabetes equal to that of the high-risk population in the DPP.[24] In the United States, over 79 million adults are at risk

TABLE 2-4. Baseline A1C Predicts 5-year Risk of Diabetes Progression

A1C (%)	5-year Risk of Diabetes Progression (%)
<5.0	<0.1
5.0–5.5	<9
5.5–6	9–25
6–6.5	25–50

From Zhang X, Gregg EW, Williamson DF, et al. A1C level and future risk of diabetes: a systematic review. *Diabetes Care.* 2010;33:1665–1673.

for progressing to T2DM based on elevated fasting glucose or A1C levels as shown in Table 2-4. An A1C of 6% to 6.5% increases the likelihood of diabetes progression 20-fold compared with those having A1C values of 5%.[20] High-risk patients should be counseled on ways to reduce their glycemic and cardiovascular risks in a timely and intensive manner.

Various professional societies have published their customized guidelines for prediabetes as shown in Table 2-5. Primary care physicians should familiarize themselves with suggestions put forth by at least one professional society. Patient counseling will be subsequently based on establishing an appropriate and timely diagnosis of prediabetes. One must also understand that the management of hyperglycemia intensifies as patients cross over the threshold into clinical diabetes.

• Risk Scores That Predict the Development of T2DM

One might argue that costly interventions and resources which may delay the onset of diabetes should be reserved for those patients who are at highest risk for disease progression. Detecting IFG identifies approximately 26% of the population as "at risk," yet the annual rate of progression to diabetes within this subset of patients is only 5.56%.[25] The OGTT for detecting IGT is more specific than IFG as an indicator of diabetes risk but is difficult to perform in clinical practice. The use of fasting glucose, OGTT, and A1C in combination identifies over 80 million Americans as being at risk for developing diabetes.[26]

The 2-page PreDx Diabetes Risk Score (DRS) (Tethys Bioscience, Inc., Emeryville, CA) is a multibiomarker blood test that may be used in patients with prediabetes to assess the 5-year risk of developing T2DM.[27] The following seven biomarkers of the PreDX DRS are quantified in a fasting blood sample:

- Plasma glucose
- Insulin
- A1C
- Adiponectin
- Interleukin-2 receptor α
- C-reactive protein
- Ferritin

An algorithm, which incorporates results of the seven biomarkers as well as gender and age, is used to generate a DRS between 1 (least risk) and 10 (highest risk) that provides a quantitative measure of a patient's likelihood of developing diabetes within 5 years. The algorithm was originally derived from a study that enrolled 6,784 persons in a 5-year diabetes outcomes study[28,29] and was then verified in two additional cohort studies involving an additional 2,837 subjects.[30,31]

The 2-page PreDx report (Fig. 2-2) provides scores in terms of absolute risk (%) of progression to diabetes over 5 years, as well as one's risk of progression relative to the general population. The results of the seven biomarkers used to calculate the DRS are also provided in the report. From

TABLE 2-5. Published Guidelines for Prediabetes Screening

Professional Society	Suggested Screening Guidelines
American Diabetes Association	• Screen all overweight adults with BMI ≥25 kg/m² with other risk factors noted in Table 2-2. • Adults with no risk factors should be screened at age 45 and then every 3 y if normal. Consider more frequent screening depending on individual risk status and initial screening testing results. • Fasting plasma glucose, A1C, or 2-h post-75 gram oral glucose challenge can be used for screening purposes.
American Association of Clinical Endocrinologists	• Those patients at high risk for developing diabetes should be screened using the 2-h post–glucose challenge or fasting plasma glucose.
International Diabetes Federation	• Identify high-risk individuals to screen such as those with central obesity (male waist circumference ≥94 cm and female ≥80 cm). (*Note, waist circumference cut-points are ethnic group and gender specific*). • An individual whose primary relative has diabetes • Individuals ≥ age 35, or ≥ age 45 for Europeans • Personal history of hypertension and/or cardiovascular disease • Personal history of gestational diabetes • Use of medications that could predispose to diabetes including nicotinic acid, glucocorticoids, thyroid hormones, β-adrenergic antagonists, thiazide diuretics, dilantin, pentamide, antipsychotic agents, and interferon-α therapy • Triglycerides >150 mg/dL • HDL-C <40 mg/dL (males) <50 mg/dL (females) • Hypertension: systolic pressure ≥130 mm Hg and or diastolic pressure ≥85 mm Hg OR previously diagnosed hypertension • Screen with fasting plasma glucose. If plasma glucose is 110–125 mg/dL, use 2-h OGTT. • A 2-h 75 gram OGTT.

From American Diabetes Association. Standards of medical care. *Diabetes Care*. 2012;35 (Suppl 1):S11–S12; Garber AJ, Handelsman Y, Einhorn D, et al. Diagnosis and management of prediabetes in the continuum of hyperglycemia—when do the risk of diabetes begin? A consensus statement from the American College of Endocrinology and the American Association of Clinical Endocrinologists. *Endocr Pract*. 2008;14(7):933–945.

a clinical perspective, results of the test may allow appropriate tailoring of intervention programs, with the most intensive interventions implemented in the highest risk individuals.

Table 2-6 summarizes the utility of tests used to screen and diagnose prediabetes, diabetes, and one's risk of progression to clinical diabetes.

▌ Is Screening for Prediabetes Cost-effective?

If the benefit of preventing or delaying diabetes can be translated into long-term health benefits by preventing diabetes complications, screening and treating prediabetes will become a worthwhile public health initiative. The costs that will be borne by individuals and society as a result of missing the opportunity to diagnose prediabetes are unclear. However, the cost-effectiveness of early screening has been examined. A study by Zhang et al. suggested that the costs for screening for prediabetes or undiagnosed diabetes are <$200, with the cost per case being lower if only patients with higher body mass indexes (BMIs) were tested.[32] Patients who screen positive for prediabetes can be introduced to cost-effective interventions such as lifestyle modification, weight loss programs, and

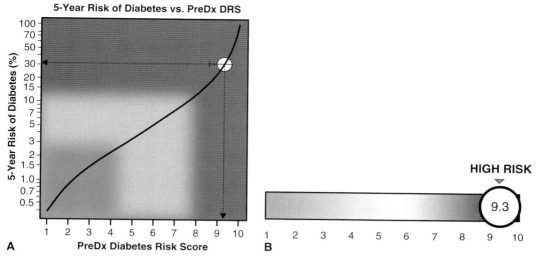

5-Year Risk of Diabetes vs. PreDx DRS

A — PreDx Diabetes Risk Score

B — HIGH RISK · 9.3

Biomarker	Result	Reference Range
Glucose	109 H	70–99 mg/dL
HbA1c[i]	5.8 H	<5.7%
Insulin	28 H	2–22 µIU/mL
CRP (High Sensitivity Assay)	3.1 H	<3.1 mg/L
Ferritin	139H	10–120 ng/mL
Interleukin 2 Receptor α*	49	22–78 IU/mL
Adiponectin*	5.4	5.2–13.1µg/mL

C

Figure 2-2 • A–C: Pre-Dx Diabetes Risk Score, Sample Report. The PreDx DRS is a quantitative diagnostic test intended to aid in the assessment of a patient's risk of progressing from prediabetes to clinical diabetes within 5 years. This 52-year-old patient has a score of 9.3, which corresponds to a 31.7% risk of progression to T2DM within 5 years, which is a 4.7-fold higher risk than an aged-match control in the general population. (Case supplied courtesy of Juan P. Frias, M.D., Tethys Bioscience, Inc., www.predxdiabetes.com.)

metformin. These noninvasive therapies will result in a per quality-adjusted life-year gained savings for screened individuals of over $8,000.[33]

The DPP projections also show clear cost-effective benefits for both lifestyle and metformin interventions implemented to delay or prevent diabetes.[34] Clearly, the benefits of early screening and lifestyle interventions outweigh the risks in patients at high risk and should be considered part of a patient's routine annual physical evaluation within the primary care setting.

Increased Complications Risks Associated with Prediabetes

Worsening glycemic control tends to impact greater risk of developing long-term diabetes-related complications. The DECODE study compared mortality rates for 25,000 subjects older than 30 years of age who had normal fasting glucose values to patients with newly diagnosed type 2 diabetes and IGT.[8] Whereas fasting glucose concentrations were not associated with increase risk of death, all-cause mortality doubled as the 2-hour postchallenge OGTT values increased from 95–200 mg per dL. Thus, the risk of mortality and cardiovascular disease approaches that of clinical diabetes as postprandial glucose values rise.

TABLE 2-6. Diagnostic and Screening Tests for Prediabetes, Diabetes, and Progression to Clinical Diabetes in Patients with Prediabetes

Lab Test	Benefits	Glitches	Recommendations for Use	Use in Screening	Approximate Unit Cost to Patient[a]
Fasting plasma glucose	• Correlated to risk of complications and disease progression • Inexpensive	• Patient must fast. • Results may be compromised by lifestyle irregularities. • Low specificity. Approximately 26% of adults have IFG while the annual incidence of diabetes among IFG patients is only 1.95%. • Progression to clinical diabetes in patients with IFG is 5.65%/y.	• If >126 mg/dL twice = diabetes • If 100–126 mg/dL twice = prediabetes	• At age 45 in asymptomatic individuals • Earlier than age 45 for patients at "high risk" for developing clinical diabetes	$29
Random plasma glucose	Component of most blood chemistry panels. Fasting not required	Value can be affected by multiple factors including concurrent illness, medication use, and relation of sampling to time of last consumed meal.	• Diagnosis can be made if glucose level is ≥200 mg/dL and patient has classic symptoms of chronic hypoglycemia (fatigue, thirst, unintentional weight lost, blurred vision).	• Test should be repeated if ≥130 mg/dL.	$29
75-g glucose challenge (OGTT)	• Most sensitive test for diagnosing IGT	• Impractical in most clinics • Requires patient to fast for 8 h, consume 75 g of glucose, and then submit to lab testing • More expensive than other tests • Capillary glucose concentrations can be 20% higher than venous plasma sampling during an OGT. World Health Organization suggests that finger sticks can be used for OGT testing, which may affect results. • High within-person variability in 2-h glucose measurements • Often not clinically practical to perform	• Glucose levels 140–199 mg/dL = IGT • Glucose levels ≥200 mg/dL = diabetes, but repeat testing is necessary	• Glucose levels 140–199 mg/dL = IGT • Glucose levels >200 mg/dL = diabetes, but repeat testing is necessary	Glucola = $6 Plasma glucose = 29 Total cost = $35

(Continued)

TABLE 2-6. Diagnostic and Screening Tests for Prediabetes, Diabetes, and Progression to Clinical Diabetes in Patients with Prediabetes *(Continued)*

Lab Test	Benefits	Glitches	Recommendations for Use	Use in Screening	Approximate Unit Cost to Patient[a]
A1C	• Does not require fasting • Predicts progression toward clinical diabetes • Predicts microvascular and macrovascular complication risk • Can be measured accurately in the vast majority of people	• Glycation of glucose to hemoglobin in nondiabetics is minimal compared with those having diabetes. • Genetic factors may influence rates of glycation • Glycation varies within ethnic populations	• 5.7–6.4% = prediabetes • ≥6.5% = diabetes	• If A1C < 6%, rescreen with A1C every 3 y. • If A1C > 6%, consider rescreening with A1C annually. • Abnormal test done during screening should be repeated.	$39
PreDx Diabetes risk score	• Testing is based on seven biomarkers predictive of disease progression • Results provide a personalized 5-year risk of progression from prediabetes to clinical diabetes	• A risk stratification test that should only be used in patients at increased risk for progression (i.e., patients with prediabetes) • This is NOT a screening test for diabetes.	• Scores range from 1 to 10, with 10 being the highest risk of developing diabetes within the next 5 y	• Useful for predicting actual progression to clinical diabetes in high-risk patients • May be used as a motivational tool (enforce healthy lifestyle choices) or integration of pharmacologic therapies sooner rather than later	

[a]Costs based on Web site: http://directlabs.com/. Accessed May 19, 2011.
From Takahashi O, Farmer AJ, Shimbo T, et al. A1C to detect diabetes in healthy adults. When should we recheck? *Diabetes Care.* 2010;33:2016–2017; Sacks DB. A1C versus glucose testing: a comparison. *Diabetes Care.* 2011;34(2):518–523; Cox ME, Edelman D. Tests for screening and diagnosis of T2DM. *Clin Diabetes.* 2009;27(4):132–138.

In the DPP, diabetic retinopathy was observed in 8% of patients with IGT compared with 13% of patients with IGT who later progressed to diabetes.[35] The IGT group has also demonstrated a progressive increase in the prevalence of hypertension and an increase in the prevalence of clinical cardiovascular disease events by approximately 50% over 4 years.[36]

In a study evaluating 77 patients with idiopathic peripheral neuropathy, 56% were found to have glucose intolerance, including 26 with IGT and 15 with clinical diabetes.[37]

Pregnancy outcomes are in part determined by the glycemic burden. The Hyperglycemia and Adverse Pregnancy Outcome Study demonstrated a continuous detrimental relationship between 1- and 2-hour after 75-g OGTT challenge elevations versus euglycemic values of <75 mg per dL during pregnancy.[38] Those mothers with 1- or 2-hour postprandial glucose levels >178 mg per dL had higher risks of primary cesarean sections, large gestational age babies, shoulder dystocia complicating delivery, preeclampsia, hyperbilirubinemia, and intensive neonatal care admissions. Thus, the ill effects of exposure to abnormal glucose tolerance on metabolic outcomes and parameters can affect individuals of all ages, even the unborn fetus.

• Pathogenesis of Prediabetes Progression

Unlike T1DM, the progression from prediabetes to T2DM occurs over a period of several years. As lean individuals gain weight and become obese over time, insulin sensitivity decreases significantly, yet glucose tolerance remains relatively normal due to a compensatory increase in insulin secretion. The higher insulin secretion is accompanied by reduced insulin activity in the liver, adipose tissue, and skeletal muscles, resulting in diminished intracellular glucose disposal. Genetically susceptible individuals progress through a spectrum of abnormal glucose states, including IFG and IGT, as β-cell function becomes impaired. Environmental factors such as poor dietary choices, inactivity, and low levels of vitamin D negatively target β-cell survivability. Over time, patients will lose not only β-cell function (as noted by the absence of first-phase insulin response) but also mass, as reflected in a rise in A1C from euglycemic values toward chronic hyperglycemia.

Declining β-cell function in the presence of increasing hyperglycemia and relatively constant insulin resistance characterizes the pathogenesis of T2DM. Achieving and maintaining recommended glycemic targets is difficult for many patients due to this progressive decline, delays in intensifying therapy, and the interplay of patient, clinician, and systemic factors impeding diabetes management in primary care. Efforts directed toward β-cell preservation *prior* to the time when insulin secretory capacity is permanently lost will allow clinicians the opportunity to introduce lifestyle interventions and cost-effective, durable pharmacologic therapies to high-risk individuals.

Although not all patients with prediabetes will progress to clinical diabetes, certainly, no clinician will be criticized for suggesting the adaptation of a healthier lifestyle to high-risk individuals. People who do not smoke, consume well-balanced meals (by consuming more fruits, vegetables, whole grains, fat-free and low-fat dairy products, and seafood while reducing consumption of salt, saturated fats, trans fats, cholesterol, and refined grains), participate in 150 minutes of moderate-intensity aerobic activity weekly, and avoid alcohol are 66% less likely to die of cancer and 65% less likely to die from cardiovascular disease.[39] Favorable nutrition behaviors include the consumption of more fruits, vegetables, whole grains, fat-free dairy products, and seafood while reducing intake of salt, saturated fat, trans fat, cholesterol, and refined grains. Adopting healthy lifestyle choices can reduce all-cause mortality by 57%.[39]

▌ The Role of the β-cell in Glucose Homeostasis and Transitioning from Prediabetes to Clinical Diabetes

Most experts believe that T2DM has a polygenic origin. A susceptible individual possesses several abnormal genes that lead to weight gain, defects in insulin secretion and action, and an increase in endogenous glucose output compromising glucose homeostasis over time.

Before the onset of glucose intolerance, a moderate degree of β-cell compensatory ability with respect to insulin resistance keeps blood glucose at near-normal levels. People with genetically susceptible β-cells are unable to produce enough insulin to maintain euglycemia targets. Even mild hyperglycemia will trigger a "downward spiral" resulting in a loss of β-cell mass and function followed by IGT and IFG.[40] Subnormal endogenouse insulin secretion coupled with heightened hepatic glucose production and reduced peripheral glucose utilization accelerates β-cell death and impaires β-cell replication.[41]

The primary defining characteristic of prediabetes is the loss of first-phase insulin secretion by the pancreatic β-cells in response to acute rises in glucose (see Fig. 10-6). One study reported declines in first-phase insulin response when fasting blood glucose exceeded 100 mg per dL and absence of first-phase response when glucose exceeded 115 mg per dL.[42] Prolonged exposure to even modestly elevated glucose has been associated with β-cell desensitization, increased apoptosis, delays in first-phase β-cell response to oral glucose, and attenuated second-phase insulin release.[43]

Not all individuals develop T2DM in response to long-term exposure to insulin resistance. The net growth rate and survival of pancreatic islets are based upon the sum of β-cell replication, size, and neogenesis (β-cell regeneration), minus the rate of β-cell apoptosis. β-cell function and mass decline when apoptosis surpasses β-cell replication and neogenesis. Obese individuals who do not develop T2DM appear to have "super β-cells." Their pancreatic islet numbers actually increase in response to glycemic stress. The β-cells in obese euglycemic individuals are also larger and more numerous than in patients who eventually progress to clinical T2DM.[44] Moreover, the islets in patients with advancing T2DM tend to be disorganized and misshapen, with secretory dysfunction exacerbated by the formation of amyloid polypeptide plaque deposition as shown in Figure 2-3.[45]

Based on clinical investigation, observation, and work with animal models, one theory of β-cell decompensation proposes five stages in the progression of diabetes, each of which reflects losses in β-cell differentiation due to changes in phenotype, function, and mass (Table 2-7).[46]

Obesity-induced insulin resistance induces chronic exposure of the β-cell to mild hyperglycemia. Stage 1 of β-cell decompensation occurs as the islets *hypertrophy* attempting to increase endogenous insulin secretion while maintaining euglycemia.[47] Moreover, β-cells in this stage have a slightly lowered set point for glucose-stimulated insulin secretion prompting them to secrete more insulin than normal at any given plasma glucose level. Animal studies have suggested this may be due to activation of glucokinase that serves as an enzymatic intracellular continuous glucose sensor.[48] Thus, an increased intracellular concentration of glucokinase favors heightened glucose-stimulated insulin secretion at subnormal set points.

As fasting glucose levels rise to the range of 89 to 130 mg per dL, β-cell dysregulation accelerates as euglycemia is no longer maintained. The excessive secretory response of insulin to ambient glycemia observed in stage 1 is no longer maintained. First-phase insulin secretion is lost, yet second-phase insulin secretion will remain preserved for a variable period of time. β-cell receptor stimulation from gut-derived incretin hormones continues to facilitate insulin secretion from islets despite progressive loss of β-cell mass and function.[47]

Fasting glucose levels in the range of 130 to 285 mg per dL herald the onset of β-cell dysregulation stage 3. Endogenous insulin production and secretion are unable to maintain euglycemia prompting the transition from prediabetes to clinical T2DM.[49] β-cell mass and function both decline rapidly as measured by glucose-stimulated insulin secretion even within what is considered the range of "normal range of glucose tolerance" (Fig. 2-4). During this transitional period, 80% of the β-cell function has been lost, and the individual is considered to be maximally insulin resistant.[50]

In stage 4, the β-cells undergo stable decompensation. Insulin secretion is considerably reduced, eventually resulting in failure of oral agents to maintain targeted glycemic control.[51] Islets become visibly damaged, as β-cells become infiltrated with amyloid fibrils, glycogen deposits, and lipid droplets.[47] When glucose levels exceed 350 mg per dL, β-cell decompensation and dysregulation are

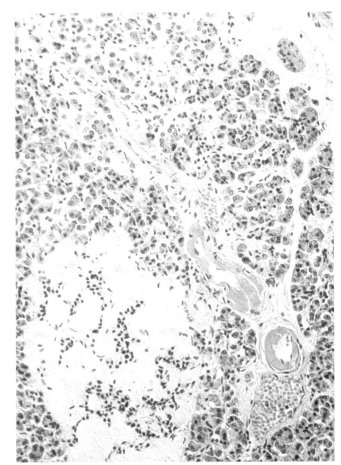

Figure 2-3 • Amyloidosis (Hyalinization) of an Islet in the Pancreas of a Patient with T2DM.
The blood vessel adjacent to the islet shows the advanced hyaline arteriolosclerosis characteristic of diabetes. This is pathologic for β-cell destruction. (Image from Rubin E, Farber JL. *Pathology.* 3rd ed. Philadelphia, PA: Lippincott Williams & Wilkins; 1999.)

complete. Exogenous insulin replacement is required to restore euglycemia and minimize the risk of long-term complications related to chronic hyperglycemia exposure.

▌ Is β-cell Failure Reversible?

Weight reduction and physical activity can improve insulin-mediated glucose disposal, reduce postprandial hyperglycemia, delay β-cell death, and slow the progression of glucose intolerance to T2DM.[5,52]

The most comprehensive clinical trial that evaluated the importance of lifestyle modification as a deterrent to diabetes in high-risk patients was the DPP[53] (see Chapter 10). Participants treated with the lifestyle-modification program experienced a 6% weight loss and 58% decrease in the incidence of diabetes compared with placebo. In subjects older than 60 years, lifestyle intervention reduced the progression to diabetes by 71%. Metformin was not as effective as lifestyle intervention in reducing diabetes risk in the population older than 60 years or in those who were less obese.

TABLE 2-7. Proposed Stages of β-cell Decompensation and Dysregulation

Stage V	Ambient Blood Glucose Values	Physiologic Changes within Islet/β-cell	Histologic Changes Noted within Islet
1	85–130 mg/dL	• Lowered "set point" for glucose-stimulated insulin secretion due to glucokinase activation	• Normal gene expression profile • β-cell hypertrophy • β-cell hyperplasia
2	89–130 mg/dL	• Loss of first-phase insulin response • Near-normal insulin stores	• Decreased expression of glucokinase, glucose transporter proteins and transcription factors
3	130–285 mg/dL	• Lose of second-phase insulin secretion • Increased ratio of proinsulin:insulin suggestive of β-cell injury • Patient is maximally insulin resistant as 80% of the β-cell function is lost.	• Reduced insulin stores within β-cell • Increased expression of genes that predispose to loss of β-cell mass and function • In obese patients, up to 40% of the β-cell mass is lost.
4	285–350 mg/dL	• β-cell apoptosis and death	• Amyloid and lipid deposits form within islets • Islets become fibrosed
5	>350 mg/dL	• Marked β-cell destruction • Loss of signaling between the α and β-cell can increase risk of hypoglycemia.	• Fibrosis

Dr. Unger expresses his appreciation to Drs. Susan Bonner-Weir and Gordon Weir for their assistance in obtaining β-cell photographs.

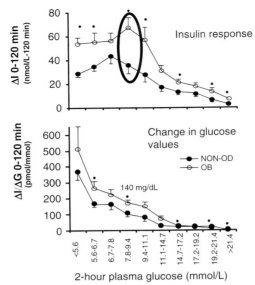

Figure 2-4 • Patients with NGT, IGT, and T2DM were evaluated using a euglycemic clamp to determine the level of glycemia at which β-cell dysfunction becomes evident clinically. Investigators noted a rise in 2-hour postprandial glucose concentration in nonobese (non-OB) patients with NGT 5.6 to 6.6 mmol per L (100 to 119 mg per dL). Between 6.7 and7.7 mmol (120 to 139 mg per dL), a progressive decline in glucose-stimulated insulin secretion was noted compared with NGT patients having a 2-hour postprandial glucose of <5.6 mmol per L. Further decline of glucose-stimulated insulin response was observed in patients with IGT having 2-hour postprandial glucose >7.8 mmol per L (140 mg per dL). Thus, a progressive decline in glucose-stimulated insulin response is observed in all patients beginning in what is considered the "normal" glucose tolerant range. Obese (OB) patients have higher glucose-stimulated insulin response than lean patients (**upper figure**). (Adapted from Gastaldelli A, Ferrannini E, Miyazaki Y, et al. β-cell dysfunction and glucose intolerance: results from the San Antonio metabolism (SAM) study. *Diabetologia.* 2004;47:31–39.)

The results of a 10-year outcomes study for DPP participants were published in 2009.[54] During the 10-year follow-up since randomization to DPP, the original lifestyle group lost and then partly regained weight. The modest weight loss with metformin was maintained. Diabetes incidence rates during the initial DPP were 4.8 cases per 100 person-years in the intensive lifestyle group, 7.8 in the metformin group, and 11.0 in the placebo group. Diabetes incidence rates in the 10-year follow-up were reduced by 34% in the lifestyle group and 18% in the metformin group compared with placebo. Thus, preservation of β-cell function and delay in progression of diabetes in high-risk individuals can persist for at least 10 years with lifestyle intervention or metformin.

Although preventing clinical diabetes progression is a noble and worthwhile pursuit, even patients with prediabetes are more likely to develop microvascular and macrovascular complications than individuals with euglycemia.[55] Therefore, true diabetes prevention must target restoration of IFG and IGT to normal glucose tolerance. In the DPP, 25% of the study participants were able to achieve normal glucose regulation (NGR) within the 3-year study window with over half achieving this important physiologic target within the first year of intervention.[56] (Fig 2-5).

Physical activity improves insulin sensitivity independent of its effect on weight loss or improvement of fat distribution in patients with IGT.[57] Unfortunately, improvement in peripheral insulin resistance reverts to levels observed in prediabetes within 1 to 2 weeks of stopping exercise training. A study of Pima Indians showed that the incidence of T2DM, as determined by oral glucose tolerance testing, was lower in more active individuals regardless of their BMI.[58]

Thus, one could determine the success of lifestyle intervention if normal glucose regulation is reestablished quickly by the high-risk patient. NGR can be attained through healthy lifestyle choices

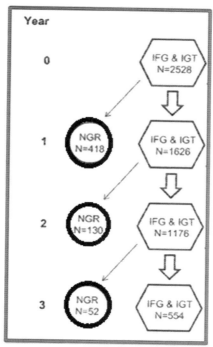

Figure 2-5 • Regression from prediabetes to normal glucose regulation (NGR) for participants of the Diabetes Prevention Program (DPP) may be enhanced via early intervention of intensive lifestyle intervention and weight loss. Each 1 kg weight loss in prediabetes is associated with a 16% reduction in diabetes risk. Of the 2,528 patients in this trial, 600 were able to achieve normal glucose regulation over 3 years via intensive lifestyle intervention that restored normal glucose regulation. The frequency of conversion to clinical diabetes increases as one ages due to reduced α-cell insulin secretory capacity. Thus, establishing healthy lifestyle choices (weight reduction, healthy meal choices, and increased activity levels) favors diabetes prevention. NGR, normal glucose regulation, IGT, impaired glucose tolerance, IFG, impaired fasting glucose. (Adapted from Perreault L, Kahn SE, Knowler WC, et al. Regression from pre-diabetes to normal glucose regulation in the Diabetes Prevention Program. *Diabetes Care.* 2009;32:1583–1588.)

independent of weight loss. However, the DPP was a clinical trial that recruited healthy volunteers who participated in a structured intervention protocol. Although lifestyle intervention might be useful in preventing or reducing diabetes risk, the adaptation of intensive interventional strategies may be expensive or unacceptable to certain ethnically, socially, and culturally diverse populations.

Pharmacotherapy has proven effective at restoring β-cell function in different high-risk population groups. Metformin appears to reestablish insulin sensitivity in obese adolescents.[59] High-risk Hispanic women with a history of gestational diabetes who took troglitazone (a thiazolidinedione) prior to its withdrawal from the market were able to preserve β-cell function and prevent T2DM, as demonstrated in the TRIPOD study.[60] Although the protective effects of troglitazone on β-cell function were effective for 8 months after the discontinuation of the drug, persistence of the improved β-cell status has not been consistently demonstrated.[61]

A randomized study of 602 patients with IGT was assigned to receive pioglitazone 45 mg or placebo to determine the rate of conversion to clinical diabetes over 48 months.[62] The annual incidence rates for T2DM conversion were 2.1% in the pioglitazone group versus 7.6% in the placebo group. As compared with placebo, pioglitazone decreased the rate of conversion to diabetes by 72% over 42 weeks. This change is slightly higher than that observed with other TZDs (52% to 62%). Pioglitazone reduced the risk of conversion to diabetes in patients with isolated IGT, IGT, and combined IFG and IGT, in both men and women as well as in all age and weight groups when compared to placebo. Unfortunately, the mean weight gain in pioglitazone-treated patients was 3.6 kg. Thus,

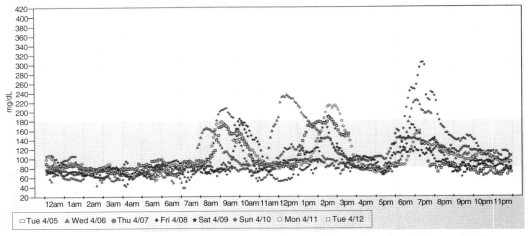

Figure 2-6 • Effects of Acarbose on Postprandial Glucose Excursions in a Patient with Prediabetes. A 66-year-old patient with a history of IGT for 2 years. Baseline A1C was 6.2%. Acarbose was titrated to 25 mg TID with meals. This graph shows 7 days of continuous glucose sensing data. Postprandial peaks persist, yet the duration of glycemic excursions is 2 to 3 hours before returning to the normal fasting range. After 2 years on acarbose, her A1C is 5.9%. (Case submitted courtesy of Jeff Unger, MD.)

one might argue that pioglitazone may be a strong candidate as a pharmacologic intervention for prediabetes. Conversely, use of pioglitazone in this patient population will likely result in weight gain, and its use in prediabetes is considered "off-label."

When compared with placebo, acarbose has been shown to reduce the progression of prediabetes to T2DM by 25% over a 3.3-year period regardless of age, sex, or BMI.[63] Unlike treatment with troglitazone, the beneficial effects of acarbose stopped as soon as the drug was discontinued. In addition, subjects in the trial experienced significant gastrointestinal (GI) side effects from the study drug, which limits its clinical usefulness. Figure 2-6 depicts the continuous glucose sensor data of a patient with IGT who has used acarbose 25 mg three times daily for 2 years.

T2DM can be prevented or delayed by pharmacologic agents that affect glucose metabolism and facilitate weight loss. Hypertensive patients are at almost 2.5 times higher risk of developing T2DM in comparison with normotensive individuals.[64]

Several studies that evaluated cardiovascular outcomes in hypertensive patients treated with angiotensin-converting enzyme (ACE) inhibitors,[65,66] calcium channel blockers,[67,68] and angiotensin II receptor blockers (ARBs)[69] noted a reduced incidence of new-onset T2DM. The Heart Outcomes Prevention Evaluation (HOPE) trial demonstrated that the ACE inhibitor ramipril reduced the incidence of macrovascular and microvascular complications in hypertensive individuals with and without T2DM.[65] Post hoc analysis of 5,720 HOPE trial participants with vascular disease but without diabetes at study entry, followed up for a mean of 4.5 years, had a 40% reduction in the diagnosis of T2DM compared with placebo-treated patients.

The results of the Nateglinide and Valsartan in Impaired Glucose Tolerance Outcomes Research (NAVIGATOR) trial showed that nateglinide (a rapid-acting sulfonylurea) was ineffective at decreasing progression of diabetes and new cardiovascular events in high-risk patients.[70] Valsartan, an angiotensin (AT-1) blocker, was ineffective at reducing cardiovascular events, yet marginally successful at reducing progression to new onset diabetes.

Although many clinical trials with antihypertensive agents have reported a positive effect on T2DM prevention, other investigations have not shown any benefit with similar drugs in delaying the onset of diabetes.[64,71] Thiazide diuretics and β-blockers may confer an increased risk of T2DM.[64,71] Speculations as to why ARBs and ACE inhibitors appear to reduce the risk of diabetes progression are listed in Table 2-8.

TABLE 2-8. Possible Links between ACE Inhibitors and ARBs in Delaying Progression of T2DM from IGT

- Hypokalemia impairs insulin secretion. ACE inhibitors and ARBs increase potassium.
- Angiotensin II can cause insulin resistance. ACE inhibitors and ARBs improve insulin sensitivity by increasing skeletal muscle blood flow.
- ACE inhibitors improve pancreatic blood flow and preserve pancreatic function.
- Biochemical evidence that adipose tissue is an endocrine organ with renin–angiotensin components. Blocking the renin–angiotensin mechanism may improve insulin sensitivity.
- Improvement of insulin sensitivity may delay or prevent onset of diabetes.

The effects of statins on diabetes risk are subject to much debate. The West of Scotland Coronary Prevention Study (WOSCOP) reported a 30% reduction in new-onset T2DM in subjects treated with pravastatin.[72] The Heart Protection Study, however, demonstrated no difference in new-onset T2DM between subjects treated with simvastatin and placebo.[73] A recently published study evaluating statin use in postmenopausal women was found to be associated with a 48% increased risk of developing diabetes.[74] The study estimated the annual diabetes incident rates of over 161,000 postmenopausal women aged 50 to 79 from 1993 through 2005. At baseline, 7.0% of women were taking statins, with 30% of women taking simvastatin, 27% taking lovastatin, 22% taking pravastatin, 12.5% taking fluvastatin, and 8% taking atorvastatin. During the study period, 10,242 incident cases of diabetes were reported. The association between statin use and diabetes progression appeared to be a class effect in this particular study. However, differences in incident rates of diabetes were noted among different cultural groups as well as in patients across a wide range of BMIs. A significantly increased risk of diabetes was observed in White, Hispanic, and Asian women (an increased risk of 49%, 57%, and 78%, respectively). Among African Americans, who made up 8.3% of the population studied, there was a nonsignificant 18% increased diabetes risk associated with statin use at baseline. Women with the lowest BMI (<25.0 kg per m²) appeared to be at higher risk of diabetes compared with obese women. The risk of diabetes progression with statin use was similar among women with and without a history of cardiovascular disease, a finding that may have important implications for balancing the risk and benefits of statins in the setting of primary prevention.

Therapeutic Options for Managing Prediabetes— A Clinical Perspective

The decision to initiate therapy for prediabetes should be undertaken with the full understanding and consent of the patient that any therapeutic intervention requires a long-term commitment. Virtually all professional societies recommend lifestyle modification as the initial intervention with consideration of pharmacologic and metabolic surgical therapy reserved for those at highest risk for progressing toward glycemic deterioration. The primary objective of intensive prediabetes management is restoration of β-cell function and preservation of β-cell mass.

Adaptation of healthy habits can delay progression of prediabetes and reduce both macrovascular and microvascular disease risk. Other metabolic disorders that confer added risk to patients with diabetes will also be minimized with lifestyle interventions, including obesity, hypertension, dyslipidemia, and depression. Reducing one's initial weight by 5% to 10% with long-term maintenance at this level is desirable based upon the findings of the DPP. Regularly planned and conducted physical activity performed at a moderately intense pace for at least 150 minutes per week is recommended.[75] Caloric restriction, increased fiber intake, and limitation of carbohydrate consumption are advisable. Lifestyle modification is recommended for all ages, although adjustment in the prescription must be made on an individual basis.

TABLE 2-9. Management/Prevention of T2DM in High-risk Individuals

Society/Association Published Guidelines	Clinical Recommendations for the Management of Prediabetes
American Diabetes Association	• Refer to effective ongoing support program targeting weight loss of 7% from baseline. • Physical activity of at least 150 min/wk of moderate activity such as walking • Consider metformin if A1C increases above the threshold of 6% despite lifestyle intervention. • Monitor for progression to clinical diabetes annually.
American Association of Clinical Endocrinologists	• Lifestyle intervention strategies include weight reduction of 5%–10% from baseline with long-term maintenance. • Moderate-intensity exercise program 30–60 min 5 d/wk • Dietary recommendations: lowered sodium intake, avoidance of excessive alcohol, caloric restriction, increased fiber intake, possible limitation on carbohydrate intake • Initiation of metformin or acarbose for "low-risk" patients, or pioglitazone in "high-risk" patients, or for those in whom lower risk therapies have not succeeded • Incretin therapies may also prove effective in β-cell preservation. • No targeted A1C is recommended. • Use statins to achieve low-density lipoprotein cholesterol (LDL-C) < 100 mg/dL non-HDL-C < 130 mg/dL (and/or apolipoprotein B ≤ 90 mg/dL). • Target blood pressure < 130/80 mm Hg • Antiplatelet therapy (low-dose aspirin) is recommended for all patients with prediabetes for whom there is no identified excess risk for GI, intracranial, or other hemorrhagic condition.
Indian Health Services	• Lifestyle intervention via a structured program and referral to a registered dietitian • Weight loss recommendation of 5%–10% with a sustained weight loss of ≥10% of initial body weight • Dietary intervention incorporates the DASH diet that can reduce blood pressure and improve lipids and insulin resistance in patients with metabolic syndrome. (*More on the DASH diet may be accessed in Chapter 3*) • Exercise 30 min 5 d a week or walk using a pedometer 10,000 steps/d. • Screen and treat for depression. • Screen and counsel for tobacco cessation. • Consider either metformin or pioglitazone for pharmacotherapy if necessary, although no targeted A1C is recommended. • Blood pressure target is <130/80 mm Hg. • Calculate the 10-y coronary heart disease risk as determined by the Strong Heart Risk Calculator, then initiate statins if patients with an intermediate 10-y risk have an LDL-C > 130 mg/dL. • Treat triglycerides > 150 mg/dL with pharmacologic agents if lifestyle intervention is ineffective. • Evaluate and treat low HDL-C with niacin. • Antiplatelet therapy (baby aspirin, 81 mg/d) is recommended for patients with a 10-y cardiovascular disease risk ≥ 10% who lack contraindications. • Risk stratification calculator can be determined at the following Web site:http://strongheart.ouhsc.edu/chdcalculator/calculator.html

From American Diabetes Association. Standards of medical care. *Diabetes Care*. 2011;34(Suppl 1):S11–S61; Garber AJ, Handelsman Y, Einhorn D, et al. Diagnosis and management of prediabetes in the continuum of hyperglycemia—when do the risk of diabetes begin? A consensus statement from the American College of Endocrinology and the American Association of Clinical Endocrinologists. *Endocr Pract*. 2008;14(7):933–945; Indian Health Service. Guidelines for care of adults with prediabetes and/or the metabolic syndrome in clinical settings. September, 2008. http://www.ihs.gov/MedicalPrograms/Diabetes/HomeDocs/Tools/ClinicalGuidelines/PreDiabetes_Guidelines_0209.pdf. Accessed April 15, 2011.

Metabolic surgery is also effective at reducing the likelihood of diabetes development in patients who have clinically severe obesity (BMI > 40 kg per m²) (see Chapter 10). However, most experts would not recommend the use of weight loss surgery to simply reduce one's risk of progressing from prediabetes to diabetes.

Pharmacotherapeutic options for use in prediabetes have not been approved by the U.S. FDA for the prevention of diabetes in children, adolescents, or adults. Therefore, any decision to initiate pharmacologic agents in prediabetes is considered as being an "off-label use." The FDA is charged with regulating the safety and sale of drugs and medical devices used in the United States. The agency does NOT regulate a doctor's practice nor are they able to dictate what they tell their patients regarding medication choices. To be fair, physicians should always discuss the off-label use of drugs with their patients prior to prescribing them. Risks and benefits of all medication use (whether or not the drugs are used on or off-label) should be detailed and noted in the medical file. Patients should be educated as to the reasons behind initiating drug therapy for a condition that may NOT progress to a more advanced disease state. Targeted glycemic and metabolic goals must be addressed and followed on subsequent visits.

Self–blood glucose monitoring should be initiated as well. Patients with prediabetes have abnormal glucose control. The objective of self–blood glucose monitoring would be to achieve glycemic patterns that are as near to normal both in the fasting and postprandial states as possible. Structured glucose testing initiated 3 days prior to each visit will be useful for evaluating glucose patterns. Patients should be instructed to check blood glucose levels seven times daily (before and after each meal and before bed) for 3 days. Forms for recording these glucose values are available for downloading at https://www1.accu-chek.com/microsites/ac_connect/pdf/ACCU-CHEK_360_ViewForm.pdf.

The recommended treatment strategies for managing prediabetes vary based on societal guidelines as displayed in Table 2-9.

Pharmacologic intervention may be considered in "high-risk" patients with A1C levels >6%. The primary targets of drug therapy should be preservation of pancreatic β-cell function and mass, minimization of hypoglycemic risk, and promotion of either weight loss or weight maintenance in nonobese individuals. When appropriate, drugs should also demonstrate favorable effects on cardiovascular biomarkers such as lipids and blood pressure. Adverse effects of medications should be minimized.

A summary of the pharmacologic effects on β-cell function and preservation is found in Table 2-10.

 TABLE 2-10. Impact of Chronic Pharmacotherapy for Prediabetes on β-cell Function and Disease Progression

Therapeutic Class	Improved Insulin Secretion	Increased β-cell Mass[a]	Diabetes Prevention[b]	Disease Modification[c]
Lifestyle	No	No	Yes	No
Metformin	No	No	Yes	No
Sulfonylurea	Yes	No	No	No
Insulin	No	No	?	No
α-Glucosidase inhibitors	Yes	No	Yes	No
Pioglitazone	No	Yes	Yes	Yes
DPP-4 inhibitors	Yes	Yes (animals only)	?	?
GLP-1 analogs	Yes	Yes (animals only)	?	?

[a]No direct means of measuring β-cell mass exists. Therefore, the effects of pharmacologic therapies are largely inferred.
[b]Randomized clinical trial evidence demonstrating a reduction in the risk of progression to T2DM.
[c]Clinical trial evidence of treatment-associated stability in glycemic control, β-cell secretory function, or both.

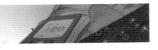

SUMMARY

Seventeen million Americans are estimated to have prediabetes, with approximately 10% of these individuals expected to convert to clinical diabetes annually. Patients with IFG or IGT are maximally insulin resistant and have lost up to 80% of the β-cell mass by the time they are diagnosed. Not surprising is the fact that many of these individuals already are afflicted with clinical evidence of neuropathy, retinopathy, chronic kidney disease, and cardiovascular disorders. Screening for prediabetes in high-risk individuals is cost-effective and can save thousands of dollars in future health-care costs when the disorder is identified and treated intensively.

Adaptation of healthy lifestyle choices with the goal of restoring NGR is key to preventing disease progression. Every 1 kg of weight lost is associated with a 16% reduction in diabetes risk.[76] Most experts would suggest introducing pharmacotherapy when the patient's A1C surpasses 6%. The goal of pharmacotherapy in patients with prediabetes is β-cell preservation.

Primary care physicians are in a unique position to screen, diagnose, and manage patients with prediabetes. By doing so, we may be able to reduce the number of individuals who ultimately progress to clinical diabetes and suffer the consequences of chronic hyperglycemia burden.

REFERENCES

1. Bonora E. The metabolic syndrome and cardiovascular disease. *Ann Med*. 2006;38(1):64–80.
2. Ford ES, Zhao G, Li C. Pre-diabetes and the risk for cardiovascular disease. A systematic review of the evidence. *J Am Coll Cardiol*. 2010;55:1310–1131.
3. Laakso M. Hyperglycemia and cardiovascular disease in type 2 diabetes. *Diabetes*. 1999;48:937–942.
4. Nielson C, Lange T, Hadjokas N. Blood glucose and coronary artery disease in nondiabetic patients. *Diabetes Care*. 2006;29:998–1001.
5. Tuomilehto J, Lindstrom J, Eriksson JG, et al. Prevention of type 2 diabetes mellitus by changes in lifestyle among subjects with impaired glucose tolerance. *N Engl J Med*. 2001;344:1343–1350.
6. Garber AJ, Handelsman Y, Einhorn D, et al. Diagnosis and management of prediabetes in the continuum of hyperglycemia: When do the risk of diabetes begin? A consensus statement from the American College of Endocrinology and the American Association of Clinical Endocrinologists. *Endocr Pract*. 2008;14(7):933–945.
7. Diabetes Prevention Program Research Group. The prevalence of retinopathy in impaired glucose tolerance and recent-onset diabetes in the Diabetes Prevention Program. *Diabet Med*. 2007;24:137–144.
8. DECODE Study Group. Glucose tolerance and mortality: comparison of WHO and American Diabetes Association diagnostic criteria. The DECODE study group. European Diabetes Epidemiology Group. Diabetes Epidemiology: collaborative analysis of diagnostic criteria in Europe. *Lancet*. 1999;354:617–662.
9. de Vegt F, Dekker JM, Jager A, et al. Relation of impaired fasting and postload glucose with incident T2DM in a Dutch population: the Hoorn Study. *JAMA*. 2001;285:2109–2211.
10. Stratton IM, Adler AI, Neil HA, et al. Association of glycaemia with macrovascular and microvascular complications of T2DM (UKPDS 35): prospective observational study. *BMJ*. 2000;321:405–412.
11. Centers for Disease Control. Number of people with diabetes increases to 24 million. http://www.cdc.gov/media/pressrel/2008/r080624.htm. Posted June 24, 2008. Accessed April 10, 2011.
12. International Diabetes Federation. Diabetes Atlas: Prevalence. http://www.eatlas.idf.org/Prevalence/. Accessed April 10, 2011.
13. American Diabetes Association. Economic costs of diabetes in the U.S. in 2007 [erratum in *Diabetes Care*. 2008;31:1271]. *Diabetes Care*. 2008;31:596–615.

14. Leal J, Gray AM, Clarke PM. Development of life-expectancy tables for people with T2DM. *Eur Heart J.* 2009;30(7) 834–839.

15. Bartnik M, Rydén L, Malmberg K, et al; Euro Heart Survey Investigators. Oral glucose tolerance test is needed for appropriate classification of glucose regulation in patients with coronary artery disease: a report from the Euro Heart Survey on Diabetes and the Heart. *Heart.* 2007;93:72–77.

16. American Diabetes Association. Standards of medical care. *Diabetes Care.* 2011;34(Suppl 1):S11–S61.

17. Mann DM, Carson AP, Shimbo D, et al. impact of A1C screening criterion on the diagnosis of pre-diabetes among U.S. adults. *Diabetes Care.* 2010;33:2190–2195.

18. Ziemer DC, Kolm P, Weintraub WS, et al. Glucose-independent, black-white differences in hemoglobin A1c levels: a cross-sectional analysis of 2 studies. *Ann Intern Med.* 2010;152:770–777.

19. Gallagher EJ, Le Roith D, Bloomgarden Z. Review of hemoglobin A1C in the management of diabetes. *J Diabetes.* 2009;1:9–17.

20. Zhang X, Gregg EW, Williamson DF, et al. A1C level and future risk of diabetes: a systematic review. *Diabetes Care.* 2010;33:1665–1673.

21. Selvin E, Steffes MW, Zhu H, et al. Glycated hemoglobin, diabetes, and cardiovascular risk in nondiabetic adults. *N Engl J Med.* 2010;362:800–811.

22. Miller WG, Myers GL, Ashwood ER, et al. State of the art in trueness and interlaboratory harmonization for 10 analytes in general clinical chemistry. *Arch Pathol Lab Med.* 2008;132:838–846.

23. Silverman RA, Thakker U, Ellman T, et al. Hemoglobin A1C as a screen for previously undiagnosed pre-diabetes in an acute-care setting. *Diabetes Care.* 2011;34:1908–1912.

24. American Diabetes Association. Diagnosis and classification of diabetes mellitus. *Diabetes Care.* 2010;33(Suppl 1):S62–S69.

25. Nichols GA, Hiller TA, Brown JB. Progression from newly acquired impaired fasting glucose to type 2 diabetes. *Diabetes Care.* 2007;30(2):228–233.

26. James C, Bullard KM, Rolka DB, et al. Implications of alternative definitions of prediabetes for prevalence in U.S. adults. *Diabetes Care.* 2011;34(2):387–391.

27. Kolberg JA, Gerwien RW, Watkins SM, et al. Biomarkers in type 2 diabetes: improving risk stratification with the PreDx Diabetes Risk Score. *Expert Rev Mol Diagn.* 2011;11(8):775–792.

28. Kolberg JA, Jorgensen T, Gerwien RW, et al. Development of a type 2 diabetes risk model from a panel of serum biomarkers from the Inter99 cohort. *Diabetes Care.* 2009;32:1207–1212.

29. Urdea M, Kolberg J, Wilber J, et al. Validation of a multimarker model for assessing risk of type 2 diabetes from a five-year prospective study of 6784 Danish people (Inter99). *J Diabetes Sci Technol.* 2009;3: 748–755.

30. Lyssenko V, Jorgensen T, Gerwien RW, et al. Validation of a multi-marker model for the prediction of incident type 2 diabetes mellitus: combined results of the Inter99 and Botnia studies. *Diab Vasc Dis Res.* 2012;9:59–67.

31. Shafizadeh TB, Moler EJ, Kolberg JA, et al. Comparison of accuracy of diabetes risk score and components of the metabolic syndrome in assessing risk of incident type 2 diabetes in Inter99 Cohort. *PLoS ONE.* 6(7):e22863. doi:10.1371/journal.pone.0022863.

32. Zhang P, Engelgau MM, Valdez R, et al. Costs of screening for pre-diabetes among U.S. adults. *Diabetes Care.* 2003;26(9):2536–2542.

33. Hoerger TJ, Hicks KA, Sorenson SW, et al. The cost-effectiveness of screening for pre-diabetes among overweight and obese U.S. adults. *Diabetes Care.* 2007;30:2847–2849.

34. The Diabetes Prevention Program Research Group. Costs associated with the primary prevention of T2DM mellitus in the Diabetes Prevention Program. *Diabetes Care.* 2003;26:36–47.

35. Ratner R, Goldberg R, Haffner S, et al. Diabetes Prevention Program Research Group. Impact of intensive lifestyle and metformin therapy on cardiovascular disease risk factors in the diabetes prevention program. *Diabetes Care.* 2005;28:888–894.

36. Chiasson JL, Josse RG, Gomis R, et al; STOP-NIDDM Trial Research Group. Acarbose treatment and the risk of cardiovascular disease and hypertension in patients with impaired glucose tolerance: the STOP-NIDDM trial. *JAMA.* 2003;290:486–494.

37. Sumner CJ, Sheth S, Griffin JW, et al. The spectrum of neuropathy in diabetes and impaired glucose tolerance. *Neurology.* 2003;60:108–111.

38. The HAPO Study Cooperative Research Group. Hyperglycemia and adverse pregnancy outcomes. *N Engl J Med.* 2008;358:1991–2002.

39. Ford ES, Zhao G, Tsai J, et al. Low-risk lifestyle behaviors and all-cause mortality: findings from the National Health and Nutrition Examination Survey III Mortality Study. *Am J Public Health*. 2011;101(10):1922–1929.

40. Leahy JL. Pathogenesis of T2DM mellitus. *Arch Med Res*. 2005;36:197–209.

41. Bagust A, Beale S. Deteriorating β-cell function in T2DM: a long-term model. *QJM*. 2003;96(4):281–288.

42. Brunzell JD, Robertson RP, Lerner RL, et al. Relationships between fasting plasma glucose levels and insulin secretion during intravenous glucose tolerance tests. *J Clin Endocrinol Metab*. 1976;42:222–229.

43. Leahy JL, Bonner-Weir S, Weir GC. β-cell dysfunction induced by chronic hyperglycemia: current ideas on mechanisms of impaired glucose-induced insulin secretion. *Diabetes Care*. 1992;15:442–455.

44. Rhodes CJ. T2DM—a matter of β-cell life and death? *Science*. 2005;307:380–384.

45. Yoon KH, Ko SH, Cho JH, et al. Selective β-cell loss and α-cell expansion in patients with T2DM mellitus in Korea. *J Clin Endocrinol Metab*. 2003;88:2300–2308.

46. Weir GC, Bonner-Weir S. Five stages of evolving β-cell dysfunction during progression to diabetes. *Diabetes*. 2004;53(Suppl 3):S16–S210.

47. Weir GC, Laybutt DR, Kaneto H, et al. β-cell adaptation and decompensation during the progression of diabetes. *Diabetes*. 2001;50:S154–S159.

48. Chen C, Hosokawa H, Bumbalo LM, et al. Regulatory effects of glucose on the catalytic activity and cellular content of glucokinase in the pancreatic β-cell. *J Clin Invest*. 1994;94:1616–1620.

49. Bell GI, Polonski KS. Diabetes mellitus and genetically programmed defects in β-cell function. *Nature*. 2001;41:788–791.

50. Gastaldelli A, Ferrannini E, Miyazaki Y, et al. β-cell dysfunction and glucose intolerance: results from the San Antonio metabolism (SAM) study. *Diabetologia*. 2004;47:31–39.

51. Wright A, Burden AC, Paisey RB, et al. Sulfonylurea inadequacy: efficacy of addition of insulin over 6 years in patients with T2DM in the UK Prospective Diabetes Study (UKPDS 57). *Diabetes Care*. 2002;25:330–336.

52. Pan XR, Li GW, Hu YH. Effects of diet and exercise in preventing NIDDM in people with impaired glucose tolerance: the Da Qing IGT and Diabetes Study. *Diabetes Care*. 1997;20:537–544.

53. Knowler WC, Barrett-Connor E, Fowler SE, et al.; the Diabetes Prevention Program Research Group. Reduction in the incidence of T2DM with lifestyle intervention or metformin. *N Engl J Med*. 2002;346:393–403.

54. Diabetes Prevention Program Research Group. 10-year follow-up of diabetes incidence and weight loss in the Diabetes Prevention Program outcomes study. *Lancet*. 2009;9702:1677–1687.

55. Zeigler D, Rathmann W, Dickhaus T, et al. Prevalence of polyneuropathy in pre-diabetes and diabetes is associated with abdominal obesity and macroangiopathy: the MONICA/KORA Augsburg Surveys S2 and S3. *Diabetes Care*. 2008;31:464–469.

56. Perreault L, Kahn SE, Knowler WC, et al. Regression from pre-diabetes to normal glucose regulation in the Diabetes Prevention Program. *Diabetes Care*. 2009;32:1583–1588.

57. Ivy JL, Zderic TW, Fogt DL. Prevention and treatment of non-insulin dependent diabetes mellitus. *Exerc Sport Sci Rev*. 1999;27:1–35.

58. Kriska AM, Saremi A, Hanson RL. Physical activity, obesity, and the incidence of T2DM in a high risk population. *Am J Epidemiol*. 2003;158:669–675.

59. Freemark M. Pharmacologic approaches to the prevention of T2DM in high risk pediatric patients. *J Clin Endocrinol Metab*. 2003;88:3–13.

60. Buchanan TA, Xiang AH, Peters RK. Preservation of pancreatic β-cell function and prevention of T2DM by pharmacological treatment of insulin resistance in high-risk Hispanic women. *Diabetes*. 2002;46:701–710.

61. The Diabetes Prevention Program Research Group. Prevention of T2DM with troglitazone in the diabetes prevention program [abstract]. *Diabetes*. 2003;52(Suppl 1):A58–A59.

62. DeFronzo RA, Tripathy D, Schwenke DC, et al. Pioglitazone for diabetes prevention in impaired glucose tolerance. *N Engl J Med*. 2011;364:1104–1115.

63. Chiasson JL, Josse RG, Leiter LA. The effect of acarbose on insulin sensitivity in subjects with impaired glucose tolerance. *Diabetes Care*. 1996;19:1191–1194.

64. Gress TW, Nieto FJ, Shahar E, et al. Hypertension and antihypertensive therapy as risk factors for T2DM mellitus: atherosclerosis risk in communities study. *N Engl J Med*. 2000;342:905–912.

65. Yusef DP, Gerstein H, Hoogwerf B, et al, for the HOPE Study Investigators. Ramipril and the development of diabetes. *JAMA*. 2001;286:1882–1885.

66. Hansson L, Lindholm LH, Niskanen L, et al. Effect of angiotensin-converting-enzyme inhibition compared with conventional therapy on cardiovascular morbidity and mortality in hypertension: the Captopril Prevention Project: (CAPPP) randomised trial. *Lancet.* 1999;353:611–616.
67. Brown MJ, Palmer CR, Castaigne A, et al. Morbidity and mortality in patients randomised to double-blind treatment with a long-acting calcium-channel blocker or diuretic in the International Mifedipine GITS study: intervention as a goal in hypertension treatment (INSIGHT). *Lancet.* 2000;356:366–372.
68. ALLHAT Officers and Coordinators for the ALLHAT Collaborative Research Group. Major outcomes in high-risk hypertensive patients randomized to angiotensin-converting enzyme inhibitor or calcium channel blocker vs. diuretic: the Antihypertensive and Lipid-Lowering Treatment to Prevent Heart Attack Trial (ALLHAT). *JAMA.* 2002;288:2981–2997.
69. Devereux RB, Dahlof B, Kjedlsen SE, et al. for the LIFE Study. Effects of losartan or atenolol in hypertensive patients without clinically evident vascular disease: a substudy of the LIFE randomized trial. *Ann Intern Med.* 2003;139:169–177.
70. McMurray JJ, Holman RR, Haffner SM, et al. Effect of valsartan on the incidence of diabetes and cardiovascular events. *N Engl J Med.* 2010;362:1477–1490.
71. Hansson L, Lindholm LH, Ekbom T, et al. Randomised trial of old and new antihypertensive drugs in elderly patients: cardiovascular mortality and morbidity the Swedish Trial in Old Patients with Hypertension-2 study. *Lancet.* 1999;354:1751–1756.
72. Freeman DJ, Norrie J, Sattar N, et al. Pravastatin and the development of diabetes mellitus: evidence for a protective treatment effect in the West of Scotland Coronary Prevention Study. *Circulation.* 2001;103:357–362.
73. Colins R, Armitage J, Parish S, et al, for the Heart Protection Study Collaborative Group. MRC/BHF Heart Protection Study of cholesterol-lowering with simvastatin in 5963 people with diabetes: a randomized placebo-controlled trial. *Lancet.* 2003;361:2005–2016.
74. Culver AL, Ockene IS, Balasubramanian R, et al. Statin use and risk of diabetes mellitus in postmenopausal women in the Women's Health Initiative. *Arch Intern Med.* 2012;172(2):144–152.
75. Handelsman Y, Mechanick JI, Blonde L, et al. American Association of Clinical Endocrinologists medical guidelines for developing a diabetes mellitus comprehensive care plan. *Endo Pract.* 2011;17(Suppl 2):1–53.
76. Perreault L, Kahn SE, Christophi CA, et al. Regression from pre-diabetes to normal glucose regulation in the diabetes prevention program. *Diabetes Care.* 2009;32(9):1583–1588.

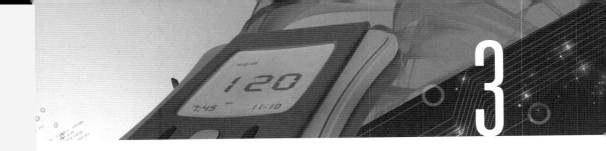

Lifestyle Interventions for Patients with Diabetes

If you decide to eat a toad, you should at least select one that is big.

—*Igbo proverb*

Introduction   Successful long-term diabetes self-management requires the integration of pharmacotherapy, proper nutrition, home blood glucose monitoring, continuing patient education, an increase in physical activity, and surveillance for and prevention of short- and long-term complications. Although physicians are eager to prescribe pharmacotherapy to their patients, discussing issues such as home blood glucose monitoring, diet, and exercise is not second nature. Most physicians have had little direct training regarding lifestyle issue management with patients, preferring instead to refer to a dietitian or certified diabetes educator (CDE). Primary care doctors must understand that they remain the "director" of the patient's management team. Although dietitians and CDEs can educate patients on lifestyle interventions, the physician is responsible for prescribing the actual dietary and activity parameters that patients follow.

Some PCPs have no access to ancillary personnel and may be their patients' only source of information regarding lifestyle modification. Physicians should encourage the adaptation of healthy and active lifestyle interventions within their patient population who have diabetes or prediabetes. Spending 3 to 5 minutes per visit on lifestyle intervention could have a positive and motivational effect on patients. If, for example, a patient has been successful in losing weight, ask what techniques were used and never forget to praise his or her efforts. One should ask about exercise and smoking cessation at each visit. The physician should make certain that the patient knows the names of his or her medications and the times they should be taken. Determine what drugs need to be refilled so that lapses in treatment will be minimized. While sitting side by side with each patient, the physician should discuss the statistical evaluations of home blood glucose monitoring. Time spent on this will most certainly encourage the patient to continue monitoring. However, a patient who does take the time to monitor and brings the meter in for downloading will certainly become discouraged if no interest is shown in the glucose readings and the efforts are ignored.

Lifestyle interventions are clearly beneficial for patients diagnosed with diabetes. Reducing caloric intake to 1,100 kcal per day has been shown to decrease fasting blood glucose levels in obese patients with T2DM and in those with normal glucose tolerance in as few as 4 days.[1] This improvement is due to decreased hepatic glucose production. Insulin sensitivity and fasting glucose levels decline further following 28 days of calorie restriction in obese patients with T2DM in association with an average weight loss of only 6 kg. Interestingly, the weight reduction does not appear to have a positive effect on pancreatic β-cell preservation or secreting capacity.[2]

In a recently published study, basal hepatic glucose production, hepatic and peripheral insulin sensitivity, and β-cell function were measured in 11 patients with T2DM at baseline as well as after 1, 4, and 8 weeks of a very-low-calorie (600 kcal per day) diet.[3] The patients had a duration of diabetes of less than 4 years and a stable BMI ranging from 25 to 45 kg per m[2]. After 1 week of caloric restriction, patients began to experience normalization of both β-cell function and hepatic insulin sensitivity as well as a decrease in pancreatic and liver triacylglycerol stores. Intrahepatic lipid concentrations decreased by 30%. Over the 8 weeks of dietary restriction, β-cell function increased toward normal and pancreatic fat decreased. As one is exposed to severe caloric restriction, intracellular free fatty acid concentrations in the liver decline resulting in mirrored decrease in hepatic export of lipoprotein triacylglycerol to the pancreas. Prolonged elevations of plasma free fatty acids decrease insulin secretion. Prior to the onset of spontaneous diabetes in rats, both total pancreatic fat and islet triacylglycerol content increase sharply.[4] Chronic saturated fatty acid exposure of β-cells also inhibits acute first-phase insulin response to glucose, whereas removal of the free fatty acids allows for recovery of this acute response as demonstrated in this study.[5] Thus, the primary pathologic abnormalities associated with T2DM can be reversed simply by reducing dietary energy intake.

Diabetes and mental illness interact in harmful ways (See Chapter 9). Patients with both diabetes and mental illness tend to be less adherent to medical care and suffer more long-term diabetes-related complications. Comorbid depression and diabetes result in worse health outcomes than other combinations of chronic diseases.[6,7] Integration of both medical and psychosocial support for such patients, although challenging, is necessary to minimize risk of premature death from suicidality or cardiovascular disease.

Improving Adherence to Diabetes Self-management Skills

Physicians can encourage patients to become active participants in their own care by simply asking how they feel about what has been prescribed to date. What efforts are working and what issues need fine tuning? Are there concepts related to the disease state of diabetes that the patient does not understand? A proactive approach to education in many cases will minimize the likelihood of patients seeking out their own sources of questionable resources from, for example, Internet chat rooms.

Behavioral changes are necessary to reduce long-term risks and maintain healthy lifestyles. By some estimates, less than 50% of patients with diabetes adhere to their recommended behavioral interventions.[8] Adherence is multidimensional in that some patients may comply with medication regimens, while ignoring dietary or exercise recommendations. Others, who "feel just fine," may exercise 2 to 3 hours a day so that they may avoid starting medications that are needed to manage hyperglycemia, hypertension, and hyperlipidemia. A study using a large national sample (National Health and Nutrition Examination Survey [NHANES]) of patients with T2DM found that 29% of insulin-treated patients, 65% of those on oral medications, and 80% of individuals managed by diet and exercise alone either never performed self–blood glucose monitoring (SBGM) or did so less than once per month.[8]

The findings from the Cross-National Diabetes Attitudes, Wishes, and Needs (DAWN) Study[9] showed patient-reported adherence rates for medication in T1DM and T2DM patients of 83% and 78%, respectively; self-monitoring blood glucose adherence was 70% and 64%, respectively; and appointment-keeping adherence was 71% and 72%, respectively. The adherence rates observed for diet for T1DM and T2DM patients were 39% and 37%, respectively, and for exercise they were 37% and 35%, respectively. Providers reported significantly better adherence for T1DM than for T2DM patients across most treatment regimens.

Several factors have been shown to influence adherence with diabetes self-care, as summarized in Table 3-1. Demographic factors such as ethnic minority, low socioeconomic status, and low

TABLE 3-1. Factors That Favor and Promote Patient Adherence to Prescribed Treatment Regimens

- Higher socioeconomic status and level of education[a,b]
- Resolution of comorbid mental illness symptomatology[c,d]
- Spousal, familial, and communal support[b]
- Satisfaction with doctor–patient relationship[e]
- Support received and availability of diabetes health-care team[b]
- Appointment reminder cards, phone calls regarding upcoming appointments, minimization of delays in seeing patients on their arrival in the office, and emphasis on the positive aspects of patient's efforts toward diabetes self-management rather than focusing on the patient's failures or oversights[f,g]
- Simplification of treatment programs[g]
- Patient adherence to medicine regimens surpasses that of lifestyle or behavioral interventions.[d]
- Comanaging "difficult" patients with a mental health worker[h]

[a]Chaturvedi N, Stephenson JM, Fuller JH. The relationship between socioeconomic status and diabetes control and complications in the EURODIAB IDDM Complications Study. *Diabetes Care.* 1996;19:423–430.
[b]Glasgow RE, Toobert DJ. Social environment and regimen adherence among type II diabetic patients. *Diabetes Care.* 1988;11:377–386.
[c]Greden JF. The burden of disease for treatment-resistant depression. *J Clin Psychiatry.* 2001;62:26–31.
[d]Rubin RR, Peyrot M. Psychological issues and treatments for people with diabetes. *J Clin Psychol.* 2001;57:457–478.
[e]Ciechanowski PS, Katon WJ, Russo JE, et al. The patient-provider relationship: attachment theory and adherence to treatment in diabetes. *Am J Psychiatry.* 2001;158:29–35.
[f]Haynes RB, Taylor DW, Sackett DL. *Compliance in health care.* Baltimore, MD: Johns Hopkins University Press; 1979.
[g]Ary DV, Toobert D, Wilson W, Glasgow RE. Patient perspective on factors contributing to non-adherence to diabetes regimen. *Diabetes Care.* 1986;9:168–172.
[h]Adili F, Larijani B, Haghighatpanah M. Diabetic patients: psychological aspects. *Ann N Y Acad Sci.* 2006;1084:329–349.

levels of education have been associated with lower regimen adherence and greater diabetes-related morbidity.[10] Lower frequency of self–blood glucose monitoring has been observed among African American and Hispanic/Latino patients when compared with non-Hispanic white patients with diabetes (10).

Patients with comorbid mental illness must have their psychological issues corrected before intensification of diabetes therapy is attempted as detailed in Chapter 9. Both treatment compliance and outcomes are linked directly to the patient's affective state.[11] PCPs should screen patients with diabetes for mental illness (schizophrenia, bipolar depression, major mood disorder, and generalized anxiety disorder) and initiate treatment when appropriate.

Family relationships play an important role in diabetes management. Greater levels of social support from spouses and other family members are associated with enhanced participation in diabetes self-management and reduce the stress associated with chronic disease management.[10]

One of the most important motivators of patient compliance is related to the amount of support received from the health-care team members. Patients who are satisfied with their doctor–patient relationship are more adherent to their treatment program and participate more fully in diabetes self-management.[12] One of the key elements to success in achieving good glycemic control for participants in the Diabetes Control and Complications Trial (DCCT) was the amount of support and availability patients received from their local health-care study site.[13]

Factors that promote adherence include reminder cards and phone calls about upcoming appointments, minimizing delays in seeing patients once they arrive at the office, and reinforcing positive attributes of the visit, rather than focusing on the negative aspects of chronic complications.[14,15]

Patients prefer simplified treatment regimens to ones that are more complex and tend to accept the need to begin pharmacotherapy for diabetes much quicker than integrating lifestyle or behavioral changes into their daily lives.[14,16]

Is the Patient "Noncompliant" or "Nonadherent"?

Physicians often relate interesting tales of patient "noncompliance." **Compliance** is best defined as "the extent to which a person's behavior coincides with medical advice."[15] **Noncompliance** implies that patients intentionally disregard or disobey the advice of their health-care provider. Noncompliance provokes negative attitudes toward patients while discouraging patients from becoming active participants in their own diabetes self-management. **Adherence** is viewed as an "active, voluntary, and collaborative effort in a mutually acceptable course of behavior prescribed to produce a positive therapeutic outcome."[15] Patients who adhere to their treatment programs do so by choice, agree to participate in self-management, understand the implications of treating all metabolic abnormalities to target, and agree to become students of their own disease states. Once presented with a treatment plan and provided with the tools necessary to become successful at self-management, a patient may voluntarily choose to adhere to the prescribed plan, offer alternative suggestions to the professional team, or, most commonly, comply with the structured plan for a short time before becoming nonadherent. Patient adherence may be multidimensional. For example, patients may have no problems using four injections of insulin daily, yet only monitor their blood glucose levels once or twice daily despite warnings that failure to monitor may result in hypoglycemia.

In an attempt to enhance patient adherence to a prescribed treatment program, health-care providers should consider the following options:

1/ Allow patient adherence to evolve over time. Weight loss and increased physical activity can prevent or delay diabetes and complications related to prolonged exposure to hyperglycemia.[17] Techniques that facilitate adherence to lifestyle changes can be adapted to primary care. Often the patient's readiness to work toward change must develop gradually. Patients facing the long-term task of adjusting their lifestyle benefit from assistance in setting highly specific behavior-outcome goals and short-term behavior targets. Individualization is achieved by tailoring goals and targets to the patient's preferences and progress, building the patient's confidence, and intensifying therapy as necessary to pursue these prescribed metabolic targets. Coach patients on ways they may achieve positive outcomes. Help them become self-reliant, and minimize their perceptions of burdensome lifestyle interventions. Patients who have multiple comorbidities (hyperlipidemia, hypertension, chronic renal failure, mental illness, severe clinical obesity, autonomic dysfunction, diabetic retinopathy) associated with their diabetes diagnosis should be referred to other specialists and ancillary personnel for intensive intervention education and management.

2/ Target a single behavioral change rather than multiple interventions at each visit. When promoting behavioral or lifestyle changes, the physician should focus on a single intervention at each visit. For example, attempting to discuss appropriate timing of home blood glucose monitoring and smoking cessation at a single 15-minute visit is unlikely to yield any positive results. Diabetes is a stressful disorder, as is nicotine abuse. A discussion of diet, weight loss, exercise, and medication timing, while arranging for specialty evaluations to monitor for retinopathy, is too overwhelming for even the most dedicated patient (Table 3-2).

3/ Praise the patient at each visit. One should offer praise to each patient at the time of the follow-up appointment. As difficult as this may be for some physicians to accept, patients often do what they can in an attempt to find favor in the eyes of their health-care team. Patients will bring in their glucose logs, their medication vials, or articles of interest that they read on diabetes management. Taking a minute to visually inspect these items means a great deal to patients. Those individuals who have been successful at weight reduction or smoking cessation or who initiated an exercise program should receive praise from the physician and a "high five."

4/ Do not be afraid to change course. Some physicians may be reluctant to intensify diabetes treatment because they may view a deterioration in the patient's condition as a reflection of their own disease state mismanagement. However, diabetes is a chronic disease that is by nature progressive and a "work in progress." Therefore, if one determines that a patient's glycemic control is not responding to the prescribed treatment, one should not hesitate to offer an alternative plan.

TABLE 3-2. CPT and ICD-9 Coding for Smoking Cessation Counseling

HCPCS/CPT Codes:
- **99406:** Smoking and tobacco-use cessation counseling visit; intermediate, greater than 3 minutes up to 10 minutes. Short descriptor: Smoke/Tobacco counseling 3-10
- **99407:** Smoking and tobacco-use cessation counseling visit; intensive, greater than 10 minutes. Short descriptor: Smoke/Tobacco counseling greater than 10
- **S9075:** Smoking Cessation Treatment
- **S9453:** Smoking Cessation Classes, non-physician provider, per session
- Various Evaluation and Management Services (associated with acute or chronic care). When providing an E/M service, if greater than 50% of face-to-face time with patient is spent in counseling, time may be used as a basis for selection of level of service.
- **99381-99397:** Preventive medicine services
- **99078:** Physician educational services in a group setting

ICD-9 diagnosis code of choice:
- **305.1:** Tobacco use disorder

The physician should remember to target success rather than accept failure. Patients do appreciate the efforts of their health-care management team as long as they can be involved in the decision-making process.

5/ Allow patients with poor glycemic control to be comfortable while intensifying their diabetes management. The patients with diabetes who are the most challenging to manage are those who have been under poor control for many years and have already experienced microvascular and macrovascular complications. These unfortunate individuals may have finally decided to get more active in their diabetes self-management, although reversal of end-stage disease is unlikely to occur. Treatment of these patients should still focus on lowering the A1C to the safest target. Patients who have spent the majority of their lives living with glucose levels in the 300 mg per dL range may not feel well when the glucose averages 150 mg per dL. They may develop adrenergic symptomatology suggestive of acute hypoglycemia. These uncomfortable symptoms tend to persist for 2 weeks before subsiding once the glycemic control is normalized. Patients who develop adrenergic symptoms should be reassured that they are simply adjusting their body sensors toward normal glycemic control. If they feel symptomatic, a blood glucose level should be obtained, and if it is 70 mg per dL or greater, no treatment should be attempted. Intensive diabetes management incorporates any modality that improves glucose control and lowers the A1C to target. Patients who feel "miserable" while treatment is intensified may become nonadherent to the prescribed protocol and linger in a state of persistent hyperglycemia.

6/ Maintain a positive attitude for all patients, even those with end-stage disease. Physicians are unable to offer patients a "cure for diabetes." Still, the physician can provide patients with many therapeutic interventions to improve and maintain glycemic control, enhance quality of life, and treat many of the long-term diabetes-related complications. From a psychological and a physiologic viewpoint, physicians should attempt to allow patients to be as comfortable as possible with their chronic disease management. There are now excellent treatments for painful diabetic peripheral neuropathy that may improve patients' symptomatology within 2 weeks of beginning medication therapy. Men with erectile dysfunction can nearly always be treated successfully with oral medications, intraurethral pellets, or intracavernosal injections. Early interventions for patients with chronic kidney disease can slow the progression of this disease process. The use of statins and aspirin can improve outcomes in patients at risk for macrovascular disease. Physicians must always work for patients in an attempt to find therapies that can improve their quality of life and minimize future long-term complication risks. Often, patients believe that having diabetes is a "death sentence." In reality, with proper education and intervention, health-care providers can always offer their patients hope for a brighter future of diabetes management. Physicians must never give up on any patient, no matter how challenging they may be.

7/ **Identify and treat patients with comorbid depression.** Identifying patients with significant psychosocial issues can improve treatment compliance. Fifteen to twenty percent of patients with diabetes have comorbid depression.[11,18] These individuals may have a difficult time adhering to self-care behaviors and display worsening of their glycemic control. Treating patients who have major depressive disorder with antidepressants may improve adherence to diabetes self-management programs.[16]

8/ **Individualize diet and physical activity treatment plans.** Individual tailoring of diet and physical activity treatment plans is recommended by major guidelines focused on diabetes, obesity, and exercise.[19,20] Placing patients on a "1,800-calorie ADA diet" is inappropriate for patients who are lean, active, adolescent, elderly, acutely ill, or incapable of following pigeon-holed recommendations. Healthy food choices and flexible meal plans should be discussed. Patients should be made aware that *diabetes is a disorder of carbohydrate metabolism*. Simply avoiding "sugar" in the diet will not improve glycemic control. One should remind patients that glucose is the central nervous system's obligate source of energy. Without carbohydrate ingestion and glucose utilization, the body cannot survive. However, excessive ingestion of carbohydrates results in the inability of the pancreatic β-cell to produce enough insulin to prevent hyperglycemia. As hyperglycemia is prolonged, glucotoxicity destroys β-cells and other important tissues including the eyes, kidneys, nerves, and endothelial cells.

Patterns of disordered eating behaviors (DEB) should also be identified in patients with both T1DM and T2DM. The incidence of DEB is estimated to range from 3%–26% of all patients with diabetes.[21] Patients with DEB are prone to extreme glycemic variability, diabetic ketoacidosis, abrupt alterations in weight, and maladaptive behavioral patterns.

Patients often are overwhelmed by large goals that seem unachievable. Target behaviors should be phased, using small increments. The physical activity target can be gradually increased from setting a 4,000 steps per day goal for walking using an inexpensive pedometer to more intense activity for longer periods, possibly with the assistance of a personal trainer. Group education sessions for patients with diabetes may be initiated with a 5- to 15-minute period of exercise. Patients should understand that any increase in physical activity is likely to improve hyperglycemia. By starting gradually, the patient can build confidence over time, with each stage having a higher likelihood of lasting success. Small advances also provide many opportunities for physician praise. Putting small steps together side by side will eventually encourage a patient to achieve the treatment target.

9/ **Use visual imagery to demonstrate the relationship between hyperglycemia and glucose toxicity.** A simple exercise in visual imagery might help patients understand the relationship between hyperglycemia and glucotoxicity. Patients who do not have diabetes have blood that is perfectly fluid in nature. Their blood is pure and fresh, similar to the water coming from a mountain stream. In contrast, hyperglycemia causes blood to become thick, sticky, and gooey, similar to maple syrup. As this hyperglycemic liquid flows through the body, the blood sticks to everything, including the eyes, kidneys, blood vessels, nerves, joints, muscles, tendons, skin, and β-cells. The longer the patient is exposed to hyperglycemia, the more likely he or she is to develop complications from kidney, nerve, eye, and heart disease. No one feels well with maple syrup running through the blood vessels. The clinician's job is to work with patients to allow them to have the syrup replaced by fresh mountain stream water.

10/ **Answer patients' questions and concerns in a relaxed and labor unintensive manner.** Imagine going to your own physician for treatment of a chronic progressive disease such as multiple sclerosis or Alzheimer's disease. Most likely, you are not an expert or thought leader in your field in this disorder, yet you understand that like many other chronic disorders we manage in primary care, MS and AD cannot be cured. With proper intensive therapy, the disease progression may be slowed and the interruption of your current quality of life will be minimal. Still, aren't there many questions that you have related to living with either disorder? What are the potential side effects of the medications prescribed, and when should they be taken—with food or on an empty stomach? Will they interfere with your blood pressure or thyroid meds? Are these new meds on my insurance formulary and if so, at what tier co-pay? Have my lab studies changed at all since the last visit? Do I need any additional studies performed at this time? Are there any clinical trials that may be appropriate for patients such as myself? How much longer will I be able to work before I am forced into retirement? Can you complete these forms for me so that I can acquire a handicapped placard for my car? OK. How would you feel if you asked these questions to your PCP while his hand was cradling the door handle as soon as he entered your exam room? After all, he only has 8 minutes to see you and he is really busy. Patients with diabetes have similar concerns. In fact, they feel frustrated that their questions are not being addressed, yet they are often being berated by providers as being "noncompliant" with their treatment plan. Spending a few extra minutes with each patient at the conclusion of each visit will solidify your relationship with them and assure that you are partnering with them toward improving their quality of life.

Lifestyle interventions that may be used to improve patient adherence with diabetes self-management are summarized in Tables 3-3 and 3-4.

 TABLE 3-3. Advanced Skills in Maintaining Lifestyle Changes

Skills	Behavior Target	Action
Keep office follow-up visits	Compliance with office visits	Praise patients for some positive aspect of their current office visit. This will encourage them to schedule and keep future visits. Do appropriate testing and evaluate for possible diabetes-related complications according to the ADA guidelines on diabetes management.
Eating out	Learn skills for eating at restaurants and the homes of others	Plan ahead, choose carefully, and assertively ask for what you want. Keep food diaries and record how much insulin is needed for eating a given meal at a particular restaurant.
Education	Learn as much about diabetes as possible	Join the ADA. Participate as a volunteer in local ADA events.
Relapse prevention	Anticipate slips and get back on track	Identify previous triggers of slips, plan ahead for likely triggers, challenge thoughts that a slip means failure (i.e., "get back on the horse"), and problem solve about how to deal with triggers. "All patients with diabetes regress on their self-management skills from time to time. Now let's work together on getting you back on the fast track to better care."
Avoiding boredom	Vary physical activity to keep motivated	Change some aspect of physical workout each month; get a personal trainer. Join a gym or fitness center. Check your blood glucose before and after exercising. You are likely to note that any activity results in improved blood glucose levels.
Self–blood glucose monitoring	Consider changing from random to paired glucose testing.	Check blood glucose levels as recommended by the physician. Always bring the meter to each visit. Physicians should spend time with each patient to analyze the meters.
Social support	Enhance support for lifestyle change	Involve significant others in activities and develop new social supports. If one person in the family makes more healthy food choices, other family members will also begin to follow a healthier lifestyle.

ADA, American Diabetes Association.

TABLE 3-4. Topics of Importance for the Successful Promotion of Diabetes Self-management

Topic	Skills to Be Learned by the Patient
Pathophysiology of diabetes	Specific diagnosis given to the patient (T1DM, T2DM, gestational diabetes, other) Progression of diabetes toward β-cell failure Comorbidities associated with diabetes (hyperlipidemia, hypertension, hypercoagulation, vascular disease, obesity, breast cancer, thyroid dysfunction, and other forms of autoimmune disease)
Rationale for intensively treating diabetes	Long-term diabetes complications (microvascular and macrovascular disease) Relationship between control and complications
Self–blood glucose monitoring	How to use the prescribed meter Schedule for performing tests Need to bring in meter on each visit for downloading data How to prick finger with minimal discomfort and ensure best accuracy of the test How one may need to use these data for adjusting premeal insulin doses, provide intelligent correction doses of insulin, fix hyperglycemia and hypoglycemia
Medications	Description Possible side effects and drug interactions Dosing instructions (what time of day, with or without food) Importance of compliance with medication regimen
Medical nutrition therapy	Importance Flexible meal planning Effects of medications on fasting or postprandial glucose levels Carb counting Effects of caffeine, fat, alcohol, and glycemic index on blood glucose control U.S. government food pyramid Using the diabetes food pyramid (Fig. 3-1) Dealing with nutrition-related fluctuations in glycemic control
Exercise	Importance of exercise on improving glycemia Pre-exercise and postexercise target blood glucose levels Anticipating, assessing, and managing exercise-induced hyperglycemia and hypoglycemia Discussion on exercises that are safe as well as potentially harmful Timing of medication (especially insulin) in relationship to exercise
Recognizing short-term diabetes-related complications	Hyperglycemia Hypoglycemia Hypoglycemic unawareness Diabetic ketoacidosis
Recognizing long-term diabetes-related complications	Microvascular (eye, kidney, nerve disease), macrovascular (cardiovascular risk, stroke, peripheral vascular disease), infection
Use of supplements	Aspirin, magnesium, folic acid, calcium, vitamin D
Instructions for special situations	Sick day rules Preconception planning Travel instructions Use of glucagon emergency kit

(Continued)

TABLE 3-4. Topics of Importance for the Successful Promotion of Diabetes Self-management (*Continued*)

Topic	Skills to Be Learned by the Patient
Preventative care	Foot care Skin care Routine Pap tests and mammograms Compliance with follow-up appointment Smoking and alcohol cessation Vaccines for seasonal influenza and pneumococcal pneumonia and hepatitis B Surveillance for complications
Psychological aspects	Screen for mental illness (depression, bipolar depression, schizophrenia, anxiety, panic disorder) Effect of diabetes on patient's intrapersonal relationships and family dynamics (See Chapter 9) Effect of diabetes on patient self-image Importance of support Denial
Instructions for family members	Management of severe hypoglycemia Ability of patient to participate in sports Assist patient with proper medication dosing
Psychosocial evaluation	Family support systems Financial (including medical insurance status), employment Changes in work schedule (i.e., currently working "graveyard shift," excessive overtime hours) Life stresses (marital status, recent move, death of a family member, increased responsibilities in the household, etc.) Evaluation for depression, bipolar disease, and other mental health disorders
Follow-up visits	Has the patient experienced any acute health problems? Have any changes occurred in any chronic health problems? Has the patient experienced any symptoms or signs suggestive of hypoglycemia, nocturnal hypoglycemia, or hypoglycemic unawareness? Does the patient have any new symptoms or signs suggestive of diabetes-related long- or short-term complications? Have any cardiac risk factors changed? Are the results of the patient's home blood glucose download data consistent with the latest A1C level?
Assessment of long-term complications	Eye (test of visual acuity—Snellen chart, funduscopic exam, intraocular pressure, eye referral) Renal (tests for microalbuminuria, creatinine clearance, GFR, serum chemistries, 24-h protein excretion) Neuropathy (peripheral sensory neuropathy evaluated with vibratory sensation, soft touch, pinprick, gait analysis, hot-cold sensation, inspection of the feet for calluses, erythema, swelling, pain, hyperalgesia, allodynia). Autonomic dysfunction identified with R-R interval evaluation and orthostatic blood pressure changes. Symptom evaluation for nocturnal diarrhea, gastroparesis, hypoglycemic unawareness, and anhidrosis. Discussion to evaluate male and female sexual dysfunction Cardiac, cerebrovascular, and peripheral vascular disease (ECG and rhythm strip, stress test, or both, based on patient's age, symptoms, duration of diabetes; lipid profile and non-HDL-C value; evaluation of peripheral pulses by physical and/or objective testing)

T1DM, type 1 diabetes mellitus; T2DM, type 2 diabetes mellitus; GFR, glomerular filtration rate; ECG, electrocardiogram; HDL-C, high-density lipoprotein cholesterol.

Delegating Patient Care Responsibilities

In any therapeutic situation, especially those involving a chronic disease state, both the physician and the patient have specific responsibilities. The medical community now knows that, although a patient may be asymptomatic, hyperglycemia in the presence of comorbid metabolic disorders such as hypertension and hyperlipidemia will result in long-term diabetes complications. Achieving normalization of glycemic control requires active participation in self-management from the asymptomatic patient with diabetes. The medical team must enlighten, nurture, and continually guide the patient toward improved diabetes control. The responsibilities of both the patient and physician are noted in Table 3-5.

 TABLE 3-5. Defining Patient and Physician Responsibilities in Diabetes Management

Patient Responsibilities for Diabetes Self-management	Physician Responsibilities for Directing the Care of Patients with Diabetes
1. Perform self–blood glucose monitoring.	1. Understand and adhere to the treatment guidelines suggested by the American Diabetes Association (ADA) and the American Association of Clinical Endocrinologists.
2. Stop smoking and minimize alcohol consumption.	2. Promote intensification of diabetes management toward the lowest A1C value that is safe to achieve for each patient while minimizing day-to-day glycemic variation.
3. Begin an exercise program for weight management and to improve physical conditioning.	3. Appropriately collect patient data so that clinical outcomes can be measured and comorbid interventions can be initiated on a timely basis.
4. Use aspirin on a daily basis if older than 18 y.	4. Determine if an insulin-requiring patient is a candidate for physiologic insulin replacement therapy using a basal-bolus regimen or even an insulin pump.
5. Make certain to have your blood pressure checked at each visit, and, if necessary, ask your doctor about beginning ambulatory or home blood pressure monitoring.	5. Discuss patient concerns about his or her diabetes self-management program at each visit.
6. Recognize and understand the psychological barriers that prevent adherence to the system of intensive self-diabetes management. Learn to express your concerns to the physician for rapid resolution.	6. Supervise the patient's diabetes education program. Make certain that the patient is a member of the ADA. As an example, make certain that you and your staff are also members of the ADA.
7. Learn foot care assessment and protection.	7. Encourage the patient to use preventive measures and risk reduction related to coexisting conditions.
8. Understand the principles behind managing hypoglycemia. Keep glucose tablets or glucose gel tubes in the home. Patients on insulin therapy should keep a glucagon emergency syringe in the home and make certain that another family member is familiar with its proper use.	8. Inspect the feet on a regular basis, identifying those individuals at risk for developing foot ulcerations.

(Continued)

TABLE 3-5. Defining Patient and Physician Responsibilities in Diabetes Management (*Continued*)

Patient Responsibilities for Diabetes Self-management	Physician Responsibilities for Directing the Care of Patients with Diabetes
9. Obtain an annual dilated funduscopic exam from an ophthalmologist.	9. Make certain that the patient's immunization schedule is current.
10. Understand the importance of targeted control of blood pressure, "glycemic variation," hyperglycemia, and hyperlipidemia.	10. Do not overlook routine testing such as Pap smears, mammograms, breast exams, prostate cancer screening, colon cancer screening, autoimmune thyroid disease evaluations, and mental illness.
11. Actively participate in continuing diabetes education programs.	11. Screen for microvascular and macrovascular disease annually or more often as needed.
12. Join the American Diabetes Association and offer your support for their many excellent programs. Share your knowledge with other patients by striving to learn as much as possible about this disease state.	12. Encourage positive lifestyle changes such as smoking and alcohol cessation, exercising, weight reduction, and compliance with the prescribed medical regimen.
13. Adhere to proper nutrition and exercise programs. Discuss any barriers to these therapies with your physician so that alternative plans may be discussed.	13. Discuss preconception planning with all female patients beginning at age 14 who have diabetes.
14. Keep your regularly scheduled appointments with your primary care physician, specialists, and other members of the diabetes treatment team.	14. Supervise the proper referral to other members of the diabetes treatment team—registered dietitians, certified diabetes educators, personal exercise trainers, cardiologist, ophthalmologist, neurologist, nephrologist, endocrinologist, and vascular surgeon.
15. Be adherent to medication regimen. Do not discontinue medications just because the prescription has expired or mild side effects are experienced. Discuss all medication changes with your doctor until you are in complete agreement with the treatment plan. Discuss any uncomfortable medication side effects with your physician prior to discontinuing them on your own.	15. Arrange for appropriate specialty care of the hospitalized patient with diabetes.
16. Understand the meaning of "A1C" and be aware of your own A1C value.	16. Document all aspects of the patient's diabetes care modules including lifestyle intervention, specialty referral, program adherence, and self–blood glucose monitoring.

(Continued)

TABLE 3-5. Defining Patient and Physician Responsibilities in Diabetes Management (*Continued*)

Patient Responsibilities for Diabetes Self-management	Physician Responsibilities for Directing the Care of Patients with Diabetes
17. Parents of children with diabetes should make certain that their schools allow them to check blood glucose levels prior to eating and, in the case of younger patients, supervise their use of insulin. Schools should maintain a copy of the patient's treatment regimen on file at all times and be familiar with managing hypoglycemia.	17. Consider screening female adolescent patients with erratic glycemic control for eating disorders. 18. Provide positive feedback to each patient during every office visit. Never take away hope. An encouraging word can go a long way. 19. Consider making your office the site for monthly community diabetes education meetings.
	20. Become the local expert in diabetes management. With more than 26 million Americans afflicted with diabetes, one could certainly build a strong practice base by being the "go to" doctor for diabetes care in the community.

Discussing Medical Nutritional Therapy with Patients

The goals of medical nutrition therapy that apply to all persons with diabetes or prediabetes may be summarized as follows:

1. Attain and maintain **optimal metabolic outcomes,** including the following:
   - Achieve blood glucose levels in the normal range or as close to normal as is safely possible to prevent or reduce the risk for complications of diabetes.
   - Minimize glycemic variability.
   - Target a lipoprotein profile that reduces the risk for macrovascular disease.
   - Lower blood pressure levels to reduce the risk for vascular disease.
2. Prevent and treat the **chronic complications** of diabetes. Nutrient intake and lifestyle should be modified as appropriate for the prevention and treatment of obesity, dyslipidemia, cardiovascular disease, hypertension, and nephropathy.
3. Improve health through **healthy food choices** and physical activity.
4. Address **individual nutritional needs,** taking into consideration personal and cultural preferences and lifestyle while respecting the individual's wishes and willingness to change.

Goals of medical nutrition therapy that apply to specific situations include the following:

1. For **youths with T1DM:** Provide adequate energy to ensure normal growth and development, integrate insulin regimens into usual eating and physical activity habits.
2. For **youths with T2DM:** Facilitate changes in eating and physical activity habits that reduce insulin resistance, promote weight loss or minimize weight gain, and improve the overall metabolic status.
3. For **pregnant** and **lactating women:** Provide adequate energy and nutrients required to attain optimal outcomes.
4. For **older adults:** Provide for the nutritional and psychosocial needs of an aging individual.
5. For individuals **treated with insulin** or insulin secretagogues: Provide self-management education for the treatment (and prevention) of hypoglycemia, acute illnesses, and anticipated exercise-related blood glucose excursions.

6. For individuals **at high risk for developing diabetes or those with prediabetes:** Decrease risk or slow disease progression by encouraging physical activity and promoting food choices that facilitate moderate weight loss or, at least, prevent weight gain.

The principles and strategies of nutrition and exercise for T1DM differ from those patients with T2DM. Patients must understand and determine the effects of diet and physical activity on their glycemic control to optimize diabetes self-management. Patients with T1DM dose insulin according to their anticipated carbohydrate intake and should be educated regarding the insulin-to-carbohydrate ratio (I/CHO). Healthy food choices, coupled with an active lifestyle, can be useful in minimizing weight gain, glycemic excursions, blood pressure elevations, and lipid levels in patients with T2DM.

Dietary Management for T1DM

To maximize success as an insulin-dependent patient, each individual must be cognizant of the following relationships between insulin and food intake:

1. The onset of action and the duration of action of the prandial (bolus) insulin dose
2. How much insulin is required to cover the expected glycemic excursions that will result from the consumption of a given amount of carbohydrates (I/CHO). This ratio may be stable throughout the day or may be variable, depending on the degree of the patient's insulin resistance.
3. The effect of fat content on carbohydrate absorption
4. How insulin resistance varies during the day. Additional insulin will be required during periods of peak insulin resistance, whereas reduced doses will be needed during times of minimal insulin resistance.
5. What level of activity is planned as a dose of insulin is being absorbed. Moderate to heavy physical activity will require a 50% reduction in prandial insulin dosing.
6. Patients with autonomic neuropathy may have gastroparesis. If insulin is dosed as the patient begins to eat, the patient may develop immediate hypoglycemia due to the delay in nutrient absorption yet will experience postprandial hyperglycemia hours later as insulin levels wane while glucose levels peak.

Although these tasks seem daunting, with practice, most patients can learn the basic principles of medical nutritional therapy. With time, dietary management of diabetes not only becomes second nature but allows patients an opportunity to challenge their own nutritional skills to improve their glycemic control. The DCCT demonstrated that patients who adjusted their food intake and insulin dosage in response to preprandial blood glucose levels achieved lower A1Cs than did patients using conventional therapy.[22] Rather than placing all patients on a "specific diet" (i.e., a 1,800-calorie ADA diet), mealtime flexibility should be encouraged, as patients dose insulin based on their carbohydrate intake. The physician should remember that patients are people too, and restricting food intake due to diabetes will lead to "closet eaters" and "cheaters." One should allow patients to eat sensibly but insist that appropriate insulin be given for each meal. Structured or paired glucose testing allows one to determine if the premeal insulin bolus is injected at the appropriate time and dose based upon the meal content.

Food contains carbohydrates, fats, and proteins as sources of energy, as well as vitamins and minerals. The carbohydrates in food have the most impact on blood glucose levels. Foods that are high in fat content can contribute to obesity and heart disease while prolonging the time of carbohydrate absorption from the gut. Dietary fat, however, plays only a minor role in glycemic control. Protein is another minor player in short-term glycemic control: 50% of consumed protein is converted into carbohydrate over 4 to 6 hours. By constituting only 10% to 20% of the total daily calorie consumption, dietary protein does not have an impact on blood glucose levels.

Generally, all carbohydrates, the preferred energy source in the body, convert to glucose within 1 to 2 hours after consumption. Variables such as fat, fiber, and the glycemic load of a meal can alter the peak excursion of blood glucose. However, these are secondary to the total amount of carbohydrate consumed. Carbohydrate consumption must be balanced with insulin production and utilization. Insulin-requiring patients must use exogenous insulin to minimize the upward drive each gram of carbohydrate has on blood glucose levels. Patients with T2DM can balance carbohydrate consumption with exercise and medications, which either enhance the release of endogenous insulin by their pancreatic β-cells or improve insulin sensitivity within skeletal muscle cells and adipose tissue.

Insulin-to-Carbohydrate Ratios and Supplemental Insulin

I/CHO is used to determine how much exogenous (injected) insulin is required to cover a given quantity of carbohydrates. Patients with T2DM who are insulin resistant and/or obese may have lower I/CHO and require more insulin; often, 1 U of rapid-acting insulin analogue is needed to cover 5 g CHO. Conversely, lean patients with T1DM may have a much higher I/CHO and may only require 1 U rapid-acting insulin analogue for each 20 g CHO consumed.

Premeal and postmeal self-monitoring is the optimal way to determine the accuracy of the patient's "carb counting" and ability to respond with an appropriate insulin dose. There may be variations in the patient's I/CHO. Each patient will have a unique response to each meal and will need to learn to calculate his or her own individual I/CHO.

Patients should to be taught the many nuances of I/CHO:

- Patients may have different meal bolus ratios for different times of the day.
- Meals with large quantities of fat result in delayed glucose availability.
- If the premeal glucose level is within normal limits, the bolus insulin covers food intake only.
- Low premeal blood glucose levels require less bolus insulin.
- High premeal levels require enough insulin to bring glucose back to normal in addition to insulin to cover food.

One should err on the side of conservative optimism when adjusting insulin doses. Excessive insulin doses should be discouraged. Some patients believe that avoiding hyperglycemia at all cost is critical to their well-being. Often, these individuals will dose themselves into hypoglycemia, only to have to consume additional carbohydrates to reverse their lows. This will result in weight gain and increased insulin resistance.

To calculate a meal bolus dose of insulin based on carbohydrate consumption, the *rule of 500* is used:

$$500/\text{total daily insulin dose} = \text{CHO covered by 1 U rapid-actinginsulin analogue (lispro, aspart, glulisine)}$$

An example of the 500 rule in use for an adult: A patient receiving a total of 50 U insulin per day:

$$500 \div 50 \text{ U insulin} = 10 \text{ g CHO per unit of rapid-acting insulin analogue}$$

Patients may need to use supplemental insulin in addition to adjusting for carbohydrate intake if the preprandial blood glucose level is greater than 150 mg per dL. Supplemental insulin can be determined by the *rule of 1,800,* which predicts how much 1 U of insulin will lower the blood glucose level: insulin sensitivity factor (1,800 per total daily dose of insulin) (Table 3-6).

Patients should be instructed on the proper interpretation of food labels, which provide information regarding nutrients, calories, and serving sizes. A can of macaroni may contain 35 g of carbohydrates per serving, which in the example described in Table 3-6 would require 4 U of insulin coverage. Should the patient eat two servings of macaroni, a total of 8 U plus supplemental insulin for preprandial hyperglycemia would be required to cover this meal.

Some patients may benefit from purchasing carbohydrate-counting books that are available through the ADA (http://www.diabetes.org/home.jsp). Carbohydrate counting does take some practice and is more reproducible in patients having the best overall glycemic control.

We can do some carb counting for two apples—one large, one medium—and determine how much insulin is needed to consume each one. Apples are 13% carbohydrate by weight. A large apple

TABLE 3-6. How to Calculate the Insulin Sensitivity Factor (1,800/Total Daily Dose of Insulin)

Patient with TDD = 50 U

Insulin sensitivity factor = 1,800/50 = 34 (1 U insulin lowers blood glucose 34 mg/dL)
  I/CHO = 1:9 (1 U covers 9 g CHO)
Preprandial glucose level = 225 mg/dL
Meal contains 50 g of CHO

- **First:** Determine how much insulin will be needed to cover the consumed carbs:
  50 g CHO/9 (I/CHO) = 5.5 U
- **Second:** Correct the premeal hyperglycemia:
  225 − 150 = 75.
  Thus, 2 U will lower the prandial glucose to the 150 mg/dL target.
- **Third:** Add the amount of insulin required to cover the carbohydrates plus the amount of insulin needed to achieve the preprandial glucose target (insulin sensitivity factor):
  5.5 + 2 = 7.5 U (can round off to 7 or 8 U)
- To determine the accuracy of the premeal insulin dose, check the blood glucose 2 h after eating. If the blood glucose is
  - Between 70 and 140 mg/dL, the dose was calculated correctly
  - <70 mg/dL, too much insulin was given for that meal
- If the **postprandial** blood glucose is >140 mg/dL, insufficient insulin was given for the meal. Remember that another correction dose can be given prior to the next meal, if the blood glucose level remains elevated. Giving another correction dose 2 h postprandially may result in insulin stacking and hypoglycemia.

TDD, total daily dose; I/CHO, insulin to carbohydrate ratio.

weighs approximately 238 g, and a medium-sized apple weighs approximately 139 g. The carbohydrate content of each apple is as follows:

Large apple: 238 × 0.13 = 30.9 g of carbs
Small apple: 139 × 0.13 = 18.1 g of carbs

A patient with an I/CHO of 1:10 would need 3.1 U to cover a large apple but only 1.8 U for a medium one. If several foods are added to this meal, the carbohydrate content of each would be determined and added to the premeal carbohydrate count. If 80 g of carbs will be consumed, the patient will need to bolus 8 U of insulin.

Most insulin pumps have "bolus wizard–type" features, allowing patients to input the type of food they will be consuming (even restaurant and fast food items are included in the wizard calculator). Based upon the patient's I/CHO ratio, the pump will determine for the patient the most appropriate amount of insulin to bolus.

For patients having an aversion to carb counting, use of a simpler prandial insulin dosing method might be considered. Bergenstal et al. compared the efficacy of a simple insulin dosing titration method with carbohydrate counting for adjusting mealtime insulin glulisine and determined

TABLE 3-7. Patient Adjustment of Prandial Rapid-acting Insulin Based upon Meal Size

Size of Meal	Rapid-acting Insulin Dose Adjustment
Very large + dessert	+3 U added to baseline dose
Large meal without dessert	+2 U added to baseline dose
Moderate size meal (larger than usual)	+1 U added to baseline dose
"Light meal." Less than usual	−1 or −2 subtracted from baseline dose
Minimal meal. Half the normal amount	−2 or −3 subtracted from baseline dose

that either method was effective at reducing A1C levels.[23] Based upon the suggestions provided in this publication, we have been initiating prandial insulin at the dose of 0.1 U per kg per meal. Thus, a 70-kg patient would inject 7 U 15 minutes prior to each meal (if the premeal glucose level is greater than 80 mg per dL. If less than 80, the insulin would be injected at the same time the meal is consumed). The dose of insulin would be adjusted as shown in Table 3-7.

Structured glucose testing should be performed 2 hours after each meal at least three times each week. If the 2-hour postprandial glucose level is either 140 to 180 mg per dL or the "delta" (difference between the baseline premeal glucose and the 2-hour postprandial glucose) is 0 to 50 mg per dL, the amount of insulin provided prior to eating is deemed appropriate. If persistent discrepancies exist, the baseline dose of prandial insulin should be reevaluated. One should also remember that basal insulin should be optimized to allow patients to achieve their fasting targeted blood glucose of 70 to 130 mg per dL.

Dietary Management for T2DM

Dietary intervention for patients with T2DM is designed to improve insulin resistance; reduce weight, when necessary; and promote adaptation of healthy food choices into the diet. Weight loss of 10 to 20 lbs can significantly improve insulin resistance and hyperlipidemia while controlling hypertension.[24–27] Reducing calorie consumption, coupled with increased energy utilization with exercise, can result in improved weight management. By monitoring the effects of different foods on blood glucose levels, patients are able to understand the effects of food consumption on glycemic control.[28]

The Diabetes Food Pyramid

The Diabetes Food Pyramid divides food into six groups (Fig. 3-1). These groups or sections on the pyramid vary in size. The largest group—grains, beans, and starchy vegetables—is on the bottom. This means that patients should eat more servings of grains, beans, and starchy vegetables than of any of the other foods. The smallest group—fats, sweets, and alcohol—is at the top of the pyramid, suggesting that fewer servings of these items should be consumed.

At the base of the pyramid are **bread, cereal, rice**, and **pasta.** These foods contain mostly carbohydrates. The foods in this group are made mostly of grains, such as wheat, rye, and oats. Starchy vegetables such as potatoes, peas, and corn also belong to this group, along with dry beans such as black-eyed peas and pinto beans. Starchy vegetables and beans are in this group because they have about as much carbohydrate in one serving as a slice of bread. Patients are advised to choose 6 to 11 servings from this group daily.

All **vegetables** are naturally low in fat and good choices to include often in meals or snacks. Vegetables are full of vitamins, minerals, and fiber. This group includes spinach, chicory, sorrel, Swiss chard, broccoli, cabbage, bok choy, brussels sprouts, cauliflower, kale, carrots, tomatoes, cucumbers, and lettuce. Starchy vegetables such as potatoes, corn, peas, and lima beans are counted in the starch and grain group for diabetes meal planning. Three to five servings of vegetables daily should be considered.

The next layer of the pyramid is **fruits**, which also contain carbohydrates. They also have plenty of vitamins, minerals, and fiber. This group includes blackberries, cantaloupe, strawberries, oranges, apples, bananas, peaches, pears, apricots, and grapes. Although two to four daily servings of fruit are suggested, their effect on blood glucose levels is greatest in the morning when insulin resistance is at its peak. Therefore, delaying fruit consumption until the afternoon when insulin resistance is reduced may help control glycemic excursions after meals.

Milk products contain a lot of protein and calcium as well as many other vitamins. The patient should choose nonfat or low-fat dairy products for the great taste and nutrition without the saturated fat. The ADA recommends two to three milk servings per day.

The **meat** group includes beef, chicken, turkey, fish, eggs, and tofu. Beans are in the starch group (1/2 cup of beans equals 15 g of carbohydrates, 3 g of protein, and no fat, unless cooked with

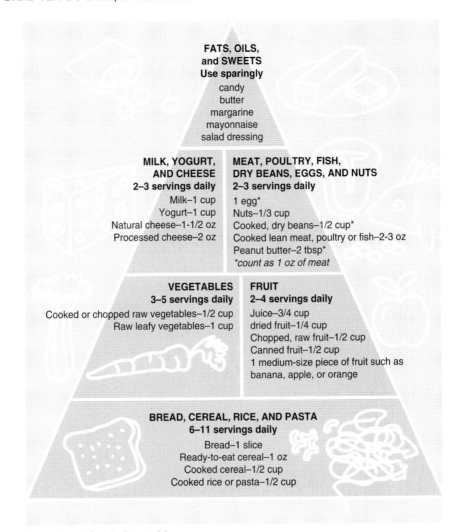

Figure 3-1 • Food Guide Pyramid.
Adapted from the National Center for Nutrition and Dietetics, the American Dietetic Association (www.aap.org), and the American Academy of Family Physicians (www.aafp.org).

bacon or ham). Other proteins in the meat group are peanut butter, cheese, and cottage cheese. Cheese is high in fat: Usually, 1 oz of cheese contains 8 g of fat. Meat and meat substitutes are great sources of protein and many vitamins and minerals. The patient should choose from lean meats, poultry, and fish and cut all the visible fat off meat. The portion sizes should be small. Three ounces is about the size of a deck of cards. Only 4 to 6 oz per day divided between meals is recommended. The long-term effects of consuming more than 20% of energy as protein on the development of nephropathy have not been determined. However, intake of protein in the usual range does not appear to be associated with the development of diabetic nephropathy.[19]

The use of **fats** and **sweets** (such as potato chips, candy, cookies, cakes, crackers, and fried foods) should be minimized and consumed on special occasions such as birthdays or anniversaries.

The effect of **alcohol** on blood glucose levels depends not only on the amount of alcohol ingested but also on the amount of alcohol consumed in relationship to food intake. Alcohol is oxidized by the liver, where gluconeogenesis may become impaired, resulting in hypoglycemia. Because both insulin and alcohol can inhibit gluconeogenesis, patients with T1DM who inject insulin and drink alcohol without eating may develop severe hypoglycemia. Alcohol also increases triglyceride levels, resulting in hyperlipidemia.[28,29] In general, the effects of alcohol on glucose metabolism are

TABLE 3-8. Calorie Content of Popular Alcoholic Beverages

Alcoholic Beverage	Calories Consumed per Drink
Martini	210
Piña colada	365
Mai tai	310
Strawberry daiquiri	150
Tom Collins	169
Bloody Mary	86
Red and rosé wine	21 per 3.5 oz
White wine	81 per 3.5 oz
Champagne	126 per 4 oz
Light beer	117 per 12 oz
Regular beer	184 per 12 oz
Tequila, gin, whiskey, vodka, rum	1–1.5 oz shot 80% proof[a] = 100 1–1.5 oz shot 100% proof[a] = 124

[a]The proof number is twice the alcohol content of the beverage. 80% proof means the liquor is 40% alcohol and 100% proof is 50% alcohol. When the shot is combined with a prepared mix such as juice or soda, the calorie counts can go much higher.
From http://www.dietbites.com/CalorieIndexSpirits.html and http://www.calorie-count.com/calories/item/14003.html.

not severe. Because insulin is not required to metabolize alcohol, no food group need be eliminated from the calculated intake. One must always remember that alcohol adds calories to the diet and, for this reason, is counted in the fat exchange group (Table 3-8). Patients with pancreatitis, dyslipidemia, or neuropathy should avoid the use of alcohol.[28]

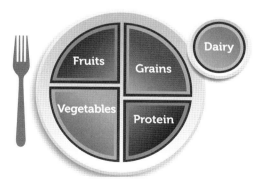

Figure 3-2 • Nutritional Guidance Related to USDA MyPlate.gov.

Balance calories:
• Enjoy food, but eat less (see example related to popcorn below)
• Avoid oversize portions

Foods to increase:
• Half of the food plate should consist of fruits and vegetables
• Half of the food plate should consist of proteins and whole grains
• Switch to fat-free or low-fat (1%) milk

Foods to reduce:
• Read food labels. Reduce foods high in sodium such as soup, bread, and frozen meals
• Avoid sugary drinks. Water is the preferred beverage

Reference: USDA: http://www.choosemyplate.gov. Accessed November 10, 2011.

In 2010, the U.S. Department of Agriculture elected to update the dietary guidelines with a graphic known as MyPlate (www.ChooseMyPlate.gov). Foods from the pyramid can be placed on the plate, which may allow the consumer to better understand the implications of their food choices. The implications of MyPlate.gov are illustrated in Figure 3-2.

Many individuals with T2DM diabetes are overweight, with 36% having a BMI of 30 kg per m^2 or greater, which would classify them as obese.[30] The prevalence of obesity is higher in women and members of minority populations with T2DM.[30] As body adiposity increases, so does insulin resistance. Obesity may also aggravate hyperlipidemia and hypertension in T2DM patients.[31]

Because of the negative effects of obesity on insulin resistance, weight loss is an important therapeutic objective for obese individuals with T2DM. Short-term studies lasting 6 months or less have demonstrated that weight loss in T2DM subjects is associated with decreased insulin resistance, improved measures of glycemia, reduced serum lipids, and reduced blood pressure.[24] Long-term data assessing the extent to which these improvements can be maintained in people with T2DM are not available.

Long-term weight loss is difficult for most people to accomplish because weight regulation is multidimensional. The genetic and neuroendocrine axis components that regulate weight are extremely complex and not well understood. Obesity is clearly a by-product of disordered energy intake and energy expenditure. In his book, Mindless Eating,[32] famed clinical obesity psychologist Brian Wansink conducted several real life experiments within various U.S. population groups. For example, a group of lucky movie patrons lined up and paid to see the Mel Gibson movie "Payback" in Chicago several years ago. Everyone who bought a ticket was given a free soft drink and either a medium-sized bucket of popcorn or a "bigger-than-your-head bucket" at no charge. Each lucky moviegoer was simply asked to remain after the show and answer a few questions about their viewing experience.

Unknown to the Mel Gibson fans and to the graduate students who conducted the postshow interviews, the free popcorn was not only prepared 5 days in advance of this show, "it was stale enough to squeak when it was eaten!" Although safe to eat, the popcorn tasted like Styrofoam or bubble wrap. Nearly everyone dipped into their free bucket of snacks throughout the 2-hour movie. Two people, thought the food tasted so disgusting that they asked for their money back, forgetting that they were provided with their 10-gallon bucket at no charge ("Oh, never mind!").

Following the movie, the graduate students began to collect their data, as many people continued to enjoy their fossil-like popcorn until they learned the real truth about the disgusting snack. Patrons who were given the largest buckets of popcorn actually consumed 53% more stale popcorn than those provided with the medium buckets. Per person caloric intake on average was 173 greater for those eating from those double-double tubs than the medium popcorn holders. On average, the large popcorn buckets induced 21 additional grabs of stale popcorn compared with the medium buckets. Perhaps this teaches us that larger plates tend to "induce" us to indulge more when consuming food. Also, simply believing that a meal will taste good will lead one to overeat.

Everyone has their own secrets to dieting success. For a less-than-expert opinion on weight loss, the reader is referred to "Last-Minute Diet Secrets-People Magazine; March 16, 2004:122–125." Excerpts from these authoritative spokespersons for the American Public are noted in Table 3-9.[33]

TABLE 3-9. Celebrities Respond to This Question: "How do movie stars like you lose those last-minute pounds before walking the runway at the Oscars?"

- Vivica Fox: "I pop herbal laxatives and drink as much coffee as I can to flush everything out."

- Melissa Rivers: "I limit my calorie intake and work out like crazy. I try to eat really clean the week prior. I always substitute one meal for just a salad with dressing on the side, and dip my fork in the dressing."

- Emma Thompson: "I try not to eat sugar, and I don't eat bread and biscuits... I really don't eat any of the things I love... But I will get back to ice cream soon, which is my favorite food."

- Bill Murray: "I did 200,000 crunches!"

Weight modulation is controlled and regulated, in part, by the central nervous system.[34] Destruction of β-cells results in the inability to secrete both insulin and amylin, which dysregulates appetite and satiety. Amylin mediates satiety mechanisms via its effects on the area postrema, an area of the brainstem that integrates hormonal and metabolic signals to regulate food consumption.[35] Amylin slows gastric emptying and glucagon secretion. Leptin, insulin, and glucagon act synergistically with cholecystokinin (synthesized by the I-cells of the small intestine and secreted from the duodenum) to reduce appetite.[36] These actions are opposed by ghrelin, concentrations of which are lower in obese and T2DM patients.[37]

In a study of other hormonal satiety mechanisms in lean and obese nondiabetic men, levels of postprandial insulin and glucose-dependent insulinotropic polypeptide (GIP) were found to be key determinants of short-term appetite regulation.[38]

A review of incretin use in patients with T1DM during the remission phase of the disease suggested that the use of GLP-1 long-acting agonists could improve satiety by allowing them to maintain a normal between-meal interval.[39]

Individuals who sleep less than 5 to 6 hours each night or who have significant sleep fragmentation (have difficulty maintaining sleep) are at high risk for gaining weight and eventually developing diabetes. The mechanism appears to be due to an imbalance between leptin and ghrelin.[40] As the body perceives more time in the "alert state," ghrelin is secreted in excess of leptin, favoring an increase in caloric intake to compensate for higher energy needs during these hours. Thus, patients who work the graveyard shift and sleep only 4 to 5 hours per day will find weight reduction very challenging, if not impossible, without improving their sleep hygiene.

The National Weight Control Registry has enrolled more than 3,000 subjects successful at long-term maintenance of weight loss.[41] A group of approximately 800 people who lost an average of 30 kg and maintained a minimum weight loss of 13.6 kg (30 lbs) for 5 years were identified from the registry. Slightly more than half lost weight through formal programs, and the remainder lost weight with a program of their own. Average energy consumption was approximately 1,400 kcal per day, with 24% of energy derived from fat. Average energy expenditure through added physical activity was 2,800 kcal per week. Importantly, nearly 77% of this sample of people who were successful in achieving and maintaining weight loss reported a triggering event that preceded the weight loss. The most common triggering events were acute medical conditions and emotional problems. Thus, a new diagnosis of T2DM could trigger lifestyle changes that result in reduced fat and energy intake and increased physical activity and associated weight loss.

The Look AHEAD (Action for Health in Diabetes) trial is a multicenter randomized clinical trial comparing the effects of an intensive lifestyle intervention program (ILI) with a diabetes support

TABLE 3-10. Interventions Assigned to the Study Arms of Look AHEAD

Arm	Assigned Interventions
Experimental: intensive lifestyle intervention (ILI)	Behavioral: Lifestyle intervention • Individual supervision and group sessions • The goal is to maintain at least a 7% decrease in weight from baseline and participate in 175 min/wk in physical activity. • Implementation over a 4-yr period • Most intensive application during year 1; less frequent attention during subsequent 3 y • Preset algorithm assists participants in achieving and maintaining weight loss (prepared meals, liquid formulas, exercise strategies, and medications).
Active comparator: diabetes support and education (DSE)	Behavioral: Diabetes support and education • Participants are offered three sessions annually in diabetes management and social support.

and education (DSE) control group on the reduction of major cardiovascular events in 5,145 over-weight or obese patients with T2DM. The study began recruiting in 2001 and is expected to report in 2014.[42] Table 3-10 depicts the interventions assigned to each study arm.

Initial 4-year data from the Look AHEAD study suggest that ILI participants experienced greater weight loss than DSE participants (–6.15% vs. 0.88%; $p < 0.001$) and greater improvement in cardiovascular fitness (12.74% vs. 1.96%; $p < 0.001$). Intentional weight loss and physical activity also statistically improved metabolic parameters within the ILI group versus the DSE cohort as follows: hemoglobin A1c level (–0.36% vs. –0.09%; $p < 0.001$), systolic (–5.33 vs. –2.97 mm Hg; $p < 0.001$) and diastolic (–2.92 vs. –2.48 mm Hg; $p = 0.01$) blood pressure, and levels of high-density lipoprotein cholesterol (3.67 vs. 1.97 mg per dL; $p <.001$) and triglycerides (–25.56 vs. –19.75 mg per dL; $p < 0.001$). Reductions in low-density lipoprotein cholesterol levels were greater in DSE than ILI participants (–11.27 vs. –12.84 mg per dL; $p = 0.009$), owing to greater use of medications to lower lipid levels in the DSE group. Thus, at 4 years, ILI participants maintained greater improvements than DSE participants in weight, fitness, A1C levels, systolic blood pressure, and high-density lipoprotein cholesterol levels.[43]

Exercise improves insulin sensitivity, can acutely lower blood glucose in patients with diabetes, and may also improve cardiovascular status. Exercise by itself has only a modest effect on weight. Exercise is to be encouraged but, like behavioral therapies, may be most useful as an adjunct to other weight loss strategies, such as dietary fat reduction. Exercise is, however, important in long-term maintenance of weight loss.

Behavioral approaches to weight loss include strategies such as self-monitoring of food intake and exercise, nutrition education, stimulus control, preplanning food intake, and self-reinforcement. Weight loss with behavioral therapy alone has been modest[31,44]; behavioral approaches may be most useful as an adjunct to other weight loss strategies.

For weight loss to be successful, focus should be placed on reducing dietary fat intake and spontaneous eating. By obtaining a nutritional history, one can estimate the number of excessive calories a patient consumes on a daily basis and offer suggestions on eliminating these "wasted calories." Figure 3-3 provides a nutritional history form that can be completed by patients within 3 minutes. Once completed, physicians should evaluate the following information:

1. If the patient is eating only once or twice daily, there is a strong likelihood that snacks are being used to reduce hunger. Snacks can be high in calories and low in nutritional value. For example, a 4-oz serving of potato chips contains more than 500 calories and a 1.5-oz candy bar will cost the patient 225 extra calories. (Caloric content for food and beverages can be found online at http://www.annecollins.com/calories/.) Patients should be advised to eat three healthy meals daily. Snacking will be reduced if hunger is better controlled. Skipping meals will not result in weight reduction.
2. Eating meals outside the home can result in excessive caloric intake, especially when patients frequent fast food restaurants. (A normal caloric meal should be equivalent to the amount of food served while traveling by air with an economy class ticket.) A Quarter Pounder with cheese, large fries, and a large shake contain 1,200 calories. To burn off these calories, the patient will need to take a brisk 5-hour walk. Eating a regular hamburger and fries contains 475 calories, requiring the patient to walk only 2 hours to balance this caloric intake. A turkey sandwich brought from home for lunch contains only 350 calories, meaning that the patient has reduced the lunch caloric consumption by 125 calories.
3. One should watch out for food consumption that may add unnecessary calories to the daily diet. For example, Starbucks coffee houses serve up more calories than caffeine. A Caramel Frappuccino will cost the patient 280 extra calories (Table 3-11).
4. The physician should be wary of the patient who consumes fruity drinks. An 8-oz cup of orange juice contains 100 calories. By using "reduced calorie fruit beverages," calories can be reduced by 50%.
5. Figure 3-4 shows the relationship between TV viewing, physical activity, and the risk of developing diabetes. Inactive individuals who view more than 15 hours of TV per week

Nutritional Assessment Form

Name: _____　**ID:** _____　**Date:** _____

1. How many meals and snacks do you eat each day? Meals _____ Snacks _____

   What types of snacks do you eat? _____

2. How many times a week do you eat the following meals away from home?

   Breakfast _____ Lunch _____ Dinner _____

3. What types of eating places do you frequently visit? (Check all that apply)

   Fast-Food _____ Diner/cafeteria _____ Restaurant _____ Other _____

   Starbucks/Coffee shop _____ Donut Shop _____

4. On average, how many pieces of fruit or glasses of juice do you eat or drink daily?

   Fresh fruit _____ Juice (8-oz cup) _____

5. On average, how many servings of vegetables do you eat each day? _____

6. How many times a week do you eat red meat? _____

7. How many times a week do you eat chicken or turkey? _____

8. How many time a week do you eat fish or shellfish? _____

9. How many hours of TV do you watch each day? _____

10. Do you usually snack while watching TV? Yes _____ No _____

11. How many times a week do you eat desserts and sweets? _____

12. How many servings of each of these drinks do you consume daily?

Water _____	Milk _____	Alcohol _____
Juice _____	Whole milk _____	Beer _____
Soda _____	2% milk _____	Wine _____
Diet soda _____	1% milk _____	Hard liquor _____
Sports drinks _____	Skim milk _____	
Iced tea _____		
Iced tea with sugar _____		

13. How many days per week do you do at least 30 minutes of continuous exercise (walking, biking, swimming, resistance training, health club, etc) _____

14. Exercise

    a) How many days a week do you exercise? _____

    b) How long does your workout last? _____

    c) What type (s) of exercise do you do? _____

Approximate daily caloric requirements for weight maintenance _____

Approximate daily calories patient is currently consuming _____

Approximate daily caloric expenditure from exercise _____

Excess calories patient is currently consuming _____

Figure 3-3 • **Nutritional Assessment Form.**

TABLE 3-11. Lisa's Nutrition Form

Source of Calories	Approximate Calories Consumed per Day
Starbucks Frappuccino	280
Fast food stop daily for lunch	300
2 snacks daily (popcorn, ice cream, chips)	350
2 glasses of orange juice/d	150
2 light beers/d	200
1 dessert daily	500
2 sodas daily	350
1 cup of whole milk with breakfast	150
3 cocktails/wk	150
Total excess calories per day (average)	**2,440**

have three times the risk of diabetes. Patients also tend to snack while watching TV, which results in situational food consumption and excessive daily caloric intake.

6. Do patients who are overweight really need to eat desserts on a daily basis? A cup of ice cream plus a slice of chocolate cake can equal 800 calories, almost one-third of the daily caloric requirement of a 70-kg man. One should suggest that the patient consider eating desserts on "special occasions," instead of as part of the daily routine. Patients who insist on eating dessert should consider eating fruit or nonfat yogurt as an alternative.

7. Simple changes in food and drink choices can reduce the daily caloric intake significantly. Skim milk has approximately 50% less calories than whole milk (150 cal per cup). Switching from regular to diet colas will eliminate 175 calories per 12 oz consumed. Light beer has 100 calories per 12-oz serving, whereas regular beer on average has 150 calories.

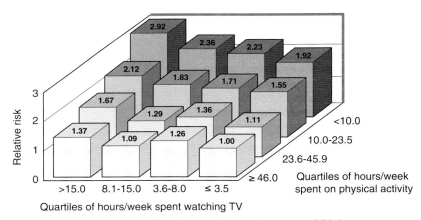

Figure 3-4 • Effects of Sedentary Lifestyle on the Development of Diabetes
This is the Health Professional's Follow-up Study (HPFS) that began in 1986 when 51,529 health professionals, ages 40 to 75 years, answered a detailed questionnaire about diet, lifestyle practices, and medical history. During 10 years of follow-up, 1,058 new cases of diabetes were diagnosed. After adjustment for age, average time spent watching TV was strongly associated with an increased risk for diabetes. This graph represents a multivariate analysis in which independent effects of watching TV and physical activity levels were observed. Reducing TV viewing and increasing physical activity can reduce the risk of developing diabetes. Adapted from Hu FB, Leitzmann MF, Stampfer MJ, et al. Physical activity and television watching in relation to risk for type 2 diabetes mellitus in men. *Arch Intern Med.* 2001;161:1542–1548, with permission.

One should be cautious about using "sports drinks" on a regular basis. Although these beverages are marketed to the general public, they basically add glucose, calories, and sodium to the diet. Elite athletes benefit more from sports drinks than persons with diabetes or prediabetes. An 8-oz bottle of Gatorade contains 50 calories, whereas a 32-oz bottle of POWERade will cost the consumer 280 extra calories. The clinician should encourage the use of "light" drinks for those who insist on using sports beverages.

8. Believe in the "power of three." Patients who can reduce caloric intake by just 100 calories per day may actually lose up to 30 lbs in 1 year! What three behaviors might eliminate 100 calories each day from one's dietary intake? Let us take a look at a few options. First, people can simply eliminate simple access to food or snacks that are hidden on or within their workspaces or desks. Second, try incorporating "food trade-offs" into one's daily routine. For example, popcorn can be consumed at a movie, but a salad with low fat dressing would be all that that person could eat for dinner. Also, go ahead and eat dessert, but this will cost the eater 45 minutes of exercise that same day. Finally, reduce calorie intake for one meal each day by simply consuming vegetables and fruit rather than bread and pasta. Not everyone will follow the power of three suggestions each day. Yet, if they are successful 70% of the time, weight loss is highly probable.

When using the Nutritional Assessment Form (Fig. 3-3), one should determine the patient's basal metabolic requirements. The **basal metabolic rate** (BMR) is the minimum number of calories required to maintain the current body weight. The BMR is calculated as follows[45]:

$$BMR = 24 \times weight\ (kg)$$

The BMR is then multiplied by a number representing the individual's activity level:

Sedentary: BMR × 1.45
Light: BMR × 1.60
Medium: BMR × 1.70
Heavy: BMR × 1.88

A patient with T2DM weighing 100 kg with a sedentary lifestyle would have a calculated BMR of 24 × 100 kg × 1.45 = 3,480. The greater the caloric restriction below 3,480 per day, the more weight that patient should lose. A pound is equivalent to 3,500 calories. Reducing the caloric consumption by 3,500 calories per week should result in a 1-lb weight loss per week. By increasing the physical activity level, a person can possibly burn 1,750 calories per week while reducing caloric consumption by a similar amount, again resulting in a net loss of 1 lb per week.

Next, one should add up all the extra calories that the patient is consuming on a near-daily basis using the nutritional intake form (Table 3-11).

Based on the fact that 3,500 calories = 1 lb, a patient who averages a weight gain of 1 lb every 10 days on their current diet should be counseled to eliminate nonessential nutrients, eat three meals a day, and choose foods from the diabetes food pyramid. Sensible meal planning and education coupled with a simple exercise program can result in weight loss in many individuals. One can also explain to patients that by simply reducing caloric intake by 150 calories per day (equal to a cookie), weight loss can be anticipated to reach 1 lb each month or 12 lbs in the first 12 months of caloric monitoring.

The following are some additional ways that physicians may promote weight reduction for their patients. Writing these instructions on an actual prescription may increase the patient's awareness of the importance of adhering to these recommendations:

- No second helpings at mealtimes
- Walk 30 minutes 5 days per week.
- Avoid all sugar-containing drinks, desserts, and high-calorie snacks.
- Drink at least four glasses of water each day.
- Stop all alcohol consumption.
- Eat three meals a day. Do not skip breakfast.

TABLE 3-12. Dietary Recommendations for Patients with Diabetes and Coexisting Metabolic Disorders

Coexisting Metabolic Disorder	Dietary Recommendations
Hypertension	• Weight reduction • Reduce sodium intake.[a] • Low-fat diet that includes fruits, vegetables (5–9 servings/d), low-fat dairy products (2–4 servings/d) • Food rich in potassium • Reduce alcohol intake to <3 drinks/d.[b]
Dyslipidemia	• For elevated LDL-C, saturated fats and trans-fatty acids should be limited to <7% of energy requirements. • For elevated triglycerides, low HDL-C, and small dense LDL-C, improve glycemic control (consider insulin), modest weight reduction, dietary saturated fat restriction, and increase physical activity
Nephropathy	• Restrict protein to 0.8 g/kg/d with the guidance of a registered dietitian (overt nephropathy). • Restrict protein to 0.8–1.0 g/kg/d for microalbuminuria.
Acute illness	• Ingest 45–50 g of carbs every 3–4 h should prevent starvation ketosis while keeping blood glucose levels at 80–180 mg/dL.

[a]For "salt-sensitive" patients. No clinical measures are available that identify patients as being salt sensitive. Salt restriction can reduce systolic blood pressure by 5 mm Hg and 2 mm Hg for diastolic blood pressure. In general, the lower the sodium intake, the greater the effect on lowering blood pressure. The goal should be to reduce sodium intake to 2,400 mg or sodium chloride (salt) to 6,000 mg/d.
[b]An association between high alcohol intake (≥3 drinks/d) and elevated blood pressure has been reported; however, there is no major difference in blood pressure between people who consume <3 drinks/d and nondrinkers.
LDL-C, low-density lipoprotein cholesterol; HDL-C, high-density lipoprotein cholesterol.
From the American Diabetes Association. Nutrition principles and recommendations in diabetes. Position Statement. *Diabetes Care.* 2004;27:S36.

Finally, patients with diabetes should shield themselves from the guilt and humiliation they feel on a daily basis brought forth by the "diabetes KGB." Also known as the "food police," these well-meaning, yet poorly informed, narcissistic, overbearing, butt-in-skies, are more frustrating than a small town speed trap. Usually your brother could care less how you eat. If your neighbor finds out you have diabetes, she will immediately morph into the mother superior of certified diabetic educators blaming "the diabetic" within your home for eating too much sugar and not enough red rice. Having neighbors or friends preach about diabetes is like being waterboarded in your own home. Soon you will become a believer in *their* own destiny agreeing to live the rest of your life eating nothing but cabbage and sugar-free jello. In reality, patients can eat meals that are nutritious and healthy. Home blood glucose monitoring after eating will help determine which foods may be problematic, rising blood glucose levels above and beyond the 180 mg per dL threshold 2 hours after eating. Patients who fail to practice sound self-management skills and instead fall victim to the KGB will soon find become "diabetes criminals." In diabetes management, bullying is never permitted!

The nutritional recommendations for patients with diabetes and coexisting metabolic conditions are summarized in Table 3-12.

 ## Comparing Popular Dietary Plans

Many times, often on a busy day, primary care doctors are asked by patients to comment on a particular dietary plan or supplement. With the explosion of smartphone apps for weight loss and Internet help sights, there is little doubt that patients will be looking for adventurous ways to weigh less and improve glycemic control. No one can be expected to take the time to learn the risks and benefits of each alleged dietary protocol, such as the world famous "Fat Loss 4 Idiots" plan that claims to guide Internet users into losing 9 lbs every 11 days.[46] With my humble apologies to all Web sites and weight loss authors who I will now offend, I will take the liberty of comparing and contrasting the most popular dietary plans with which most physicians have some limited knowledge (see Table 3-13).

TABLE 3-13. Comparing Diets of Interest for Patients with Diabetes

Diet Name	Description	Advantages	Disadvantages
South Beach Diet	Allows the consumption of the right type of carbs using the glycemic index[a] while reducing saturated fat content of consumed foods OK to eat whole grains, fruits, and veggies (as suggested by the MyPlate.com U.S. Dept. of Agriculture Web site) Phase 1 results in rapid weight loss (up to 13 lbs) over 2 wk by restricting many foods. Phase 2 allows the reintroduction of certain foods and weight loss will slow. Phase 3 reintroduces moderate amounts of the initially restricted foods allowing patient's to maintain their weight.	Nutritionally balanced after phase 1 May be useful to reverse prediabetes acutely No fat or calorie counting required 1,000 simple recipes are provided. Patients learn to use the glycemic index.[a] Encourages regular meals and snack consumption	Can be expensive and time consuming Many people find this diet too restrictive. Due to extensive carb restriction, exercisers may find this diet difficult to follow.
Sugar Busters Diet	Prohibits refined sugar and starches that rank high in the glycemic index[a] such as potatoes and pasta In theory, sugar is toxic to bodies. Sugar causes an increase in insulin production resulting in weight gain. Daily calorie intake is split into 40% fat, 30% protein, and 30% carbohydrates. Provides an average intake of 1,200 calories/d (approximately 50% of what is normally consumed by a healthy 70-kg male adult)	No carb or calorie counting Eliminates many foods that are clearly unhealthy Focuses on healthy eating (whole grains and fresh fruits and vegetables, beans, lentils, fish or lean meat, and low-fat or fat-free dairy products) Encourages exercises as part of the dietary plan	Not suitable for vegetarians. Additional protein supplementation may be needed based on weight of the patient. Eliminates some valuable minerals and nutrients. Vitamin supplements should be encouraged. Weight loss is probably due to caloric restriction, not the 40:30:30 ratio the plan encourages patients to follow.

(Continued)

Diet Name	Description	Advantages	Disadvantages
Weight Watchers Points Diet	Patients may eat what they want as long as they do not exceed their daily "point limit." All foods are assigned points. Participants are weighed weekly and are then advised on how many points they should eat on a daily basis until the next weigh in.	Does not exclude major food groups Teaches portion control Participants encouraged to dine out Behavioral support is provided in the form of weekly meetings. Encourages the use of self–blood glucose monitoring to evaluate the effect of food on glucose excursions	Expensive membership over time Weight loss is slow for many participants. Participants must know the exact serving size to calculate point values. Participants can spend those points on unhealthy foods!
The Zone Diet	Weight loss will occur if insulin levels can be managed while dieting. If one is adherent to the daily dietary consumption recommendations, insulin levels will improve, which should, in turn, speed up "fat burning." The meal plate is divided into "zones." Lean proteins (fish, skinless chicken, egg whites, tofu) should total 33% of what is eaten. Fruits and vegetables should total the other 66%.	Teaches good eating habits such as portion control Encourages fruit- and vegetable-rich diet By restricting carbs, cravings disappear after several days. Rapid weight loss can occur with the Zone Diet. Exercising 3–5 d a week is encouraged. Omega-3 supplements should be used.	Some feel that the diet unscientifically suggests that vascular inflammation is reduced. Some carbohydrates such as whole grains are restricted, which has been criticized. Rapid weight loss is often followed by rapid weight gain. Required use of nutritional supplements will be expensive.
Atkins Diet	Excess carbohydrate consumption causes weight gain and may exacerbate diabetes. Favors high protein intake over carbs Initially, participants reduce carb and increase protein intake.	Tends to favor rapid weight loss Has been proven to be effective in the short term Inexpensive	Restrictive diet Not supported by the American Diabetes Association Condones high consumption of saturated fats Patients complain of bad breath, nausea, headaches (due to induction of ketosis) as the diet is initiated. Vitamin supplements should be provided. Not suitable for vegetarians Long-term effects of high protein and fat on vital organs have been questioned.

(Continued)

TABLE 3-13. Comparing Diets of Interest for Patients with Diabetes *(Continued)*

Diet Name	Description	Advantages	Disadvantages
Jenny Craig	Provides a personalized consultant who educates patients on balancing a healthy lifestyle with proper nutrition	Foods are low in calories yet highly nutritious. Special foods on menus are available for people with diabetes and for those who keep kosher.	May be expensive to many. The "consultants" at many centers are not RDs or CDEs. As a result, a patient who enrolls weighing 300 lbs may be inappropriately informed that their weight goal will be set at "150 lbs." This could add to a patient's frustration!
DASH Diet (Dietary Approaches to Stop Hypertension)	Diet has been found to be very effective at lowering blood pressure while slightly improving glycemia. Favors meals that are rich in fruits, vegetables, and low-fat or nonfat dairy. Provides calcium, potassium, and magnesium, which can lower blood pressure. Nutritionally sound foods benefit glycemic control.	Diet favors the use of grains, especially whole grains; lean meats, fish and poultry, nuts and beans. Meal planning is flexible enough to meet the lifestyle and food preferences of most people. Diet plan endorsed by many professional organizations such as the American Heart Association; the National Heart, Lung, and Blood Institute; and the U.S. Dept. of Agriculture. Exercise and lifestyle modification are encouraged.	This is NOT a specific weight loss diet. Daily intake will be between 1,600 and 3,200 cal/d. DASH is of primary benefit to patients who want to reduce their blood pressure using "natural means." More weight is likely to be reduced if participant lives a healthy lifestyle and exercises more.

[a]The glycemic index (GI) is not universally accepted; critics argue that it does not reflect the way that most people actually eat and that the ratings can be deceiving, since each food is rated individually, not combined in a meal. Foods that are cooked differently may have a different GI rating.

The Exercise Prescription for Diabetes

Exercise in the days before insulin we regarded as useful, but by no means did we appreciate it as vital in the care of diabetes… We should return to it to help us in the treatment of all of our cases…
—*Eliot P. Joslin, Treatment of Diabetes Mellitus, 1959*

Eliot Joslin, the first master clinician of diabetes, envisioned that not all of the mysteries of diabetes would be solved by the 1922 discovery of insulin. Historically, exercise has been a mainstay of diabetes treatment since the 1700s, when physicians advised their patients to ride long distances on horseback, believing that the friction of the body against the saddle would reduce the need to urinate and minimize dehydration. One could only imagine how many of these hyperglycemic jockeys with blurry vision survived their trail rides. Although most patients today do not cite their fear of horseback riding as one of their many excuses to avoid exercising, motivating anyone to increase his or her physical activity presents a major challenge for PCPs.

The most common reasons why patients do not engage in regular exercise as part of their comprehensive diabetes self-management treatment plan include lack of time, health-related reasons (i.e., pain, fatigue, joint stiffness), boredom, lack of convenient exercise locations, and expense. Failure to exercise may also reflect a long history of obesity and inactivity, which is shared not only among people with diabetes but also in patients with schizophrenia.[47,48] Patients who have developed diabetes-related complications, despite their previous attempts at behavioral interventions, may be reluctant to engage in any physical activity, especially as they become more symptomatic.

PCPs are well aware of the beneficial role exercise has on improving metabolic abnormalities related to hypertension, diabetes, hyperlipidemia, obesity, chronic pain disorders, and mental illness. Although anyone, even a nonphysician, can advise a patient about the benefits of exercise, physicians must assess their patients' general medical condition, determine any risks associated with exercising, and prescribe an individualized exercise regimen that is practical, safe, and likely to improve metabolic parameters. How can physicians best implement and integrate exercise into the overall treatment plan of diabetes?

Not all patients believe that reducing long- and short-term diabetes-related complications is the primary reason to initiate an exercise program. Some may view exercise as yet another burden imposed on them by their physicians or as "punishment" for being overweight. Other patients may consider exercise as being inherently unpleasant or stressful. To change a patient's perception regarding exercise, four principles should be followed:

1. Exercise participation becomes more likely when the patient perceives the **individual benefits** of increasing activity on his or her own diabetes control. The option to exercise is ultimately patient driven. Exercise must be viewed as being a valuable tool in allowing one to achieve their personalized metabolic targets.
2. Exercise is likely to be sustained if the specific activity chosen has few barriers to implementation. Exercise must integrate easily within the patient's lifestyle, beliefs, and attitudes. Physicians can help patients clarify their choices.
3. Physicians should express the positive outcomes associated with exercise rather than reinforce the negative consequences of inactivity. Which statement would a patient prefer to hear during a routine 8-minute office visit: (1) "I am so happy that you are beginning to exercise 3 days a week. If you check your blood glucose level prior to and 30 minutes after the concluding the exercise you should notice an improvement in your sugars. Then you'll understand how your body responds to sustained activity." Or (2) "Look, Mr. Speedy, your idea of exercise is a nice brisk sit! You are going to simply gain more weight, your blood pressure will go up and I will not be able to get your A1C to 7%." Patients should always be educated regarding potential negative consequences associated with exercise (joint and muscle pain, fatigue, shortness of breath, and even hypoglycemia).
4. Exercise is more likely to be sustained if consistently reinforced by the health-care management team and staff.

When initiating a discussion about exercise, one should consider how a patient may benefit from these positive attributes that are associated with increasing physical activity levels:

1. *Health benefits*, such as improvements in glucose regulation, weight control, lipid profiles, hypertension, and increased work capacity
2. *Social benefits*, such as increased interaction with family members, "social others" (i.e., training partners), and participation in organized, community-based activities

3. *Psychological benefits*, most notably *reduced* anxiety and depression, stress reduction, and enhanced feelings of well-being

In addition to the benefits of exercise, the following key points should also be discussed:

1. Exercise does not have to be done at Olympic levels while wearing spandex or designer clothing. More modest levels of activity can be quite effective. Ample research suggests that 30 minutes a day of moderate-intensity physical activity, such as brisk walking, performed 5 days a week will confer the majority of exercise-related benefits.[17] Although 30 uninterrupted minutes is the ideal, three shorter, modest levels of activity will also be beneficial.

2. Exercise should be viewed as part of a lifelong management program. The patient should not attempt to begin exercising at high intensity. A good program is one that progresses through a series of stages until an effective and acceptable level is achieved. Together, providers and patients should select a series of goals that are safe and effective over time in allowing patients to achieve their goals.

3. Patients will have to learn how to exercise properly (i.e., to perform the activity so that they avoid discomfort, injury, and problems with their diabetes). Proper stretching and warm-up activities are important. This will require them to be willing to experiment a bit with new behaviors, including adjusting their diabetes regimen. Patients should be instructed to wear proper fitting shoes (which should be replaced every 3-4 months) and stockings, which are completely stretched upward across the foot and ankle to avoid friction ulcers.

4. Patients do not have to determine how to appropriately initiate an exercise program on their own. Health-care professionals and others in their communities are there to help. The physician should consider establishing introductory group exercise classes at the office led by a certified personal trainer. A good trainer could make exercise an enjoyable, challenging, and rewarding experience for patients with limited exercise tolerance.

5. Patients should select activities that they are likely to continue in the long run. For example, if a patient is unable to swim, prescribing a water aerobics class may be unreasonable. Older patients may enjoy "mall walking" with other senior citizens. Martial arts studios offer a variety of cardiovascular classes for all age groups and also motivate and challenge participants to accelerate their levels of expertise.

6. Exercise should be a part of the patient's daily schedule. Although all patients have "hectic lifestyles," taking time out for themselves is critical to maintaining a healthy mind and body. Many patients with diabetes enjoy participating in yoga, kickboxing, pilates, and Tai Chi workouts. Zumba, Insanity, and PD90 exercise can be performed in groups or at home through streamed videos via the internet.

Having laid this foundation, clinicians can now prescribe an exercise program that is likely to be a source of enjoyment and will be sustained over time. Exercise prescriptions should not be generalized. If advised to "go out and start an exercise program today," a patient who is poorly conditioned is likely to finish a 5-minute jog feeling worse than yesterday when the day was spent watching football on TV. Exercise will immediately be viewed negatively, similar to having an emergency root canal procedure performed.

One should start exercise prescribing by discussing the following questions with the patient:

• What are your **goals** for exercise? Do you want to lose weight, improve your blood pressure, improve your A1C, improve your physical conditioning, prevent heart disease, improve your chance of fertility, or become a world-class swimmer? A patient's goals may parallel or be totally at odds with those of the clinician. Whatever the goals, one should not be judgmental. The clinician should remember that the rationale might not reflect what the clinician feels is most important, but it may result in achieving the same end point.

• What **types of physical activity** do you like to do or think you would like to try? This question is designed to help guide patients in selecting an appropriate activity that they are motivated to do. If they do not have a strong sense for what they want, a useful strategy is to ask them to indicate their preference between the following options: (a) long- or short-duration exercise, (b) high- or low-intensity exercise, (c) exercising alone or with others, (d) exercising at home or at a facility, (e) exercising indoors or outdoors, and (f) participating in a competitive or cooperative sport.

If a patient is unable to list any types of physical activities that may be suitable, suggestions should be offered based on the completed patient-directed daily activity profile (Table 3-14). The clinician should seriously consider establishing group exercise programs that may introduce patients to safe and inexpensive forms of physical activity. Highly motivated physicians may even consider participating or leading these classes themselves. Once patients have narrowed down the possibilities or even selected specific exercise activities, the physician should help them address the second axiom: Physical activity must be realistic and feasible in order for it to be sustained.
Questions that should next be considered include the following:

- Does the chosen activity require special **facilities?** A variety of activities (swimming, martial arts, tennis) can only be performed at dedicated facilities. Perhaps joining a local health club, fitness center, or YMCA will allow the patient to have access to multiple activities under one roof. Are the facilities easily accessible and in proximity to the patient's home?
- Does the physical activity require special **equipment?** Is the necessary equipment available and affordable?
- Does the physical activity require special **training?** Are training opportunities readily available, scheduled at convenient times, easy to get to, and affordable? Physicians may wish to solicit discounted memberships from local gyms, YMCAs, martial arts studios, and health clubs for use by patients.
- Does the physical activity require **group involvement?** Several sports require one or more additional people to play. Will patients always be able to find partners when they want or need to play?
- Is the physical activity **seasonal?** To maintain a regular exercise program, patients choosing these will need to have alternate activities that they enjoy in the off-season. For example, cross-country skiing can be replaced by mountain biking.

The physical limitations related to diabetes comorbidities should be addressed individually (Table 3-15).

After beginning an exercise program, helping patients stay motivated to continue their physical activity is critical to successful diabetes lifestyle management. Motivational tips that might help patients stay on track with their exercise program include the following[49]:

1. One should advise patients to **avoid** the temptation to do **too much too fast.** Patients should gradually build up their level of physical conditioning to avoid injury, fatigue, pain, and discouragement and always use proper equipment while exercising.
2. The patient should **monitor blood glucose levels** before, during, and after exercise to understand the effects of physical activity on individual glycemic control. Some patients may experience hypoglycemia 12 to 16 hours after completing their training session. The patient should be aware of the symptoms of hypoglycemia (weakness, lethargy, confusion, loss of muscle strength, increase sweating, blurred vision—all of which may also be symptoms of excessive exercise intensity). If symptomatic, the patient should check the blood glucose levels and treat the hypoglycemia appropriately.
3. The patient should know the **pre-exercise targets** for **safe glycemic control** while exercising. If the blood glucose level is outside of the safe range, what interventions should be used to prepare for exercise? The patient should learn to adjust medications (especially insulin) prior to exercise. (One useful method to recommend is keeping a training log that includes monitoring results to help patients remember what did and did not work for them.)
4. The patient should **schedule exercise in advance.** Setting a schedule will help patients avoid conflicting activities. A regular exercise schedule for patients with T1DM will also help them more effectively adjust their regimen so that they better control their diabetes.

TABLE 3-14. Patient-directed Daily Activity Profile

1. My typical day includes:
   - ___ Hours of sleep
   - ___ Hours of low-intensity activity (such as driving, reading, watching television)
   - ___ Hours of moderate-intensity activity (such as walking, gardening, housework)
   - ___ Hours vigorous activity (such as aerobic exercise, heavy labor, competitive sports)

2. The physical activities I enjoy most are:
   (a)
   (b)
   (c)

3. The physical activities I would like to try or learn are:
   - Swimming ___
   - Jogging ___
   - Martial arts ___
   - Kickboxing ___
   - Tennis ___
   - Soccer ___
   - Baseball ___
   - Weight training ___
   - Cardiovascular exercises (treadmill, stationary cycle, Stairmaster, elliptical machine) ___
   - Circuit training at a women's gym ___
   - Tennis ___
   - Racquetball ___
   - Yoga ___
   - Pilates ___
   - Insanity workouts ___
   - P90X workouts ___
   - Zumba ___
   - Tai Chi ___
   - I don't know ___
   - Other: ___

4. I see the following as obstacles to exercising (check all that apply):
   - ___ Lack of time
   - ___ Fear of hypoglycemia
   - ___ Poor skills/coordination
   - ___ Age
   - ___ Boredom
   - ___ Low energy
   - ___ Cost
   - ___ Lack of family support
   - ___ Lack of child care
   - ___ Lack of facilities
   - ___ Arthritis
   - ___ Other medical conditions
   - ___ Pain during or after exercise
   - ___ No interest in exercise at this time
   - ___ No obstacles at this time toward exercise
   - ___ Laziness

5. Are you interested in participating in a monthly group exercise program? Yes/No

6. Do you have a membership at any local health clubs or gyms? Yes/No

7. Do you have a partner in mind with whom you might be able to exercise? Yes/No

8. Do you prefer exercising alone or with others. (circle your preference)

Adapted from Marrero DG. Time to get moving: helping patients with diabetes adopt exercise as part of a healthy lifestyle. *Clin Diabetes.* 2005;23:154–159.

TABLE 3-15. Exercising with Diabetes Comorbidities: Risks and Recommendations

Comorbidity	Retinopathy	Nephropathy[a]	Autonomic/Peripheral Sensory Neuropathy
Risks	Increase blood pressure Increase retinal hemorrhages	Hemodynamic changes Exacerbated hypertension Coexisting retinopathy is likely	Impairment of temperature control Orthostatic hypotension Diarrhea Dehydration Foot ulcerations Callus formation on feet Difficulty maintaining balance Higher risk of sudden death due to acute MI
Recommendations for exercise	Walking Swimming Low-impact aerobics Stationary cycling Endurance exercises	Low-impact, non–weight-bearing activities (swimming)	Swimming Bicycling Rowing Chair exercises
Contraindicated exercises	Power lifting Valsalva Boxing maneuvers Martial arts Jogging Racquet sports Strenuous trumpet playing High-impact aerobics	Weight training Valsalva maneuvers Calisthenics in patients with left ventricular dysfunction	Treadmill Prolonged walking or jogging Step aerobics
Medical evaluations	DR every 12 mo Mild NPDR every 6–12 mo Severe NPDR every 2–4 mo PDR every 1–2 mo	Ambulatory blood pressure monitoring during exercise might be considered	Comprehensive cardiovascular exam should be performed on all patients with autonomic dysfunction prior to initiating exercise. Always promote adequate hydration and blood glucose monitoring before, during, and after exercise. Avoid exercising in extreme heat or cold environments.

[a]Specific physical activity recommendations have not been developed for patients with incipient (microalbuminuria >20 mg/min albumin excretion) or overt nephropathy (200 mg/min). Patients with overt nephropathy often have a reduced capacity for physical activity, which leads to self-limitation in activity level. Although there is no clear reason to limit low- to moderate-intensity forms of activity, high-intensity or strenuous physical activity should probably be discouraged in these individuals unless blood pressure is carefully monitored during exercise.

MI, myocardial infarction; DR, diabetic retinopathy; NPDR, nonproliferative diabetic retinopathy; PDR, proliferative retinopathy. From American Diabetes Association. Physical activity/exercise and diabetes. Position Statement. *Diabetes Care.* 2004;27:S58–S62 and Marrero DG. Time to get moving: helping patients with diabetes adopt exercise as part of a healthy lifestyle. *Clin Diabetes.* 2005;23:154–159.

5. Getting a **training partner** may be motivational. If the training partner is not a family member, the physician should counsel the patients to discuss their diabetes with their partner, managing suspected hypoglycemia and dehydration.

6. The patient should set **realistic exercise goals.** Exercise goals need to be precisely defined and realistically attainable. It is also important that the goals be defined by exercise behavior (e.g., "walk for 30 minutes three times per week") rather than defined by an outcome of exercise behavior (e.g., "lose 20 lbs").

7. To reduce boredom, the physician should help patients identify **alternative exercise activities.** The patient should learn to cross-train using different activities. After performing the same physical activity for several months, the skeletal muscles involved with that exercise become extremely efficient at performing those movements. Although sports-specific exercises may be an excellent way to prepare for participating in certain types of sporting events, such as skiing, the level of physical conditioning will not be increased if the same exercise is performed during each session. Rather than continuing to improve, patients may become bored as they simply maintain a certain level of fitness. Cross-training also reduces the risk of developing painful overuse syndromes as different exercises work different muscle and tendon groups. Participants in cross-training conditioning can choose from a long list of activities that they may choose to perform several times a week:

Cardiovascular Exercise
- Running, treadmill
- Swimming
- Cycling (recumbent, stationary, mountain biking)
- Rowing
- Stair climbing, elliptical machines
- Racquetball, basketball, tennis
- Kickboxing, Zumba dance, P90X and Insanity workouts
- Mixed martial arts training

Resistance Training
- Calisthenics (push-ups, crunches, pull-ups)
- Free weights
- Weight machines, cable machines
- Circuit training

Flexibility
- Stretching (should be done prior to each exercise session to prevent injury)
- Yoga
- Pilates
- Tai Chi (excellent for patients with muscle and joint pain)

8. The physician should explain the **difference between** "**failure**" and "**backsliding**." Any deviation from a schedule or failure to meet expectations is viewed as failure. Even world-class athletes will experience burnout and need to take time off from conditioning. This should be considered as a temporary backslide rather than a permanent failure. Most patients will get back on track quickly, possibly after taking on a different form of physical activity. Patients should be told to "tackle the future and not haggle over the past."

9. The physician should **reinforce the patient's efforts** for lifestyle intervention at each office visit. One can comment on parameters such as weight loss, body fat reduction, reduction of the BMI or waist circumference, improvement in A1C or lipid values, and emotional affect since the previous visit. Simply telling the patient that he or she "looks great" when compared with the previous office visit will go a long way to maintain the patient's motivation toward a positive change. One should make certain to inquire about the patient's current exercise program and suggest ways in which the activity level may be safely intensified or adjusted. If the patient is experiencing burnout, suggest alternative exercises such as yoga, Pilates, or

martial arts. Jogging on a treadmill can become boring for some patients after just a few weeks. A change in "scenery" would be welcomed by most patients who are losing interest in their prescribed physical activity.

Dr. Bill Polonsky (Director of the Diabetes Behavioral Institute in San Diego) tells the story of one of his patients with T2DM employed as a structural engineer. One week after beginning his daily walking program, the patient called for an "urgent appointment." While still wearing his jogging shorts and appearing sweaty, the patient spoke as if he had just discovered the "cure for diabetes." The anxious patient pulled 15 pages of downloaded, computer analyzed, color coded glucose logs from his brief case and handed them to Dr. Polonsky. "Dr. did you know that walking just 20 minutes a day will lower your blood glucose values on average 76 points from baseline?" Appearing stunned at the revelation, Dr. Polonsky responded, "Oh, my gosh. This is totally impressive. I wonder what would happen if you walked 45 minutes EVERY day." The patient grabbed the papers from Polonsky's hands and took off running down the street, stopping once to monitor his blood glucose level as he headed toward work.

Clinicians should always remember that despite their best efforts and motivational discussions, not all patients will have any intention or desire to become more active. Directing one's personal frustration toward these patients would only be counterproductive. Those patients who do increase their activity level will undoubtedly appreciate the time and efforts put forth by their primary care doctor. Physicians who can successfully motivate patients into becoming more active will enjoy coaching them toward having a better mind and body.

Pre-exercise Evaluation

A detailed medical evaluation with appropriate diagnostic studies is indicated for patients having any macrovascular or microvascular complications, which may be worsened by exercise. Identification of at-risk patients will allow the physician to design an individualized exercise prescription capable of minimizing risks. The pre-exercise history and physical examination should focus on symptoms and signs of diseases affecting the heart, vascular system, eyes, kidneys, feet, and nervous system.

Patients who require a graded exercise test prior to prescribing an exercise program include the following[50]:

1. Patients with diabetes who are planning to initiate moderate- to high-intensity physical conditioning
2. Patients at risk for underlying cardiovascular disease:
   - Age greater than 35 years
   - Age greater than 25 years
     - T2DM greater than 10 years' duration
     - T1DM greater than 15 years' duration
3. Presence of any additional risk factors for coronary artery disease (CAD) (smoking, hypertension, hyperlipidemia, proteinuria, family history of CAD, hyperuricemia, obesity, and laboratory evidence of elevated highly sensitive C-reactive protein, B-type natriuretic peptide, homocysteine, renin, or urinary albumin-to-creatinine ratio)[51]
4. Presence of microvascular disease (proliferative retinopathy, nephropathy, microalbuminuria, peripheral sensory neuropathy)
5. Peripheral vascular disease
6. Autonomic neuropathy

Patients who exhibit nonspecific electrocardiogram (ECG) changes in response to exercise, or who have nonspecific ST and T wave changes on resting ECG, should undergo alternative testing such as dobutamine–atropine stress myocardial perfusion imaging radionuclide stress testing,[52] stress echocardiogram,[53] or single-photon emission computed tomography (SPECT) scan.[54]

Patients planning to participate in low-intensity forms of physical activity, such as walking, should have additional pre-exercise studies performed based on sound clinical judgment

TABLE 3-16. Classification of Physical Activity Intensity Based on Exercise Lasting up to 60 Minutes

Exercise Intensity	Maximal Heart Rate (%)[a]	RPE[b]
Very light	>35	>10
Light	35–54	10–11
Moderate	55–69	12–13
Hard	70–89	14–16
Very hard	>90	17–19
Maximal[c]	100	20

[a]Maximal heart rate = 220 – age. (Preferably the maximum heart rate should be determined during a maximal graded exercise test.)
[b]Borg 6–20 relative perceived exertion (RPE) scale rating (see Table 3-17).
[c]Maximal values are mean values achieved during maximal exercise by healthy adults.

(Tables 3-16 and 3-17). Patients with known CAD or left ventricular dysfunction should be referred to a cardiologist for pre-exercise testing.

Preparing to Exercise

A proper exercise session should include a warm-up, endurance phase, and cool-down period. The warm-up should consist of 5 to 10 minutes of aerobic activity (walking, cycling, and/or stretching) at a low-intensity level. Following the warm-up, muscles should be gently stretched for another 5 to 10 minutes. Focus should be placed on stretching those muscles that will be worked maximally during the endurance phase. The endurance phase of exercise requires the patient to attain and maintain the desired heart rate (Table 3-16) continuously for 15 to 20 minutes. Thus, a 50-year-old patient who desires to pursue hard physical activity will need to maintain a heart rate of 220–50 = 170 × 0.85 = 144 beats per minute for 15 to 20 minutes. The cool-down and warm-up phases are similar in their intensity and duration. The cool-down phase is designed to gradually bring the heart rate down to the pre-exercise level.

TABLE 3-17. Borg 6–20 Relative Perceived Exertion Scale[a]

Rate of Perceived Exertion (RPE)	Verbal Description of RPE
6–7	Very, very light
8–9	Very light
10–12	Fairly light
13–14	Somewhat hard
15–16	Hard
17–18	Very hard
19–20	Very, very hard

[a]The Borg RPE scale is a valid method for monitoring and prescribing exercise intensity in adults, children, and adolescents. Perceived exertion may be used as an adjunct to heart rate monitoring and can be used to predict heart rates in patients who are not monitored with telemetry. For example, an RPE of 13 correlates with a percentage of maximal heart rate of 55% to 69% or moderate-intensity exercise (see Table 3-16). Ten percent of patients tend to select inappropriate RPE scores when exercising and may require a different tool for exercise prescribing.
Adapted from the Centers for Disease Control and Prevention. Physical activity for everyone: measuring physical activity intensity: perceived exertion (Borg Rating of Perceived Exertion Scale). http://www.cdc.gov/nccdphp/dnpa/physical/measuring/perceived_exertion.htm. Accessed and verified February 25, 2007.

The basic principles of safely exercising with diabetes include the following:

1. The clinician should encourage aerobic conditioning.
2. The patient should make certain that foot care is proper (wear socks, keep feet dry, use orthotics when necessary).
3. The patient should wear a diabetes identification bracelet or shoe tag.
4. Proper hydration is necessary before, during, and after exercising. At least 17 ounces of fluid should be consumed 2 hours before exercising. During physical activity, fluids should be taken early and often in an amount sufficient to compensate for loses in sweat reflected in body weight loss or the maximum amount of fluid tolerated.
5. The patient should avoid exercising in extremely hot or cold environments.
6. Free weight training may be acceptable for young individuals with diabetes but not for older patients or those with long-standing diabetes. Patients with microvascular and macrovascular complications should avoid resistance training.
7. Moderate weight training programs using light weights, cables, and Nautilus-like machines using light weights with frequent repetitions can be used for maintaining or enhancing upper body strength in nearly all patients with diabetes.

Exercise and Type 1 Diabetes

The primary concern of patients with T1DM who participate in exercise is to avoid hypoglycemia. This requires that the patient understand the metabolic and hormonal responses to physical activity and is well trained in diabetes self-management skills (home blood glucose monitoring, carb counting, hydration, management of hypoglycemia, detection of urinary or serum ketones, and sick day protocols). The increasing use of intensive insulin therapy has provided patients with the flexibility to make appropriate insulin dose adjustments for various activities. The rigid recommendation to use carbohydrate supplementation—calculated from the planned intensity and duration of physical activity, without regard to glycemic level at the start of physical activity, the previously measured metabolic response to physical activity, and the patient's insulin therapy—is no longer appropriate. Such an approach not infrequently neutralizes the beneficial glycemic-lowering effects of physical activity in patients with T1DM.

General guidelines that may prove helpful in regulating the glycemic response to exercise include the following:

1. Metabolic control before exercise:
   • The patient should avoid exercise if fasting glucose levels are higher than 250 mg per dL and ketosis is present and use caution if glucose levels are higher than 300 mg per dL and no ketosis is present.
   • The patient should ingest an additional 15 g of carbohydrate if glucose levels are less than 100 mg per dL.
2. Blood glucose monitoring before, immediately following the conclusion of the exercise session, and 4 to 12 hours after ending heavy physical conditioning. The patient should identify when changes in insulin or food intake are necessary:
   • The patient should learn the glycemic response to different exercise conditions.
3. Food intake:
   • The patient should consume added carbohydrate as needed to avoid hypoglycemia.
   • Carbohydrate-based foods should be readily available during and after exercise.

As opposed to patients with T2DM, studies have failed to show any long-term improvement in A1C levels associated with exercise performance in patients with T1DM. However, because physical activity can improve cardiovascular fitness, lower blood pressure, and improve lipid profiles, exercise should be strongly encouraged in patients with T1DM. The process of physical conditioning through exercise training can result in a 20% to 30% reduction in daily insulin requirements.[55]

Exercising with an Insulin Pump

Using an insulin pump is advantageous for people who desire to participate in regular physical activity, especially when the exercise is at a moderate or intense level for more than 30 minutes. If exercise times are consistent, the pump basal rate can be reduced by 50% 60 to 90 minutes before the anticipated start physical exertion. Patients with well-controlled T1DM who use insulin pumps can perform 30 minutes of mild to moderate exercise beginning 2 to 3 hours after breakfast without risking hypoglycemia.[56]

The increased metabolic demands that accompany exercise require an increase in fuel mobilization from sites of storage (liver and adipose tissue) and an increase in fuel utilization by the skeletal muscles. These physiologic accompaniments to exercise are controlled by precise endocrine responses to physical activity. Unfortunately, these methods of endocrine control are lost in patients with T1DM, and the glycemic response to exercise depends on the following factors:

- Exercise intensity, duration, and type (aerobic or anaerobic training)
- Fitness level and nutritional status of the patient
- Temporal relationship between physical activity and mealtime
- Temporal relationship to previous insulin bolus and basal insulin level
- Site of insulin administration
- Overall level of glycemic control
- Presence of diabetes-related complications

During the transition from rest to exercise, the skeletal muscles shift from using free fatty acids to glucose and glycogen for the primary energy source.[57] As exercise duration exceeds 60 to 90 minutes, glycogen levels are depleted, leaving free fatty acids and glucose to supply skeletal muscles with energy. Glucose becomes the primary source of energy during exercise as hepatocytes shift from glycogenolysis to gluconeogenesis. Circulating insulin levels play a major role in maintaining glucose homeostasis during prolonged exercise (Fig. 3-5). When free insulin levels are elevated, glycogenolysis and gluconeogenesis will both be impeded. Free fatty acid levels will also be reduced, and exercising skeletal muscles will have no source of energy. The athlete will develop hypoglycemia

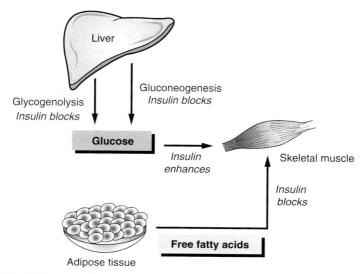

Figure 3-5 • Blood Glucose Homeostasis in Response to Exercise. Sources of energy during exercise include free fatty acids (FFAs) originating from adipose tissue and glucose derived from hepatic gluconeogenesis and glycogenolysis. Glucose uptake by skeletal muscle cells is insulin independent yet enhanced by circulating insulin levels. Some insulin is needed during exercise to overcome elevated levels of FFAs and counterregulatory hormones (glycogen and glucagons), which can induce hyperglycemia and ketosis.

and weakness in response to exercise. Higher levels of insulin will also block glucagon release from the pancreatic α cells, further reducing the body's ability to respond to hypoglycemia.

If the circulating insulin levels are low, free fatty acid production, glycogenolysis, and gluconeogenesis will all be accelerated. Glucagon levels will also rise, resulting in hyperglycemia and possible diabetic ketoacidosis (DKA).

The principles to safely exercising with an insulin pump include the following:

1. The patient should understand the **association between metabolism and physical activity.** Some activities, such as resistance or high-intensity interval training, stress mainly anaerobic energy sources and can have a markedly different effect on glycemia compared with prolonged or mild aerobic exercise.
2. The patient should establish **glycemic patterns.** Patients should be knowledgeable about their usual glycemic response to exercise. For example, mild exercise may require no adjustment in pre-exercise basal rates, whereas moderate to heavy exercise will necessitate a 50% basal rate reduction. Patients will need to adjust their pump parameters based on their individual response to exercise.
3. The patient should understand **carbohydrate requirements** for exercise. Carbohydrate consumption should be made according to the predicted glycemic response to physical activity. The patient should monitor glucose levels frequently during sustained exercise lasting more than 30 minutes and provide additional carbohydrates to maintain blood glucose levels in the range of 120 to 180 mg per dL.
4. The patient should **expect a training response to glycemic control over time.** Active patients should notice a glycemic training response occurring after exercising consistently for 2 to 3 weeks. Training increases fat utilization and potentially spares blood glucose. This response may reduce the need for regimen changes during prolonged aerobic activities. In addition, as muscle mass increases in response to training, an individual's overall insulin sensitivity may increase, which may allow for lower basal and bolus insulin doses.
5. If the **blood glucose level is lower than 100 mg per dL**, the patient should suspend or reduce the basal insulin rate during exercise. However, physical activity lasting more than 30 minutes may require consumption of additional carbohydrates to prevent exercise-induced hypoglycemia.
6. Patients may exercise if the blood **glucose level is less than 250 mg per dL** and no ketones are present in the urine. If blood glucose levels are greater than 250 mg per dL and no ketones are present, a small bolus of insulin may allow the patient to safely exercise. If ketones are found and the pre-exercise level is greater than 250 mg per dL, exercise is ill advised.
7. Use of a real-time continuous glucose monitoring system (CGMS) is beneficial for predicting and detecting hypoglycemia in patients with T1DM. The symptoms of acute hypoglycemia and fatigue from exercise might be difficult to determine. Both conditions can result in dizziness, confusion, sweating, blurred vision, and decreased strength or endurance. A recently published randomized, controlled 26-week study evaluated two groups of well-controlled patients with T1DM using either multiple daily injections or insulin pumps. The baseline A1C of the participants, ages 10 to 65, was 7.5%. The conventional group performed traditional home blood glucose monitoring and wore a "masked" continuous glucose sensor every other week. The interventional group wore unmasked CGMS daily for 26 weeks. The primary outcome was to determine the amount of time each group spent in a predefined hypoglycemic range less than 63 mg per dL based upon the interstitial glucose readings. The time spent per day in hypoglycemia was approximately 50% shorter in the CGMS group than in the control group ($p = 0.03$). The A1C was 0.27% lower in the CGMS group at 26 weeks ($p = 0.008$) and the number of hours spent per day in the target blood glucose range of 70 to 180 mg per dL was 17.6 versus 16 hours, favoring the CGMS cohort ($p = 0.009$). Thus, use of CGMS can minimize time spent in hypoglycemia while improving A1C levels in both children and adults with intensively controlled T1DM.[58]

Exercising at Very High Altitude

An increasing number of people with T1DM are participating in intensive physical activity at altitudes between 11,000 and 18,000 feet above sea level. This "high-altitude" exercise tends to alter one's anticipated physiologic insulin requirements compared with what is normally observed at sea level. Euglycemic individuals experience an increase in both glucose and insulin requirements during exercise at low altitude.[59] After 3 weeks at 13,000 feet, resting glucose and glucose levels during exercise decrease compared with sea level values, whereas insulin levels return to and remain at sea level values.[60] This suggests decreased glucose mobilization or increased insulin sensitivity as a result of acclimatization to high altitude. In patients with T1DM, the increase in glucose uptake by skeletal muscle in response to aerobic conditioning at sea level is comparable to that in subjects without diabetes. However, because individuals with T1DM lack the ability to automatically adjust insulin secretion to match glycemic excursions and overcome defective counterregulatory mechanisms, exercise response at high altitude is different than that observed in healthy subjects. In addition, high altitude presence can cause acute mountain sickness (AMS) characterized by headache, anorexia, diarrhea, fatigue, and sleep disorders. AMS increases sympathetic activity, resulting in further deterioration of glycemic control.[61]

A study published by de Mol et al. suggested mountain climbers with T1DM who exercise above 11,000 feet should be counseled to maintain or only slightly decrease insulin doses.[62] (Patients should be told that despite their extremely strenuous and labor-intensive exercise, as well as their reduced caloric intake, their glucose counterregulation becomes inflated, resulting in mild insulin resistance.) Finally, although the use of acetazolamide is not recommended in patients with T1DM because of the perceived risk for ketoacidosis, six of eight patients who used the drug in this study had no ill effects.[62]

Exercise and T2DM

Habitual aerobic fitness and/or physical activity are associated with significantly lower cardiovascular and overall mortality to a much greater extent than could be explained by glucose lowering alone. Wei et al.[63] reported on 1,263 men with T2DM who underwent a detailed examination, including a maximal treadmill exercise test with ECG monitoring, physical exam, and blood tests between 1970 and 1993. Mortality over the course of their study participation was the primary end point. After nearly 12 years of follow-up, mortality in the "moderate-fit" group was approximately 60% lower than in "low-fit men." Low-fit men had a 2.2-fold greater mortality risk compared with men having moderate or high fitness levels. Mortality rates in men with T2DM who did not participate in any physical activity were 1.8-fold higher than in men who were active participants in exercise. Interestingly, low-fit men also tended to have multiple cardiac risk factors including nicotine abuse, hyperlipidemia, hypertension, and obesity.[64]

The recommended exercise prescriptions for patients with T2DM from the American College of Sports Medicine (ACSM) and the American Diabetes Association are listed in Table 3-18.

Because of the increased evidence for health benefits from resistance training, the ACSM now recommends that resistance training be included in fitness programs for adults with T2DM.[65] With advancing age, there is a tendency for progressive declines in muscle mass, increased adiposity, and increased insulin resistance, all of which can be improved with resistance training.[66] Resistance exercise improves insulin sensitivity to about the same extent as aerobic conditioning.[67] Patients with T2DM who exercise can improve the following metabolic parameters:

1/ **Carbohydrate metabolism and insulin sensitivity.** Moderate exercise three to four times a week lasting 30 to 60 minutes improves A1C levels 10% to 20% from baseline. Patients with the most severe insulin resistance show the greatest improvement in A1C levels.[50]

2/ **Prevention of cardiovascular disease.** Patients with T2DM and metabolic syndrome are at risk for premature CAD, hypertension, hypercoagulation, hyperinsulinemia, central adiposity,

TABLE 3-18. Recommendations of Major Professional Associations on Types and Amounts of Physical Activity

Patient Type	Aerobic Conditioning			Resistance Training[a]		
	Frequency	Intensity	Duration/Mode	Frequency	Number of Exercises	Sets/Repetitions
Healthy Adults						
ACSM Position Stand (2000)[b]	3–5 d/wk	65%–90% maximum heart rate Start lower intensity if unfit	20–60 min continuous aerobic activities; 20–30 min minimum	2 d/wk	8–10 exercises involving major muscle groups	1 set, 8–12 reps
T2DM						
ACSM (2000)[b]	Minimum of three nonconsecutive days/week	40%–75% maximum heart rate	10–15 min continuous physical activity, increasing to 30-min sessions	2 d/wk	Minimum of 8–10 exercises involving major muscle groups	Minimum set, 10–15 reps
ADA Guidelines (2006)[c]	Exercise should be distributed over 3 d with no more than two consecutive days being exercise free.	50%–70% maximum heart rate >70% maximum heart rate	30 min 5 d/wk 45 min 2 d/wk	3 d/wk targeting all major muscle groups	Progress to three sets of 8–10 repetitions that cannot be lifted more than 8–10 times	

[a]Resistance training recommendations assume that the patient with T2DM has no microvascular or macrovascular complications.
[b]Data compiled from Albright A, Franz M, Hornsby G, et al. American College of Sports Medicine Position Stand: exercise and type 2 diabetes. *Med Sci Sports Exerc.* 2000;32:1345–1360.
[c]Data compiled from Sigal RJ, Kenny GP, Wasserman DH, et al. Physical activity/exercise and type 2 diabetes. A consensus statement from the American Diabetes Association. *Diabetes Care.* 2006;29:1433–1438.
ACSM, American College of Sports Medicine; T2DM, type 2 diabetes mellitus; ADA, American Diabetes Association.

and atherogenic dyslipidemia. Poor aerobic fitness levels are associated with many of the same cardiovascular risk factors. Exercise will lower plasma insulin levels and improve insulin sensitivity at the site of the skeletal muscle and adipose tissue, thus benefiting the cardiovascular status of physically active individuals.[68,69]

3/ **Hyperlipidemia.** Regular physical activity reduces triglycerides and may improve high-density lipoprotein cholesterol (HDL-C) levels in patients with diabetes.[68]

4/ **Hypertension.** Reducing circulating insulin levels in patients can reduce blood pressure.[68]

5/ **Obesity.** Although data suggest that physical activity may enhance weight loss, weight reduction and weight maintenance are best accomplished when calorie-restricted diets are used in conjunction with regular physical activity. Exercise appears to reduce levels of intra-abdominal fat, which can increase levels of adiponectin, and reduce insulin resistance.[68]

6/ **Prevention of T2DM.** Weight reduction combined with regular moderate exercise has been found to delay or prevent diabetes in three published trials.[17,70,71]

▌ Adjusting Doses of Insulin for Travel

Frequent blood glucose monitoring, avoidance of alcoholic beverages, and adequate hydration with noncaffeinated beverages are good general rules for safe travel. Caffeine can cause headaches, palpitations, perspiration, and anxiety, all of which are symptoms of hypoglycemia. Insulin pumpers should keep their pump clocks set to their original times while traveling. Patients using multiple daily injections (MDI) should keep their wristwatches set to correspond to the time at their original point of departure to make timing of insulin injections related to mealtimes easier.

The flexibility of insulin pump therapy allows for the safest and most stress-free travel, especially when unexpected travel delays occur. Prior to any long-distance travel, MDI patients should be placed on a basal-bolus regimen consisting of glargine or detemir plus a fast-acting insulin analogue. NPH and regular insulin have such unpredictable rates of absorption that hyperglycemia or hypoglycemia is much more likely to occur.

In general, adjustments to insulin doses are unnecessary if patients are crossing **fewer than 5 time zones.** Patients on basal-bolus insulin who are using glargine should be advised to maintain their same injection schedule when traveling cross-country. For example, a patient from Los Angeles who injects glargine at 10 PM nightly should inject at 7 PM while visiting New York. On return to Los Angeles, the 10 PM dosing resumes.

When traveling **west to east**, the day becomes shorter and mealtimes may be closer together. Doses of premeal short-acting insulin analogues may need to be slightly lowered if injected within 4 to 5 hours of the previous meal to avoid insulin stacking (see Chapter 5). Patients need to be aware of insulin absorption pharmacokinetics principles and predict how much insulin remains at their previous subcutaneous depot to accurately dose insulin for their next meal.

For travel across **more than five time zones**, patients on basal-bolus insulin may take 50% of their prescribed basal insulin dose prior to landing at their destination and 50% at their bedtime on the first day. Thus, a patient who is taking glargine 50 U daily would take 25 U on landing and 25 U at 10 PM on day 1 and 50 U at 10 PM on day 2. The bolus doses of short-acting insulin analogues would remain based on preprandial blood glucose levels and carbohydrate content of each meal.

As a reminder, patients should be advised to stretch their legs and walk around the cabin periodically to avoid developing a deep venous thrombosis on long plane trips.

Pump patients should carry **supplies of basal insulin** in case their pump malfunctions. Basal insulin can be administered in a dose equivalent to the total daily basal dose. If, for example, the patient's pump basal rate is 1 U per hour, glargine 24 U may be administered once daily until the pump is functioning again. Some patients may wish to take a "pump holiday" and not use their pumps when on vacation. Reverting back to basal-bolus insulin therapy using glargine plus a Novo-Log or lispro pen injector is perfectly acceptable for these patients.

Patients on daily GLP-1 agonists such as exenatide or liraglutide, may continue the use of these medication while flying as they are unlikely to result in hypoglycemia. Dosing adjustments for weekly exenatide are also not necessary. However, pramlintide is a known inducer of postprandial hypoglycemia. Therefore, some patients prefer to withhold premeal injections of this drug while flying. Once at their destination, the usual doses of these drugs may be continued.

Open insulin vials retain their potency at room temperature for at least 1 month, but in warm climates, insulin should be stored either in a refrigerator or in thermal insulated bags. Halozyme vials, used enhance dispersion of insulin products, should be utilized within 12 hours of being removed from the refrigerator.

Extreme temperatures and **humidity** can also affect glucose meters and test strips. Meters generally perform best within temperature ranges of 59°F to 95°F. High-altitude physical exertion may result in retinal hemorrhages, DKA, and hypoglycemia for patients with T1DM.[72] Blood glucose meters are also inaccurate above 10,000 feet. A quality control check with the control solution is the best way to verify that the meter and strips are working together properly. Control solutions are solutions of known glucose concentrations. Every meter has at least one control solution, and some have three levels of control solutions (low, normal, and high) so patients can test the meter at the extremes. Control solution is used with the meter the same way a patient tests a drop of blood. Using control solution on the first strip out of a new vial or package is a great way to ensure the accuracy of results. One should not use strips that are bent, outdated, or damp.

For patients with T2DM, the **timing** of oral medications is not as critical as that of insulin. If the patient is on twice-daily metformin, a thiazolidinedione (TZD), or sulfonylurea, skipping a dose and having slight hyperglycemia for 6 to 8 hours is preferable to taking two doses too close together and risking hypoglycemia. Insulin Degludec has a 42-hour duration of action and allows for more flexible dosing than insulin glargine and detemir. Omitting a dose for up to 42 hours will have minimal effects on fasting blood glucose control.

Self–Blood Glucose Monitoring

SBGM allows patients to evaluate their individual response to lifestyle and pharmacologic interventions and to assess whether short-term glycemic targets are being achieved. SBGM can also be used to detect extreme changes in blood glucose levels, including hypoglycemia, hyperglycemia, and DKA. Patients who successfully use SBGM can learn to adjust insulin doses, alter activity levels, and learn the correlation of food intake with pharmacologic therapy. For patients using MDI of insulin or pregnant women on insulin, SBGM at least four times daily should be encouraged. The positive correlation between frequent blood glucose testing and A1C levels and reduction in hospital admissions due to DKA is well known for patients with T1DM.[73] However, the optimal frequency and timing of SBGM for patients with T2DM are unknown and should be dependent on assisting patients to achieve targeted fasting and postprandial glycemic control[74] listed in Table 3-19.

Patients with diabetes have two different options for SBGM. Random glucose testing allows the patient to assimilate the information obtained by a single capillary blood sample to acutely adjust an elevated or low blood glucose value. Patients who use insulin pumps may perform SBGM 8 to 10 times daily, attempting to micromanage every glucose excursion that occurs throughout the day. Excessive

 TABLE 3-19. Glycemic and Blood Glucose Targets

Glycemic Target	Blood Glucose Target[a]
Fasting and preprandial glucose	<110 mg/dL
2-h postprandial glucose	<140 mg/dL

[a]Consensus panel recommendations from the American Association of Clinical Endocrinologists. ACE guidelines for glycemic control. *Endocr Pract.* 2002;8(Suppl 1):7–8.

random glucose testing may result in insulin stacking and hypoglycemia in which rapid-acting insulin is bolused while previously administered rapid-acting insulin remains to be absorbed. A recently published Internet survey demonstrated that patients who experienced an episode of nocturnal hypoglycemia used an average of 5.6 extra test strips the week following the event and reduced their insulin dose by 25%.[75] Hypoglycemia is known to increase anxiety, prompt more frequent doctor visits and phone calls, and increase ED visits and hospitalizations due to syncope, confusion, or chest pain related to hypoglycemia. Frequent hypoglycemia could increase health-care costs for all of society.[76]

Structured glucose testing is useful for recognizing specific problematic glycemic patterns such as hypoglycemia, fasting hyperglycemia, and postprandial hyperglycemia. Identifying the most likely cause of these patterns can assist the patient in altering behaviors and changing medications to improve overall glycemic control.[77] Structured glucose testing has been used very effectively in basal insulin treat to target protocols, allowing patients with poorly controlled T2DM to attain targeted A1Cs of less than 7%.[78–82]

Although A1C is used to assess long-term glycemic control, intraday glycemic control can be assessed either by SBGM or continuous glucose monitor systems (CGMS). Unlike random blood glucose testing, structured sampling allows the patient and clinician to identify significant and consistent patterns of glycemic excursions that are amenable to therapeutic interventions.

Paired or structured testing can be performed before and after meals to determine the effect of food intake on glycemic excursions. Patients who check pre- and postexercise will learn how insulin resistance at the peripheral muscle sites appears to improve with mild to moderate activity preformed 5 days a week. In addition, one could even determine what time of day exercise appears to have the most glucose-lowering effect by testing pre- and postprandial blood glucose at breakfast for 2 or 3 days before initiating exercise. Once the exercise program begins in earnest, the paired testing is simply repeated and the reductions in blood glucose values can be identified. This pattern testing can be repeated for each meal.

The International Diabetes Federation guidelines specify that the timing and frequency of SBMG regimens should be customized and address each patient's specific educational, behavioral, and specific educational requirements. The clinicians must also be able to monitor the impact of prescribing a specific therapy to that individual.[83]

SBMG is useful only when patients and clinicians possess the ability and willingness to accurately assess the significance of the blood glucose data generated and use the information to make appropriate and effective treatment changes (pharmacologic and/or behavioral) that can lead to positive outcomes. The ultimate goals of structured testing are to (a) minimize hypoglycemia event frequency, (b) reduce postprandial hyperglycemia and glycemic variability, and (c) lower A1C over time. These outcome measurements should be accomplished in a timely manner and should be continued indefinitely, as diabetes self-management is a lifelong endeavor.

Structured testing provides patients with immediate feedback regarding the safety and efficacy of pharmacologic therapies as well as the roles that foods, stress, illness, and physical activity play on their glycemic control. Thus, patients are able to visualize and connect their daily decision-making processes to control their diabetes with components of their behavioral and prescribed therapies. Soon, patients become empowered to adhere to their regimens or be more accepting of strategies that are likely to positively improve their glycemic control. The goal will always be for patients to be able to control their diabetes rather than for diabetes to control the lives of those patients who have the disorder.

Structured SBGM has shown to be beneficial for patients with both T1DM and T2DM.[84,85]

The Step study is a large, 12-month, multicenter, primary care–based clinical trial that evaluated the impact of a structured SBGM regimen in poorly controlled, insulin-naive patients with T2DM. Utilizing a structured data collection form (ACCU-CHECK 360-degree View tool—https://www.accu-chek.com/us/data-management/360-view-printable-tool.html), patients were instructed to record and plot a seven-point SBGM profile on 3 consecutive days. Physicians and patients worked together to interpret and act upon the data presented at the time of their quarterly office visits. Based upon the patterns suggested by these simple testing parameters, treatment modifications were suggested and implemented when necessary. At the conclusion of the trial, patients in the structured testing cohort showed a significantly greater improvement in A1C than those in the control group. Significant reductions in postprandial glucose excursions and glycemic variability were also noted. Nearly three times more patients in the structured testing group received a treatment change recommendation at the month 1 visit compared to

A. Patient 1

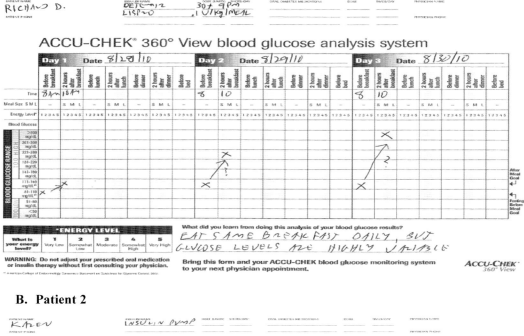

B. Patient 2

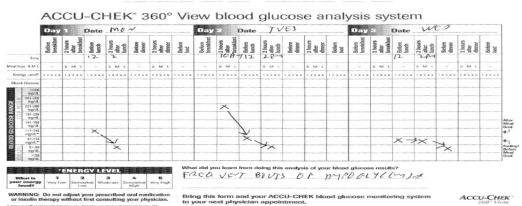

Figure 3-6 • A. Patient 1. A 45-year-old man with T1DM. A1C = 8.5. Fasting glucose levels appear to be within the target range of 80 to 140 mg per dL. However, the 2-hour postprandial glucose levels are high for breakfast, rising greater than 180 mg per dL on 2 of 3 days. Patient was advised to inject the rapid-acting insulin at least 15 minutes prior to mealtime (which he was not doing consistently) and to reduce the amount of carbs he was consuming for breakfast. Insulin dose was not changed initially. Repeat A1C after 2 months was 7.3%. **B. Patient 2.** A 33-year-old patient with an A1C of 5.5%. The patient has a history of hypoglycemic unawareness and experiences frequent bouts of hypoglycemia and refuses to wear a continuous glucose sensor because this device is not covered by her insurance. Structured testing demonstrates that she becomes hypoglycemic 3 days in a row 2 hours after eating lunch. Based on the pattern observed above, the patient agreed to make the following adjustments in her insulin regimen: (a) Reduce the meal-time bolus by 25%. (b) Increase the duration of her extended bolus from 90 minutes to 3 hours. (c) Continue checking the blood glucose levels 2 hours after each meal. Any negative change from baseline is predictive of hypoglycemia. For example, if a premeal blood glucose is 120 mg per dL and 2-hour postprandial glucose is 90 mg per dL, the "delta" is a minus 30 mg per dL. Because rapid-acting insulin has a duration of action of 4 hours, a blood glucose level taken at 2 hours after eating reflects what the patient's glucose level is, while 60% of the insulin bolused at mealtime remains "on board."

C. Patient 3

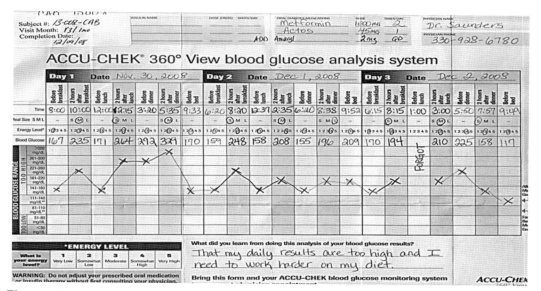

Figure 3-6 • *(Continued)* Thus, if this patient took 4 U for lunch (2 U as an immediate bolus and 2 as an extended bolus over 2 hours), she would have approximately 1.6 U remaining to be absorbed with another 1 U remaining in the extended bolus to be delivered; (d) the basal rate of the pump was adjusted to slow the rate of insulin delivery. The idea is to raise the patient's ambient glucose level to between 140 and 200 mg per dL for 2 to 3 weeks, allowing her to recover her ability of hypoglycemia awareness. Three months later, the patient returned with an A1C of 6.8%. A download of her glucose meter demonstrated that 85% of her total readings were in the target range (80–180 mg per dL), 20% were above target, and 5% were in the range of hypoglycemia (less than 60 mg per dL). **C. Patient 3.** A 44-year-old obese female with a 5-year history of T2DM, BMI is 42 kg per m². The patient refuses to exercise. Current medications include metformin 1 g BID with food and pioglitazone 45 mg Q AM. The structured glucose testing performed before and after meals as well as at bedtime (7 times daily) for 3 days prior to her scheduled office visit demonstrates a pattern of fasting and postprandial hyperglycemia. Her A1C was 8.9%. Patient was symptomatic at the time this 360-degree view was initially performed (distal paresthesias, fatigue, and nocturia). She agreed to continue metformin and begin insulin detemir 10 U at bedtime, increasing by 1 U each night until the fasting glucose level reached less than 110 mg per dL. After 3 months, her A1C was 7.6%. Prandial insulin was then added at dinner (0.1 U per kg) and titrated to keep the 2-hour postprandial glucose level to less than 180 mg per dL. Three months after starting the rapid-acting prandial insulin, her A1C was 6.8% and her BMI was 39 kg per m². Because she was feeling more energetic, she agreed to initiate an exercise program at a local kickboxing club.

patients in the control group. Patients in the paired glucose monitoring group also continued to receive significantly more therapeutic adjustments throughout the 12-month study versus the controlled group to "fine-tune" their diabetes care regimen. Equally important to the investigators was that structured testing patients felt that the use of the data collection tool provided a focal point for more meaningful discussions with their physicians who had also been trained on the use and interpretation of the tool.

Figure 3-6 displays four patient 360-degree view profiles and customized treatments suggested based on their structured glucose testing profiles.

Blood Glucose Monitoring Results Are Subject to User Error!

Because the accuracy of SBGM is user dependent, physicians should evaluate each patient's monitoring technique at regular intervals.

D. Patient 4

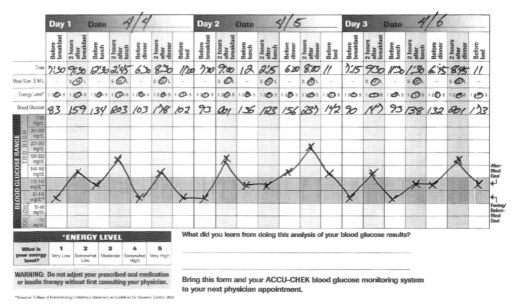

Figure 3-6 • *(Continued)* **D. Patient 4.** A 56-year-old man with an 8-year history of T2DM. There is no personal or family history of diabetes-related complications. However, this patient is concerned that he is unable to get his A1C below 7.5% despite exercising intensively 5 days each week, and using metformin 1 gram BID. He is not overweight. The doctor suggested that he perform 7-point glucose testing for 3 consecutive days via the 360-degree view protocol and bring the graph into the office on the following week. The patient generated data collection clearly demonstrates normal fasting glucose values and no evidence of hypoglycemia. However, his postprandial glucose levels are consistently elevated despite exercising every day after dinner. The patient agreed to begin using a DPP-4 inhibitor and continue his current dose of metformin. In 4 months his A1C declined to 6.7% and there was no further evidence of postprandial hyperglycemia on his monthly 360-degree view records.

Suggestions for proper use of SBGM include the following:

1. The patient should not use alcohol prior to sampling, as alcohol may dilute the blood specimen and provide an inaccurate reading. Patients should wash their hands thoroughly prior to sampling. If a blood glucose level appears unusually "out of line" with prior testing values, patients should repeat the test before acting on that value. A patient who handled a piece of cake or some fruit prior to sampling without washing their hands could obtain a very high false elevation in their blood glucose value.

2. The patient should pick "two favorite fingers" from each hand and use those fingers exclusively for testing. The patient should sample from the middle of the fingertips, not the sides of the finger, to minimize pain. Over time, a callus will develop. Sampling from the area of the callus will be painless.

3. If the glucose result obtained is thought to be in error, the patient should not retest from the same finger but use the other hand to retest.

4. Patients who participate in activities at high altitudes or in low temperatures should check the accuracy of their meter at the manufacturing Web site for their individual testing environment.

5. Make certain that each strip container is correctly coded to the meter. Regulatory agencies such as the FDA encourage built-in safety features such as no-coding strip technology to reduce common operator errors.

6. Increases in hematocrit will lower blood glucose values because higher number of red blood cells impedes diffusion of the plasma through the strip, reducing the volume available to the enzymatic reaction.

7. Although alternative site testing (thigh, forearm, palm of hand) is available on most meters, the most accurate readings remain at the patient's fingertips, especially when hypoglycemia is suspected. The patient should avoid alternative site testing immediately after exercise or eating.[86]

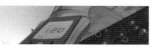

SUMMARY

Both public health and clinical interventions are needed to stem the tide of obesity and diabetes. Although there is an important emphasis at a public health level on prevention, more than 20 million adults in the United States will seek treatment for diabetes.[87] Most of these individuals are overweight or obese. If this population is treated without a sustainable lifestyle component, they are likely to gain additional weight, increase their waist circumference, worsen their insulin resistance, become hypertensive, and increase their risk of cardiovascular and microvascular-related mortality. As health deteriorates, more medications are likely to be prescribed in an attempt to intensify therapy and treat patients' metabolic parameters to target. Unfortunately, symptomatic patients often experience a deterioration in their quality of life. They lose confidence and desire to participate in any diabetes self-management programs. As exercise becomes a painful challenge, patients are likely to develop depression, which is exacerbated and prolonged by the physical symptoms of diabetes.[88]

Strategies and suggestions regarding behavioral interventions should be discussed with patients at each visit. Early intervention using medical nutrition therapy, exercise, and a home blood glucose monitor will have a positive impact on patients' futures. Patients have so many questions and fears about diabetes, yet physicians spend little time discussing their concerns during their regular office visits. Physicians should find something positive to say about each patient at every visit. The clinician should sit down with him or her side by side and explain that "Yes, having diabetes is a bummer, but by including you in our diabetes treatment team we can make your life so much better. Let me show you how!"

REFERENCES

1. Markovic TP, Jenkins AB, Campbell LV, et al. The determinants of glycemic responses to diet restriction and weight loss in obesity and NIDDM. *Diabetes Care.* 1998;21:687–694.

2. Maggio CA, Pi-Sunyer FX. The prevention and treatment of obesity: application to type 2 diabetes. *Diabetes Care.* 1997;20:1744–1766.

3. Lim EL, Hollingsworth KG, Aribisuala BS, et al. Reversal of type 2 diabetes: normalization of beta cell function in association with de creased pancreas and liver triacylglycerol. *Diabetologia.* 2011;54: 2506–2514.

4. Carpentier A, Zinman B, Leung N, et al. Free fatty acid mediated impairment of glucose-stimulated insulin secretion in nondiabetic Oji-Cree individuals from the Sandy Lake community of Ontario, Canada: a population at very high risk for developing type 2 diabetes. *Diabetes.* 2003;52:1485–1495.

5. Lee Y, Lingvay I, Szczepaniak LS, et al. Pancreatic steatosis: harbinger of type 2 diabetes in obese rodents. *Int J Obes (Lond).* 2010;34:396–400.

6. Harkness E, Macdonald W, Valderas J, et al. Identifying psychosocial interventions that improve both physical and mental health in patients with diabetes: a systematic review and meta-analysis. *Diabetes Care.* 2010;33(4):926–930.

7. Renn BN, Feliciano L, Segal DL. The bidirectional relationship of depression and diabetes: a systematic review. *Clin Psychol Rev.* 2011;31(8):1239–1246.

8. Harris MI. National Health and Nutrition Examination Survey (NHANES III). Frequency of blood glucose monitoring in relation to glycemic control in patients with type 2 diabetes. *Diabetes Care.* 2001;24:979–982.

9. Peyrot M, Rubin RR, Lauritzen T, et al. Psychosocial problems and barriers to improved diabetes management: results of the Cross-National Diabetes Attitudes, Wishes and Needs (DAWN) Study. *Diabetes Med.* 2005;22:1379–1385.

10. Glasgow RE, Toobert DJ. Social environment and regimen adherence among type II diabetic patients. *Diabetes Care.* 1988;11:377–386.

11. Unger J. Managing mental illness in patients with diabetes. *Practical Diabetol.* 2006;25:44–53.

12. Ciechanowski PS, Katon WJ, Russo JE, et al. The patient-provider relationship: attachment theory and adherence to treatment in diabetes. *Am J Psychiatr.* 2001;158:29–35.

13. The DCCT Research Group. Resource utilization and costs of care in the Diabetes Control and Complications Trial. *Diabetes Care.* 1995;18:1468–1478.

14. Haynes RB, Taylor DW, Sackett DL. *Compliance in Health Care.* Baltimore, MD: Johns Hopkins University Press; 1979.

15. Ary DV, Toobert D, Wilson W, et al. Patient perspective on factors contributing to non-adherence to diabetes regimen. *Diabetes Care.* 1986;9:168–172.

16. Rubin RR, Peyrot M. Psychological issues and treatments for people with diabetes. *J Clin Psychol.* 2001;57:457–478.

17. Pan XR, Li GW, Hu YH, et al. Effects of diet and exercise in preventing NIDDM in people with impaired glucose tolerance. The DaQing IGT and Diabetes Study. *Diabetes Care.* 1997;20:537–544.

18. Gonder-Redenick LA, Cox DJ, Ritterband LM. Diabetes and behavioral medicine: the second decade. *J Consult Clin Psychol.* 2002;70:611–625.

19. Franz MJ, Bantle JP, Beebe CA, et al. Evidence-based nutrition principles and recommendations for the treatment and prevention of diabetes and related complications. *Diabetes Care.* 2003;26(Suppl 1):S51–S61.

20. American Association of Clinical Endocrinologists. Medical guidelines for the management of diabetes mellitus: the AACE system of intensive diabetes self-management—2002 update. *Endocr Pract.* 2002;8(Suppl 1):40–82.

21. Young-Hyman DL, Davis CL. Disordered eating behavior in individuals with diabetes: importance of context, evaluation and classification. *Diabetes Care.* 2010;33(3):683–689.

22. Delahanty LM, Halford BN. The role of diet in behaviors in achieving improved glycemic control in intensively treated patients in the Diabetes Control and Complications Trial. *Diabetes Care.* 1993;16:1453–1458.

23. Bergenstal RM, Johnson M, Powers MA, et al. Comparison of a simple algorithm with carbohydrate counting for adjustment of mealtime insulin glulisine. *Diabetes Care.* 2008;31(7):1305–1310.

24. Amatruda JM, Richeson JF, Welle SL, et al. The safety and efficacy of a controlled low energy (very-low-calorie) diet in the treatment of non-insulin dependent diabetes and obesity. *Arch Intern Med.* 1988;148:873–877.

25. Greco AV, Mingrone G, Giancaterini A, et al. Insulin resistance in morbid obesity: reversal with intramyocellular fat depletion. *Diabetes.* 2002;51:144–151.

26. Raitakari M, Ilvonen T, Ahotupa M. Weight reduction with very-low-caloric diet and endothelial function in overweight adults: role of plasma glucose. *Arterioscler Thromb Vasc Biol.* 2004;24:124–128.

27. Goldstein DJ. Beneficial health effects of modest weight loss. *Int J Obes Relat Metab Disord.* 1992;16:397–415.

28. American Diabetes Association. Nutrition recommendations and principles for people with diabetes mellitus (position statement). *Diabetes Care.* 1999;22(Suppl-1):S42.

29. Pownall HJ, Ballantyne CM, Kimball KT, et al. Effect of moderate alcohol consumption on hypertriglyceridemia: a study in the fasting state. *Arch Intern Med.* 1999;159:981–987.

30. Cowie CC, Harris MI. Physical and metabolic characteristics of persons with diabetes. In: National Diabetes Data Group, eds. *Diabetes in America,* 2nd ed. Bethesda, MD: NIH, NIDDK; 1995:117–164 (NIH publ. no. 95-1468).

31. Albu J, Konnaaarides C, Pi-Sunyer FX. Weight control: metabolic and cardiovascular effects. *Diabetes Rev.* 1995;3:335–347.

32. Wansink B. *Mindless Eating.* New York, NY: Bantam Books; 2007.

33. *Last-Minute Diet Secrets*-People Magazine; March 16, 2004:122–125.

34. Rosenbaum M, Leibel RL, Hirsch J. Obesity. *N Engl J Med.* 1997;337:396–407.

35. Mack C, Wilson J, Athanacio J, et al. Pharmacological actions of the peptide hormone amylin in the long-term regulation of food intake, food preference, and body weight. *Am J Physiol Regul Integr Comp Physiol.* 2007;293:1855–1863.

36. Lutz TA Pancreatic amylin as a centrally acting satiating hormone. *Curr Drug Targets.* 2005;6:181–189.

37. Higgins SC, Gueorguiev M, Korbonits M. Ghrelin: the peripheral hunger hormone. *Ann Med.* 2007;39:116–136.

38. Verdich C, Toubro S, Buemann B, et al. The role of postprandial releases of insulin and incretin hormones in meal-induced satiety-effect of obesity and weight reduction. *Int J Obes Relat Metab Disor.* 2001;25:1206–1214.

39. Dupre J. Glycaemic effects of incretins in type 1 diabetes mellitus: a concise review with emphasis on studies in humans. *Regul Pept.* 2005;128:149–157.

40. Cappuccio FP, D'Elia L, Strazzullo P, et al. Quantity and quality of sleep and incidence of type 2 diabetes: a systematic review and meta-analysis. *Diabetes Care.* 2010;33(2):414–420.

41. Wing RR, Hill JO. Successful weight loss maintenance. *Annu Rev Nutr.* 2001;21:323–341.

42. http://www.clinicaltrials.gov/ct2/show/NCT00017953?term=Look+AHEAD&rank=1. Accessed May 3, 2011.

43. The Look AHEAD Research Group. Long-term effects of a lifestyle intervention on weight and cardiovascular risk factors in individuals with type 2 diabetes mellitus. *Arch Intern Med.* 2010;170(17):1566–1575.

44. Brown S, Upchurch S, Anding T, et al. Promoting weight loss in type 2 diabetes. *Diabetes Care.* 1996;19:613–624.

45. Alfonzo-Gonzalez G, Doucet E, et al. Estimation of daily energy needs with the FAO/WHO/UNO 1985 procedures in adults: comparison to whole-body indirect calorimetry measurements. *Eur J Clin Nutr.* 2004;58:1125–1131.

46. http://fatloss4idiots.com/?hop=dozeman. Accessed November 11, 2011.

47. Wirshing DA, Meyer JM. Obesity in patients with schizophrenia. In: Meyer JM, Nasrallah H, eds. *Medical Illness and Schizophrenia.* Washington, DC: American Psychiatric Press; 2003:39–58.

48. Thakore JH, Mann JN, Vlahos I, et al. Increased visceral fat distribution in drug-naive and drug-free patients with schizophrenia. *Int J Obes Relat Metab Disord.* 2002;26:137–141.

49. Botelho RJ. *Beyond Advice: Developing Motivational Skills.* Rochester, NY: Motivate Healthy Habits; 2002.

50. American Diabetes Association. Physical activity/exercise and diabetes. Position Statement. *Diabetes Care.* 2004;27:S58–S62.

51. Wang TJ, Gona P, Larson MG, et al. Multiple biomarkers for the prediction of first major cardiovascular events and death. *N Eng J Med.* 2006;355:2631–2639.

52. Schinkel AFL, Elhendy A, van Domburg RT, et al. Prognostic value of dobutamine-atropine stress myocardial perfusion imaging in patients with diabetes. *Diabetes Care.* 2002;25:163–1643.

53. Marwick TH, Case C, Sawada S, et al. Use of stress echocardiography to predict mortality in patients with diabetes and known or suspected coronary artery disease. *Diabetes Care.* 2002;25:1042–1048.

54. Wackers FJT, Young LH, Inzucchi SE, et al. Detection of silent myocardial ischemia in asymptomatic diabetic subjects: the DIAD study. *Diabetes Care.* 2004;27:1954–1961.

55. Trovati M, Anfossi G, Vitali S, et al. Postprandial exercise in type 1 diabetes patients on multiple daily insulin injection regimen. *Diabetes Care.* 1988;11:107–110.

56. Trovati M, Carta Q, Cavalot F, et al. Continuous subcutaneous insulin infusion and postprandial exercise in tightly controlled type 1 (insulin-dependent) diabetic patients. *Diabetes Care.* 1984;7:327–330.

57. Sato Y, Iguchi A, Sakamoto N. Biochemical determination of training effects using insulin clamp technique. *Horm Metab Res.* 1984;16:483–486.

58. Battelino T, Phillip M, Bratina N, et al. Effect of continuous glucose monitoring on hypoglycemia in type 1 diabetes. *Diabetes Care.* 2011;34(4):795–800.

59. Baker PL. Adventure travel and type 1 diabetes: the complicating effects of high altitude. *Diabetes Care.* 2005;28:2563–2572.

60. Larsen JJ, Hansen JM, Olsen NV, et al. The effect of altitude hypoxia on glucose homeostasis in men. *J Physiol.* 1997;504:241–249.

61. Moore K, Vizzard N, Coleman C, et al. Extreme altitude mountaineering and type 1 diabetes; the Diabetes Federation of Ireland Kilimanjaro Expedition. *Diabetes Med.* 2001;18:749–755.

62. de Mol P, de Vries ST, de Koning EJP, et al. Increased insulin requirements during exercise at very high altitudes in type 1 diabetes. *Diabetes Care.* 2011;34(3):591–595.

63. Wei M, Gibbons LW, Kampert JB, et al. Low cardiorespiratory fitness and physical inactivity as predictors of mortality in men with type 2 diabetes. *Ann Intern Med.* 2000;132:605–611.

64. Church TS, Cheng YJ, Earnest CP, et al. Exercise capacity and body composition as predictors of mortality among men with diabetes. *Diabetes Care.* 2004;27:83–88.

65. Albright A, Franz M, Hornsby G, et al. American College of Sports Medicine Position Stand: exercise and type 2 diabetes. *Med Sci Sports Exerc.* 2000;32:1345–1360.

66. American College of Sports Medicine. American College of Sports Medicine Position Stand: exercise and physical activity for older adults. *Med Sci Sports Exerc.* 1998;30:992–1008.

67. Ivy JL. Role of exercise training in the prevention and treatment of insulin resistance and non-insulin-dependent diabetes mellitus. *Sports Med.* 1997;24:321–336.

68. Myers J. Cardiology patient pages: exercise and cardiovascular health. *Circulation.* 2003;107:e2–e5.

69. Buse JB, Ginsberg HN, Bakris GL, et al. Primary prevention of cardiovascular diseases in people with diabetes mellitus: a scientific statement from the American Heart Association and the American Diabetes Association. *Circulation.* 2006. Abstract published online ahead of print article: http://circ.ahajournals.org/cgi/content/abstract/CIRCULATIONAHA.106.179294vl. Accessed and verified, January 1, 2011.

70. Diabetes Prevention Program Research Group. Reduction in the incidence of type 2 diabetes with lifestyle intervention or metformin. *N Engl J Med.* 2002;346:393–403.

71. Tuomilehto J, Lindstrom J, Eriksson JG, et al. Prevention of type 2 diabetes mellitus by changes in lifestyle among subjects with impaired glucose tolerance. *N Engl J Med.* 2001;344:1343–1350.

72. Moore K, Vizzard N, Coleman C, et al. Extreme altitude mountaineering and Type 1 diabetes; the Diabetes Federation of Ireland Kilimanjaro Expedition. *Diabetes Med.* 2001;18:749–755.

73. Levine BS, Anderson BJ, Butler DA, et al. Predictors of glycemic control and short-term adverse outcomes in youth with type 1 diabetes. *J Pediatr.* 2001;139:174–176.

74. American Diabetes Association. Position Statement. Standards of medical care in diabetes *Diabetes Care.* 2005;28:S10.

75. Brod M, Christensen T, Thomsen TL, et al. The impact of non-severe hypoglycemic events on work productivity and diabetes management. *Value Health.* 2011;14(5):665–671.

76. Heaton B, Martin S, Brejle T. The economic effects of hypoglycemia in a health plan. *Managed Care Interface.* 2003;16(7):23–27.

77. Polonsky WH, Jelsovsky MS, Panzera S, et al. Primary care physicians identify and act upon glycemic abnormalities in structured, episodic blood glucose monitoring data from non-insulin-treated type 2 diabetes. *Diabetes Technol Therap.* 2009;11(5):283–291.

78. Blonde L, Merilainen M, Karwe V, et al. Patient directed titration for achieving glycaemic goals using a once-daily basal insulin analogue: an assessment of two different fasting plasma glucose targets—the TITRATE study. *Diabetes Obes Metab.* 2009;11:623–631.

79. Gerstein HC, Yale J-F, Harris SB, et al. A randomized trial of adding insulin glargine vs avoidance of insulin in people with type 2 diabetes on either no oral glucose-lowering agents or submaximal doses of metformin and/or sulphonylureas. The Canadian INSIGHT (Implementing New Strategies with Insulin Glargine for Hyperglycaemia Treatment) Study. *Diabetes Med.* 2006;23:736–742.

80. Zinman B, Fulcher G, Rao PV, et al. Insulin degludec, an ultra-long-acting basal insulin, once a day or three times a week versus insulin glargine once a day in patients with type 2 diabetes: a 16-week, randomised, open-label, phase 2 trial. *The Lancet.* 2011. Doi:10.1016/S0140-6736(10)62305-7.

81. Riddle MC, Rosenstock J, Gerich J. The treat-to-target trial: randomized addition of glargine or human NPH insulin to oral therapy of type 2 diabetic patients. *Diabetes Care.* 2003;26:3080–3086.

82. Davies M, Storms F, Shutler S, et al. Improvement of glycemic control in subjects with poorly controlled type 2 diabetes: comparison of two treatment algorithms using insulin glargine. *Diabetes Care.* 2005;28:1282–1288.

83. International SMBG Working Group/International Diabetes Federation: Global guideline on self-monitoring of blood glucose in non-insulin related type 2 diabetes, 2009 [article online]. www.idforg. Available from http://www.idf.org/guidelines/self-monitoring. Accessed November 10, 2011.

84. Kato N, Kato M. Use of structured SMBG helps reduce A1C levels in insulin-treated diabetic patients. Poster presentation (881-P), 71st Annual Scientific Sessions of the American Diabetes Association. San Diego, CA. June 26, 2011.

85. Polonsky WH, Fisher L, Schikman CH, et al. A structured self-monitoring of blood glucose approach in type 2 diabetes encourages more frequent, intensive and effective physician interventions: results from the Step study. *Diabetes Technol Ther.* 2011;13:797–802.

86. Fedele D, Corsi A, Noacco C, et al. Alternative site blood glucose testing: a multicenter study. *Diabetes Technol Therap.* 2003;5:983–989.

87. Centers for Disease Control and Prevention. *National Diabetes Fact Sheet: General Information and National Estimates on Diabetes in the United States, 2005.* Atlanta; U.S. Department of Health and Human Services, Centers for Disease Control and Prevention; 2005. Available online: http://www.diabetes.org/uedocuments/NationalDiabetesFactSheetRev.pdf. Accessed July 5, 2006.

88. Greden JF. The burden of disease for treatment-resistant depression. *J Clin Psychiatry.* 2001;62:26–31.

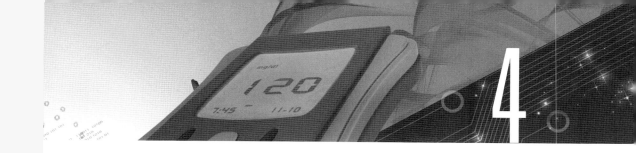

Polycystic Ovary Syndrome

It's not how much you have that makes people look up to you, it's who you are.
—*Elvis Presley, American rock "n" roll icon (1935–1977)*

Introduction Poetically described as "the thief of womanhood,"[1] polycystic ovary syndrome (PCOS) was first diagnosed in 1935 by two Chicago obstetricians in seven women with a constellation of symptoms including hirsutism, amenorrhea, infertility, and large polycystic ovaries.[2] PCOS remains characterized by irregular and chronic anovulation, signs and symptoms related to elevated androgens (hirsutism and acne), and polycystic ovaries. Additionally, PCOS is strongly associated with metabolic disorders and comorbidities including insulin resistance, prediabetes, diabetes, dyslipidemia, hypertension, obesity, endometrial carcinoma, depression, cardiovascular disease (CVD), and obstructive sleep apnea.[3–5] PCOS can cause infertility, irregular menses, severe acne, and hirsutism. Women with PCOS constitute the largest group of women at risk for developing CVD and diabetes. The cardiovascular and metabolic risk factors associated with PCOS are potentially reversible. Although the patient's immediate problems and concerns necessitate sensitive attention and prompt therapy, PCPs should view this disorder as an opportunity to practice proactive preventive medicine for this chronic, progressive disease. Early diagnosis, lifestyle interventions, and appropriate pharmacotherapy can result in a reduction in serious associated metabolic sequelae and restore fertility.

Prevalence and Pathogenesis of Polycystic Ovary Syndrome

PCOS is the most common endocrine abnormality in American reproductive-aged females resulting in menstrual irregularity and infertility.[6] The prevalence of PCOS in adult women is estimated to be between 6% and 10%.[6] PCOS symptomatology usually begins at the time of menarche. Environmental modifiers, such as weight gain, may delay the clinical presentation of PCOS until women reach puberty. Premature pubarche (appearance of pubic hair growth), the result of early secretion of adrenal steroids, may be a harbinger of the syndrome.[7] Genetic studies support the increased frequency of PCOS in first-degree relatives of affected women.[8]

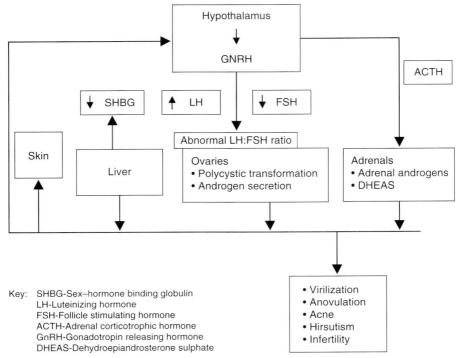

Figure 4-1 • PCOS neuroendocrine dysfunction.

Because of the heterogeneity of this disorder, multiple interrelated endocrine pathways have been implicated in the pathogenesis of PCOS (Fig. 4-1). A normally functioning hypothalamic–pituitary–ovarian axis supports the maturation of ovarian follicles via the release of luteinizing hormone (LH) from the anterior pituitary gland. Follicle-stimulating hormone (FSH) stimulates the production of the ovarian follicles and is also secreted from the anterior pituitary gland. Within the ovarian follicle, theca cells synthesize androgen. Once formed, the androgens diffuse into the ovarian granulosa cells where they are converted into estrogen.

Patients with PCOS experience **increased ovarian androgen biosynthesis** as a result of abnormalities occurring at all levels of the hypothalamic–pituitary–ovarian axis:

1. LH hypersecretion is a characteristic hallmark of PCOS. LH is secreted in a pulsatile manner. Women with PCOS have an increase in both the LH pulse frequency and amplitude resulting in increased 24-hour secretion. LH hypersecretion is thought to occur secondary to an increased frequency of hypothalamic gonadotropin-releasing hormone (GnRH) pulsation. Higher circulation levels of LH stimulate the production of androgens by the ovarian theca cells. (GnRH) must be accelerated in PCOS.[9]
2. Increasing the GnRH pulse generator favors the synthesis and release of LH over FSH.
3. When the concentration of LH increases relative to FSH, the ovaries preferentially synthesize testosterone.
4. Insulin acts synergistically with LH to increase androgen production within the theca cell.
5. Insulin also inhibits the hepatic synthesis of SHBG, which normally binds testosterone. The higher levels of unbound or "free" testosterone increase the biologic activity of the circulating hormone. The concentration of free testosterone is often elevated, whereas the total testosterone level may be only slightly increased.[10]
6. Testosterone further inhibits (whereas estrogen stimulates) the hepatic synthesis of SHBG.[11]

An increase in free and total serum **testosterone** levels results in androgenization, the most obvious features of which are hirsutism, acne, and diffuse alopecia. Hyperandrogenemia interferes

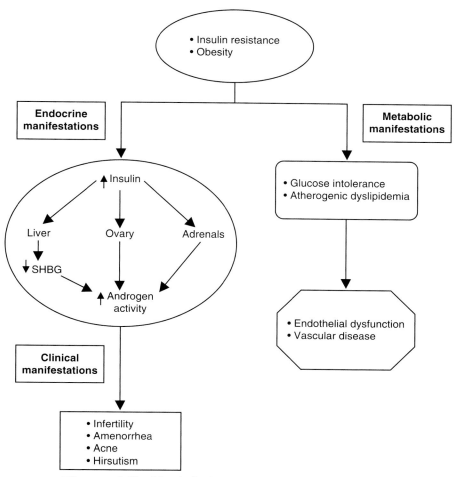

Figure 4-2 • Metabolic abnormalities associated with PCOS.

with the hypothalamic–pituitary axis, leading to anovulation (Fig. 4-1). The absence of a dominant follicle prevents development of nondominant follicles, resulting in the formation of multiple ovarian cysts.[12] Androgen excess also affects other metabolic parameters such as lipid concentrations. A recently published study demonstrated reduced levels of glucagon-like peptide-1 (GLP-1) and glucose-dependent insulinotropic polypeptide (GIP) in patients with PCOS.[13] In normal subjects, these incretin hormones are responsible for 70% of the insulin response during a meal. However, in patients with T2DM and in other insulin-resistance conditions, the incretin effect is impaired. The reduced physiologic levels of incretin hormones in patients with PCOS may have pharmacologic and therapeutic implications warranting future investigations.

Women with PCOS typically have hyperinsulinemia and insulin resistance.[14] Insulin resistance is known to precede the development of T2DM. Studies have shown that 30% to 40% of women with PCOS have impaired glucose tolerance (IGT), and as many as 10% develop T2DM mellitus by the age of 40.[10] Figures 4-1 and 4-2 summarize the pathogenesis and clinical outcomes associated with PCOS.

Diagnostic Criteria for Polycystic Ovary Syndrome

The 2003 Rotterdam PCOS Consensus Conference, held by the European Society of Human Reproduction and Embryology in conjunction with the American Society for Reproductive Medicine, developed the following diagnostic criteria for PCOS.[15]

1. A history of irregular menstrual cycles and anovulation with onset at puberty. *Twenty-five percent of women with PCOS have regular menstrual cycles.*
2. Elevated total and free testosterone levels.
3. The presence of polycystic ovaries and the **exclusion** of other hormonal disorders with similar clinical features such as adult-onset congenital adrenal hyperplasia, hyperprolactinemia, adrenal or ovarian androgen-producing adenomas, hyperthecosis, and Cushing syndrome. The term hyperthecosis refers to the presence of nests of luteinized theca cells in the ovarian stroma secondary to differentiation of the ovarian interstitial cells into steroidogenically active luteinized stromal cells. These nests or islands of luteinized theca cells are scattered throughout the stroma of the ovary, rather than being confined to areas around cystic follicles as in PCOS. The end result is greater androgen production of androgens. The clinical features of hyperthecosis are similar to those of PCOS. However, women with hyperthecosis have more hirsutism and are much more likely to be virilized.[16] Hyperthecosis results in elevations of both estrogen and androgen production, increasing the risk of endometrial hyperplasia and endometrial carcinoma, especially in postmenopausal women.

The Rotterdam PCOS Consensus Panel suggested that tests of insulin resistance are not necessary to make the diagnosis of PCOS or to select the type of treatment. Obese women with PCOS should be screened for metabolic syndrome and T2DM.

The Androgen Excess Society stresses the importance of hyperandrogenism as the cardinal feature of PCOS, placing less emphasis on ovarian morphology. Thus, *the cardinal diagnostic features of PCOS are based on a patient's dysfunctional reproductive and metabolic endocrine access rather than on the physical appearance of the ovaries.* The clinical manifestations of PCOS are listed in Table 4-1.

Clinical Evaluation of Polycystic Ovary Syndrome

Figure 4-3 summarizes the historical and clinical features that should be evaluated in patients suspected of having PCOS. The typical history reveals a patient whose menarche begins as anticipated at the average age of 12 to 13 years. Shortly after menarche, the periods become irregular. Physicians may prescribe oral contraceptives to help regulate the menstrual cycles. Oral contraceptives lower serum androgen levels, improve menstrual cycle regularity, and reduce hirsutism and acne. Although beneficial for the treatment of PCOS, the use of oral contraceptives can result in a delay in one's clinical diagnosis. Early, intensive lifestyle and pharmacologic management of the metabolic disorders associated with PCOS is essential for reducing one's risk of diabetes and CVD progression.

Clinical Features Associated with Polycystic Ovary Syndrome

• Hirsutism, Alopecia, and Acne

Hirsutism is the most common manifestation of androgen excess associated with PCOS. Approximately 10% of reproductive-aged women without PCOS are hirsute, versus 70% of patients with PCOS.[17,18] Hair growth occurs on the chin, cheek, sideburns, neck, chest (Figs. 4-4 and 4-5) and between the breasts, on the periareolar area and upper arms, and below the umbilicus. Distribution of hair with dark hairs spreading onto the thighs may be observed in some patients. An increase in "terminal" or "androgenic" hair supersedes the appearance of short, fine, light-colored vellus hair, which is normally found throughout the body. The onset of hirsutism in PCOS follows menarche, although some girls have earlier onset of pubic hair development and some degree of hirsutism. As patients gain more weight, the hirsutism intensifies.

Diffuse alopecia occurs in 40% to 70% of women with PCOS. Poor nutrition (particularly related to low protein intake), anemia, genetic predisposition, and zinc deficiencies in association with androgen excess increase the risk of developing alopecia[19] (Fig. 4-6).

TABLE 4-1. Clinical Manifestations of PCOS

Manifestation	Comment
Menstrual dysfunction and/or infertility	PCOS, an entity of chronic anovulation, is associated with the most frequent cause of anovulatory infertility.
Hirsutism	Hirsutism in association with menstrual dysfunction is often the most common finding in PCOS.
Acne	Biochemical evidence of hyperandrogenism may occur in the absence of hirsutism or acne.
Alopecia	Alopecia is common and often associated with other features of PCOS.
Visceral (android) fat distribution and obesity	Obesity particularly associated with a visceral fat distribution may further perpetuate the symptoms and risks for metabolic and cardiovascular risks.
Insulin resistance	Possibly related to increase in body iron stores (serum ferritin levels) which result in β-cell dysfunction. Insulin sensitizers (metformin) lower serum ferritin level in obese and overweight women with PCOS.[a]
Miscellaneous	
Sleep apnea	Obstructive sleep apnea in PCOS is a serious symptom that must be looked for particularly in those with increased visceral fat.
Acanthosis nigricans and skin tags	The severity of skin findings may parallel the degree of insulin resistance, and a partial resolution may occur with weight reduction and treatment of the insulin-resistant state.

[a]Luque-Ramirez M, Alvarez-Blasco F, Botella-Carretero JI, et al. Increased body iron stores of obese women with polycystic ovary syndrome are a consequence of insulin resistance and hyperinsulinism and are not a result of reduced menstrual loss. *Diabetes Care* 2007;30:2309–2313.

The PCOS-associated acne often precedes the development of hirsutism. Forty percent of girls with severe acne who are resistant to oral and topical agents (including isotretinoin) have PCOS.[20] Severe or moderate acne persists and even worsens in women ages 20 to 40 (Fig. 4-5). The clinical finding of acne may be the sole manifestation of androgen excess in women with PCOS.[20]

Generally, the androgenic-induced dermatologic anomalies observed in PCOS proceed from acne in the peripubertal period to hirsutism as a young adult to androgenic alopecia in the mature adult.

• Central Obesity

Women with PCOS may relate a sudden onset of weight gain over 6 to 18 months, further complicating symptoms associated with menstrual irregularities, infertility, acne, and hirsutism. The weight gain is often associated with a significant carbohydrate craving. Because of the exaggerated pancreatic β-cell secretion of insulin following the consumption of carbohydrate-rich meals, patients may experience postprandial symptoms suggestive of hypoglycemia such as loss of concentration, hunger, sweating, tremor, and insomnia. Weight gain is associated with an increase in visceral fat distribution, contributing to the development of IGT, atherogenic dyslipidemia, and proinflammatory markers, which constitute the components of metabolic syndrome.[21] The central obesity favors progression to T2DM and increases the risk of CVD in patients with PCOS (Fig. 4-7).

Obese PCOS women are more insulin resistant than lean PCOS patients and lean controls. Although lean women with PCOS appear to secrete higher levels of basal insulin compared to age-matched controls, they do not exhibit signs of insulin resistance.[22] Increased serum ferritin levels, indicating increased body iron stores, have been noted in obese and overweight women with PCOS. Insulin favors the intestinal absorption and tissue deposition of iron. β-cell dysfunction may be induced by

History
   Age at menarche:
   Menstrual pattern:
      Date of last menstrual period:
      Menstrual interval:
      Menstrual duration:
      Are periods regular: Yes   No
   Current form of contraception:
   Obstetrical history: Gravida Para Abortion (Elective Spontaneous)
   Family history of female relatives with irregular periods, severe acne, excessive hair growth, and
   infertility: Yes   No
      Which relatives?
   Family history of type 2 diabetes in parents, aunts, uncles, siblings?
                                         Yes   No
      Which relatives?
   Current medications, including oral contraceptives:
   Review of systems:
      Acne or hirsutism
      Headaches
      Breast discharge

Physical Examination
   Vital signs:
      BMI:
      Blood pressure:
      Waist circumference:
   Skin:
      Acanthosis nigricans: Yes   No   Location:
      Hirsutism: Chin Cheek   Sideburns   Neck
      Between breasts Periareolar
   Upper arms   Between umbilicus and pubic triangle
   Androgenic alopecia (male pattern baldness) yes   no
   Acne   None   Mild   Moderate   Severe

Pelvic exam:
      Vulva and vagina
      Cervix
      Uterus
      Adnexa
      Rectal-vaginal exam
   Thyroid exam: evidence of enlargement or nodularity
   Breast exam: check for galactorrhea

Laboratory Assessment of PCOS*
   1. Total and free testosterone levels
   2. Dehydroepiandrosterone sulphate (DHEAS) levels
   3. Sex-hormone binding globulin
   4. Fasting lipid profile
   5. Fasting plasma glucose level
   6. 17 α-hydroxyprogesterone (elevated in late-onset congenital adrenal hyperplasia)
   7. Fasting insulin level
   8. Urinary free cortisol (if indicated to rule out Cushing syndrome)
   9. Serum ferritin level
   10. Transvaginal ultrasonography[†]

*Blood tests should be performed after a patient has been off oral contraceptives for at least 6 weeks.
Hormone levels should be obtained in the early morning for patients with regular menses, between days 3
and 8 of their cycle.
[†]Test is not needed if patient does not wish to conceive and if other diagnostic criteria for PCOS are
present.

Figure 4-3 • History, physical, and laboratory workup of patients with PCOS.

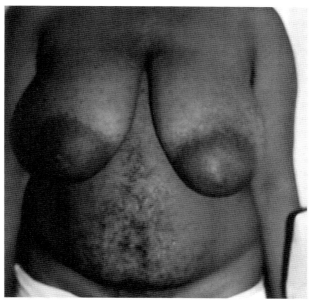

Figure 4-4 • Patient with PCOS displaying diffuse hirsutism on abdomen and chest. (Photo provided courtesy of Walter Futterweit, MD.)

iron deposits in pancreatic islets similar to mechanistic models observed in hemochromatosis. The use of insulin sensitizers, such as metformin, might be useful in reversing elevated iron stores.[22a]

• Sleep Apnea

In comparison with healthy subjects, patients with PCOS have a 4- to 30-fold increased prevalence of sleep apnea.[23] Major symptoms of sleep apnea include snoring, daytime somnolence, and fatigue. Sleep apnea increases the risk of developing hypertension, myocardial infarctions, stroke, and diabetes.[24] The Epworth Sleepiness Scale may be used to screen patients for excessive sleepiness (Fig. 4-8).

Sleep dysfunction can be an independent risk factor toward the development of T2DM. A meta-analysis of sleep literature by Cappuccio et al.[25] concluded that there is an "unambiguous increased

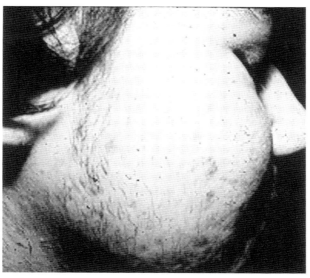

Figure 4-5 • Severe facial acne and hirsutism in a patient with PCOS. (Photo provided courtesy of Walter Futterweit, MD.)

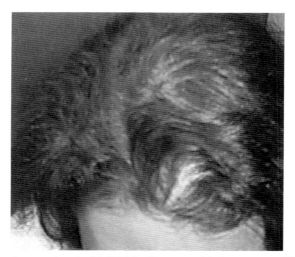

Figure 4-6 • Alopecia associated with PCOS. (Photo provided courtesy of Walter Futterweit, MD.)

risk of developing T2DM at either end of the distribution of sleep duration and with qualitative disturbances of sleep." Subjects averaging less than 5 to 6 hours per night of sleep have a 28% chance of developing T2DM, whereas those with difficulty maintaining sleep have an 84% likelihood of developing the disorder.

The mechanisms by which sleep apnea may potentiate insulin resistance implicate an imbalance between two hormones known to regulate food intake. Leptin is a peptide released by adipocytes

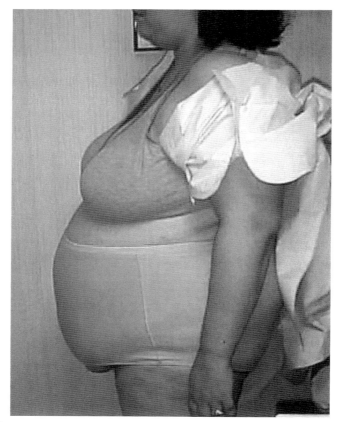

Figure 4-7 • Central obesity, a hallmark of PCOS and insulin resistance, is strongly associated with CVD risk. (Photo provided courtesy of Walter Futterweit, MD.)

The Epworth Sleepiness Scale

How likely are you to doze off or fall asleep in the following situations in contrast to just feeling tired? This refers to your usual way of life in recent times. Even if you have not done some of these things, try to work out how they would have affected you.

Use the following scale to choose the most appropriate number for each situation:

> 0 = would never doze
> 1 = slight chance of dozing
> 2 = moderate chance of dozing
> 3 = high chance of dozing

Situation	Chance of dozing
Sitting and reading	
Watching TV	
Sitting inactive in a public place (e.g., a theater or a meeting)	
As a passenger in a car for an hour without a break	
Lying down to rest in the afternoon when circumstances permit	
Sitting and talking to someone	
Sitting quietly after a lunch without alcohol	
In a car, while stopped for a few minutes in traffic	
TOTAL (max. 24)	

An Epworth score ≥ 10 indicates that the patient is experiencing significant sleepiness. From Johns MW. New method for measuring daytime sleepiness: the Epworth Sleepiness Scale. *Sleep* 1991;14:540–545 with permission.

Figure 4-8 • The Epworth Sleepiness Scale.

that provides information related to one's energy expenditure to hypothalamic regulatory centers. In humans, circulating leptin levels rapidly decrease or increase in response to acute caloric shortage or surplus. Elevated plasma leptin levels *decreases* hunger and vice versa. Ghrelin is produced predominantly by the stomach and is also involved in energy balance regulation. However, in contrast to leptin, elevation in plasma ghrelin *stimulates* appetite. (See Chapter 8, Comanaging Associated Disorders of Diabetes).[26,26a] Individuals with insomnia, sleep fragmentation, and sleep apnea have a physiologic state that favors ghrelin secretion and leptin resistance. As the body spends more time in the "awake state," additional nutritional intake and fat storage are needed to insure an adequate energy source for 20 hours of activity. Individuals who sleep 7 to 8 hours per night require enough energy intake and storage for only 16 to 17 hours of daily activity. The short night sleep patterns associated with insomnia, sleep fragmentation, and obstructive sleep apnea increase ghrelin secretion and favors leptin resistance. Although an individual may remain in bed for 10 to 12 hours a day, he or she is not sleeping efficiently. Ghrelin levels rise as the body strives to provide additional nutritional and energy stores to be used for during the 20 hours per day of wakefulness. The tendency for these patients is toward weight gain and insulin resistance. CPAP (continuous positive airway pressure) usage in young, obese patients with PCOS and sleep apnea has been found to improve insulin sensitivity, reduce diastolic blood pressure, and reduce sympathetic output. Patients with a BMI > 35 kg per m^2 who used CPAP for 8 hours per night demonstrated the best improvement in metabolic parameters.[26b]

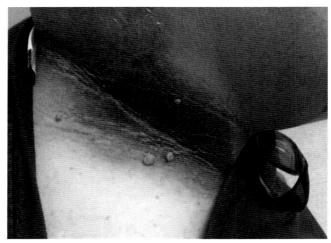

Figure 4-9 • Acanthosis nigricans and skin tags. (Photo courtesy of Jeff Unger, MD.)

• Acanthosis Nigricans and Skin Tags

The findings of acanthosis nigricans (Fig. 4-9) with or without skin tags are clinical markers of insulin resistance.[27] In the absence of a paraneoplastic syndrome, acanthosis nigricans is an epiphenomenon of dermal hyperplasia seen mostly in the nape of the neck, axillae, groin, inner lips of vulvae, periumbilical and inframammary areas, and the dorsum of the fingers and knuckles. They are characterized as brownish-grey, velvety, or verrucous hyperparakeratotic pigmented areas, more commonly seen in obese women of Hispanic or African American descent, although they may be also noted in lean and white populations. Parents of children with acanthosis nigricans often express their frustration in their inability to "wash off the brown dirt with soap, water, and even bleach." Skin tags are not often seen in women before the age of 40 years, and if present earlier, the tags are an important clinical clue to the presence of hyperinsulinism or impaired insulin sensitivity. Weight loss can improve both insulin resistance and the dark appearance of acanthosis nigricans.

▌Laboratory Studies and Radiographic Evaluation of Polycystic Ovary Syndrome

• Laboratory Studies

Hormonal studies are performed on patients with PCOS to determine the presence and severity of hyperandrogenism as well as whether the primary source is adrenal or ovarian. Although laboratory studies may be helpful in confirming the diagnosis of PCOS, no consensus statement has been published for the workup of these patients. Because of the circadian cyclicity of many of the hormones being evaluated, one should make note of the time the laboratory studies are obtained and when they are performed in relation to the patient's menstrual cycle. Reference should also be made as to what medications the patient is taking at the time the tests are done, as some (such as oral contraceptives) may result in an inaccurate interpretation of the test results.

Hormonal testing should be performed in the early morning hours due to their circadian cyclicity. Patients with regular menstrual cycles should have their blood samples obtained between days 3 and 8 of the menstrual cycle. All initial blood tests on patients suspected of having PCOS should be performed at least 6 weeks after the cessation of oral contraceptives. Blood values obtained while the patient uses oral contraceptives are not useful in diagnosing PCOS because oral contraceptives lower circulating androgen levels.[28]

Although elevations in androgen levels are frequently observed with PCOS, some patients have normal free testosterone and total testosterone values.[29] Standardized normal serum androgen levels for adolescents and older women have not been determined. Notwithstanding these limitations, measurement of the free testosterone is thought to be a sensitive method of assessing hyperandrogenemia.[30] A total testosterone value greater than 50 ng per dL is considered elevated.[31] The optimal value for serum testosterone in women is unknown. Most women with a level greater than 50 ng per dL will have irregular menses and clinical symptoms related to hyperandrogenism. The level of free (unbound) testosterone is usually elevated in patients with PCOS.

Dehydroepiandrosterone sulfate (DHEAS) is a major androgen precursor secreted from the adrenal gland. Patients having elevations of both DHEAS and total testosterone should be evaluated for an androgen-secreting tumor.[32] Additional tests, such as 17-ketosteroids (measuring androgen metabolites in the urine) and 17-OH progesterone, are useful in determining if the patient has an adrenocortical tumor, adrenal cancer, or adrenal hyperplasia. These tests should be obtained in patients with a DHEAS level greater than 700 ng per dL. Normal DHEAS levels range from 200 to 300 ng per dL (Table 4-2).

TABLE 4-2. Interpretation of Laboratory and Radiographic Studies in Patients Suspected of Having PCOS

Laboratory Test	Normal Range[a]	Comment
Free testosterone	0–9.5 ng/mL	Hallmark feature of PCOS when elevated >50 ng/mL The "free" testosterone is unbound to SHBG and reflects the patient's biologically active level of testosterone. Draw in early morning. Repeat test to confirm abnormal values.
Dehydroepiandrosterone sulfate	35–430 µg/dL	Androgen precursor secreted from the adrenal gland Elevated in cases of infertility, amenorrhea, hirsutism, hyperandrogenemia, adrenal tumors, and congenital adrenal hyperplasia Elevated DHEAS requires further diagnostic testing to determine source of androgen excess.
17-ketosteroids (KS)	6–12 mg/24 h	Measures androgen metabolites in the urine In association with elevated DHEAS may indicate adrenal tumor or adrenal hyperplasia Spironolactone can raise levels of 17-KS.
17-OH progesterone	**Day 3:** 200–100 ng/dL **Midcycle:** 100–250 ng/dL **Luteal phase:** 100–500 ng/dL	Measures serum androgen levels. Deficiencies are noted with hyperandrongenemia. In association with elevated DHEAS may indicate adrenal tumor or adrenal hyperplasia
Sex-hormone binding globulin (SHBG)	18–114 nmol/L	SHBG levels are low in obesity and hyperandrogenemia and with insulin resistance. If SHBG is low, more free testosterone becomes metabolically active and induces the signs of hyperandrogenemia.

(Continued)

TABLE 4-2. Interpretation of Laboratory and Radiographic Studies in Patients Suspected of Having PCOS *(Continued)*

Laboratory Test	Normal Range[a]	Comment
Urinary cortisol	10–100 mg/24 h	Measured in patients having cushingoid features. Levels exceeding 100 mg/24 h are suggestive of Cushing disease.
Luteinizing hormone (LH)	On day 3, the normal LH level is <7 mU/mL.	In PCOS, both the level of circulating LH and its relation to FSH levels are elevated due to an increase in amplitude and frequency of LH pulses from the pituitary gland.
	On LH surge day, the LH level may increase to >20 mU/mL.	Elevated LH concentrations occur in 60% of PCOS patients. The LH/FSH ratio is >2:1 or 3:1 in up to 95% of PCOS patients.
Follicle-stimulating hormone (FSH)	3–20 mU/mL	Normally, the LH/FSH ratio is close to 1:1 A higher ratio is suggestive of PCOS.
Prolactin	<24 ng/mL	Increased prolactin levels can interfere with ovulation. If elevated, consider further testing (MRI) to evaluated patient for pituitary adenoma. May be elevated in PCOS
Screening tests for metabolic syndrome	Lipids Fasting glucose 2-h post glucose challenge	Fasting plasma glucose levels of 100–126 mg/dL indicate IFG. Plasma glucose drawn 2 h after a 75-g glucose challenge between 140–199 mg/dL is indicative of IGT. Plasma glucose >200 mg/dL is diagnostic of diabetes. Normal lipid values are: Total cholesterol ≤ 200 mg/dL HDL-C ≥ 55 mg/dL LDL-C ≤ 130 mg/dL Triglycerides ≤ 150 mg/dL
Ultrasound imaging	Optimally performed during the early follicular phase (days 3–6) of the menstrual cycle in women with regular menses Anovulatory women should be scanned at random or 3–5 d after a progestin-induced withdrawal bleed.	Pelvic imaging is indicated only if the ovaries are palpable on physical examination or the total testosterone concentration is >200 ng/mL. 23% of "normal women" have characteristics of polycystic ovaries. Polycystic ovaries are observed in many other disease states (see text). Evaluate development of large cysts, effects of therapy on reducing cysts, and changes in the endometrium. High frequency of fatty liver disease on ultrasonography

[a]Most hormone levels should be obtained on day 3 of menstrual cycle. Several determinations of plasma total and free testosterone levels are made.
HDL-C, high-density lipoprotein cholesterol; LDL-C, low-density lipoprotein cholesterol; MRI, magnetic resonance imaging.

Patients with cushingoid features should have a urine cortisol determination. Levels greater than 100 µg per 24 hours are strongly suggestive of Cushing syndrome.

If the 17-hydroxyprogesterone level at 8:00 AM (measured in the follicular phase of the menstrual cycle) is greater than 4 ng per mL, the patient probably has nonclassic adrenal hyperplasia resulting from a 21-hydroxylase deficiency. This diagnosis can be confirmed by a 60-minute ACTH stimulation test. Approximately 2% of women who present with hyperandrogenism and oligo-ovulation or anovulation have nonclassic adrenal hyperplasia resulting from a 21-hydroxylase deficiency. The prevalence of this congenital disorder varies markedly among different ethnic groups, from below 1% in Hispanic populations to as high as 5% to 8% in Ashkenazi Jewish populations.[33]

A normally cycling premenopausal woman has an LH/FSH ratio of 1:1. Although a normal LH/FSH ratio does not exclude the diagnosis of PCOS, a ratio of 2:1 or 3:1 is found in 95% of patients with PCOS.[12,34] An isolated rise in LH levels occurs in 60% of patients with PCOS.[29] SHBG values are low in hyperandrogenemic and hyperinsulinemic states and in obesity.[35]

Patients suspected of having PCOS should have advanced lipid profiling performed to determine their cardiovascular risk. VAP (vertical auto profile) testing may be superior to routine lipid analysis as subfractionation allows assessment of low-density lipoprotein (LDL) particle size, subclasses, and atherogenic lipoprotein phenotype. (See Chapter 7, Acrovascular Complications.) VAP testing does not require the patient to fast prior to sampling. Patients with PCOS may demonstrate a reduction in LDL size with a concomitant increase in the more atherogenic types III and IV LDL particle subclasses. Four major subspecies, large LDL-I, medium LDL-II, small LDL-III, and very small LDL-IV, and the predominance of small and very small LDL has been accepted as an emerging CV risk factor by the National Cholesterol Education Program Adult Treatment Panel III.[36] In addition, PCOS patients have lower levels of high-density lipoproteins (HDL-C), apolipoprotein A-1, and insulin levels versus. age-matched controls.[37]

IGT is present in 30% to 40% of women with PCOS, and in as many as 10%, T2DM develops by age 40.[38] These prevalence rates are among the highest known in women of similar age.[39] Insulin resistance is more common in patients with PCOS than in unaffected counterparts matched for body mass index (BMI), fat-free mass, and body fat distribution.[40] Insulin resistance alone cannot fully account for the predisposition to and development of T2DM diabetes in PCOS patients. Most women with PCOS are able to fully compensate for their insulin resistance by increasing pancreatic secretion of insulin. However, those with a first-degree relative with T2DM have a disordered and insufficient β-cell response to meals or a glucose challenge.[41] Patients may develop clinical diabetes in response to pregnancy or glucocorticoid administration.[42] A fasting plasma glucose level lower than 100 mg per dL is considered normal. Impaired fasting glucose (IFG) is diagnosed when the fasting glucose levels are 100 to 125 mg per dL. Fasting glucose levels greater than 126 mg per dL are diagnostic of diabetes. IGT is diagnosed if plasma glucose levels are greater than 140 mg per dL or less than 200 mg per dL at 2 hours after a 75-g glucose challenge is performed. A patient has diabetes if either her random or 2-hour postchallenge blood glucose level exceeds 200 mg per dL.

Freeman et al.[43] assessed patients with PCOS for both IGT and insulin resistance using a "muffin test." In this prospective study, 13 patients who had previously been screened for IGT and insulin resistance using the standard 2-hour oral glucose tolerance test were provided with a meal consisting of a large Costco chocolate chip muffin and 8 oz of orange juice. This "mixed-meal tolerance test," following a 10-hour fast, contained 800 kcal (105 g of carbohydrates, 38 g of fat, and 12 g of protein). The meal was consumed within 15 minutes. Glucose and insulin levels were drawn at baseline, 30, 60, 90, and 120 minutes following ingestion of the muffin. The area under the insulin curve (AUC) during the mixed-meal tolerance test was computed using the following formula: AUC = 0.25 (fasting value) + 0.5 (½-hour value) + 0.75 (1-hour value) + 0.5 (2-hour value). An insulin AUC above 100 mIU per mL was used as the cutoff value for insulin resistance. Of the 13 participants, 3 (23%) had normal insulin AUC values and 10 (77%) had evidence of insulin resistance and IGT.

Glucola (50 to 100 g liquid glucose) contains 37% glucose, 11% maltose, and 10% triose.[44] This mixture is commonly associated with adverse effects such as nausea, vomiting, heartburn, and reactive hypoglycemia, which can be attributed to glucose's increased osmolarity, sweetness, and increased absorption with early insulin release. Glucola costs $6 per unit, whereas Costco muffins cost $0.50 each, making the test "media" more cost effective and palatable. Patients with PCOS who are insulin resistant are more likely to progress toward clinical diabetes regardless of their BMI, waist circumference, waist-to-hip ratio, or degree of central adiposity.[43] Therefore, performing a mixed-meal tolerance test appears to be a simple, well-tolerated, and cost effective means by which one may screen for insulin resistance and IGT in this high-risk population.

• Ultrasonographic Imaging

Transvaginal ultrasonography is necessary for infertility evaluation and management. If a patient does not wish to conceive and meets the Rotterdam criteria for PCOS, ultrasonography is not necessary. In these cases, confirmation of the morphologic characteristics of the patient's ovaries would not affect management. The specificity of morphologic evidence of polycystic ovaries on ultrasonography is limited by the fact that 23% of apparently normal women have characteristic findings of polycystic ovaries[45] (see Fig. 4-10). Polycystic ovaries may also be observed in Cushing syndrome, idiopathic hirsutism, and hyperprolactinemia and with the use of medications such as valproic acid and ovulation-inducing agents.[46] The best time to perform an ultrasound of the pelvis is in the early follicular phase (days 3 to 6 of the menstrual cycle) in women with regular menses. Anovulatory women with oligomenorrhea may be scanned at random or 3 to 5 days after a progestin-induced withdrawal bleed.

The criteria that suggest PCOS on ultrasound include the presence of 12 or more follicles measuring 2 to 9 mm in diameter in each ovary and/or increased ovarian volume of greater than 10 mL.[47] Ultrasound may also be useful in identifying women who have endometrial hypertrophy, which may be diagnostic of endometrial carcinoma. Table 4-3 lists the technical recommendations for performing transvaginal ultrasonography in patients suspected of having PCOS.

Ultrasonography of the liver in patients with PCOS may identify patients with fatty liver infiltration.[48] Despite the radiographic evidence, only 15% of patients with PCOS and nonalcoholic steatohepatitis (NASH) have abnormal liver chemistries.[49] NASH is strongly associated with insulin resistance and is considered a precursor to clinical diabetes.[50]

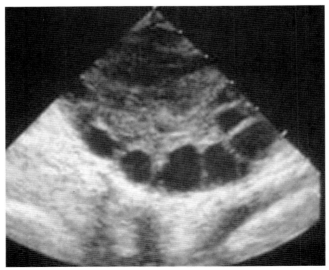

Figure 4-10 • Polycystic ovary. A 32-year-old patient with polycystic ovary syndrome, yet no other clinical or hormonal evidence of PCOS. (Photo courtesy of Jeff Unger, MD.)

TABLE 4-3. Technical Recommendations for Performing Ultrasonography on Patients Suspected of Having PCOS

1. Use state-of-the-art equipment and appropriately trained personnel.
2. Transvaginal approach should be used whenever possible, especially in obese patients.
3. Regularly menstruating women should be scanned during the follicular phase of the cycle (cycle days 3–5). Oligomenorrheic or amenorrheic women should be scanned 3–5 d after a progestin-induced withdrawal bleeding or at random.
4. Follicle number should be estimated both in longitudinal and anteroposterior cross sections of the ovary. The size of follicles <10 mm should be expressed as the mean of the diameters on the two sections.

From Rotterdam ESHRE/ASRM-Sponsored PCOS Consensus Workshop Group. Revised 2003 consensus on diagnostic criteria and long-term health risks related to polycystic ovary syndrome. *Fertil Steril.* 2004;81:19–25.

Polycystic Ovary Syndrome Associated with the Metabolic Syndrome, Insulin Resistance, Cardiovascular Disease, and T2DM

• Linking Polycystic Ovary Syndrome with the Metabolic Syndrome

Women with PCOS are at high risk for developing T2DM and CVD related to metabolic syndrome. Therefore, PCPs must identify patients with PCOS not just as part of a routine workup for anovulation or infertility but to identify individuals with increased risk for cardiovascular morbidity and mortality. Of the 5 to 6 million women in the United States who have both PCOS and the metabolic syndrome, less than two-thirds are aware of either their diagnosis or their increased cardiovascular risk.[51] Approximately 50% of all women with PCOS have clinical characteristics that qualify them as having metabolic syndrome.[52]

Metabolic syndrome is a constellation of interrelated risk factors that favor the development of atherosclerotic CVD and an increased risk for the development of T2DM. The National Cholesterol Education Program Adult Treatment Panel guidelines (NCEP–ATP III)[36] defining metabolic syndrome were based on data from the Third National Health and Nutrition Examination Survey (NHANES III).[53] Metabolic syndrome was defined as having three or more of the characteristics listed in Table 4-4. The 2003 American College of Endocrinology Position Statement also added IGT as a component of the syndrome, with a glucose level of 140 to 199 mg per dL obtained 120 minutes after a 75-g glucose challenge.[54]

TABLE 4-4. Criteria for the Metabolic Syndrome in Women with PCOS[a]

Risk Factor	Cutoff
Waist circumference	>35 inches
Triglycerides	≥ 150 mg/dL
HDL-C	<50 mg/dL
Blood pressure	≥ 130/≥ 85 mm Hg
Fasting and 2-h glucose from a 75-g oral glucose challenge test	110–126 mg/dL (fasting) and/or a 2-h glucose challenge 140–199 mg/dL

[a]Women having three of five criteria qualify for the syndrome.
HDL-C, high-density lipoprotein cholesterol.
From Rotterdam ESHRE/ASRM-Sponsored PCOS Consensus Workshop Group. Revised 2003 consensus on diagnostic criteria and long-term health risks related to polycystic ovary syndrome. *Fertil Steril.* 2004;81:19–25.

• Linking Polycystic Ovary Syndrome with Insulin Resistance

Insulin resistance is defined as a subnormal response to a given concentration of endogenous insulin. Insulin resistance is present in metabolic disorders such as obesity, physical stress (i.e., postsurgical, post-trauma), sepsis, acromegaly, pregnancy, hypertriglyceridemia, and Cushing syndrome. Patients with prediabetes eventually develop T2DM when the pancreatic β-cells become unable to produce enough insulin to keep fasting blood glucose levels less than 126 mg per dL and postprandial glucose levels less than 200 mg per dL. Whereas metabolic syndrome is present in 50% of patients with PCOS, insulin resistance is present in nearly all such women.[55] Insulin resistance is associated with other metabolic abnormalities such as hypertension and dyslipidemia. The obvious need for evaluation and aggressive management of these comorbidities in patients with PCOS cannot be understated.

A simple and inexpensive way to assess the likelihood of a patient being insulin resistant is to calculate the triglyceride-to-HDL-C ratio. A normal ratio is considered to be 3.5:1 or lower. A ratio of 3.5:1 or greater is suggestive of insulin resistance. For example, a patient whose triglyceride level is 350 mg per dL and whose HDL-C is 35 mg per dL would have a ratio of 10:1, favoring insulin resistance.[56] In 2005, The American Association of Clinical Endocrinologists (AACE) published a position statement suggesting that all patients diagnosed with PCOS should be considered as having insulin resistance and increased risks for developing T2DM and CVD.[57]

Patients with PCOS rapidly progress from normal glucose tolerance through prediabetes and into T2DM. Approximately 15% of PCOS patients convert from normal glucose tolerance to IGT yearly, and 50% of PCOS patients develop T2DM by age 30.[58] The incidence of T2DM in patients with PCOS is 13%, with a mean age of 42 years in comparison with 1.4% of a control population.[59] The more irregular the menses, the more likely women with PCOS are at risk for developing T2DM, particularly in obese patients.[59]

Cardiovascular risk is increased in women with PCOS who have additional metabolic abnormalities often seen in association with obesity. Seventy percent of obese women with PCOS have dyslipidemia.[60]

Although not clinically apparent, initially, patients with PCOS are at risk for developing hypertension later in life.[61] Inflammatory markers such as C-reactive protein (CRP), homocysteine, and microalbuminuria are associated with endothelial cell dysfunction and increased CVD risk. Patel et al.[62] demonstrated a threefold increase of metabolic syndrome in women with PCOS having an albumin-to-creatinine ratio (ACR) greater than 7 mg per g (premicroalbuminuria) in comparison to patients having an ACR less than 7 mg per g. Screening factors associated with premicroalbuminuria include hypertension and an elevation in alanine aminotransferase (ALT) with levels greater than 40 U per L. These results suggest that even low levels of albuminuria in women with PCOS may be a useful marker of cardiovascular dysfunction.

• Polycystic Ovary Syndrome Increases Risk of Coronary Artery Disease

PCOS is associated with a high prevalence of coronary artery calcification as determined by electron-beam computed tomography and[63] most likely due to an increased level of plasminogen activator inhibitor (PAI-1).[64] Improvement in insulin sensitivity lowers PAI-1 levels. Metabolic abnormalities common to PCOS patients include hypertriglyceridemia, increased levels of very-low-density lipoproteins (VLDLs), decreased levels of HDL-C, and abnormal glucose levels. Insulin resistance coupled with hyperandrogenemia contributes to the atherogenic lipid state in PCOS. Testosterone decreases lipoprotein lipase activity in visceral fat cells, which favors an atherogenic dyslipidemic metabolic environment.

A risk factor model analysis has calculated that patients with PCOS have a four- to sevenfold higher risk of myocardial infarction in comparison with age-matched controls.[65] This study also determined that women with PCOS had a sevenfold increased progression to T2DM (15% vs. 2.3% in control subjects).

A study evaluating 143 patients younger than age 60, whose complaint of chest pain required cardiac catheterization, determined that 42% had radiographic evidence of PCOS, double the

TABLE 4-5. Summary of Data Linking PCOS to CVD

1. The prevalences of both T2DM and a myocardial infarction–equivalent state and IGT are substantially increased in patients with PCOS. The AACE and American College of Endocrinologists recommend screening for diabetes in all patients with PCOS by age 30.

2. Multiple recognized cardiovascular risk factors are present in excess in women with PCOS. The result is a higher than usual prevalence of the Adult Treatment Panel III–defined metabolic syndrome in women with PCOS.

3. Imaging studies in women with PCOS have uniformly identified a higher prevalence of anatomic and functional abnormalities indicative of existing underlying CVD or dysfunction in comparison with age-matched controls.

Data from American Association of Clinical Endocrinologists position statement on metabolic and cardiovascular consequences of polycystic ovary syndrome. Polycystic ovary syndrome writing committee. *Endocr Pract.* 2005;11:126–134.

frequency in the general population.[66] Patients with PCOS exhibit more coronary artery segments with more than 50% stenosis and significantly greater clinical heart disease than do women with normal ovaries as detected by ultrasound.[67]

Using oligomenorrhea as a surrogate marker for PCOS, a 2- to 2.5-fold increase in the incidence of T2DM was noted in the prospective Nurses' Health Study of more than 101,000 women. In a mean follow-up of 14 years, a history of oligomenorrhea was associated with a 100% increased prevalence of fatal and 50% increased incidence of nonfatal coronary artery disease after adjusting for age, smoking history, and BMI.[59] Eighty percent of women with oligomenorrhea are thought to have PCOS.[57,66,68] Table 4-5 summarizes the cardiovascular risks associated with PCOS.

The data relating to CVD with PCOS can be summarized as follows:

- The prevalence of T2DM (a myocardial infarction–equivalent state) and IGT (a prediabetes condition associated with cardiovascular risk) are both increased in women with PCOS.
- Many recognized cardiovascular risks are significantly increased in women with PCOS.
- Women with PCOS have insulin resistance, which increases the risk for CVD.
- Fifty percent of women with PCOS have diagnostic criteria that qualify them as having metabolic syndrome. This constellation of metabolic risk factors tends to increase the likelihood of developing CVD.
- Imaging and cardiac studies in young women with PCOS have demonstrated a higher incidence of anatomic and functional abnormalities indicative of underlying CVD when compared with age-matched controls.

Although all studies evaluating the link between CVD, PCOS, and insulin resistance are not uniform in their conclusions, most consistently predict an increased risk for adverse cardiovascular events in patients with PCOS. Collectively, the data suggest that PCPs recognize these patients as being at high risk for developing T2DM and CVD. They should therefore undergo a comprehensive evaluation for recognized CVD and metabolic risk factors. Aggressive treatment to reduce cardiovascular risk and to slow the rate of progression to T2DM should be encouraged.

• Cancer Risk Associated with Polycystic Ovary Syndrome

Endometrial carcinoma is more prevalent in patients with PCOS.[69] This association has been attributed to the persistent stimulation of endometrial tissue by unopposed estrogen release. Ovarian progesterone secretion is minimized in PCOS, as patients do not ovulate. Endometrial carcinoma is also associated with T2DM and obesity.[69] Breast and ovarian carcinomas may be more common in PCOS patients. However, the specific risk factors associated with breast and ovarian carcinomas are difficult to determine. Obesity, anovulation, infertility, and hormonal treatments for infertility may all have some influence on the development of breast and ovarian carcinomas.

Additional information related to the link between diabetes and cancer may be found in the macrovascular complications chapter.

• Polycystic Ovary Syndrome and Mood Disorders

Women with PCOS are at increased risk for diminished quality of life and mood disorders.[70] A recent study noted that women with PCOS were at an increased risk for depressive disorders (new cases) compared with controls (21% vs. 3%).[71] A large study of over 100 women with PCOS evaluated from a female patient population of 1,359 found a high prevalence of low quality of life in those with PCOS.[70] Women with PCOS had lower quality of life on all seven factors of the modified PCOSQ (emotional disturbance, weight, infertility, acne, menstrual symptoms, menstrual predictability, and hirsutism). Weight gain remains the greatest concern of patients with PCOS regardless of their prescribed treatment regimen.[70]

A PubMed search of major relevant articles published from 1985 to 2009 dealing with both PCOS and psychological morbidity showed frequent references to eating disorders and a sevenfold increased suicide rate in this patient population.[72] The symptoms most often associated with PCOS comorbid psychological dysfunction include hirsutism, obesity, amenorrhea, and subfertility. Physicians should consider screening all patients with PCOS for major depression and suicidality. The Columbia Suicide Severity Rating Scale is widely used in primary care to assess patients at risk for suicide. The scale is available online at: http://www.cssrs.columbia.edu/docs/C-SSRS-Risk_Assessment_Version_2-1-12.pdf. The PHQ-9 self-reporting questionnaire may be administered to patients to assess one's likelihood of having depression as well as the severity of their disorder. The form may be downloaded at: http://www.integration.samhsa.gov/images/res/PHQ%20-%20Questions.pdf.

• PCOS and Infertility

Women with PCOS should be considered as being "subfertile" rather than absolutely infertile based upon the unpredictability of their ovulation. As a general rule, PCOS women represent one of the most difficult groups to induce ovulation both successfully and safely. Opinion differs as to which therapeutic options are the safest and most effective at allowing patients to become pregnant and carry their pregnancy to term. Most experts would agree that because PCOS is a medical disorder, lifestyle intervention including weight reduction and exercise therapy should be the foundation of care for those patients desiring to become pregnant. Pharmacotherapy and surgical interventions can be used for those who fail to respond to more conservative management.

• Treatment of Polycystic Ovary Syndrome

An opportunity exists to reverse some of the associated metabolic, endocrine, and oncologic outcomes that are associated with PCOS, especially in younger women.[73] Lifestyle modification with weight reduction, exercise, smoking cessation, and pharmacotherapy all are helpful in managing PCOS patients. Table 4-6 summarizes the treatment strategies for PCOS.

As with all primary care patients, therapy for PCOS should be customized and based on the particular patient's metabolic, gynecologic, and cosmetic concerns. For example, a woman who desires to become pregnant might have the most success when treated with an insulin-sensitizing drug rather than oral contraceptives, which may reduce hirsutism and acne. Hirsutism might be addressed using spironolactone or oral contraceptives.

• Restoring the Menstrual Cycle

Restoring natural menstrual cycling with oral contraceptives has both psychological and physiologic benefits. Oral contraceptives increase hepatic production of SHBG, which, in turn, binds free testosterone, making testosterone less likely to target androgen receptors. As a result, acne, hirsutism, and alopecia may subside. The estrogenic component of the oral contraceptive suppresses LH, resulting in decreased ovarian androgen production. The choice of oral contraceptive is important

TABLE 4-6. Management Strategies for Patients with PCOS

- Recognition of PCOS is essential.
- Lifestyle modification emphasizing the need for nutritional balance, weight reduction, exercise, and smoking cessation should be the cornerstone of therapy in all patients with PCOS. Referral to a registered dietitian may be beneficial.
- Screen for diabetes, especially in obese women with PCOS who have a family history of T2DM.
- Diagnose and treat lipid disorders with medical nutrition therapy as well as lipid-lowering drugs.
- Check blood pressure on each visit and manage hypertension with appropriate lifestyle interventions and pharmacotherapy.
- Consider measuring inflammatory markers such as high-sensitivity C-reactive protein (CRP-hs), which when elevated may impart a high cardiovascular risk to the PCOS patient.
- Consider use of metformin therapy as the initial intervention, particularly if the patient is obese. Metformin improves many metabolic abnormalities in PCOS and may help regulate menstrual cyclicity. Metformin can also reverse infertility. (Metformin has not been FDA approved for use in PCOS although abundant medical literature supports its efficacy.)
- Use pioglitazone (a TZD) in patients with IGT or frank diabetes. TZDs are Category C drugs; their use is contraindicated during pregnancy.
- Off-label use of incretin therapies may be useful in *some* patients
- Use nonandrogenic oral contraceptives and an antiandrogen agent (spironolactone) to treat the skin manifestations of PCOS. Ancillary use of electrolysis and laser therapy may be beneficial.
- Screen for major depression and suicidality in all patients with PCOS. Treat or refer when appropriate.

FDA, Food and Drug Administration.

because most progestins also possess androgenic effects. Contraceptives containing nonandrogenic progestins such as norgestimate and desogestrel are preferred.[74] Drospirenone, an analogue of spironolactone with unique antimineralocorticoid and antiandrogenic activities, is available for use in combination with ethinyl estradiol, thus potentially becoming the ideal oral contraceptive for women with PCOS.[75] Oral contraceptives do not improve the metabolic abnormalities associated with PCOS and may increase insulin resistance.[35] If insulin resistance deteriorates with the use of oral contraceptives, metformin may be added to the treatment regimen.

• Antiandrogens

Spironolactone possesses moderate antiandrogenic effects when large doses (100 to 200 mg per day) are used.[76] Patients who desire cosmetic improvements for their hirsutism, acne, and alopecia may be treated successfully with a combination of oral contraceptives and spironolactone. Women desiring pregnancy should use both spironolactone and a combination of an estrogen and a progestin. The drug's effects on improving hirsutism may not become clinically apparent for up to 9 months. Cessation of spironolactone therapy often results in the recurrence of acne and hirsutism or worsening of alopecia within 3 months. Side effects of spironolactone include gastrointestinal discomfort, postural hypotension, increased urination, decreased libido, irritability, mastodynia, hyperkalemia, and muscle pain. Midcycle bleeding resulting from progestin-like properties at high doses of spironolactone may occur. Whether or not spironolactone is secreted in breast milk is uncertain.

Spironolactone and oral contraceptives are synergistic and can be used concomitantly for the following reasons: (a) spironolactone has a minimal effect on improving hirsutism, acne, and alopecia when compared with the combined effects of both drugs, (b) spironolactone cannot be used during pregnancy and has a Category D rating (risk to the fetus, but drug benefits may outweigh the risk), and (c) 50% to 70% of women who use spironolactone experience midcycle bleeding.

5-α-reductase inhibitors suppress the conversion of testosterone to dihydrotestosterone (DHT) in the prostate. In the skin and other tissues, the effect of finasteride is mediated by inhibition of type 1 5-α-reductase. Dosages of 2.5 to 5.0 mg daily have been used to suppress hirsutism in women with PCOS[65] with minimal side effects. A 32% to 78% reduction in hirsutism was associated with a decrease in plasma DHT.[77] Finasteride is not approved by the U.S. Food and Drug Administration (FDA) for treating hirsutism in patients with PCOS.

Eflornithine hydrochloride, an inhibitor of the enzyme ornithine decarboxylase in human skin, has been approved for topical use in treating facial hirsutism. The inhibition of hair growth is its primary action, but clinical data are too limited to recommend its routine use.

• Insulin Reducers

A reduction in insulin levels ameliorates sequelae associated with hyperinsulinemia and hyperandrogenemia. Therapies that normalize insulin levels can effectively treat the metabolic abnormalities associated with PCOS.

Metformin inhibits hepatic glucose production, thereby reducing the androgen production of theca cells.[78] Metformin may also directly influence ovulation. A meta-analysis of 13 studies in which metformin was used by 543 patients reported that those taking metformin had an odds ratio for ovulation of 3.88 as compared with placebo and an odds ratio for ovulation of 4.41 for metformin plus clomiphene, when compared with clomiphene alone.[79] Metformin also improved fasting insulin levels, blood pressure, and levels of LDL-C.

In women with PCOS, metformin tends to increase the endogenous secretion of both GIP and GLP-1.[13] Although insulin sensitivity was not improved in patients using metformin, the drug did lower the total plasma testosterone levels of both lean and obese patients with PCOS.[13] Metformin appears to increase plasma concentrations of GLP-1 by increasing GLP-1 biosynthesis and secretion as well as by inhibiting dipeptidyl-peptidase-4 further inhibiting GLP-1 degradation.[80–82]

Women with PCOS who conceive while taking metformin have a lower likelihood of developing gestational diabetes or suffering a spontaneous abortion when compared with PCOS women who are not prescribed metformin.[83] A 30% to 40% reduction in the incidence of spontaneous abortions throughout pregnancy has been reported in patients using metformin.[83] Metformin is a Category B drug whose use in pregnancy has not been shown to cause an increased rate of birth defects. Metformin should not be used while breastfeeding.

Because metformin can cause previously anovulatory women to ovulate, unplanned pregnancies may occur. Caution should be used in prescribing metformin as sole therapy in adolescents and young adults without using some form of contraception and offering preconception planning. This is especially important when metformin is used in obese patients with T2DM. Most women with PCOS can have successful pregnancies without a dramatic increase in health risk.[84] There are no guidelines for dosing metformin in patients with PCOS. However, a total daily dose of 2,000 mg is recommended. The drug should be taken with meals. Side effects include bloating, diarrhea, and nausea. When initiating metformin, one should begin with a low dosage of 500 mg daily taken with food for 7 to 10 days, then increased to twice daily with breakfast and dinner. Every 2 weeks, the dose should be increased to a maximum of 2,000 mg as tolerated. After 6 to 8 weeks, the side effects of metformin become minimal with the exception of occasional diarrhea. Folic acid supplements should be prescribed, as metformin reduces the gastrointestinal absorption of this vitamin. Women taking metformin should discontinue use of the drug within 24 hours of undergoing any intravenous contrast study. Resumption of the drug is safe once renal function is retested and documented as normal. A serum creatinine level greater than 1.4 mg per dL might increase the risk of developing lactic acidosis when using metformin. (For further information on use of metformin, see chapter on T2DM.)

The chronic use of metformin in women with PCOS is an important area of debate. Whereas 10% of patients with PCOS have T2DM, nearly all women have insulin resistance and are at high risk for progressing rapidly toward clinically apparent T2DM. Nearly 30% to 50% of obese patients with both PCOS and IGT convert to T2DM by age 30 years.[85] In these women, PCOS should be viewed less as an infertility or cosmetic disorder and more as a disorder that is likely to cause premature CVD and diabetes.[85] In the obese cohort of the Diabetes Prevention Program, patients using metformin had a 31% reduction in progression to diabetes from IGT over 3 years when compared with patients taking placebo.[86]

The **thiazolidinediones** (TZDs) improve insulin action in the liver, skeletal muscle, and adipose tissue. TZDs, like metformin, affect ovarian steroid synthesis.[87] TZDs improve the chances of ovulation, reduce free testosterone levels, increase levels of SHBG, reduce levels of PAI-1, and improve glycemia.[88,89] TZDs have an FDA pregnancy Category C (a known teratogen in animal studies) rating. Oral contraceptives or barrier methods to prevent pregnancy should be prescribed when patients with PCOS use TZDs. Because of concern about using TZDs during pregnancy, metformin is more commonly used to treat PCOS.

TZDs improve the frequency of menstrual cycles while reducing hyperinsulinemia and hyperandrogenism in PCOS. TZDs have proven beneficial in reducing the risk of progression to T2DM and in decreasing a number of inflammatory markers associated with the metabolic syndrome (see Table 4-7). In a head-to-head study, metformin tended to improve the frequency of menstrual cyclicity slightly more than rosiglitazone.[90] TZDs may also be helpful in managing NAFLD, which may be present in 50% of women with PCOS.[91]

Patients who desire fertility should be placed on metformin rather than TZDs. Patients with respiratory failure, congestive heart failure, hypoxia, or liver transaminase levels exceeding three times the upper limit of normal at baseline should not be started on a TZD. Liver function testing should be monitored quarterly during the first year of TZD use and periodically thereafter. Fifteen percent of women who use a TZD will experience weight gain and edema. Initial dosages are 15 mg daily of pioglitazone, increasing to 30 mg after 6 to 8 weeks.

• Inducers of Ovulation

Two classes of ovulation drug treatments are available in the United States, clomiphene citrate and human gonadotropins. Clomiphene citrate is usually the first treatment step in anovulatory, infertile patients who desire to become pregnant. Clomiphene is an estrogen-like hormone that acts on the hypothalamus, pituitary gland, and ovary to increase levels of FSH and LH, thereby improving the likelihood of growing an ovarian follicle and triggering ovulation.[10]

A study by Legro randomly assigned 626 infertile women with PCOS to receive clomiphene plus placebo, metformin extended-release plus placebo or a combination of metformin extended-release and clomiphene for up to 6 months.[92] Medication was discontinued when pregnancy was confirmed and subjects were followed until delivery. The conception rate among subjects who ovulated was significantly lower in the metformin group (21.7%) than in either the clomiphene group (39.5%, $p = 0.002$) or the combination-therapy group (46.0%, $p < 0.001$). With the exception of pregnancy complications, adverse-event rates were similar in all groups, although gastrointestinal side effects were more frequent and vasomotor and ovulatory symptoms were less frequent in the metformin group than in the clomiphene group. Among pregnancies, the rate of multiple pregnancies was 6.0% in the clomiphene group, 0% in the metformin group, and 3.1% in the combination-therapy group. Clomiphene was superior to metformin in achieving live birth in infertile women with the PCOS, although multiple births is a complication. However, the authors also made the following observations based on their data: (a) randomized trials should be performed to determine the risks and benefits of continued use of metformin throughout pregnancy as their study did not address this question, (b) women with PCOS do have an increased rate of complications such as gestational diabetes (12% in this study, vs. 2% to 5% in the general U.S. population) and preeclampsia (12% in this study vs. 3% to 8% in the general U.S. population), (c) obesity contributes to the risk of pregnancy complications, and (d) subjects in the Legro study received extended-release metformin, which may be less efficacious in women with PCOS than is immediate-release metformin.[93]

• GLP-1 Analogues

Because GLP-1 levels are reduced in patients with PCOS, the use of a GLP-1 agonist would appear to be a reasonable pharmacologic choice for reversing many of the metabolic anomalies associated with the disorder.[13] However, randomized placebo-controlled clinical trials evaluating safety and efficacy of incretin mimetics have not been performed in large numbers of patients.

TABLE 4-7. Pharmacotherapy for Patients with PCOS

Agent	Mechanism of Action	Examples	Uses			
			Acne	Restores Menses	Ovulation Insulin	Lowers Induction Levels
Oral contraceptives (combined estrogen and progestin)	Increase SHBG. Suppress LH and FSH Decrease ovarian androgen production Progestin is an antiandrogen.	EE + norgestimate (Ortho-tryclin) EE + desogestrel (Ortho-Cept) EE + drospirenone (Yasmin)	+	+		
Antiandrogens	Decreases binding affinity of androgens at receptors	Spironolactone	+			
Metformin	Decreases HGP Reduces ovarian steroidogenesis	Metformin (Glucophage) Metformin XR (Fortamet)	+	+	+	+
Thiazolidinediones	Insulin sensitizer Direct effect on ovarian steroidogenesis	Pioglitazone (Actos)	+	+	+	+

SHBG, sex-hormone binding globulin; LH, luteinizing hormone; FSH, follicle-stimulating hormone; EE, ethinyl estradiol; HGP, hepatic glucose production.

GLP-1 secretion from the L-sells of the distal small intestines occurs in response to food intake. GLP-1 accentuates glucose-dependent insulin production and secretion by the pancreatic β-cell, and inhibits glucagon secretion in a glucose-dependent manner. GLP-1 also suppresses appetite, reduces energy intake, and delays gastric emptying.[94] All of these actions favor maintenance of the euglycemic state. Patients with T2DM appear to have either reduced levels of circulating GLP-1 or GLP-1 resistance secondary to chronic hyperglycemia. Individuals treated with GLP-1 analogues demonstrate a favorable reduction in A1C, fasting plasma glucose levels, and weight, as well as improvement in cardiovascular risk biomarkers.

In a 24-week randomized controlled trial in women with PCOS, exenatide plus metformin was found to be superior to exenatide or metformin monotherapy in reducing weight (mean weight loss of 6 ± 0.5 kg) while improving menstrual cycles, ovulation rate, free androgen index, and insulin sensitivity.[95]

Liraglutide has not been studied specifically in patients with PCOS. However, a subset of PCOS patients was included in weight loss studies involving nondiabetic obese subjects. Whether liraglutide had any positive effects on weight loss, restoration of normal menstrual cycles, or return to fertility is unclear.

• Bariatric Surgery

Although bariatric surgery may be considered as an effective therapy in patients with severe clinical obesity, few studies have shown any significant improvement in weight, hirsutism, insulin resistance, or fertility in women with PCOS.[96]

The pharmacologic therapies used for PCOS are summarized in Table 4-7.

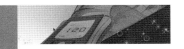

SUMMARY

Patients with PCOS present with overt symptoms of infertility, menstrual irregularities, hirsutism, and acne. Many patients also possess metabolic and hormonal abnormalities that can significantly increase their risk for developing coronary artery disease, T2DM, and endometrial carcinoma. Many patients have obstructive sleep apnea, which may aggravate insulin resistance and weight gain. PCPs should screen patients suspected of having PCOS. Early recognition of this disorder may reverse the physical signs associated with the disease, while correcting the metabolic abnormalities that can pose a significant health risk for untreated individuals. Although lifestyle modification and pharmacotherapy are used to treat PCOS, there remains a paucity of long-term outcome data regarding the benefits of metabolic interventional strategies for patients with PCOS. Insulin sensitizers can improve ovulatory function, lower insulin resistance, lower androgen levels, and increase the likelihood of becoming pregnant. The use of clomiphene citrate has also been found to be effective at inducing ovulation in women with PCOS desiring pregnancy. Patients with PCOS should be screened for major depression and suicide risk.

REFERENCES

1. Kitzinger C, Willmott J. "The thief of womanhood:" women's experience of polycystic ovarian syndrome. *Soc Sci Med.* 2002;54:349–361.
2. Stein I, Leventhal N. Amenorrhea associated with bilateral polycystic ovaries. *Am J Obstet Gynecol.* 1935;29:181–191.
3. Hardiman P, Pillay OC, Atiomo W. Polycystic ovary syndrome and endometrial carcinoma. *Lancet.* 2003;361:1810–1812.
4. Svatikova A, Wolk R, Gami AS, et al. Interactions between obstructive sleep apnea and the metabolic syndrome. *Curr Diabetes Rep.* 2005;5:53–58.
5. Coviello AD. Polycystic ovary syndrome: multiple pathways to a common phenotype? *Endocr Pract.* 2009;15(4):387–389.
6. Hart R, Hickey M, Franks S. Definitions, prevalence and symptoms of polycystic ovaries and polycystic ovary syndrome. *Best Prac Res Clin Obstet Gynaecol.* 2004;18:671–683.
7. Ibanez L, Valls C, Potau N, et al. Polycystic ovary syndrome after precocious pubarche: ontogeny of the low-birthweight effect. *Clin Endocrinol (Oxf).* 2001;55:667–672.
8. Kahsar-MillerMD, Nixon C, Boots LR, et al. Prevalence of polycystic ovary syndrome (PCOS) in first-degree relatives of patients with PCOS. *Fertil Steril.* 2001;75(1):53–58
9. Waldstreicher J, Santoro NF, Hall JE, et al. Hyperfunction of the hypo-thalamic-pituitary axis in women with polycystic ovary disease: indirect evidence for partial gonadotroph desensitization. *J Clin Endocrinol Metab.* 1988;66:165–172.
10. Ehrmann DA. Medical progress: polycystic ovary syndrome. *N Engl J Med.* 2005;352:1223–1236.
11. Nelson VL, Qin KN, Rosenfield RL, et al. The biochemical basis for increased testosterone production in theca cells propagated from patients with polycystic ovary syndrome. *J Clin Endocrinol Metab.* 2001;86:5925–5933.
12. Sherif K. Polycystic ovary syndrome in primary care. *Female Patient.* 2005;30:24–28.
13. Svendsen PF, Nilas L, Madsbad S, et al. Incretin hormone secretion in women with polycystic ovary syndrome: roles of obesity, insulin sensitivity, and treatment with metformin. *Metab Clin Exp.* 2009;(58):586–593.
14. Legro RS, Castracane VD, Kauffman RP. Detecting insulin resistance in polycystic ovary syndrome: purposes and pitfalls. *Obstet Gynecol Surv.* 2004;59:141–154.
15. Rotterdam ESHRE/ASRM-Sponsored PCOS Consensus Workshop Group. Revised 2003 consensus on diagnostic criteria and long-term health risks related to polycystic ovary syndrome. *Fertil Steril.* 2004;81:19–25.
16. Geist SH, Gains JA. Diffuse luteinization of the ovaries associated with masculinization syndrome. *Am J Obstet Gynecol.* 1942;43:975.
17. Legro RS. Diagnostic criteria in polycystic ovary syndrome. *Semin Reprod Med.* 2003;21:267–275.

18. Hunter MH, Carek PJ. Evaluation and treatment of women with hirsutism. *Am Fam Physician.* 2003;67:2565–2572.

19. Carmina E. Prevalence of idiopathic hirsutism. *Eur J Endocrinol.* 1998;139:421–423.

20. Timpatanapong P, Rojanasakul A. Hormonal profiles and prevalence of polycystic ovary syndrome in women with acne. *J Dermatol.* 1997;24:223–229.

21. DeNino WF, Tchernof A, Dionne IJ, et al. Contribution of abdominal adiposity to age-related differences in insulin sensitivity and plasma lipids in healthy nonobese women. *Diabetes Care.* 2001;24:925–932.

22. Vrbíková J, Cibula D, Dvoráková K, et al. Insulin sensitivity in women with polycystic ovary syndrome. *J Clin Endocrinol Metab.* 2004;89(6):2942–2945.

22a. Luque-Ramirez M, Alvarez-Blasco F, Botella-Carretero JI, et al. Increased body iron stores of obese women with polycystic ovary syndrome are a consequence of insulin resistance and hyperinsulinism and are not a result of reduced menstrual loss. *Diabetes Care* 2007;30:2309–2313.

23. Fogel RB, Malhotra A, Pillar G, et al. Increased prevalence of obstructive sleep apnea syndrome in obese women with polycystic ovary syndrome. *J Clin Endocrinol Metab.* 2001;86:1175–1180.

24. American Academy of Sleep Medicine. Sleep-related breathing disorders in adults: recommendations for syndrome definition and measured techniques in clinical research. The Report of an American Academy of Sleep Medicine Taskforce. *Sleep.* 1999;22:667–689.

25. Cappuccio FP, D'elia L, Strazzullo P, et al. Quantity and quality of sleep and incidence of type 2 diabetes: a systematic review and meta-analysis. *Diabetes Care.* 2010;33:414–420.

26. Chin-Chance C, Polonsky KS, Schoeller DA. Twenty-four-hour leptin levels respond to cumulative short-term energy imbalance and predict subsequent intake. *J Clin Endocrinol Metab.* 2000;85:2685–2691.

26a. van der Lely AJ, Tschop M, Heiman ML, et al. Biological, physiological, pathophysiological, and pharmacological aspects of ghrelin. *Endocr Rev.* 2004;25:426–457.
Tasali E, Chapotot F, Leproult R, et al. Treatment of obstructive sleep apnea improves cardiometabolic function in young obese women with polycystic ovary syndrome. *J Clin Endocrinol Metab* 2011;96:365–374.

26b. Tasali E, Chapotot F, Leproult R, et al. Treatment of obstructive sleep apnea improves cardiometabolic function in young obese women with polycystic ovary syndrome. *J Clin Endocrinol Metab.* 2011;96:365–374.

27. Hermanns-Le T, Scheen A, Pierard GE. Acanthosis nigricans associated with insulin resistance: pathophysiology and management. *Am J Clin Dermatol.* 2004;5:199–203.

28. Vermeulen A, Verdonck L, Kaufman JM. A critical evaluation of simple methods for the estimation of free testosterone in serum. *J Clin Endocrinol Metab.* 1999;84:3666–3672.

29. Laven JS, Imani B, Eijkermans MJ, et al. New approach to polycystic ovary syndrome and other forms of anovulatory infertility. *Obstet Gynecol Surv.* 2002;57:755–767.

30. Cibula D, Hill M, Starka L. The best correlation of the new index of hyperandrogenism with the grade of increased hair. *Eur J Endocrinol.* 2000;143:405–408.

31. Luthold WW, Borges MF, Marcondes JA, et al. Serum testosterone fractions in women: normal and abnormal clinical states. *Metabolism.* 1993;42:638–643.

32. Meldrum DR, Abraham GE. Peripheral and ovarian venous concentration of various steroid hormones in virilizing ovarian tumors. *Obstet Gynecol.* 1979;53:36–43.

33. Redmond GP. Clinical evaluation of the woman with an androgenic disorder. In: Redmond GP, ed. *Androgenic Disorders.* New York: Raven Press; 1995:1–20.

34. Taylor AE, McCourt B, Martin K, et al. Determinants of abnormal gonadotropin secretion in clinically defined women with PCOS. *J Clin Endocrinol Metab.* 1997;82:2248–2256.

35. Sherif K. Benefits and risks of oral contraceptives. *Am J Obstet Gynecol.* 1999;180(6 Pt 2):S343–S348.

36. 2002 Third Report of the National Cholesterol Education Program (NCEP) Expert Panel on Detection, Evaluation, and Treatment of High Blood Cholesterol in Adults (Adult Treatment Panel III) final report. *Circulation.* 2002;106:3143–3421.

37. Berneis K, Rizzo Manfredi R, Lazzaroni V, et al. Atherogenic lipoprotein phenotype and low-density size and subclasses in women with polycystic ovary syndrome. *Clin Endocrin and Metab.* 2007;92(1):186–189.

38. Legro RS, Kunselman AR, Dodson WC, et al. Prevalence and predictors of risk for type 2 diabetes and impaired glucose tolerance in polycystic ovary syndrome: a prospective, controlled study in 254 affected women. *J Clin Endocrinol Metab.* 1999;84:165–169.

39. Krosnick A. The diabetes and obesity epidemic among the Pima Indians. *N Engl J Med.* 2000;97:31–37.

40. Dunaif A. Insulin resistance and the polycystic ovary syndrome (PCOS): mechanism and implications for pathogenesis. *Endocr Rev.* 1997;18:774–800.

41. Dunaif A. Finegood DT. beta cell dysfunction independent of obesity and glucose intolerance in the polycystic ovary syndrome. *J Clin Endocrinol Metab.* 1996;81:942–947.

42. Kousta E, Cela E, Lawrence N. The prevalence of polycystic ovaries in women with a history of gestational diabetes. *Clin Endocrinol (Oxf)*. 2000;53:501–507.

43. Freeman R, Pollack R, Rosenbloom E. Assessing impaired glucose tolerance and insulin resistance in polycystic ovarian syndrome with a muffin test: an alternative to the glucose tolerance test. *Endocr Pract*. 2010;1(5):810–817.

44. Harano Y, Sakamoto A, Izumi K, et al. Usefulness of maltose for testing glucose tolerance. *Am J Clin Nutr*. 1977;30:924–931.

45. Polson DW, Adams J, Wadsworth J, et al. Polycystic ovaries: a common finding in normal women. *Lancet*. 1988;1(8590):870–872.

46. Yeh HC, Futterweit W, Thornton JC. Polycystic ovarian disease: U.S. features in 104 patients. *Radiology*. 1987;163:111–116.

47. Balen A. Ovulation induction for polycystic ovary syndrome. *Hum Fertil (Camb)*. 2003;3:106–111.

48. Dewailly D, Ardaens Y, Robert Y. Ultrasound for the evaluation of PCOS. In: Azziz A, Nestler JE, Dewailly D, eds. *Androgen Excess Disorders in Women*. Philadelphia, PA: Lippincott-Raven. 1997:269–278.

49. Kinkhabwala S, Schiano TD, Futterweit W, et al. Prevalence of non-alcoholic fatty liver disease in polycystic ovary syndrome. *Program of the 87th Annual Meeting of the Endocrine Society*, San Diego, CA, June 5, 2005; p 445 (Abstract P2-365).

50. Marchesini G, Brizi M, Morselli-Labate AM, et al. Association of nonalcoholic fatty liver disease with insulin resistance. *Am J Med*. 1999;107:450–455.

51. Peppard HR, Marfori J, Iuomo MJ, et al. Prevalence of polycystic ovary syndrome among premenopausal women with type 2 diabetes. *Diabetes Care*. 2001;24:1050–1052.

52. Ford ES, Giles WH, Dietz WH. Prevalence of the metabolic syndrome among U.S. adults: findings from the third National Health and Nutrition Examination Survey. *JAMA*. 2002;287:356–359.

53. U.S. Department of Health and Human Services (DHHS). National Center for Health Statistics. *Third National Health and Nutrition Examination Survey (NHANES III), 1988–1994*. Hyattsville, MD: Center for Disease Control and Prevention; 1996.

54. Insulin Resistance Syndrome Task Force. American College of Endocrinology Position Statement on the Insulin Resistance Syndrome. *Endocr Pract*. 2003;9;236–252.

55. Nestler JE. Insulin resistance syndrome and polycystic ovary syndrome. *Endocr Pract*. 2003;9 (suppl 2):86–89.

56. Laws A, Reaven GM. Evidence for an independent relationship between insulin resistance and fasting plasma HDL-cholesterol, triglyceride and insulin concentrations. *J Intern Med*. 1992;231:25–30.

57. American Association of Clinical Endocrinologists Polycystic Ovary Syndrome Writing Committee. American Association of Clinical Endocrinologists Clinical Position Statement on Metabolic and Cardiovascular Consequences of Polycystic Ovary Syndrome. *Endocr Pract*. 2005;11:126–134.

58. Legro RS, Gnatuk CL, Kunselman AR, et al. Changes in glucose tolerance over time in women with polycystic ovary syndrome: a controlled study. *J Clin Endocrinol Metab*. 2005;90:3236–3242.

59. Solomon CG, Hu FB, Dunaif A, et al. Long or highly irregular menstrual cycles as a marker for risk of type 2 diabetes mellitus. *JAMA*. 2001;286:2421–2426.

60. Legro RS, Kunselman AR, Danaif A. Prevalence and predictors of dyslipidemia in women with polycystic ovary syndrome. *Am J Med*. 2001;111:607–613.

61. Wild S, Pierpoint T, Jacobs H, et al. Long-term consequences of polycystic ovary syndrome: results of a 31 year follow-up study. *Hum Fertil (Camb)*. 2000;3:101–105.

62. Patel AA, Bloomgarden ZT, Futterweit W. Premicroalbuminuria in women with polycystic ovary syndrome: a metabolic marker. *Endocr Pract*. 2008;14(2):193–200.

63. Christian RC, Dumesic DA, Behrenbeck T, et al. Prevalence and predictors of coronary artery calcification in women with polycystic ovary syndrome. *J Clin Endocrinol Metab*. 2003;88:2562–2580.

64. Atiomo WU, Bates SA, Condon JE, et al. The plasminogen activator system in women with polycystic ovary syndrome. *Fertil Steril*. 1998;69:236–241.

65. Dahlgren E, Janson PO, Johansson S, et al. Polycystic ovary syndrome and risk for myocardial infarction: evaluated from a risk factor model based on a prospective population study of women. *Acta Obstet Gynecol Scand*. 1992;71:599–604.

66. Polson DW, Adams J, Wadsworth J, et al. Polycystic ovaries: a common finding in normal women. *Lancet*. 1988;1:870–872.

67. Birdsall MA, Farquhar CM, White HD. Association between polycystic ovaries and extent of coronary artery disease in women having cardiac catheterization. *Ann Intern Med*. 1997;126:32–35.

68. Solomon CG, Hu FB, Dunaif A. Menstrual cycle irregularity and risk for future cardiovascular disease. *J Clin Endocrinol Metab*. 2002;87:2013–2017.

69. Balen A. Polycystic ovary syndrome and cancer. *Hum Reprod Update.* 2001;7:522–525.
70. Barnard L, Ferriday D, Guenther N, et al. Quality of life and psychological well being in polycystic ovary syndrome. *Hum Reprod.* 2007;22:2279–2286.
71. Hollinrake E, Abreu A, Maifeld M, et al. Increased risk of depressive disorders in women with polycystic ovary syndrome *Fertil Steril.* 2007;87:1369–1376.
72. Bishop SCB, Basch S, Futterweit W. Polycystic ovary syndrome, depression and affective disorders. *Endocr Pract.* 2009;15(5):475–482.
73. Gu K, Cowie CC, Harris MI. Diabetes and decline in heart disease mortality in heart disease mortality in U.S. adults. *JAMA.* 1999;281:129–1297.
74. Kuhl H. Comparitive pharmacology of newer progestogens. *Drugs.* 1996;51:188–215.
75. Guido M, Romualdi D, Giuliani M. Drospirenone for the treatment of hirsute women with polycystic ovary syndrome: a clinical, endocrinological, metabolic pilot study. *J Clin Endocrinol Metab.* 2004;89:2817–2823.
76. Spritzer PM, Lisboa KO, Mattiello S, et al. Spironolactone as a single agent for long-term therapy of hirsute patients. *Clin Endocrinol (Oxf).* 2000;52:587–594.
77. Tartagni M, Schonauer MM, Cicinelli E, et al. Intermittent low-dose finasteride is as affective as daily administration for the treatment of hirsute women. *Fertil Steril.* 2004;82:752–756.
78. Mansfield R, Galea R, Brincat M, et al. Metformin has direct effects on human ovarian steroidogenesis. *Fertil Steril.* 2003;79:956–962.
79. Lord JM, Flight IHK, Norman RJ. Insulin-sensitising drugs (metformin, troglitazone, rosiglitazone, pioglitazone, D-chiro-inositol) for polycystic ovary syndrome. *Cochrane Database Syst Rev.* 2003;3:CD003053.
80. Yasuda N, Inoue T, Nagakura T, et al. Enhanced secretion of glycagon-like peptide 1 by biguanide compounds. *Biochem Biophys Res Commun.* 2002;298:779–784.
81. Lenhard JM, Croom DK, Minnick DT. Reduced serum dipeptidyl peptidase-IV after metformin and pioglitazone treatments. *Biochem Biophys Res Commun.* 2004;324:92–97.
82. Mannucci E, Tessi F, Bardini G, et al. Effects of metformin on glucagon-like peptide-1 levels in obese patients with and without type 2 diabetes. *Diabetes Nutr Metab.* 2004;17:336–342.
83. Glueck CJ, Wang P, Goldenberg N, et al. Pregnancy outcomes among women with polycystic ovary syndrome treated with metformin. *Hum Reprod.* 2002;17:2858–2864.
84. Sharpless JL. Polycystic ovary syndrome and the metabolic syndrome. *Clin Diabetes.* 003;21:154–161.
85. Nestler JE. Should patients with polycystic ovary syndrome be treated with metformin? An enthusiastic endorsement. *Hum Reprod.* 2002;17:1950–1953.
86. Knowler WC, Barrett-Connor E, Fowler SE, et al. Reduction in the incidence of type 2 diabetes with lifestyle intervention or metformin. *N Engl J Med.* 2002;346:393–403.
87. Mitwally MF, Witchel SF, Casper RF. Troglitazone: a possible modulator of ovarian steroidogenesis. *J Soc Gynecol Investig.* 2002;9:163–167.
88. Belli SH, Graffigna MN, Oneto A, et al. Effect of rosiglitazone on insulin resistance, growth factors, and reproductive disturbances in women with polycystic ovary syndrome. *Fertil Steril.* 2004;81:624–629.
89. Romualdi D, Guido M, Ciampelli M. Selective effects of pioglitazone on insulin and androgen abnormalities in normo- and hyperinsuinaemic obese patients with polycystic ovary syndrome. *Hum Reprod.* 2003;18:1210–1218.
90. Baillargeon JP, Jakubowicz DJ, Iuorno MJ, et al. Effects of metformin and rosiglitazone, alone and in combination, in nonobese women with polycystic ovary syndrome and normal indices of insulin sensitivity. *J Clin Endocrinol Metab.* 2004;82:893-902.
91. Bloomgarden ZT. Thiazolidinediones. *Diabetes Care.* 2006;28:488–493.
92. Legro RS, Barnhart HX, Schlaff WD, et al. Clomiphene, metformin, or both for infertility in the polycystic ovary syndrome. *N Engl J Med.* 2007;356:551–566.
93. Gusler G, Gorsline J, Levy G, et al. Pharmacokinetics of metformin gastric-retentive tablets in healthy volunteers. *J Clin Pharmacol.* 2001;41:655–661.
94. Unger J, Parkin C. Type 2 diabetes: an expanded view of pathophysiology and therapy. *Postgrad Med.* 2010;122(3):145–157.
95. Elkind-Hirsch K, Marrioneaux O, Bhushan M, et al. Comparison of single and combined treatment with exenatide and metformin on menstrual cyclicity in overweight women with polycystic ovary syndrome. *J Clin Endocrinol Metab.* 2008;93(7):2670–2678.
96. Escobar-Morreale HF, Botella-Carretero-Botella JI, Blasco-Ivarez FA, et al. The polycystic ovary syndrome associated with morbid obesity may resolve after weight loss induced bariatric surgery. *J Clin Endocrinol Metab.* 2005;90(12):6364–6369.

Prevention, Diagnosis, and Treatment of Microvascular Complications

PART 1/DIABETIC NEUROPATHY

News flash: Well-managed diabetes is the
leading cause of …NOTHING.
—*Bill Polonsky, PhD, CDE. Director, Diabetes*
  Behavioral Institute, San Diego, CA

■ Historical Perspective

When insulin was discovered in 1922 by Fredrick Banting and Charles Best, only 2% of the population of industrialized countries had diabetes. Patients managing to survive the effects of severe calorie-restricted diets prescribed as the only means of treatment for diabetes often suffered from cataracts, blindness, severe foot and leg infections, sterility, boils, and tuberculosis. Infectious diseases that could be managed successfully in nonimmune compromised patients proved fatal to diabetics. Patients with gangrene or postoperative infections would often be left to linger until death because little could be done to promote acceptable wound healing or reduce their emotionally charged neuropathic pain. Women who were able to conceive rarely were able to carry the fetus to term. Diabetes became a death sentence to those afflicted by the disease. The life expectancy of patients with T1DM diabetes was between 6 and 12 months from the time of diagnosis. Most patients died in hospital wards where medical personnel offered only starvation as a therapeutic option to those who were already emaciated and dehydrated from acute diabetic ketoacidosis.

Death from diabetic ketoacidosis in 1900 overstimulated the senses of patients and health-care providers alike as described in "The History of Insulin" by Michael Bliss.[1]

"When the doctors found an abundance of ketones in the urine, they knew the diabetes was entering the final states. They could smell it, too, for some ketone bodies were also volatile and were breathed out. It was a sickish-sweet smell, like rotten apples, that sometimes pervaded whole rooms or hospital wards."

There is little doubt that the discovery of insulin has had the most significant effect on global health than any other drug in history. For the first time, physicians had a truly effective and powerful weapon against a mortal disease. Yet insulin was not a "cure" for diabetes. Following the awarding of the Nobel Prize in medicine (1923) to the discoverers of insulin, Dr. Elliott Joslin predicted that the era of the coma as the central problem of diabetes would give way to the era of complications.[1] The miracle of insulin has been to multiply the life expectancy of patients with diabetes 25-fold. No longer are patients dying of diabetic ketoacidosis but of the complications related to chronic exposure to hyperglycemia.

Historians view the success of insulin with stunning irony. Insulin has allowed patients with diabetes to live longer and to propagate. The number of people worldwide with diabetes began and is continuing to rise. Many patients with diabetes who are not aggressively managed, especially from the onset of their disease, develop complications that are costly to themselves as well as to society. Although so many people worldwide were celebrating the discovery of insulin, others were prophesying that the introduction of insulin as a life-saving treatment for diabetes would cause society to bear a financial burden for patients who become long-term survivors. In 1923, Dr. Otto Leyton of London urged that insulin "be given free to poor diabetics *only* on the condition that they have no progeny."[2]

The prediction in the 1920s that prolonging the lives of patients with diabetes would result in economic hardship has certainly become a modern reality. Thus, with the discovery of insulin, the true complexity of the diabetic state was beginning to unfold. The era of death from coma was transformed into an era of death from complications. When Banting received his standing ovation upon being presented with his Nobel Prize for medicine in 1923, the attendees at the ceremony honestly believed that the mystery of diabetes had been solved. Little did they know that the true complexity of diabetes would become apparent only when patients lifespans approached those of euglycemic individuals.

As patients diagnosed with diabetes are living years longer than those diagnosed only 10 to 20 years ago, exposure to "cumulative glycemic burden" favors the activation of microvascular and macrovascular complications pathways.[3,4] Prior to 2004, the American Diabetes Association (ADA) recommended that the A1C not be allowed to exceed 8% and that patients be treated to a goal of 7%.[5] By dropping the 8% "action threshold" in favor of a general recommendation to treat "most patients" to less than 7% in 2004, the ADA for the first time acknowledged the importance of reducing one's exposure to chronic hyperglycemia.[6] Yet not all patients with excessive glycemic burdens will develop complications while others with minimal exposure to hyperglycemia may lose their vision. Thus, physicians who manage patients with diabetes must be fully aware of one's customized metabolic targets, family history, environmental factors, which may trigger complication pathways (obesity, smoking, alcohol use, physical inactivity) and duration of disease in order to minimize one's complication risk. Compassionate care for primary care providers is defined by one's ability to assist patients navigate safely through a "minefield laden with complication pathway triggers" while balancing one's quest to achieve metabolic normalcy.

Risk Factors for Developing Microvascular Disease Extend beyond Glycemic Control

The basic tenet that targeted glycemic control minimizes one's risk of developing long-term complications appears to be well established based on epidemiologic observations and prospective clinical trials. Published standards of care suggest maintaining A1C levels as close to normal as possible.[7] Unfortunately, some patients with well-managed diabetes may still develop long-term complications, while others with poor control appear to be immune from any ill effects of chronic hyperglycemia.[8] How can this inequity of diabetes-related complications be explained to patients who are doing all they can to minimize risk as well as to those who are nonadherent to all therapeutic interventions?

The Joslin Gold Medalists comprise 351 U.S. residents who have survived with T1DM for greater than 50 years.[9] A high proportion of Medalists remain free from proliferative diabetic retinopathy (42.6%), nephropathy (86.9%), neuropathy (39.4%), or cardiovascular disease (51.5%).

Why would patients who for so long were using only one to two injections of insulin per day who had no access to intensive glucose monitoring, blood pressure (BP) or lipid management have exceeded all expectations by minimizing their prevalence of complications? Other patients with T1DM develop proliferative retinopathy and chronic kidney disease despite remaining vigilant in maintaining their prescribed A1C levels. Clearly, factors other than simple glycemic control factor into long-term outcomes for all patients with diabetes.

One of the most important contributors to diabetes complications are the accumulation of advanced glycation end products (AGEs). AGEs develop as a result of nonenzymatic, irreversible glycation of proteins, lipids, and nucleic acids.[10] Chronic hyperglycemia, glycemic variability, and oxidative stress drive the formation of AGEs, which bind to receptors (RAGE) on endothelial cells. Once receptor bound, AGEs contribute to vascular injury by increasing procoagulant activity, adhesion molecule expression, monocyte influx, altered endothelial cell signaling, vascular stiffness, and oxidative stress.[10]

In the Joslin Gold Medalist population, AGE levels had an *inverse* relationship to microvascular complication rate. Could these unique individuals have a genetically expressed self-defense mechanism, which protected them against long-term microvascular events? After all, AGEs are not "user friendly" and tend to upregulate complications.[11] As shown in Figure 5-1, the binding of AGEs to AGE receptors would normally upregulate the expression of multiple complication pathways.[12] The

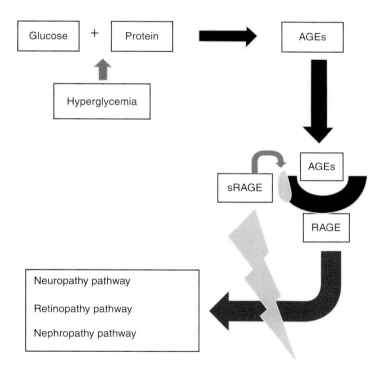

Figure 5-1 • Protective Mechanism of the Advanced Glycation End Product (AGE) Pathway.
AGEs form via nonenzymatic glycation of proteins, lipids, and nucleic acids. Once formed, AGEs promote vascular stiffness and alter cellular receptor signaling by binding with AGE receptors (RAGE). The greater the number of AGEs bound to RAGE, the more enhanced oxidative stress becomes resulting in a downstream cascade of events, which, over a number of years, will often result in a number of microvascular complications. However, in patients who "escape" microvascular disease despite having a history of prolonged hyperglycemia and elevated AGEs, binding of AGEs to RAGE induces the release of a soluble receptor ligand known as sRAGE. sRAGE competitively reduces activation of AGE complication pathways, thereby blocking the downstream cascade mechanism which would otherwise induce microvascular complications. Patients who are genetically prone to producing the sRAGE ligand may be spared complications. Those who cannot produce the sRAGE ligand may be at higher risk of developing microvascular disease. (Adapted from Yan SF, Ramasamy R, Schmidt AM. The RAGE axis: a fundamental mechanism signaling danger to the vulnerable vasculature. *Circ Res.* 2010:106:842–853.)

more AGEs become receptor bound, the greater the likelihood of developing a complication over time. However, patients, such as the Joslin Gold Medalists, appear to have been provided with a truly unique gift from their parents known as a "soluble" AGE. As the AGE binds to the RAGE, a small protein ligand breaks free of the receptor effectively "blocking" the complication pathway from progressing forward. Patients who can produce the "soluble RAGE" are likely to be symptom free, whereas those patients who lack the soluble component are prone to develop the complications.

From a clinical perspective, the lessons learned from the Joslin Gold Medalist suggest that patients who demonstrate few if any microvascular and macrovascular complications 15 to 20 years after being diagnosed with diabetes may be at lower risk of complications. Targeting an A1C of 6% to 7% in these individuals may not be necessary and could increase the likelihood of developing hypoglycemia. However, patients who develop complications within 5 to 10 years of being diagnosed with diabetes may not have protective mechanisms to minimize the progression of retinopathy, neuropathy, and nephropathy. These patients should be identified and treated ambitiously, making certain that they achieve all of their metabolic targets. In addition, such individuals should be screened for macrovascular complications. Lifestyle interventions, such as weight loss, smoking and alcohol cessation, exercise, and self-blood glucose monitoring should be emphasized.

Although HEDIS Quality Assurance programs stress the importance of treating patients' A1Cs to target, scientific evidence suggest that glycemic control may play only a minor role in the progression of *some* complications.[13] Hirsch and Brownlee have suggested that the A1C and the duration of diabetes explained only 11% of the variation in retinopathy risk for the entire Diabetes Control and Complication Trial (DCCT) study population.[14] The remaining 89% of the risk should be attributed to environmental factors, lipids, BP, glycemic variability, and genetics. Much remains to be explored to help clinicians and patients minimize their long-term complication risks.

Primary care physicians face a daunting task striving to reverse modifiable risk factors, which have been implicated in promoting complications. The percentage of U.S. adults who report themselves as being smokers, inactive, obese, overweight, and having hypertension or elevated cholesterol is shown in Figure 5-2.[15] Fortunately, the percentage of patients with diabetes who smoke has

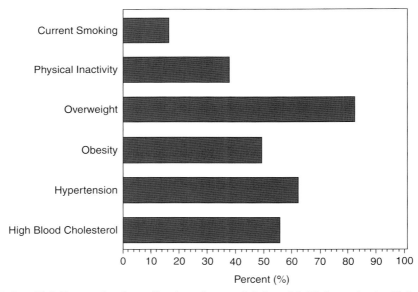

Figure 5-2 • Risk Factors for Complications Among Adults with Diabetes in the United States—2007. According to the CDC, 15.1% of U.S. adults with diabetes smoked, 38.2% reported being physically inactive, 83.5% were overweight or obese, 51.1% were obese based on self-reported height and weight, 67% had hypertension, and 62.6% said that they were diagnosed with high cholesterol. Centers for Disease Control and Prevention Data and Trends. http://www.cdc.gov/diabetes/statistics/comp/fig10.htm. Accessed December 12, 2011.

declined from 21.7% in 1994 to 20% in 2007. All other risk factor trends have been increasing during this same reporting period.[15] Duration of diabetes and exposure to glycemic burden also impact the risk of complications.[16]

Biochemical and Molecular Pathways That Trigger Diabetes-related Complications

The sequelae of chronic hyperglycemia in diabetes of all phenotypes are divided into microvascular and macrovascular complications. The consequences of microvascular disease include loss of vision, renal insufficiency, and neuropathy (distal sensory neuropathy and diabetic autonomic neuropathy [DAN]). Macrovascular complications include myocardial infarction (MI), stroke, and peripheral arterial disease (PAD). The link between glycemic burden and induction of disease-specific complication pathways has been established by four independent biochemical abnormalities: increased polyol pathway flux, increased formation of AGEs, activation of protein kinase C (PKC), and increased hexosamine pathway flux. These seemingly unrelated pathways have an underlying common denominator: an increase in oxidative stress caused by the overproduction of superoxide by the mitochondrial electron transport chain.

• Oxidative Stress

The microvascular and macrovascular complications of diabetes are believed to be caused by oxidative stress. Intracellular oxidative stress occurs when the production of reactive oxygen species (by-products of normal metabolism) exceeds the capacity of the cells' antioxidants to neutralize them, resulting in cellular dysfunction and damage.[17] Oxidative stress may be minimized by maintaining optimal control of metabolic parameters such as glucose, lipids, and BP. Endothelial cells chronically exposed to oxidative stress activate multiple complication pathways (Fig. 5-3).

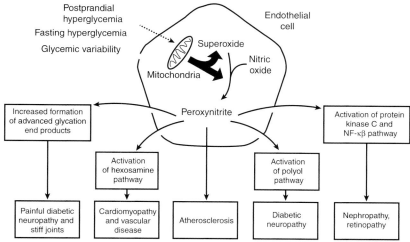

Figure 5-3 • The "Downstream Effects" of Oxidative Stress–Induced Diabetes Complication Pathways. Postprandial and fasting hyperglycemia and glycemic variability result in the production of superoxide within the mitochondria of endothelial cells. NO regulates vascular tone and minimizes adhesion molecule penetration of the vascular walls. When superoxide interacts with peroxynitrate, the endothelial cell's mitochondrial electron transport system becomes impaired, resulting in endothelial dysfunction. Transcription of endothelial-derived cytokines induces pathways known to activate microvascular complications. Peroxynitrate also favors lipid oxidation leading to atherosclerosis and macrovascular disease. NF-kβ, nuclear factor kappa B. (Adapted from Unger J. Reducing oxidative stress in patients with type 2 diabetes mellitus: a primary care call to action. *Insulin.* 2008;3:176–184.)

Endothelial cells maintain the barrier between the blood and the vascular wall. Nitric oxide (NO), which is produced within the endothelial cell, regulates vascular tone, while keeping the vessel walls smooth and free of adhesion molecules. Peroxynitrite (PN) (an NO derivative) is formed when NO interacts with superoxide produced within the mitochondria of oxidatively stressed endothelial cells. PN inhibits the endothelial cell's mitochondrial electron transport system, induces endothelial dysfunction, and activates the expression of endothelial-derived cytokines. These cytokines act like a fuse on a stick of dynamite igniting a series of pathways that, over time will promote the development of microvascular and macrovascular disease.[17,18]

Oxidative stress is triggered more powerfully by postprandial glucose fluctuations than by sustained hyperglycemia.[19] The effects of oxidative stress on long-term diabetes outcomes have important implications in clinical practice. Why do some patients who have "normal" "A1C" levels lower than 6% develop retinopathy, whereas others who have "poorly controlled diabetes" (A1C greater than 9%) remain retinopathy-free their entire lives?

In the DCCT, the diabetic retinopathy (DR) risk at identical sustained levels of A1C was significantly reduced by intensive treatment.[20] For example, in the group of patients who had a sustained A1C of 9% for the entire study duration, the risk of retinopathy was reduced by more than 50% in the intensive control group, even though both the conventional and intensively treated patients had identical A1C levels. Intensively managed patients had less DR due to improved daily glycemic variability when compared with glucose profiles of the conventionally treated patients. This study demonstrates the importance of hyperglycemia, hypoglycemia, and "malglycemia" in promoting complications. Figure 5-4A,B show a patient with chronic kidney disease and retinopathy whose initial "malglycemia" improved with the addition of a GLP-1 analogue.

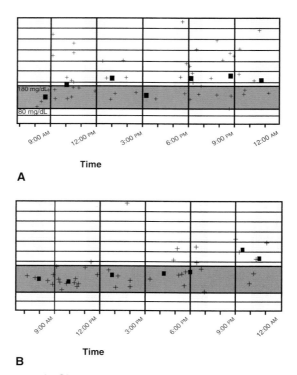

Figure 5-4 • Improvement in Glycemic Variability. A 52-year-old school teacher with stage 4 chronic kidney disease and nonproliferative retinopathy. Despite being on an insulin pump, the patient's self–blood glucose monitoring suggests wide glycemic variability as shown in panel **A.** (Each + symbol represents a glucose value obtained during that time over a 2-week interval.) The *square* represents the average fasting and postprandial glucose values over 2 weeks. After the patient was placed on liraglutide (off label with concurrent use of insulin), his glycemic control and variability were significantly improved. Although this case is *suggestive* of glycemic variability, MAGE as determined by continuous glucose sensing is the most appropriate model for measuring daily variability as shown in panel **B.** (Case courtesy of Jeff Unger, MD.)

Acute glucose fluctuations and hyperglycemia both at fasting and during the postprandial periods result in accelerated advanced glycation and the generation of oxidative stress. Chronic hyperglycemia is best assessed by measuring A1C, whereas acute fluctuations (also known as MAGE—mean amplitude of glycemic excursions) may be determined mathematically by continuous glucose monitoring.[19] Thus, both acute glycemic variability and measures of chronic hyperglycemia (A1C) are important factors in upregulating oxidative stress (Fig. 5-5). Some experts believe that glucose variability (MAGE) greater than 40 mg per dL, as measured by continuous glucose sensors, should be targeted for intensive intervention to minimize oxidative stress.[21] One should note that oxidative stress is considered the unifying mechanism, which drives all complication pathways related to diabetes.[22]

Hyperglycemia, whether acute (postprandial) or chronic, has tissue-damaging effects on cell types such as capillary endothelial cells of the retina, mesangial cells in the renal glomerulus, and peripheral neurons. Why are some cells prone to develop complications, whereas others appear to be immune to the effects of similar exposure to chronic hyperglycemia? The answer lies in a cell's ability to assimilate the amount of glucose required as an energy source before transporting nonessential glucose out of the cell. Cells (such as neurons and nephrons) that are inefficient interstitial transporters of glucose undergo oxidative stress, which induces endothelial dysfunction, vascular inflammation, and activation of pathways that trigger complications.[17] Other cells [such as those in the gastrointestinal (GI) tract] are more efficient at transporting excessive glucose from inside the cell externally, thereby minimizing the risk of oxidative stress.

Vascular endothelial cells form physical and biologic barriers between the vessel wall and the circulating blood cells, with the endothelium playing an important role in the maintenance of vascular homeostasis. Central to this role is the endothelial production of NO, which is synthesized by the constitutively expressed endothelial isoform of NO synthase. Vascular diseases, including hypertension, diabetes, and atherosclerosis are characterized by impaired endothelium-derived NO bioactivity that may contribute to clinical cardiovascular events. Endothelial cells exposed to oxidative stress generate high levels of reactive oxygen species via their mitochondrial electron-transport chain. Susceptible cells will activate biochemical pathways likely to progress toward long-term microvascular and macrovascular complications unless metabolic stability is restored.

Endothelial dysfunction drives atherosclerosis. Endothelial cell protective mechanisms (e.g., NO and prostacyclin), which are derived vasodilators, favor antiatherogenic mechanisms within the vasculature. Expression of endothelium-derived vasoconstrictors (e.g., endothelin-1 and thromboxane) has been associated with proatherosclerotic events.[23,24]

Just as a town's department of public works is responsible for repairing potholes that plague city streets, the body has the capacity to form a cellular "patch" over a site of acute endothelial injury. Derived from bone marrow, endothelial progenitor cells (EPCs) are mobilized to the peripheral

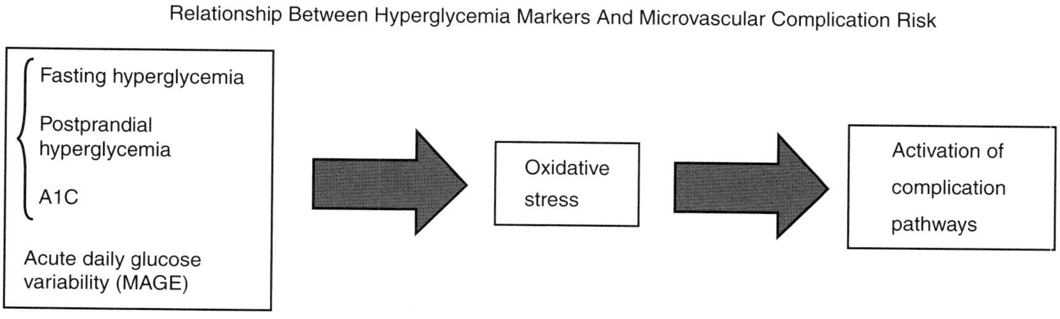

Relationship Between Hyperglycemia Markers And Microvascular Complication Risk

Figure 5-5 • Relationship between Hyperglycemia Markers and Microvascular Complication Risk. Fasting hyperglycemia and postprandial hyperglycemia both contribute to excessive glycation, resulting in a rise in A1C. Acute fluctuations in daily glycemia, as measured by continuous glucose sensors, like A1C will result in a rise in oxidative stress. Complication pathways are activated in response to oxidative stress. Therefore both chronic and acute hyperglycemic abnormalities should be targeted and controlled in order to minimize one's risk for developing long-term complications. (Adapted from Monnier L, Colette C. Glycemic variability. Should we and can we prevent it? *Diabetes Care.* 2008;(Suppl 2):S150–S154.)

circulation in response to tissue ischemia through the release of growth factors and cytokines. The EPCs hone into the ischemic or damaged tissue and stimulate endothelial repair. In addition to traditional cardiovascular risk factors, oxidative stress has been associated with reduction in the number and function of circulating EPCs, whereas an expanded EPC pool decreases cardiovascular mortality.[25]

Oxidative stress may even be induced in individuals without diabetes. Using a hyperglycemic clamp, euglycemic subjects exposed to ambient glucose levels greater than 200 mg per dL for just 2 hours were found to have increased levels of urinary F2 isoprostanes (a surrogate marker of oxidative stress).[26] Exposure to blood glucose levels greater than 180 mg per dL results in prolonged endothelial cell dysfunction and vascular inflammation, which persist for 7 days, even once the acute episode of hyperglycemia is reversed.[4] Thus, patients with both acute and chronic hyperglycemia live in a constant state of oxidative stress, a metabolic status that favors progression toward microvascular and macrovascular endpoints. From a clinical perspective, a patient who records a *fasting* blood glucose of 200 mg per dL has likely been exposed to activated oxidative stress–related metabolic pathways during their entire resting hours. Failure to recognize and reverse this glycemic burden will put patients at risk for complications that can have a profound effect on their longevity and quality of life.

Table 5-1 lists therapeutic approaches a patient may employ to reduce oxidative stress.

• Advanced Glycosylation

Nonenzymatic glycosylation and oxidation of proteins are natural phenomena of aging that occur very slowly. As glucose becomes incorporated into proteins, AGEs are formed in an irreversible chemical reaction. During this process, reactive oxygen species, such as superoxide and hydrogen peroxide, are also produced. When ambient glucose levels are elevated, the extent of glycosylation increases as sugars become attached to free amino groups on proteins, lipids, and nucleic acids, thereby altering the function and metabolism of these macromolecules. AGE receptors (RAGEs) on macrophages induce monocytes and endothelial cells to increase the production of inflammatory cytokines and adhesion molecules[27] (Fig. 5-6). The resulting basement membrane thickening can cause symptoms such as joint stiffness and diffuse pain in response to light touch. AGEs can also bind to AGE receptor sites on endothelial cell surfaces, leading to increased inflammatory responses, vascular permeability, and procoagulant activity. The ability to form and detoxify AGE by-products may be genetically predetermined, explaining why some patients who have poor glycemic control

 TABLE 5-1. Practical Approaches to Reducing Oxidative Stress

1. Use insulin analogues preferentially over human insulin because their pharmacokinetic profiles mimic physiologic pharmacokinetic profiles more closely.

2. Advise patients to inject prandial rapid-acting insulin analogues 15 min prior to meals if their baseline glucose levels are >80 mg/dL. This will allow the absorption of insulin to match up more precisely with the onset of carbohydrate absorption from the gut

3. Reducing carbohydrate intake will lessen postprandial glucose excursions

4. Exercising will improve peripheral insulin resistance and help reduce postprandial hyperglycemia

5. Use incretin therapies such as GLP-1 analogues or DPP-4 inhibitors where appropriate. These drugs work to reduce postprandial excursions.

6. Pramlintide, a synthetic analogue of human amylin, has been shown in clinical trials to reduce surrogate markers of oxidative stress

Adapted from Unger J. Reducing oxidative stress in patients with type 2 diabetes mellitus: a primary care call to action. *Insulin.* 2008;3:176–184.

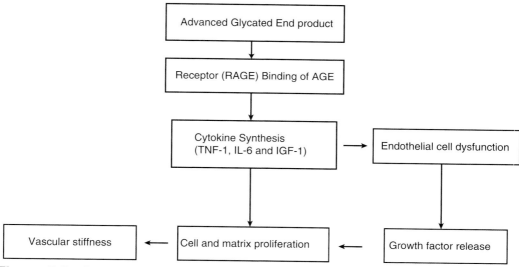

Figure 5-6 • Pathway Linking Advanced Glycation to Diabetes Complications. (See text for explanation of pathway.)

are fortunate to experience no diabetes-related complications, whereas those less fortunate with prediabetes may develop retinopathy or painful diabetic neuropathy (Fig. 5-1).

• Activation of the Polyol Pathway

During hyperglycemia, glucose levels rapidly increase in tissues, such as the kidneys, nerves and retina that are insulin-independent for glucose uptake. Excess glucose enters the polyol pathway activating aldose reductase, which increases intracellular levels of fructose and sorbitol in these complication prone target sites.[22] (Fig. 5-7). The resulting alteration in osmotic gradient favors penetration of water, protein precipitation, and cataract formation within ocular lenses. In peripheral nerves, elevated sorbitol levels leads to axonal edema, altered neurologic function and neuropathic pain. The effects of polyol pathway activation within the kidneys are debated, but may ultimately result in dysfunction of the proximal tubules.

• Activation of the Protein Kinase C Pathway

Hyperglycemia activates production of diacylglycerol (DAG), a second messenger protein that relays signals from receptors on the cell surface to target molecules within the cell (Fig. 5-8). Second messengers not only alter the normal activity of a cell, but amplify the signal, which induces the change. Among the signals induced by second messaging, DAG's primary role is activation of the PKC pathway. PKC production initiates a complex intracellular signaling cascade, affecting gene expression in many organs and tissues throughout the body.[28] The effects of the PKC enzyme within plasma membranes are cell specific. In patients with diabetes, PKC activation has been linked with retinopathy and nephropathy.

• Hexosamine Pathway

Hyperglycemia results in a diversion of glucose metabolism from glycolysis to the pathologic hexosamine pathway. The shift in normal metabolism causes a change in gene transcription within affected cells favoring the production of inflammatory cytokines as shown in Figure 5-9. Rising plasma concentrations of transforming growth factor-β1 (TGF-β1) and plasminogen activator inhibitor type-1 (PAI-1) adversely affect the kidneys and the vasculature.[22]

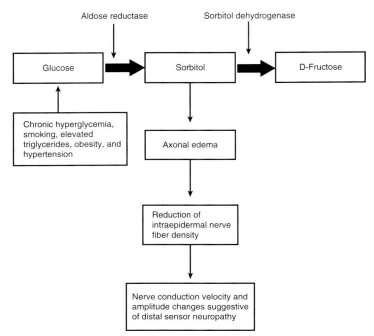

Figure 5-7 • Relationship of the polyol pathway to activation of diabetic neuropathy hyperglyce-mia results in an increased accumulation of sorbitol and fructose in cells such as neurons and retina tissue, which are unable to eliminate the excess sugars. This changes the osmotic gradient within these susceptible cells, resulting in neuronal dysfunction.

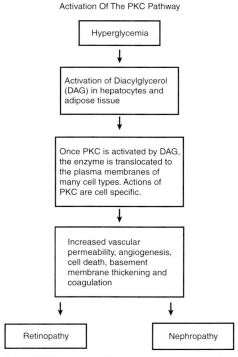

Figure 5-8 • **Activation of the PKC Pathway.** Chronic hyperglycemia induces the activation of the PKC pathway, which, when combined with increasing oxidative stress and inflammatory cytokine production, results in thickening of the renal arteriolar walls, glomerular basement membrane, and tubular basement membrane. Retinal vessels are also affected by an increase in hyperglycemia-induced PKC signaling.

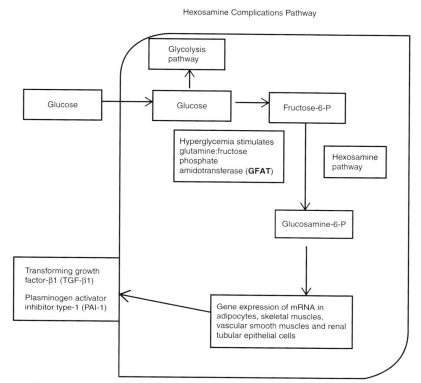

Hexosamine Pathway

Hexosamine Complications Pathway

Figure 5-9 • Hexosamine Pathway and Hexosamine Complications Pathway. The normal route of glucose metabolism is through glycolysis. During hyperglycemia, glucose is diverted into the hexosamine pathway in which an enzyme called GFAT (glutamine fructose-6 phosphate amidotransferase) converts the fructose-6 phosphate into glucosamine-6 phosphate. This results in pathologic changes in gene expression within the cell nucleus. Inflammatory cytokines, PAI-1 and TGF-β1 are produced by the cells resulting in vascular disease affecting the kidneys and arteries. (From Schleichler ED, Weigert C. Role of hexosamine biosynthetic pathway in diabetic nephropathy. *Kidney Int.* 2000;58(Suppl 77):S13–S18.)

• Neuroinflammation

Autoimmune mechanisms may play a role in both the initiation and rate of deterioration of neuropathy. The production of free radicals and superoxide can disrupt the normal neuroprotection achieved by the neurovascular unit.[29] The neurovascular unit consists of a neuron surrounded by astrocytes and microglial cells (Fig. 5-10A). Astrocytes maintain extracellular ion homeostasis within neurons.[30]

Microglial cells (Fig. 5-10A) are the resident macrophages of the central nervous system.[31] As biologic sensors, these cells continually survey the neurons, making certain that normal neurophysiologic protective mechanisms are active. Microglial cells are capable of mounting both an inflammatory and reparative response when they become "activated." Once the microglial cells become activated, through physical stress or pharmacologic interference with their protective mechanisms, they produce inflammatory cytokines [interleukin-6 (IL-6)], damage neuronal segments, and alter neurologic activity (Fig. 5-10B).[31] Opioid use has been found to activate microglial cells, causing them to produce inflammatory cytokines, which result in chronic, disabling pain.[32]

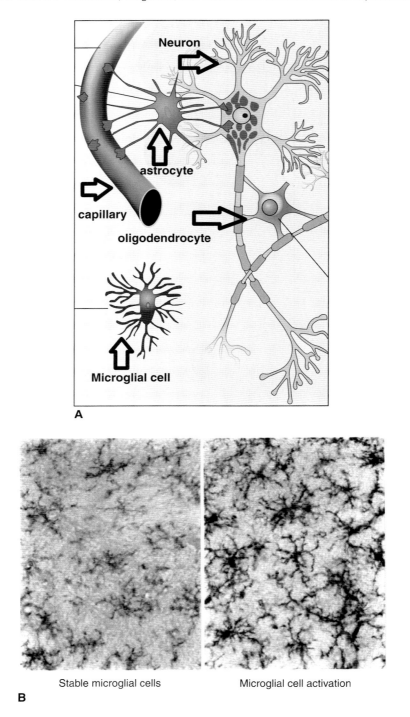

Figure 5-10 • Neuroinflammation. A. Anatomy of the neurovascular unit. **B.** Microglial cell activation. The neurovascular unit consists of astrocytes, which are modulators of ions and glutamate within neurons and microglial cells. Microglial cells are living sensors, which protect a given neuronal segment. Stable microglial cells (pictured on the left of **B**) produce a cytokine IL-10, which protect the neuron from inflammation. Microglial cell activation will occur when patients are exposed to physical or emotional stress. Certain medications, such as opioids, will also trigger microglial cell activation (shown on the right of **B**). Once activated, the microglial cells shift cytokine production to IL-6 and glutamine, both of which are inflammatory and injurious to the neuron. (Adapted from Unger J. Diabetic neuropathy: early clues, effective management. *Appl Neurol.* 2005:23–30.)

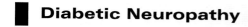

Diabetic Neuropathy

This chapter will discuss screening, diagnosis, and management of diabetic neuropathy. Microvascular disorders related to chronic kidney disease and retinopathy will be presented in Chapter 6.

• Introduction to Neuropathic Disease

The neuropathies are among the most common of the long-term complications of diabetes, affecting up to 50% of patients.[33] The clinical features of diabetic neuropathy vary immensely. Patients may present to a wide spectrum of specialists including dermatology, podiatry, urology, cardiology, psychiatry, gynecology, cardiology, family medicine, rheumatology, pain management, orthopedics, ophthalmology, audiology, ENT, and gastroenterology. Neuropathies are characterized by a progressive loss of nerve fibers and nerve fiber density, resulting in altered nerve conduction velocity. There is increasing evidence that measures of neuropathy, such as electrophysiology and quantitative tests, are predictors of not only endpoints, including foot ulceration, but also mortality.[34] Screening, diagnosing, and managing patients for both sensory and autonomic neuropathies are well within the realm of primary care. Recognizing that patients have cardiac autonomic dysfunction warrants specialty referral.

An expert panel has defined diabetic neuropathy as "the presence of symptoms and/or signs of peripheral nerve dysfunction in people with diabetes after the exclusion of other causes."[35] Neuropathy cannot be diagnosed without an appropriate neurologic examination. Because up to 75% of patients may be asymptomatic, all patients with diabetes must be screened frequently to determine the presence of signs suggestive of diabetic peripheral and autonomic neuropathies.

Neuropathy is one of the most common complications of diabetes, with a lifetime prevalence between 25% and 50% in persons with diabetes.[36] In developed countries, diabetic neuropathy accounts for 50% to 75% of nontraumatic amputations.[37] Mortality in patients with autonomic neuropathy is 25% to 50% within 10 years of the onset of symptoms.[38]

Approximately 50% of patients with diabetes experience symptomatic diabetic peripheral neuropathy (DPN), yet only 15% to 25% have symptoms severe enough to warrant treatment.[39] Estimates of the number of people in the United States with diabetic peripheral neuropathic pain (DPNP) range from 600,000 to 3.6 million.[40]

Diabetic neuropathy can be identified in patients with prediabetes and impaired glucose tolerance (IGT). A study evaluating 77 patients with idiopathic peripheral neuropathy found that 33% were diagnosed with IGT and 19% had clinical diabetes.[41] Up to 35% of patients with IGT (prediabetes) have painful neuropathy.[42]

Perkins et al. demonstrated a 30% reduction in sural nerve fiber density in patients with diabetic neuropathy in comparison to nondiabetic individuals.[43] Prolonged hyperglycemia (A1C greater than 9%) not only reduces nerve fiber density but also results in delayed nerve conduction velocity.[44] Alterations in normal nerve conduction velocity will be perceived as neuropathic pain and may contribute to autonomic dysfunction.

• Risk Factors for Developing Diabetic Neuropathy

Of the 1,172 patients with T1DM who participated in the DCCT, neuropathy developed in 23% who had no evidence of neuropathic disease at baseline.[45] The highest rates of neuropathy in patients with T2DM occur in those who have had hyperglycemia for more than 25 years. Factors other than glycemic control appear to be influential in determining risk for developing neuropathy. Elucidating the risk factors for neuropathy is important, given the association between the risk factors and increased diabetes-related morbidity and mortality. Mortality in patients with neuropathy is high, and the cause of death is often coronary heart disease.[46] Risk factors for the development of neuropathy may be categorized as modifiable and nonmodifiable (see Table 5-2).

• Definition and Classification

The typical DPN is a chronic, symmetrical, length-dependent sensorimotor polyneuropathy. DPN develops in association with a background of chronic hyperglycemia and comorbid metabolic

TABLE 5-2. Risk Factors for Diabetic Neuropathy

Neuropathy Modifiable Risk Factors	Neuropathy Nonmodifiable Risk Factors
• Obesity	• Family history
• Hypertriglyceridemia	• Advancing age
• Cigarette smoking	• Duration of diabetes
• Hypertension	
• Glycemic variability	
• A1C	

Adapted from Tesfaye S, Chaturvedi N, Eaton SEM. Vascular risk factors and diabetic neuropathy. *N Engl J Med.* 2005;352:341–350.

derangements related to hypertension and hyperlipidemia. DPN is statistically associated with other microvascular complications such as DR and diabetic neuropathy.[46]

Many proposed classifications for diabetic neuropathy have been published. For point of discussion, Table 5-3 lists a means by which the neuropathy may be localized as well as categorized. Figure 5-11 shows the pain distribution common to the sensorimotor neuropathies.

Sensorimotor Neuropathies

Diabetic amyotrophy typically occurs in patients aged 50 to 60 years who have T2DM. Presenting symptoms include severe pain and unilateral or bilateral muscle weakness associated with atrophy of the proximal thigh muscles. The cause, although unknown, may be related to infarctions in the lumbosacral plexus. Diabetic amyotrophy results in severe and debilitating pain. Patients experience difficulty in climbing stairs or simply getting up from seated positions.

TABLE 5-3. Classification of Diabetic Neuropathy

Sensorimotor Neuropathies

Examples Based Upon "Disease Localization"	Sensorimotor (Disease Location/Description)
Mononeuropathy (confined to a single nerve)	• Carpal tunnel syndrome • Tarsal tunnel syndrome • Ulnar neuropathy • Peroneal nerve entrapment syndrome • Lateral femoral cutaneous nerve entrapment syndrome
Mononeuritis multiplex (may involve the distribution of several peripheral nerves)	• Painful, simultaneous, or sequential involvement of individual nerve trunks • Evolves over days or years • Presents with acute or subacute loss of sensory and motor function of individual nerves • Pattern is initially asymmetric. • Over time symptoms may become symmetrical. • Common locations are in the low back, hip, and leg.
Plexopathy	• Diabetic amyotrophy • Diabetic truncal radiculoneuropathy
Distal sensory symmetric polyneuropathy	• Bilateral, symmetrical painful paresthesias, worse at rest and improves with activity. Most often starting in feet, then progressing to hands
Focal neuropathy	• Confined to the distribution of a single cranial or peripheral nerve

(continued)

TABLE 5-3. Classification of Diabetic Neuropathy *(Continued)*

Diabetic Autonomic Neuropathies

Classification	Clinical Concerns
Hypoglycemia awareness autonomic failure	• Loss of hypoglycemia counterregulation • May result in immediate loss of consciousness without warning that blood glucose levels are falling • Frequent episodes of hypoglycemia including exercise-induced, nocturnal and recurrent mild events occurring within the same 24-h period
Cardiac autonomic neuropathy	• Impaired autonomic control of the cardiovascular system • Associated with high risk of all-cause mortality, silent ischemia, coronary artery disease, stroke, diabetic nephropathy, and perioperative morbidity • Orthostatic hypotension common • Have abnormalities in BP regulation
Diabetic gastropathy	• Results in disordered gut motility in patients with T1DM primarily • Patients may experience impaired oral drug absorption, erratic glycemic control due to mismatch between normal absorption of insulin and delayed nutrient absorption from the gut. • Abdominal bloating, early satiety, fecal incontinence, nocturnal diarrhea, and constipation are common features. • Poor postprandial regulation of BP. Patients experience postprandial hypoglycemia • Patients express poor quality of life.
Sexual dysfunction	• Men experience loss of erectile function and loss of libido. • ED is a predictor of silent MI for patients with T2DM. • ED prevalence varies between 35% and 90% within males having diabetes. • Women have vaginal dryness and dyspareunia.
Diabetic uropathy	• Secondary to alteration of the detrusor smooth muscle, neuronal dysfunction, and urothelial dysfunction • Affects 43%–87% of patients with T1DM and 25% of T2DM • Difficulty with delayed and complete bladder emptying • Frequent urinary tract infections • Nocturia
Sudomotor dysfunction	• Sweat glands are innervated by unmyelinated cholinergic sympathetic C-fibers, which become dysfunctional in some patients with diabetes. • May result in dryness of the skin in the feet increasing one's risk of foot ulceration and infections • Loss of sweating may impair exercise function, resulting in dehydration on hot days. • High risk for Charcot arthropathy • Patients with severe sudomotor dysfunction sweat only from the neck down, not on the forehead. • Some patients may experience hyperhidrosis or gustatory sweating timed to occur within minutes of eating.

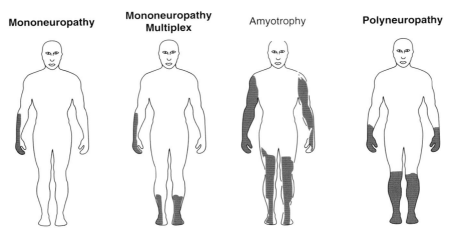

Figure 5-11 • **Pain Distribution Associated with Sensorimotor Neuropathies.** (Modified from presentation by Charles Argoff at American Conference on Pain Medicine, New York. June 16, 2007.)

Mononeuropathies

- **Focal** and **multifocal neuropathies** are confined to the distribution of a single peripheral nerve (mononeuropathy) or multiple peripheral nerves (mononeuropathy multiplex). Mononeuropathies are caused by vasculitis, ischemia of the capillaries supplying the neurons, or nerve infarcts.[47] **Cranial neuropathy** in diabetic patients is rare, typically affecting older persons with a long history of diabetes.[48] Cranial nerves III, IV, or VI may be involved (Fig. 5-12). The classic presentation of a cranial neuropathy is acute-onset diplopia with ptosis and papillary sparing associated with ipsilateral headache. Neurologic deficits resolve on average within 2½ months. Recurrence rates are 25% in patients with diabetes. Advise patients with a cranial neuropathy to wear a patch over the affected eye and to adhere to strategies that improve glycemic control.
- **Nerve entrapment syndromes** begin gradually and may become disabling over time without intervention. Most often, the median, ulnar, peroneal, lateral femoral cutaneous, or tibial nerve within the tarsal tunnel is involved. Entrapment syndromes affect up to 30% of patients with diabetes and should be evaluated carefully in all those with signs and symptoms of neuropathy.[49]
- **Carpal tunnel syndrome** (median neuropathy) is a clinically relevant problem in 6% of patients with diabetes.[50] Painful paresthesias of the fingers may progress to a deep-seated ache, which radiates proximally through the forearm. Symptoms are worse at night. Motor weakness can become progressive, and thenar wasting occurs over time.

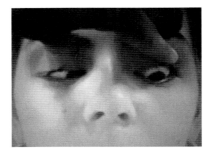

Figure 5-12 • **Left VI Nerve Palsy.** Left-sided cranial nerve VI palsy in a patient with poorly controlled T1DM (A1C = 9.6%) who recovered spontaneously within 12 weeks after the onset of her symptoms of dyplopia and unilateral headaches. (Photo courtesy of Jeff Unger, MD.)

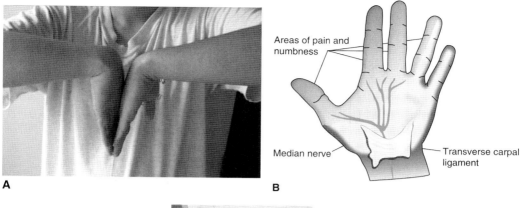

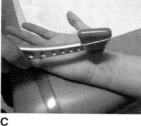

Figure 5-13 • Demonstrates Distribution of Paresthesias in a Patient with a Positive Phalen Test. A. The Phalen test—forearms held vertically and hands held in complete flexion for 1 minute—is positive if paresthesia develops in the median nerve. **B.** Distribution within 30 seconds. **C.** The Tinel sign—percussion over the median nerve that induces paresthesia over the distribution of the nerve—is suggestive of carpal tunnel syndrome.

Two clinical tests (Phalen and Tinel signs) may be used to screen for carpal tunnel syndrome as shown in Figure 5-13. The Phalen test—forearms held vertically and hands held in complete flexion for 1 minute—is positive if paresthesia develops in the median nerve distribution within 30 seconds. The Tinel sign—percussion over the median nerve that induces paresthesia over the distribution of the nerve—is suggestive of carpal tunnel syndrome. However, nerve conduction studies are required to confirm the diagnosis. Treatment options include wrist splints for nocturnal symptoms. Cortisone injections in the carpal tunnel may provide symptomatic relief; however, they often need to be repeated. Surgical intervention is required for pain relief and to prevent the acceleration of muscle wasting.

- **Ulnar neuropathy** occurs in 2% of diabetic patients as a result of nerve compression immediately distal to the ulnar groove beneath the edge of the flexor carpi ulnaris aponeurosis in the cubital tunnel. Alcoholism is a risk factor. Typical symptoms include painful paresthesias in the fourth and fifth digits associated with hypothenar and interosseous muscle wasting. Treatment is conservative. Patients with motor loss and muscle wasting may require surgical intervention.
- **Compression** of the **lateral femoral cutaneous nerve** (meralgia paresthetica), although uncommon in diabetes, can result in pain, paresthesias, and sensory loss over the lateral aspect of the thigh. Most cases resolve spontaneously. In cases associated with severe pain, allodynia, and disability, corticosteroid injections using focal nerve blocks at the inguinal ligament or surgical decompression may be required.
- **Tarsal tunnel syndrome** is a painful lower limb entrapment syndrome that involves the tibial nerve, as it traverses the tarsal tunnel. The tibial nerve innervates only the muscles of the soles. Walking or standing triggers severe burning pain over the plantar aspect of the foot. A positive Tinel sign on the underside of the medial malleolus with atrophy of the sole muscles are typical

clinical observations. Sensation over the dorsum of the foot is normal. Ankle reflexes are maintained. Nerve conduction studies demonstrate asymmetry compared with the normal leg.

Treatment options include nighttime splinting in a neutral position and targeted injections of local anesthetics and corticosteroids into the tarsal tunnel. Surgical decompression remains a controversial option in patients with diabetes who have severe pain and abnormal nerve conduction studies.[49]

- Diabetic **truncal radiculoneuropathy** affects middle-aged and elderly men. The primary feature is pain of acute onset that resolves spontaneously within 4 to 6 months. The pain—which is worse at night—is described as an aching or burning sensation with superimposed lancinating stabs. Patients describe the location of pain as being in a girdle-like distribution along the lower thoracic or abdominal wall. The pain may be unilateral or bilateral. Patients may experience profound weight loss associated with the onset of their symptoms. Clinical findings range from no abnormalities to sensory loss and painful hyperesthesia in a complete dermatomal pattern.

Diabetic truncal radiculoneuropathy shares many features with diabetic amyotrophy, except the latter is more painful and occurs in patients whose glycemic control is much worse.

Sensorimotor Neuropathy

Chronic sensorimotor distal symmetric polyneuropathy is the most common form of neuropathy observed in patients with diabetes. Afflicted patients typically experience burning, tingling, and lancinating pain. Some may complain only of numbness or tingling. Pain is typically worse at rest and decreases with activity. Table 5-4 lists several questions, which may be used to promptly and efficiently screen patients for the presence of sensorimotor distal symmetric polyneuropathy.

The neuropathic pain associated with diabetes is chronic and progressive, unlike acute pain, which most often results from tissue damage and serves a protective function. The chronic pain of diabetic neuropathy serves no protective function, degrades health and functioning, and leads to comorbidities such as depression or sleep disturbances. Neuropathic pain may be stimulus evoked (e.g., allodynia) or stimulus independent (spontaneous) as well as continuous or intermittent. Spontaneous pain is paroxysmal and described by patients as sharp, stabbing, or shock-like in nature. An exaggerated response to a typically non-painful stimulus may be provoked by simply wearing stockings, shoes, or sleeping with bed sheets touching one's feet. Patients with sensory neuropathy will perceive any pressure against their feet as a noxious, painful stimulus, which may affect their sleep and balance. Neuropathy also elicits painful allodynia defined as a painful response to a non-painful stimulus. Allodynia occurs ONLY in response to a innocuous stimulus. For example, the pain from a sunburn becomes acutely exacerbated when one attempts to take a shower. Since when should taking a shower be uncomfortable? The shower is an innocuous stimulus, yet the damaged nerves in patients with neuropathy are highly sensitized. Thus, the act of bathing (an nonpainful stimulus) elicits pain.

 TABLE 5-4. Questions which When Answered Affirmatively Strongly Suggest a Diagnosis of Diabetic Sensorimotor Distal Symmetric Polyneuropathy

- Do your feet burn, hurt, or tingle?
- Is your pain worse at rest and relieved with activity?
- Are you having difficulty with your balance?
- Does wearing socks or shoes bother you?
- Is your pain causing you to feel helpless or disabled?
- Is your pain interfering with your sleep?
- Is your pain affecting your quality of life?

• Clinical Recognition and Diagnosis of Diabetic Neuropathy

Although complex electrophysiologic, histologic, and autonomic function tests are required to confirm the diagnosis of diabetic neuropathies, a simple neurologic examination in the primary care office often can be used for screening purposes. Once the diagnosis is made, appropriate treatment may be initiated.

Screening for diabetic neuropathy is an important component of routine diabetes care. Most patients with mild sensory neuropathy have no detectable clinical findings. Many patients will not voluntarily discuss symptoms related to diabetic neuropathy without direct questioning by the physician. Most cases of neuropathy may be easily diagnosed based on the patient's review of systems, validated neuropathic pain questionnaires, and a simple neurologic examination.

Current recommendations suggest that providers screen all patients for distal symmetric polyneuropathy at diagnosis and at least annually thereafter using the simple clinical tests listed below.[51] Electrophysiologic testing is needed only when the clinical features of the patient are atypical. Skin biopsies may also be used to diagnose distal sensory neuropathy as well as progression of neuropathy over time. Patients should also be carefully evaluated for clinical evidence of autonomic dysfunction.

Validated Neuropathic Pain Questionnaires

Although neuropathic pain can be diagnosed clinically based on historical data and the patient's physical examination, well-validated questionnaires may also be used to rule out other pain disorders in the differential diagnosis (Table 5-5). Pain scales that may be of most benefit to primary care physicians are listed in Table 5-6.

• Physical Examination of Patients with Diabetic Neuropathy

The physical examination of a patient with diabetes can be performed in less than 5 minutes and requires only a 128-Hz tuning fork, a reflex hammer, and the examiner's hand. An annual neurologic exam should include the following steps:

1/ **Inspection of the feet.** This is mandatory for all patients with diabetes at the time of their initial visit and annually thereafter. Dry skin, distended veins, callosity, and multiple deformities (such as claw foot and prominent metatarsal heads) may suggest Charcot arthropathy (Fig. 5-14). In this condition, increased pressure on the plantar surface may lead to ulceration. Foot ulceration and amputation are the most common consequences of diabetic neuropathy and are major causes of morbidity and disability in persons with diabetes. Table 5-7 lists risk factors for amputation.

2/ **Monofilament test.** This is the most commonly used method for assessing foot ulcer risk. Most screening is performed with the 10-g monofilament. The device is placed perpendicular to a foot surface until it bends, and the patient is asked whether sensation is perceived. Protocols differ as to the number of sites on the foot that are tested and the criteria for a positive test for ulcer risk. The most common algorithm recommends four sites per foot: generally the hallux and metatarsal heads 1, 3, and 5. However, there may be little advantage gained from multiple site assessments. There is also no universal agreement as to what constitutes an abnormal result (i.e., one, two, three, or four abnormal results from the sites tested). Despite these problems, the 10-g monofilament is widely used for the clinical assessment of neuropathy.[39] When reporting the results of monofilament testing, one should mention the number of times the patient was able to perceive the sensation of each foot. For example, "patient perceived 3/5 monofilament tests on the left foot and 1/5 on the right foot."

Patients who are insensate are at an inherently higher risk of developing ulcerations and infections that may require amputation. Simply advising patients to inspect their feet each day may not motivate patients to perform this visual inspection. Instead, the clinician should give a monofilament to each patient who is insensate and advise him or her to "check the feet each night and contact the

TABLE 5-5. Differential Diagnosis of Diabetic Peripheral Neuropathic Pain

- Heavy metal poisons, environmental toxins
- Alcohol use/abuse
- Medications (e.g., amiodarone, vincristine, cisplatin, metronidazole, statins, isoniazid, phenytoin, HIV drugs, and gemfibrozil)
- Pernicious anemia (vitamin B_{12} deficiency)
- Multiple sclerosis
- Chronic renal failure (uremia)
- Hypothyroidism
- Syphilis
- Collagen vascular disease
- Porphyria
- Hereditary neuropathy
- Myeloma
- >250 mg/d of vitamin B_6
- Neoplasms
- Restless legs syndrome
- Spinal cord injuries
- Lupus
- Sjögren syndrome
- Amyloidosis
- Sarcoidosis
- HIV
- Absolute vitamin D deficiency (defined as a serum 25-hydroxyvitamin D level < 20 ng/mL)
- Low free testosterone

TABLE 5-6. Validated Neuropathic Pain Scales

Leeds Assessment of Neuropathic Symptoms and Signs[a]

- 7-item questionnaire
- Differentiates between neuropathic and non-neuropathic pain
- Score >25 is suggestive of neuropathic pain

Neuropathic Pain Questionnaire[b]

- 12-item questionnaire
- Assesses pain qualities distinct to neuropathic pain
- Useful in assessing treatment efficacy

Brief Pain Inventory for DPN[c]

- 11-item questionnaire (4-item pain severity scale and 7-item pain interference scale)
- Assesses the severity of pain, its impact on daily functioning, pain location, and efficacy of treatment

[a]From Bennett M. The LANSS Pain Scale: the Leeds assessment of neuropathic symptoms and signs. *Pain.* 2001;92:147–157; with permission.
[b]From Krause SJ, Backonja MM. Development of a neuropathic pain questionnaire. *Clin J Pain.* 2003;19:306–314.
[c]From Zelman DC, Gore M, Dukes E, et al. Validation of a modified version of the brief pain inventory for painful diabetic peripheral neuropathy. *J Pain Symptom Manage.* 2005;29:401–410.

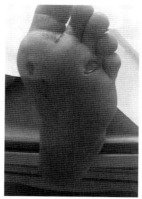

Figure 5-14 • Charcot Arthropathy. Charcot arthropathy affects up to 7.5% of patients with diabetes. The Charcot foot is deformed, mechanically unstable, and prone to ulceration. The etiology of the Charcot process is unknown but may be triggered by a pathologic vascular response following a traumatic insult such as a fall. Increased perfusion to the injured extremity may lead to bone resorption, which, in association with sensory and autonomic neuropathies, increases one's risk of developing foot ulcerations and deep wound infections. Any ulcerations or foot deformities associated with loss of sensation in a patient who has diabetes increase the risk of amputation 32-fold. Charcot arthropathy may present initially with a minimally painful foot with intact pulses and exuberant erythema. As the joint becomes unstable, a rocker bottom deformity ensues. (From Farber DC, Farber JS. Office-based screening, prevention, and management of diabetic foot disorders. *Prim Care.* 2007;34(4):873–885.)

doctor whenever any sensation returns to the feet." Physicians are encouraged to call their insensate patients 1 week after they receive their monofilament to ask if they "have noticed any change in sensation." This reinforces the importance of using the instrument. In reality, return of sensation will not occur. However, the use of the monofilament essentially forces the patient to make a visual examination of the feet. When a small blister or ulcer is seen, the patient will most likely contact the health-care provider at which time a detailed foot inspection can be performed. This technique may save limbs through early detection of neuropathic ulcers.

3/ **Plantar foot temperature monitoring.** Limb salvation may be further enhanced with the use of plantar foot temperature-guided avoidance therapy. Insensate patients are given infrared temperature sensors, which are placed on six locations on the soles of the feet twice daily. When a temperature difference of greater than 4°F between the same locations of the two feet are noted, the patient is advised to *reduce* the activity of the foot with the higher temperature. Several days or weeks may pass until

TABLE 5-7. Risk Factors for Amputation Associated with DPN

Loss of protective sensation (altered biomechanics)
Evidence of increased pressure (erythema and hemorrhage under a callus) foot deformities
Duration of diabetes for more than 10 y (male gender)
Prolonged poor glycemic control
Cardiovascular, retinal, or renal complications
Alcohol abuse
Peripheral vascular disease
Obesity
Elevation of the forefoot-rear foot pressure ratio

Adapted from Unger J. Diabetic neuropathy: early clues, effective management. *Appl Neurol.* 2005;9:23–30; and Sosenko J. The epidemiology of neuropathic foot ulcers in individuals with diabetes. *Curr Diab Rep.* 2002;2:477–481, with permission.

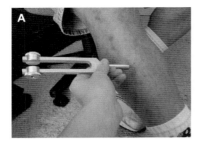
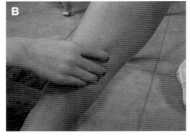
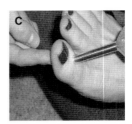
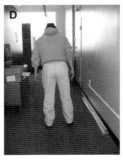
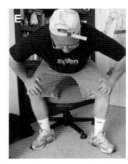

Figure 5-15 • Performing the Diabetic Peripheral Neuropathic Pain Examination. A. When testing for allodynia (a painful response to a nonpainful stimulus) place a vibrating 128-Hz tuning fork on the patient's lower extremity. Normally, the vibration would not illicit a painful response. However, if the vibration is perceived as being sharp, stabbing or burning, the patient is diagnosed as having "allodynia." **B.** Hyperalgesia is defined as having an exaggerated response to pain. Thus, if one were to lightly squeeze a patient's leg, no pain response would be generated. Patients with DPN have nerves, which are inflamed and dysfunctional. Any light touch is likely to be perceived as pain. **C.** The vibrating 128-Hz tuning fork placed on the patient's hallux. A patient who fails to appreciate any vibration is considered as being insensate. **D.** Observe the patient's gait. Patients with DPNP have lost their position sense and proprioception. The have difficulty maintaining their balance. As such, they tend to walk shuffling their feet close to the ground. Before making a turn, the patient will pause briefly, correct for any balance deficiencies and slowly proceed forward. **E.** Gower sign. Patients with diabetic amyotrophy have severe weakness in their proximal hip and leg muscles. They are unable to stand up without placing their hands on their knees and using their shoulder muscles for support. After standing up, patients will demonstrate a significant tremor in their hands and walk with a wide-based gait. (Photos courtesy of Jeff Unger, MD.)

temperatures equate once again. However, two studies have proven that such therapies are the most effective means to prevent limb loss in high-risk patients.[52,53] Self-measurement of sole temperature, followed by off-loading when temperature differences are detected, is currently the only scientifically supported tool for the prediction and prevention of diabetic foot ulcers in an insensate foot.[54]

4/ Check for loss of **ankle reflexes**— a sign of advanced peripheral neuropathy.

5/ Figure 5-15 displays additional features of a comprehensive neurologic examination for patients with diabetes.

• Skin Biopsies

Skin biopsies are becoming recognized as an important tool for diagnosing DPNP.[55] The technique quantitates the number of small epidermal nerve fibers within a 3-mm-diameter skin punch biopsy (Fig. 5-16). Intraepidermal nerve fiber density (INFD) correlates with the duration of diabetes more so than the patient's A1C, suggesting that skin biopsies might be useful as a marker of neuropathy progression.[56] Patients with diabetic neuropathy may demonstrate a normal INFD skin biopsy. In such cases, the skin biopsy should be repeated after 3 months in the same location because a change

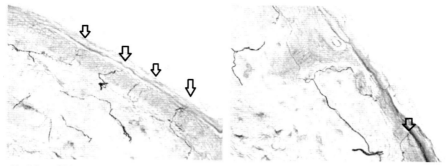

Figure 5-16 • **Skin Biopsy of a Patient with Distal Sensory Neuropathy. Arrows** represent the intraepidermal nerve fibers branching above the dermal-epidermal junction in two patients. The patient in panel **A** has normal neurologic function. The patient in panel **B** has diabetic sensory neuropathic pain and paresthesias. Note the difference in intraepidermal nerve fiber densities in the two patients. The patient in panel **A** has had T2DM for just 2 years, whereas the patient in panel **B** has had T2DM for over 14 years.

in fiber density over time is highly suggestive of progressive neuropathy. A skin biopsy should also be performed in symptomatic patients in whom a nerve conduction study reveals no abnormalities.[57]

Prior to performing a 3-mm punch biopsy, physicians should contact their local pathologist to make certain that they have the appropriate expertise to interpret the specimen.

• Automated Point-of-Care Nerve Conduction Studies for Primary Care

Portable devices have been developed to provide point-of-care nerve conduction studies within the primary care office setting. The devices use computational algorithms that are able to drive an electrical stimulus, measure a neurologic response, and provide an accurate report of the study results. Specialized training is not required for using the equipment, and the procedures are reimbursed by some third-party payers, including Medicare, using the 2010 CPT code 95905.[58]

The NC-stat by NeuroMetrix (Fig. 5-17) comprises a single use biosensor, an electronic monitor, and a remote report generating system. A chip embedded in the biosensor panel measures skin

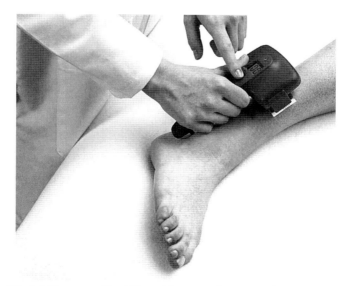

Figure 5-17 • NC-stat Biosensor. The NC-stat biosensor detects sural nerve conduction velocity and amplitude. The results are read directly from the screen on the device. (Photo courtesy of NeuroMetrix.)

surface temperature. The analysis algorithm adjusts for differences in skin surface temperature and will not report a reading if the patient's leg surface is less than 73°F.

According to the FDA, the intended use for the NC-stat device, which measures sural nerve conduction velocity and amplitude, is "to stimulate and measure neuromuscular signals that are useful in diagnosing and evaluating systemic and entrapment neuropathies."

The sensitivity and specificity of the NC-stat for diagnosing diabetic sensorimotor polyneuropathy, as defined by clinical and conventional electrophysiologic evaluation are 92% and 82%, respectively.[59] Point-of-care testing should be considered as a screening tool for diabetic sensorimotor polyneuropathy. Standardized nerve conduction velocity studies, if warranted, remain the standard of care for rendering the specific diagnosis.[60]

• Pharmacologic Management of Diabetic Peripheral Neuropathic Pain (DPNP)

Observational studies suggest that neuropathic symptoms improve with optimization of glycemic control and improvement in glycemic variability. As with other diabetes-related complications, patients should be encouraged to stop smoking and reduce their weight while ambitiously managing their lipids and BP.

Successful management of DPNP should target individualized outcomes, based upon the patient's presentation as shown in Table 5-8.

Nearly 25% of patients with painful neuropathy receive no treatment for their disorder.[61] In this study, which included almost 6,000 patients, 53% received a short-acting opioid and 40% were treated with a nonsteroidal anti-inflammatory agent, neither agent having been shown to be efficacious agents versus neuropathic pain. Providers must recognize and treat patients' neuropathic pain, although many individuals have difficulty describing their symptoms and assessing their improvement in response to therapies.

 TABLE 5-8. Individualized Goals of Distal Sensory Neuropathy (DPNP) Management

DPNP Associated Symptom/Sign	Primary Treatment Target
Pain	Reduce pain by 50% within the first 4 wk of initiating a pharmacotherapeutic intervention Improve function and quality of life of patients with chronic neuropathic pain
Loss of balance	Minimize risk of falls Screen male patients for low testosterone, which may cause secondary osteoporosis and muscle weakness Screen and treat patients for vitamin D deficiency, B_{12} deficiency and thyroid disorders
Fatigue	Use pharmacotherapy, which may improve both sleep and painful neuropathy Screen for sleep apnea and circadian rhythm sleep disorders. Treat where appropriate. Encourage weight loss, alcohol and nicotine cessation
Amputation surveillance for high-risk patients	Consider daily foot inspections coupled with plantar foot temperature monitoring Use home monofilament testing to "force" self-foot inspection
Psychiatric comorbities	Screen for major depression, which, if undiagnosed and inadequately managed may affect adherence to treatment regimens

TABLE 5-9. Recommendations for First- and Second-tier Agents for the Treatment of DPNP

Drug Type	Reason For Recommendation	Drug Names
First tier	≥2 RCTs in DPNP	Duloxetine, oxycodone CR, pregabalin, TCAs
Second tier	1 RCT in DPNP ≥1 in other painful neuropathies	Carbamazepine; gabapentin lamotrigine, tramadol, venlafaxine ER
Topical agent	Mechanism of action	Capsaicin, lidocaine
Other	≥1 RCTs in other painful neuropathies or other evidence	Bupropion, citalopram, methadone, paroxetine

CR, controlled release; DPNP, diabetic peripheral neuropathic pain; ER, extended release; RCT, randomized controlled trials; TCAs, tricyclic antidepressants.
Adapted from Argoff CE, Backonja M-M, Belgrade MJ, et al. Consensus guidelines: treatment planning and options. *Mayo Clin Proc.* 2006;81(4, Suppl):S12–S25.

Many drugs have been investigated for the treatment of DPNP, but few have demonstrated good efficacy in larger, long-term randomized clinical trials with placebo comparators. No drug relieves 100% of one's symptoms, and the mechanisms of efficacious actions of current pharmacotherapy are unclear. DPNP cannot be cured with any drug that is currently marketed. However, the patient's symptoms may certainly be improved when therapy is chosen conscientiously and appropriately. Only two agents, duloxetine and pregabalin, have received specific FDA approval for the treatment of DPNP.[62]

In 2006, the American Society of Pain Educators published their Consensus DPNP Treatment Guidelines and Advisory Board recommendations for first- and second-tier agents.[33] The recommendations (Table 5-9) were based on the level of evidence available from clinical trials and the expert committee's clinical experience. Table 5-10 lists the specific dosing recommendations for drugs used to treat DPNP, drug interactions, and dosing precautions.

One may be successful in augmenting neuropathic pain response with the use of several inexpensive and safe alternative medications. In an observational trial, Lee and Chen studied 51 patients with T2DM who experienced neuropathic pain (burning, tingling, numbness, and throbbing sensations in their lower extremities).[63] The mean serum 25-hydroxyvitamin D concentration in this cohort was 18 ng per mL. Normal vitamin D levels should be greater than 30 ng per dL. Therefore, the symptomatic patients in this study were considered as being "severely vitamin D deficient." McGill pain questionnaires and a visual analogue self-reporting scale were administered prior to patients initiating vitamin D replacement. At 3 months, the mean serum 25-hydroxyvitamin D concentrations increased to 30 ng per dL and the pain scores improved by 48%. When using vitamin D one should target a serum 25-D concentration of greater than 24 ng per mL according to this study. However, improvement in neuropathy is best observed when the serum 25-D concentration ranges from 30 to 50 ng per mL. In our patient population, such levels can be achieved by providing patients with 4,000 to 6,000 IU of vitamin D_3 daily. Symptomatic improvement is usually observed within 2 to 4 weeks.

Observational studies suggest that intracellular magnesium deficiency in patients with diabetes may account for abnormal nerve conduction studies.[64] Oral magnesium oxide supplements (250 to 750 mg) taken on an empty stomach at bedtime have been shown to improve the acute and chronic painful paresthesias of diabetic neuropathy within 2 weeks.[65] Magnesium is a noncompetitive N-methyl D-aspartate (NMDA) receptor antagonist that affects the perception of pain within the spinal cord in animal models.[66] Diarrhea is the most common adverse effect associated with magnesium use.

Metanx is a prescription vitamin supplement indicated for patients with "loss of protective sensation and neuropathic pain associated with DPN." Unlike other drugs, which are approved for the treatment of DPNP, the use of Metanx appears to target discomfort associated with neuropathic paresthesias. The drug, which combines active forms of vitamin B_6, folate, and vitamin B_{12}, doubles NO

TABLE 5-10. First-line Medications for Neuropathic Pain

Medication	Starting Dose	Titration	Maximum Dose	Duration of Adequate Trial	Potential Drug Interactions	Precautions
α₂δ ligands						
Gabapentin	300 mg tid	Increase 300 mg tid q7d	1,200 mg tid	3–8 wk for titration + 1–2 wk at maximum dose	Antacids reduce bioavailability. Therefore, take gabapentin 2 h after using an antacid. May significantly increase norethindrone levels	Category C—pregnancy safety rating has not been established. Use with caution in patients with severe renal disease.
Pregabalin	50–75 mg tid or b.i.d	Increase to 300 mg/d after 3–4 d, then by 150 mg/d as tolerated	600 mg/d	2–4 wk	May increase sedative effects of ethanol and lorazepam	Pregnancy safety category rating pending. Side effects include dizziness, somnolence, and peripheral edema without cardiovascular implications. Can induce sedation. Reduce dose by 50% for creatine clearance <60 mL/min.
Antidepressants						
Duloxetine	30 mg q d with breakfast	After 1 wk increase to 60 mg q d with breakfast	120 mg q d	2–4 wk	Coadministration of drugs that inhibit CYP2D6 (paroxetine, fluoxetine, quinidine) may increase duloxetine blood levels. Duloxetine moderately inhibits elimination of CYP2D6 substrates (TCAs, type 1C antiarrhythmics). Duloxetine + monoamine oxidase inhibitors can cause malignant hyperthermia.	Category C—pregnancy safety rating has not been established. Titration from 30 to 60 mg minimizes nausea. Other side effects include somnolence, agitation, dizziness, and constipation.

TCAs	10–100 mg taken—2 h before bedtime	25 mg every 7 d as tolerated	75–150 mg daily; if blood level of active drug and its metabolite is below 100 mg/mL, continue titration with caution.	6–8 wk with at least 1–2 wk at maximum tolerated dose	Use with cimetidine, quinidine, and duloxetine may increase levels of TCAs. May interact with thyroid medications and alcohol	Rated Category D (unsafe) for use during pregnancy. Side effects include cardiac conduction disturbances, arrhythmias, seizures, glaucoma, urinary retention, syncope, dry mouth. Avoid in patients >60.
Venlafaxine	37.5–75 mg/d	Increase by 75 mg/d weekly	375 mg/d standard venlafaxine or 225 mg/d extended release formulation	2–4 wk	Contraindicated with concomitant use of MAOI	May raise BP 10–15 mm Hg. Pregnancy Category C
Topical medications						
Capsaicin cream		Apply to painful area on limb b.i.d × 2 wk. Rub in with vigor.	Discontinue at 2 wk, even if no improvement seen	None	None	OTC. Category C—pregnancy safety rating has not been established. Warn patient that drug will burn when applied to skin surface. Exercising immediately after application may exacerbate burning sensation.
Lidoderm patch	5%	Apply to painful area for 12 h daily	Can apply to multiple areas of the body if needed. OK to cut patches in halves as well. This saves money.	2–4 wk	None	Category B pregnancy safety rating

(Continued)

Table 5-10. First-line Medications for Neuropathic Pain *(Continued)*

Medication	Starting Dose	Titration	Maximum Dose	Duration of Adequate Trial	Potential Drug Interactions	Precautions
Anticonvulsants						
Topiramate	25 mg at hs	Increase by 25 mg at hs weekly as tolerated	400 mg/d	2–4 wk	Dose adjustments are necessary when used with carbamazepine, phenytoin, and ethinyl estradiol. Reduce dose for renal dysfunction.	Side effects include increase in paresthesias, cognitive difficulty, weight loss, glaucoma, kidney stones, and metabolic acidosis. Pregnancy Category C
Lamotrigine	Weeks 1–2 = 25 mg/d	Weeks 3–4 = 50 mg/d Week 5 = 100 mg/d Week 6 = 200 mg/d	400 mg/d	4–6 wk	Titrate dose very slowly. Dose adjustments needed for patients taking phenytoin, phenobarbital, primidone, rifampin, and valproate	Risk of Stevens-Johnson syndrome and toxic epidermal necrolysis. Most common side effects include nausea, epigastric pain, headache, drowsiness, and dizziness.
Analgesics						
Tramadol	12.5 mg qid		200 mg/d	2 wk	Common side effect: nausea (23%), constipation (21%), headache (17%), somnolence (12%)	Four-times daily dosing is a drawback. Increased risk of seizures in patients taking concomitant SSRIs, TCAs, and opioids. Higher risk of seizures in patients with head trauma, coexisting seizure disorders, and substance abuse
Oxycodone CR	10 mg every 12 h	60 mg every 12 h	60 mg	4 wk	Side effects: constipation (42%), nausea (36%), dizziness (32%); may exacerbate preexisting DAN.	If long-term use is prescribed, an opioid agreement should be signed with the patient.

tid, three times daily; b.i.d, twice daily; TCAs, tricyclic antidepressants; MAOI, monoamine oxidase inhibitor; OTC, over-the-counter; qid, four times daily; hs, bedtime dosing; SSRI, selective serotonin reuptake inhibitor; DAN, diabetic autonomic neuropathy.

production within smooth muscle cells, resulting in increasing blood flow to peripheral nerves.[67] A small double-blind, placebo-controlled study demonstrated that the use of Metanx (two tablets per day for 2 weeks then one tablet daily) for 1 year improved vibratory sensation in patients with neuropathic symptoms and established sensory loss.[68] Randomized,double blind placebo controlled studies supporting the coadministration of Metanx with allopathic medications for DPNP have not been published

• Evidence-based Treatment Recommendations for Diabetic Peripheral Neuropathic Pain

Upon reviewing the evidence-based consensus treatment guidelines published by the American Society of Pain Educators[33] and the ADA Standards of Medical Care[51] the following recommendations are suggested as a framework for managing symptomatic and disabling DPNP:

1. One should improve glycemic control and glycemic variability.
2. First-tier drugs should include duloxetine and pregabalin.
3. Second-tier drugs should include venlafaxine ER, TCAs, gabapentin, and lamotrigine.
4. Third-tier drugs should include topiramate, paroxetine, topical lidocaine, and topical capsaicin.
5. Adding magnesium oxide 250 to 500 mg at bedtime will reduce paresthesias in many patients + vitamin D_3 4,000 IU daily. (Note: This is anecdotal and not supported by evidence-based guidelines.)

Patients who are being actively treated for DPNP should be asked at each visit whether their pain is improved, stable, or getting worse. Use of a "pain index" might be helpful in monitoring therapy. To calculate a pain index, one should ask the following questions at each visit:

- "On how many of the past 30 days have you experienced any pain?"
- "On average, how would you rate the intensity of your typical daily pain from 0 to 10, where 0 is no pain and 10 is excruciating and disabling pain?"
- "On average, over the past 30 days, how many hours per day do you perceive any pain?" (The maximum answer would be 24 hours.)

To determine the pain index, one should use the following formula:
For example, if a patient, prior to initiating pharmacologic therapy, reports daily pain with an average intensity of 7 and duration of 12 hours, the pain index = 7 × 12 + 30 = 114. If the patient returns for follow-up and reports daily pain with an intensity of 3 and duration of 3 hours, the pain index has been reduced to 3 × 3 + 30 = 39, representing a nearly 70% reduction in total pain.

$$\text{Pain index} = \text{Pain intensity} \times \text{duration} + \text{frequency}$$

Patients should experience at least a 50% reduction in pain from baseline from the first-tier drugs by week 3. If no improvement is seen, modification of therapy may be warranted. Doses of the first-tier drugs may be increased if the medication is well tolerated. Rational polypharmacy may be considered. Patients on serotonin and norepinephrine reuptake inhibitors (SNRIs) should not use concomitant TCAs or tramadol. Patients on tramadol should avoid using other opioids as this may increase the risk of seizures. However, patients using duloxetine may safely use topical agents, antiepileptic drugs, and opioids. Those on pregabalin may use TCAs, opioids, topical agents, and tramadol.

• Treatment of Refractory DPNP Pain

Methadone, a potent μ (mu) agonist, has several unique properties, which may be useful in managing patients with persistent neuropathic pain. Methadone displays antagonism to NMDA receptors, known modulators of neuropathic pain and important in the attenuation of the development of morphine tolerance.[69] NMDA is an excitatory amino acid that has been implicated in the development of neuropathic pain and opioid tolerance. Similar to the mechanism of action for

TCAs, methadone inhibits the reuptake of norepinephrine and serotonin, thus facilitating relief from neuropathic pain. Methadone has no active metabolites, thereby decreasing the incidence of adverse side effects such as confusion, sedation, myoclonus, and seizures, which may occur with other opioids. Side effects associated with methadone use include nausea, constipation, vomiting, sweating, pruritus, and, rarely, respiratory depression. Discontinuation of methadone should be carried out similar to stopping any long-acting opioid, with a slow taper over a period of days to weeks to prevent withdrawal symptoms and cessation of the taper if pain reappears. Methadone's analgesic effect begins within 20 minutes of drug administration, peaks in 3 to 4.5 hours, and has a duration of action of 4 to 6 hours.[70] The drug is inexpensive with the cost of sixty 10-mg tablets averaging $34. Dosing may begin at 5 mg daily and increased according to the patient's response to therapy.

When managing patients on chronic opioids for diabetic neuropathy, one should follow the guidelines published by individual state medical boards. The American Pain Society has also published guidelines for chronic opioid use, which offer specific recommendations prior to initiating

 TABLE 5-11. American Pain Society Guidelines for Effective Pain Management of Controlled Substances

1. Prescribing controlled substances for chronic pain should only be accomplished within an established physician–patient relationship and should be based on clearly diagnosed and documented unrelieved pain.

2. A patient evaluation including physical examination and comprehensive medical history shall be conducted prior to the initiation of treatment.

3. Pain evaluation should also include assessment of the pain, physical and psychological function, diagnostic studies, previous interventions including pharmacotherapy, substance abuse history, and underlying coexisting conditions.

4. Complex pain patients warrant consultation by a physician specializing in pain medicine, addiction, or substance abuse counseling.

5. Treatment plans should be customized with specific objectives of care clearly discussed with the patient.

6. Patients should receive controlled substances from a single prescriber and from a single pharmacy whenever possible.

7. Documentation of informed consent with the patient should be charted. Informed consent includes a discussion of the risks and benefits of chronic opioid use.

8. Periodic review of the efficacy of drug therapy and the etiology of the patient's pain should be performed. Physicians should consider appropriateness of continuing drug therapy or using alternative interventions if needed. Long-term opioid therapy is associated with the development of tolerance to the drug's analgesic effects and may induce neuroinflammation. Therefore, increasing doses of opioids may not be effective in chronic pain management.

9. Consider using a pain management agreement with each patient that specifies the rules for medication use and the consequences for misuse. Pain management agreements are not needed for hospice or nursing home patients. A sample pain management agreement can be downloaded from the www.medicalboard.iowa.gov website.

10. A physician who prescribes controlled substances to a patient for more than 90 d for the treatment of chronic pain shall consider utilizing drug testing to ensure that the patient is receiving appropriate therapeutic levels of prescribed medications or if the physician has reason to believe that the patient is at risk for drug abuse for diversion.

11. The physician shall consider termination of patient care if there is evidence of noncompliance with the rules for medication use, drug diversion, or a repeated pattern of substance abuse.

From American Pain Society http://www.aapainmanage.org/literature/Advocacy/Iowa_Pain_Management_Rules07_19_11.pdf

and while following chronic pain patients (Table 5-11). Patients on chronic opioids should be treated to a daily pain intensity level of less than or equal to 4. This is considered to be "functional pain," meaning that the patient's pain is unlikely to interfere with their daily routine.

The combination of gabapentin plus morphine has also been demonstrated in a double-blind, placebo-controlled study to improve symptomatic neuropathic pain better than either of the drugs used alone.[71] In this study, the most effective combination dose of the drugs for treating neuropathic pain was approximately morphine 30 mg per day and gabapentin 1,800 mg per day.

Diabetic Autonomic Neuropathy (DAN)

DAN is a serious and common complication of diabetes. The reported prevalence of DAN varies widely depending on the cohort studied and the methods of assessment. In randomly selected cohorts of asymptomatic individuals with diabetes, approximately 20% had abnormal cardiovascular autonomic function.[72] DAN frequently coexists with other peripheral neuropathies and diabetic complications or may be isolated. The major clinical manifestations of DAN are listed in Table 5-12.

The 5-year mortality rate for patients with DAN is three times higher than in diabetic patients without autonomic involvement.[73] The leading cause of death in patients with either symptomatic or asymptomatic autonomic neuropathy is heart disease.

Although peripheral and autonomic neuropathies are often considered to have similar risk factors and etiologies, DAN may be linked to a neuronal autoimmune disorder. The presence of autonomic nerve autoantibodies (ANabs) have been found in over 50% of patients with T1DM who have progressive DAN. In a prospective observational study, Granberg et al. followed 41 patients with T1DM over 14 years while intermittently performing tests of autonomic function on all patients.[74] Periodic measurements of ANabs were performed. The 56% of patients who tested positive for ANabs demonstrated significantly higher frequencies of at least one abnormal cardiac autonomic nerve function test. No direct association between A1C and the presence of ANabs has been determined, suggesting that susceptibility to autoantibody formation is unrelated to advanced glycation.[74]

Cardiac Autonomic Neuropathy (CAN)

Cardiac autonomic neuropathy (CAN) is defined as the impairment of autonomic control of the cardiovascular system. The prevalence of CAN varies widely from 2.5% to 50%. Predictors of CAN include patient age, duration of diabetes, glycemic control, presence of sensorimotor neuropathy and retinopathy, hypertension, obesity, smoking, and hypertriglyceridemia.[75] Improved glycemic and metabolic control tend to mitigate the effects of CAN in patients with T1DM and T2DM.[76,77]

CAN occurs in 17% of patients with T1DM and 22% of patients with T2DM.[78] CAN causes abnormalities of heart rate control and vascular dynamics. Patients experience postural hypotension, exercise intolerance, and silent myocardial ischemia.

Resting tachycardia is an early sign of CAN as is a lack of heart rate increase to mild exercise. Patients with postural hypotension also experience an abnormal circadian pattern of BP, the opposite of what is seen in the normal physiologic state. Ambulatory BP monitoring of patients with DAN demonstrate a rise in BP overnight and a fall in BP in the early morning.[79] Lack of nocturnal BP fall (nondipping) or an increase in BP during the night (reverse dipping) is observed in 30% of patients with T2DM and is considered a marker for DAN[80] (see Chapter 7 for further details on ambulatory BP abnormalities in patients with CAN). Ambulatory monitoring is able to provide information on BP variability, expressed as a standard deviation of average 24-hour daytime or nighttime BP values. This parameter is frequently increased in patients with diabetes, a sign of deranged autonomic control of circulation and/or increased vascular thickness. Orthostatic hypotension may also be detected by ambulatory monitoring. An excessive BP surge in the morning is associated with an

TABLE 5-12. Clinical Manifestations of DAN

Affected Organ/System	Clinical Findings
Cardiovascular	• Sinus tachycardia/bradycardia • Systolic and diastolic dysfunction • Decreased exercise tolerance • Orthostatic hypotension • Abnormal circadian rhythm of BP • Sleep apnea • Loss of ischemic pain response • Silent ischemia • Intraoperative and perioperative cardiovascular instability
Sudomotor	• Gustatory sweating • Decreased thermoregulation • Dehydration in response to exercise • Anhydrosis • Hyperhydrosis • Heat intolerance • Dry, cracked skin • Pathologic fungal infections • Decreased sweating especially on the forehead and in the extremities • Altered blood flow • Edema
GI	• Esophageal dysmotility • Gastroparesis • Nocturnal diarrhea • Alternating diarrhea and constipation • Fecal incontinence
Uropathy	• Retrograde ejaculation • Erectile dysfunction • Dyspareunia • Frequent urinary tract infections • Neurogenic bladder
Metabolic	• Hypoglycemia associated autonomic failure (HAAF) • Erratic glycemic control due to unpredictable gastric emptying
Ocular	• Pupillomotor function impairment (e.g., decreased diameter of dark adapted pupil) • Pseudo Argyll-Robertson pupil[a]

[a]Argyll-Robertson pupils are typically small (2 mm), irregular in shape and react poorly to light. Response to accommodation and convergence remains intact. Visual acuity is normal. Dilation with mydiatic agents is typically poor. Diabetes causes Argyll-Robertson pupils via a vasculopathy, which affects the pupillary fibers. Argyll-Robertson pupils are also associated with neurosyphilis, alcohol abuse, and multiple sclerosis. The classic Argyll-Robertson pupil does not respond to light stimulus. Pseudo Argyll-Robertson pupils do display some light response.

increased cardiovascular risk in patients regardless of their glycemic status.[81] Morning hypertension in diabetic patients can increase the rate of progression to diabetic nephropathy.[82]

Perhaps the most frightening consequence of CAN is silent ischemia. In the Framingham study, 39% of patients with diabetes had an asymptomatic MI documented by electrocardiography.[83] Silent ischemia is dangerous because patients cannot sense pain associated with an acute coronary event and are less likely to seek medical care. The mortality rate from a silent infarct is 47% versus 35% in patients able to perceive pain.[84] Physicians should consider pain in any part of the chest in a patient with diabetes as being of myocardial origin until proven otherwise. Other signs of silent MI include fatigue, edema, hemoptysis, nausea and vomiting, diaphoresis, arrhythmias, and dyspnea.

The widespread use of currently available modalities for detection of structural heart disease in patients with T2DM is limited by high costs and low accessibility. A simple blood test, brain natriuretic peptide (BNP) may be useful as a potential screening tool. The cardiac ventricles secrete BNP in response to an increase in wall stress.[85] Higher plasma BNP and NT-proBNP have been detected in patients with T2DM without overt cardiovascular disease compared with matched controls. Elevated BNP has also been linked with increased mortality and a higher prevalence of silent ischemia.[86] Still, debate remains regarding the routine application of BNP as a screening test for silent ischemia in patients with T2DM. Cut-off values for BNP, which may be used for screening high-risk patients, have not been established. The frequency, timing, and impact of screening-directed interventions on long-term health outcomes remain to be clarified by randomized controlled trials. One might consider performing an inexpensive screening BNP study on patients with CAN who may be at risk for developing silent ischemia. The cost of a BNP is approximately $100. If the BNP is elevated, left ventricular function should be assessed via echocardiography.[87]

Orthostatic Hypotension

Orthostatic hypotension is diagnosed when a patient's systolic BP falls more than 30 mm Hg upon standing from a supine position. Patients may also experience dizziness, weakness, visual impairment, headache, and loss of consciousness. Orthostatic hypotension may be exacerbated in patients who are volume depleted from taking diuretics or who experience excessive sweating, diarrhea, or polyuria. Medications such as β-blockers, TCAs, and phenothiazines can also contribute to orthostatic changes. Interestingly, patients often become abruptly hypotensive when eating or within 10 minutes of injecting insulin. Because the symptoms of orthostatic hypotension and hypoglycemia are similar, one should be advised to monitor blood glucose levels if they do become symptomatic.

Insulin-provoked orthostatic hypotension occurs quickly after the injection is given. Exogenous insulin may mediate hypotension by increasing capillary permeability and causing a mild intravascular depletion. Insulin may also stimulate the release of NO—a potent vasodilator from endothelial cells.[72]

Orthostatic hypotension is difficult to treat because the upright BP must be raised without inducing hypertension when the patient becomes supine. Symptomatic patients should be advised to wear supportive stockings to increase venous return from the lower extremities, removing them at bedtime.[88] Patients should become proactive when changing from a supine to a standing position. Holding on to a chair or bed for 30 seconds after standing may minimize one's fall risk. Bathing in hot water should be avoided and insulin injections should be administered while in the supine position.

Fludrocortisone acetate (florinef) can increase BP in patients with orthostatic hypotension but may also potentiate congestive heart failure (CHF), edema, and hypertension. Antihypertensive drugs may produce a paradoxical increase in BP by activating or antagonizing α- or β-adrenergic receptors that are inappropriately expressed as a result of autonomic denervation or dysfunction.[47]

Subcutaneous octreotide (sandostatin) may be used in patients with orthostatic hypotension refractory to other therapies. Octreotide has a pressor effect on patients with DAN. Dosages of 1 μg per kg per day may cause abdominal cramping and nausea.[89]

Sudomotor Dysfunction

Extremes of anhidrosis and hyperhidrosis occur in 10% to 75% of people with DAN.[90] Sweat glands are innervated by the sudomotor, postganglionic, and unmyelinated cholinergic sympathetic C-fibers. Thus, vascular flow within the dermis is regulated by the autonomic nervous system. Patients with

DAN may experience changes in skin temperature, heat regulation, and skin texture. Defective sweat formation will likely favor the development of cracked, dry surfaces, which become a haven for the growth pathogenic bacteria and fungi. The quantitative sudomotor axon reflex test (QSART) is capable of detecting distal small fiber polyneuropathy with a sensitivity of greater than 75% and is considered the primary reference method for detecting sudomotor dysfunction for clinical and research purposes.[91] QSART measures sweat output in response to acetylcholine, which reflects the function of postganglionic sympathetic unmyelinated sudomotor nerve fibers. Electrodes are placed on the patient's arms and legs while the sweat volume produced by acetylcholine iontophoresis is determined. A mild electrical stimulation on the skin surface allows the acetylcholine to activate the sweat glands.

Some individuals with significant sudomotor dysfunction sweat only from the chest down and produce no sweat around their face or head. These individuals are prone to heat stroke and dehydration. They should be extremely cautious while exercising, as they may experience rapid dehydration. Exercising on warm days should be avoided, and frequent oral electrolyte fluid replacement should be followed.

Patients may also experience *gustatory sweating* characterized by profuse sweating of the face, scalp, and neck during or immediately after ingestion of food or drink. While no single test confirms the diagnosis of diabetic gustatory sweating, supporting evidence may be obtained by documenting the presence and distribution of sweating in response to meals. The increased moisture should appear during or after eating and be restricted to the head and neck region. No specific foods have been found to consistently trigger gustatory sweating, which may become a source of embarrassment for any patient with DAN. Gustatory sweating occurs when previously denervated sweat glands become reinnervated with sympathetic or parasympathetic nerve fibers.[90] Axonal regeneration results in overcompensation of cholinergic sympathetic nerves triggered by direct stimulation of the taste buds. Placing food directly into the stomach does not evoke gustatory sweating.[90] Glycopyrrolate, an antimuscarinic compound, may benefit some patients with gustatory sweating.[92] Botulinum toxin has been used for refractory gustatory sweating with limited success.[93]

Diabetic Gastropathy

GI dysfunction is common in patients with diabetes. Diabetic gastropathy results in intermittent diarrhea and constipation. Diarrhea may be nocturnal. Sixty percent of patients with diabetes experience constipation.[72] Before attributing constipation to DAN, hypothyroidism, colon cancer, and side effects from drugs such as TCAs and calcium channel blockers (CCBs) should be ruled out as possible causes. Additional hydration and use of fiber products are useful in managing chronic constipation. Patients may also find relief with minocycline 50 mg twice daily with breakfast and dinner. The mechanism of minocycline 50 mg efficacy on stabilizing and reversing gastropathy is uncertain.

Gastroparesis occurs in 25% of patients with T1DM.[88] True gastroparesis is rarely seen in patients with T2DM. Hyperglycemia delays gastric emptying, whereas hypoglycemia results in rapid passing of gastric contents into the small intestine. Dosing insulin becomes problematic in patients with gastroparesis because the insulin is administered based on the time when the drug absorption is likely to coincide with the rise in blood glucose after nutrients pass into the plasma from the small intestine. One can never be certain when nutrients are being absorbed in patients with gastroparesis. In addition, patients may give a prescribed dose of insulin prior to eating, only to develop early satiety and abdominal pain after eating a small amount. The administered insulin will likely result in postprandial hypoglycemia. As the nutrient absorption is delayed for several hours, the patient will experience hyperglycemia 3 to 4 hours after eating as insulin peak absorption wanes while glucose levels rise. The postprandial hyperglycemia will result in persistent gastroparesis in time for the following meal.

Gastroparesis should always be suspected in patients with glycemic variability and chronic hyperglycemia. Although radiographic studies may be helpful in confirming a diagnosis of gastroparesis, they do not always correlate well with the degree of symptoms. In fact, some severely symptomatic patients may have normal radiographic studies.

Improvement in overall glycemic control is the primary goal of treatment of diabetic **GI autonomic neuropathy.** Hyperglycemia retards gastric emptying and reduces GI motility, whereas hypoglycemia speeds nutrient delivery into the periphery.[94] Management of insulin therapy can be challenging in patients with delayed gastric emptying because matching the timing of the injection with the anticipated rise in postprandial glucose absorption is difficult, if not impossible, to predict. One should advise patients with delayed gastric emptying who use an insulin pump to take an "extended wave bolus" at mealtime (see chapter 13 on Insulin Pump Therapy). Extended administration allows insulin to be absorbed over 3 to 4 hours rather than as a large dose with a meal. This reduces the incidence of postprandial hypoglycemia in patients with GI autonomic neuropathy.[95]

Those patients who cannot use an insulin pump should consider injecting their insulin 30 to 45 minutes *after* finishing their meal rather than at the onset of eating to avoid immediate postprandial hypoglycemia. Some patients may experience relief of symptoms within 1 to 2 weeks of using twice daily minocycline or erythromycin. In theory, these antibiotics reduce excessive bacterial overgrowth in the GI tract, allowing the normal GI flora to become stabilized. Patients who do not notice improvement in the GI symptoms within 2 weeks of starting antibiotics should be prescribed an alternative treatment.

Neurogenic Bladder

Bladder complications in patients with diabetes may be secondary to an alteration of the detrusor smooth muscle as well as neuronal and urothelial dysfunction. Estimates of the prevalence of bladder dysfunction are 43% to 87% of type 1 diabetic patients and 25% of type 2 diabetic patients.[91] The correlation between coexisting diabetic cystopathy and peripheral neuropathy ranges from 75% to 100%.

The symptoms of neurogenic bladder (cystopathy) include difficulty urinating, urinary incontinence, pyelonephritis, and chronic urinary tract infections. The dysfunctional bladder may become distended up to three times its normal size. Ironically, as patients have diminished pain sensation, bladder distention is asymptomatic. Voiding frequency is diminished and the process is incomplete, which may lead to urinary tract infections and pyelonephritis. Dribbling and overflow incontinence are common.

A postvoid residual volume (PVR) of more than 150 mL is diagnostic of cystopathy.[72] Measurement of peak urinary flow rate and PVR should be considered in patients with lower urinary tract symptoms when diagnosis remains doubtful.[96]

Patients with cystopathy should be instructed to palpate their bladder and attempt to urinate when their bladder is full. If unable to start the urine flow, they can massage the abdomen just above the pubic bone applying firm pressure downward against the bladder to initiate urine flow (Crede maneuver). Self-catheterization may be needed in some patients and has a low risk of infection. Pharmacotherapy is directed at improving bladder emptying and reducing the risk of urinary tract infections (Table 5-13).

Hypoglycemia-associated Autonomic Failure

Hypoglycemia occurs when blood glucose concentrations fall below the level necessary to properly maintain the body's requirement for energy and stability. Approximately 6% of all deaths in patients with T1DM aged less than 40 years are due to hypoglycemia-associated autonomic failure (HAAF).[97] Research also suggests that the incidence of hypoglycemia is particularly high among patients treated with insulin over extended periods of time, again reinforcing the idea that advanced disease progression and increased insulin use subsequently increase the risk of hypoglycemia. The UK Hypoglycemia Study Group found that the incidence of severe hypoglycemia in patients with T1DM treated with insulin for greater than 15 years was three times higher than in those treated for less than 5 years. In patients with T2DM, the prevalence of severe hypoglycemia increased from 7% to 25% when comparing patients treated with insulin for less than 2 years to those treated for greater than 5 years, respectively.[98]

TABLE 5-13. Pharmacologic Therapies for DAN

Condition	Suggested Drug Therapy	Comments
Orthostatic hypotension	• 9-α fluorohydrocortisone 0.5–2 mg/d • Clonidine 0.1–0.5 mg at bedtime • Octreotide 0.1–1.0 µg/kg/d	• May cause volume overload, CHF, hypertension • May cause paradoxical hypertension, hypotension, sedation, and dry mouth • Injection site pain and diarrhea but helpful for refractory cases
Gastroparesis	• Erythromycin 250 mg with breakfast and dinner • Minocycline 50 mg with breakfast and dinner • Insulin pump therapy	• Usually effective within the 1st wk. Stop either drug if ineffective within 14 d of starting therapy. Long-term use often necessary. Tetracycline is associated with sun sensitivity reactions. Erythromycin may cause diarrhea, abdominal cramps, or nausea. • Patients on insulin pumps should use an "extended wave bolus." As hyperglycemia improves, so will the symptoms.
Diarrhea	• Metronidazole 250 mg three times daily for at least 3 wk • Minocycline 50 mg with breakfast and dinner indefinitely • Octreotide 50 µg three times daily	
Cystopathy	• Bethanechol 10 mg four times daily • Doxazosin 1–2 mg two to three times daily	• Hypotension, headache, palpitations
ED	• PDE-5 drugs	• See Table 5-14
Female sexual dysfunction	• Vaginal lubricants (over the counter) • Vaginal estrogen cream	• Women experience dyspareunia, postcoital bleeding, and reduced sexual arousal.

CHF, congestive heart failure; PDE-5, phosphodiesterase-5.

Repeated hypoglycemic events can lead to hypoglycemia unawareness, whereby hormonal, autonomic, sympathetic neural, and adrenomedullary responses are attenuated, such that the warning symptoms of developing hypoglycemia are essentially lost. This subsequently compromises natural behavioral defenses against hypoglycemia, such as the ingestion of food, so that instead of an episode of mild hypoglycemia developing that can be easily self-managed by the patient, more serious episodes of hypoglycemia may occur that require external intervention. Indeed, studies have shown that adults with T1DM who have impaired awareness of hypoglycemia are much more likely to be exposed to asymptomatic hypoglycemia and are at higher risk of developing severe hypoglycemia than those with normal awareness. Hypoglycemia unawareness occurs as a result of a physiologic response to recurrent hypoglycemic events known as HAAF (Fig. 5-18).

Over time, repeated episodes of mild hypoglycemia cause the normal glycemic thresholds for initiating sympathoadrenal, symptomatic, and cognitive responses to subsequent hypoglycemia to shift to lower blood glucose concentrations. This impairs the natural defense mechanisms required for prevention and reversal of hypoglycemia. HAAF creates a vicious circle because T1DM patients already have a defective glucose counterregulatory response. Hypoglycemia unawareness ultimately leads to a significantly reduced detection of hypoglycemia in the clinical setting and further, more severe episodes of hypoglycemia (Fig. 5-19). Multiple studies have shown that as little as 2 to 3 weeks of scrupulous avoidance of hypoglycemia can reverse hypoglycemia unawareness.[99,100]

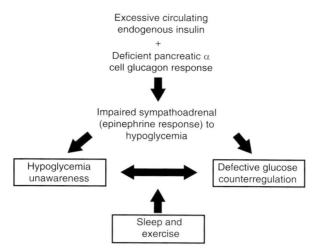

Figure 5-18 • Diagrammatic Representation of the Concept of Hypoglycemia-associated Autonomic Failure (HAAF). (Reprinted from Unger J, Parkin C. Recognition, prevention, and proactive management of hypoglycemia in patients with type 1 diabetes mellitus. *Postgrad Med.* 2011;123(4):71–80, with permission.)

Strategic Management of DAN

DAN is best treated by targeting metabolic control of the patient's blood glucose, lipids, and BP. Smoking and alcohol use should be immediately discontinued, and patients should be encouraged to reduce their weight, when appropriate. The overall risk of CAN may be reduced by 70% with physiologic management of hyperglycemia, hyperlipidemia, and hypertension, as well as with the use of ACE inhibitors.[38] Unless contraindicated, patients should be placed on aspirin. The response to therapeutic intervention is dependent on the patient's baseline degree of autonomic dysfunction. Intensive glycemic control can reverse deterioration in heart rate variability in as little as 1 year.[101] Often, symptomatic DAN may stabilize soon after glycemia improves.[102]

The pharmacotherapeutic agents used for the treatment of DAN are listed in Table 5-13.

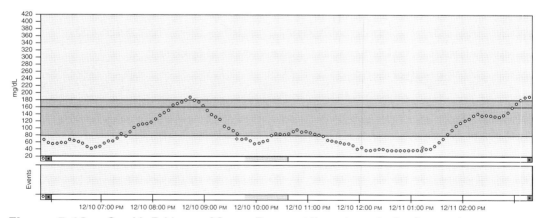

Figure 5-19. • Graphic Evidence of Severe Recurrent Hypoglycemia. Continuous glucose sensor of a 38-year-old patient with T1DM and hypoglycemic unawareness on an insulin pump. Each dot represents an interstitial blood glucose reading taken at a 5-minute interval. The *darkened area* in the middle of the graph represents the targeted glucose control zone of 80 to 180 mg per dL. The patient is noted to have multiple episodes of prolonged hypoglycemia lasting between 30 and 120 minutes over a 9-hour period. Note that some of his glucose levels are as low as 40 mg per dL. The patient slept through multiple auditory sensor alarms from 11:15 PM until 1 AM until awakened by his wife who gave him 4 oz of apple juice. His wife did confirm his hypoglycemia with a finger stick at 1:15 AM (as shown by dot) after which his glucose levels rose in response to the juice. (Case courtesy of Jeff Unger, MD)

Erectile Dysfunction

Erectile dysfunction (ED) is defined as the inability to maintain a sufficiently rigid erection for vaginal penetration and ejaculation.[103] Risk factors for men likely to experience ED include physical inactivity, obesity, smoking, watching more than 20 hours of TV each week, depression, diabetes, hyperlipidemia, hypertension, stroke, and the presence of cardiovascular disease.[104] Concomitant medication use, such as antidepressants and antihypertensive medications may also increase one's risk of experiencing ED.

ED is an independent risk factor for coronary artery disease.[105] ED often coexists in patients with hypertension, cerebrovascular disease, peripheral arterial disease, and diabetes. Both ED and endothelial dysfunction share a common pathologic pathway affecting impairment of NO–induced vasodilation. Thus, patients with ED, especially those with diabetes, should undergo a comprehensive proactive workup for cardiovascular disease.[106]

Sixty percent of men with diabetes experience ED.[107] Owing to the high prevalence of this diabetes-related and often significant complication, primary care physicians should identify patients who suffer from ED and offer them counseling on therapeutic interventions. Direct inquiry can be made regarding the patient's erectile performance using the questions listed in Table 5-14. The laboratory workup for men with ED should include an A1C, lipid profile, thyroid-stimulating hormone, free thyroxin, prostate-specific antigen (PSA), serum prolactin, free testosterone, and sex hormone–binding globulin (SHBG).[108]

Penile erection is a hemodynamic process initiated by the relaxation of smooth muscle in the corpus cavernosum and its associated arterioles (Fig. 5-20). During sexual stimulation, NO is released from nerve endings and endothelial cells within the corpus cavernosum. NO activates the enzyme guanylate cyclase, which, in turn, increases synthesis of cyclic guanosine monophosphate (cGMP) in the smooth muscle cells of the corpus cavernosum. The cGMP triggers smooth muscle relaxation, allowing increased blood flow into the penis resulting in an erection. The tissue concentration of cGMP is regulated by the rates of both synthesis and degradation via phosphodiesterases (PDEs), the most abundant of which in the corpora cavernosum is PDE-5. Thus, inhibition of PDE-5 enhances erectile function by increasing the amount of cGMP available in the corpora cavernosum. Because sexual stimulation is required to initiate the local release of NO, the inhibition of PDE-5 has no effect in the absence of sexual arousal.[108]

TABLE 5-14. Sexual History Questions for Men with ED

Question Related to Sexual Performance	Interpretation of Response
How long have you had problems with erections?	Acute onset is more often related to a functional disorder, whereas chronic ED is secondary to organic disease.
How many times per month do you attempt intercourse?	Patients having intercourse more than twice weekly may benefit from daily dosing of a PDE-5 inhibitor.
Are you having difficulty with premature ejaculation (PME)?	PME may be treated off label with selective serotonin reuptake inhibitor (SSRI) drugs, which have the side effect of delayed ejaculation.
Are you able to obtain and maintain an erection with sexual stimulation?	If patients can obtain and maintain erections with sexual stimulation more than 50% the time, they may still benefit from PDE-5 drugs, yet their ED may be less severe than they anticipated.
In the past 30 d have you had any nocturnal or early morning erections?	Nocturnal erections may occur more often in men with psychogenic ED yet will be absent in those with organic disease.

(Continued)

TABLE 5-14. Sexual History Questions for Men with ED
(Continued)

Have you noticed any changes in the sensation of your penis over the past 6 mo?	Any pain or tingling in the tip of the penis may indicate a prostate disorder, such as acute or chronic prostatitis
Have you noticed a curvature to your erections?	This would be observed in patients with Peyronne plaque. Examination and palpation of the shaft of the penis would reveal a fibrous plaque surrounding the area from where the penis is normally curved during an erection.
Would you rate your sexual desire as being normal, decreased, or increased over the past 6 mo?	Men with gonadal dysfunction, (low testosterone) may experience a reduced libido associated with ED. Patients should be screened with total, free and % free testosterone via an early morning lab sampling. Obesity, nephrotic syndrome, hypothyroidism, Graves disease, HIV, aging, cirrhosis, and certain medication (steroids, anticonvulsants, hormones) may alter the level of sex hormone-binding globulin (SHBG). Testosterone is highly bound to SHBG and albumin. Therefore, SHBG levels may also need to be tested. The lower limit of normal when discussing free testosterone is typically 50 pg/mL.
Over the past 3 mo, what percentage of your erections has been satisfactory for successful intercourse?	Frequent attempts with low success rate could suggest a number of pathologic events, including increased pelvic outflowing of blood from the penis during intercourse, and the inability of the penis venous system to collect and trap blood during sexual stimulation. Urology referral is indicated.
Have you had a prior evaluation for sexual dysfunction in the past? If so, what, if anything, was prescribed and what was successful?	Most often, drugs that worked in the past will work again subsequently. Interestingly, many men may obtain their first PDE-5 drug from a "friend" rather from their physician. Some men may experience adverse events associated with certain drugs—visual or hearing loss, myalgias, headaches, orthostatic hypotension, penile burning. (This information is critical so that appropriate medication adjustments may be prescribed.)
What medications are you taking at this time, both prescribed and over the counter?	Drug interactions may occur when using prescription medications for ED. Therefore, one must be clear as to what concomitant medications the patient is using prior to prescribing any drugs.
How much do you smoke and drink? Do you use any illicit drugs?	Cessation of smoking, drinking and use of illicit drugs will often minimize the likelihood of having ED. Weight loss and sleep apnea also contribute to a higher risk of ED.
Do you ride a bicycle long distances?	Pressure placed on the pudendal nerve is a common cause of ED in younger men.

Adapted from Unger J. How to assess and treat erectile dysfunction. *Emerg Med.* 2004;36:28–37, with permission.

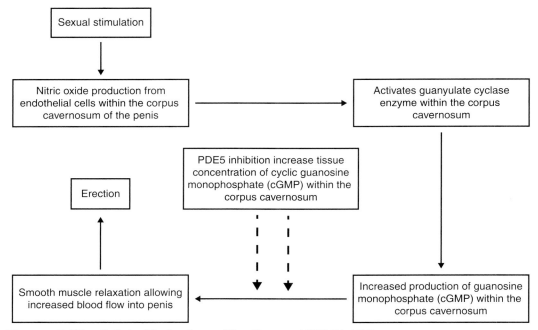

Figure 5-20 • **Cellular Mechanisms of Erections and PDE-5 Inhibitors.**

ED can be successfully managed with a variety of oral medications (PDE-5 inhibitors), transurethral alprostadil pellets, and intracavernosal injections. Table 5-15 lists the pharmacodynamics of the oral medications. Table 5-16 lists recommendations for use of PDE-5 drugs in patients with cardiac disease, and Table 5-17 suggests dose alterations of PDE-5 drugs for patients with renal insufficiency.

The newest member of the PDE-5 inhibitor class is avanafil. This drug has a 30 minute time to onset of action and a relatively short half-life of just 3 to 5 hours. Available in doses of 50, 100 and 200 mg, the drug should be administered at least 30 minutes prior to initiation of sexual

 TABLE 5-15. Pharmacodynamics of the Phosphodiesterase-5 (PDE-5) Inhibitors

Drug	Available Doses (mg)	Onset of Action (minutes)	Duration of Action (h)	Comment
Sildenafil	25, 50, 100	14–20	8–12	Contraindicated with nitrates Take on empty stomach.
Vardenafil	2.5, 5, 10, 20	30–120	8–12	Contraindicated with nitrates Take on empty stomach. Caution with α-blockers because of risk of orthostatic hypotension
Taldalafil	2.5[a], 5[a], 10, 20	30–120	36	Coadministration with nitrates contraindicated Longest half-life of all PDE-5 drugs
Avanafil	50, 100, 200	30–40	3–5 hours	Contraindicated with nitrates. Use with caution with α-blockers May work and allow some patients to have successful erections within 15 minutes after usage

[a]The 2.5- and 5-mg tablets may be used for daily administration.

TABLE 5-16. Recommendation for Use of Phosphodiesterase-5 (PDE-5) Inhibitors in Men with Heart Disease

- PDE-5 inhibitors are absolutely contraindicated with the concomitant use of nitrates.
- Coadministration of a PDE-5 inhibitor and a nitrate within 24 h of each other may result in hypotension or death.
- The risks and benefits of using PDE-5 inhibitors should be discussed with all cardiac patients whether or not they are using nitrates.
- Consider monitoring BP for 1 h in patients with heart failure or hypotension after a PDE-5 inhibitor is administered in the office setting.

activity regardless of food intake. Coadministration with antihypertensive medications such as enalapril and amlodipine may result in a slight reduction in supine systolic and diastolic blood pressures. However, concomitant use of avanafil and α-blockers may result in clinically significant orthostatic changes in blood pressure. Avanafil 200 mg has been shown to potentiate the hypotensive effect of nitrates. Thus, the use of avanafil in patients taking any form of nitrates is contraindicated.

PDE-5 inhibitors are generally safe and effective when used for the treatment of ED in men with heart disease. However, these drugs are potent vasodilators, and physicians should carefully consider whether their high-risk patients [unstable or refractory angina, uncontrolled hypertension, New York Heart Association (NYHA) Functional Class IILTV, recent MI less than 2 weeks prior to consultation, hypertrophic cardiomyopathy, moderate/severe valvular disease] could be adversely affected by these vasodilatory effects.[109]

Recent labeling changes to sildenafil (Viagra), tadalafil (Cialis), and vardenafil (Levitra) reflect a small number of cases of sudden vision attributed to nonarteritic ischemic optic neuropathy (NAION). Although stating that a direct link between NAION and PDE-5 has not been found, the FDA has advised patients on these drugs to notify their physicians immediately in the event of any sudden vision loss in one or both eyes. Physicians should inquire about a history of prior severe vision loss prior to prescribing PDE-5 drugs to any patients with ED.

TABLE 5-17. Phosphodiesterase-5 (PDE-5) Inhibitor Dosing Adjustments for Patients with Chronic Kidney Disease (CKD Stage 4–5)

Medication	Dose Adjustment
Sildenafil	Start dose of 25 mg when creatinine clearance is <30 mL/min.
Tadalafil	Start dose of 5 mg once daily (maximum 10 mg once every 48 h) when creatinine clearance is 31–50 mL/min. Maximum dose of 5 mg when creatinine clearance is <30 mL/min and patient is on hemodialysis.
Vardenafil	No dose adjustment required for CKD 4. Vardenafil has not been evaluated in patients on renal dialysis.
Avanafil	Dose adjustment of doses up to 200 mg are not required for patients with a creatinine clearance > 30 mL/min. Avanafil pharmacokinetics has not been determined in patients with severe renal disease or those individuals on dialysis.

Sources: Viagra (sildenafil citrate) Prescribing Information. http://www.fda.gov/cder/foi/label/2005/020895s021lbl.pdf. Accessed January 9, 2007.
Levitra (vardenafil HCl) Prescribing Information. http://www.umvgraph.com/bayer/inserts/levitra.pdf. Accessed January 9, 2007.
Cialis (tadalafil) Prescribing Information. http://pi.lilly.com/us/cialis-pi.pdf. Accessed January 9, 2007.
Stendra Prescribing Information: http://www.stendra.com/assets/pdf/STENDRA-avanafil-tablets-full-PI.pdf. Accessed June 17, 2012.

Sudden sensorineural hearing loss (SSHL) in association with PDE-5 inhibitor use has resulted in an FDA requirement for more stringent labeling. Although there is currently no direct evidence for a mechanism, some experts postulate acute hearing loss is related to the prolonged effects of intracellular cGMP within the cochlea.[110]

Tadalafil and vardenafil can be coprescribed at 50% maximum doses in patients with benign prostatic hypertrophy (BPH) receiving α-blockers. Daily tadalafil is now indicated for the treatment of BPH and ED as well as the signs and symptoms of both disorders.[111] The new indications for tadalafil for once daily use are based on a clinical trial program of three placebo-controlled efficacy and safety studies that included 1,989 men. Two of these studies were in men with BPH, and one study was specific to men with both ED and BPH. In the ED+BPH study, Cialis 5 mg for once daily use significantly improved scores on the International Index of Erectile Function-Erectile Function Domain (IIEF-EF), a questionnaire evaluating sexual function, and the International Prostate Symptom Score (IPSS), a questionnaire evaluating symptoms of BPH.[112]

Women with sexual dysfunction attributable to diabetes may also experience a reduction in libido, pain with intercourse, and difficulty achieving orgasm. One should encourage women with vaginal dryness to use vaginal lubricants before sexual intercourse. Vaginal estrogens, when appropriate, may be beneficial for patients experiencing dyspareunia, incontinence, and atrophic vaginitis.

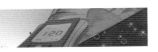

SUMMARY

Physicians must recognize the contribution of A1C, postprandial glucose levels, glycemic variability, and oxidative stress in patients at risk for developing diabetes related complications. Genetics appears to play both a protective and promotional role in patients exposed to chronic hyperglycemia. Oxidative stress activates the polyol, PKC-kinase, hexosamine, neuroinflammation, and advanced glycation pathways, which, over time favor the development of diabetes-related complications. Patients who appear to have minimal protection against various microvascular and macrovascular complications should be ambitiously screened and treated for complications as soon as they become clinically apparent. Any patient with complications should be intensively treated to customized metabolic targets in an attempt to reverse existing anomalies while minimizing the likelihood of developing others.

Diabetic neuropathies are the most common long-term complications observed in patients with diabetes. The diagnosis and management of most patients with sensory and autonomic neuropathy are within the realm of primary care medicine. Arguably the most critical of all neuropathic disorders are cardiac autonomic neuropathy and hypoglycemia awareness autonomic failure, both of which may result in sudden death.

Early detection of hyperglycemia followed by targeted reduction in one's glycemic burden should provide patients with diabetes a life devoid of complications, which may impact both their quality of life and longevity.

REFERENCES

1. Bliss M. *The Discovery of Insulin.* Chicago, IL: University of Chicago Press; 1982:21.
2. Leyton O. Insulin and diabetes mellitus [letter]. *BMJ.* 1923;882.
3. Brown JB, Nichols GA, Perry A. The burden of treatment failure in type 2 diabetes. *Diabetes Care.* 2004;27:1535–1540.
4. Brownlee M. Biochemistry and molecular cell biology of diabetic complications. *Nature.* 2001;414:813–820.

5. American Diabetes Association. Standards of medical care for patients with diabetes mellitus (Position Statement). *Diabetes Care*. 2003;26(Suppl 1):S33–S50.

6. American Diabetes Association. Standards of medical care for patients with diabetes mellitus (Position Statement). *Diabetes Care*. 2004;27(Suppl 1):S15–S35.

7. Diabetes Control and Complications Trial/Epidemiology of Diabetes Interventions and Complications (DCCT/EDIC) Research Group. Modern-day clinical course of type 1 diabetes mellitus after 30 years' duration: the diabetes control and complications trial/epidemiology of diabetes interventions and complications and Pittsburgh epidemiology of diabetes complications experience (1983–2005). *Arch Intern Med*. 2009;169(14):1307–1316.

8. The Diabetes Control and Complications Trial/Epidemiology of Diabetes Interventions and Complications (DCCT/EDIC) Study Research Group. Intensive diabetes treatment and cardiovascular disease in patients with type 1 diabetes. *N Engl J Med*. 2005;353:2643–2653.

9. Vinik A. The question is, my dear Watson, why did the dog not bark? The Joslin 50-Year Medalist Study. *Diabetes Care*. 2011;34(4):1060–1063.

10. Goh SY, Cooper ME. Clinical review: the role of advanced glycation end products in progression and complications of diabetes. *J Clin Endocrinol Metab*. 2008;93:1143–1152.

11. Genuth S, Sun W, Cleary P, et al. DCCT Skin Collagen Ancillary Study Group. Glycation and carboxymethyllysine levels in skin collagen predict the risk of future 10-year progression of diabetic retinopathy and nephropathy in the diabetes control and complications trial and epidemiology of diabetes interventions and complications participants with type 1 diabetes. *Diabetes*. 2005;54:3103–3111.

12. Yan SF, Ramasamy R, Schmidt AM. The RAGE axis: a fundamental mechanism signaling danger to the vulnerable vasculature. *Circ Res*. 2010;106:842–853.

13. National Committee for Quality Assurance. www.ncqa.org. Accessed December 4, 2011.

14. Hirsch IB, Brownlee M. Beyond hemoglobin A1c: need for additional markers of risk for diabetic microvascular complications. *JAMA*. 2010;363(22):2291–2292.

15. Centers for Disease Control and Prevention Data and Trends. http://www.cdc.gov/diabetes/statistics/comp/fig10.htm. Accessed December 4, 2011.

16. Fowler MJ. Microvascular and macrovascular complications of diabetes. *Clinical Diabetes*. 2011;29(3):116–122.

17. Unger J. Reducing oxidative stress in patients with type 2 diabetes mellitus: a primary care call to action. *Insulin*. 2008;3:176–184.

18. Moriel P, Abdalla DS. Nitrotyrosine bound to beta-VLDL-apopoproteins: a biomarker of peroxynitrite formation in experimental atherosclerosis. *Biochem Biophys Res Commun*. 1997;232:332–335.

19. Monnier L, Mas E, Ginet C, et al. Activation of oxidative stress by acute glucose fluctuations compared with sustained chronic hyperglycemia in patients with type 2 diabetes. *JAMA*. 2006;295:1681–1687.

20. The Diabetes Control and Complications Trial Research Group. The relationship of glycemic exposure (HbA1c) to the risk of development and progression of retinopathy in the Diabetes Control and Complications Trial. *Diabetes*. 1995;44:968–983.

21. Monnier L, Colette C. Glycemic variability. *Diabetes Care*. 2008;(Suppl 2):S150–S154.

22. Brownlee M. The pathobiology of diabetic complications: a unifying mechanism. *Diabetes*. 2005;54(6):1615–1625.

23. Kuhlencordt PJ, Gyurko R, Han F, et al. Accelerated atherosclerosis, aortic aneurysm formation, and ischemic heart disease in apolipoprotein E/endothelial nitric oxide synthase double-knockout mice. *Circulation*. 2001;104:448–454.

24. Hirsch IB, Brownlee M. Should minimal blood glucose variability become the gold standard of glycemic control? *J Diabetes Complications*. 2005;19:178–181.

25. Fadini GP, Sartore S, Agostini C, et al. Significance of endothelial progenitor cells in subjects with diabetes. *Diabetes Care*. 2007;30:1305–1313.

26. McGowan TA, Dunn SR, Falkner B, et al. Stimulation of urinary TGF- and isoprostanes in response to hyperglycemia in humans. *Clin J Am Soc Nephrol*. 2006;1:263–268.

27. Vlassara H, Palace MR. Diabetes and advanced glycation endproducts. *J Intern Med*. 2002;251:87–101.

28. Meier M, King GL. Protein kinase C activation and its pharmacological inhibition in vascular disease. *Va Med*. 2000;5:173–185.

29. Watkins LR, Milligan ED, Maier SF. Glial activation: a driving force for pathological pain. *Trends Neurosci*. 2001;24:450–455.

30. Koehler RC, Gebremedhin D, Harder DR. Role of astrocytes in cerebrovascular regulation. *J Appl Physiol*. 2006;100:307–317.

31. Watkins LR, Maier SF. Glia: a novel drug discovery target for clinical pain. *Nat Rev Drug Discov.* 2003;2:973–985.

32. Vallejo R, de Leon-Casasola O, Ramsun B. Opioid therapy and immunosuppression: a review. *Am J Ther.* 2004;11:354–365.

33. Argoff CE, Backonja M-M, Belgrade MJ, et al. Consensus guidelines: treatment planning and options. *Mayo Clin Proc.* 2006;81(4 Suppl):S12–S25; doi:10.4065/81.4_Suppl.S12.

34. Carrington AL, Abbott CA, Shaw JE, et al. Can motor nerve conduction velocity predict foot problems in diabetic neuropathy over a 6-year outcome period? *Diabetes Care.* 2002;25:2010–2015.

35. Boulton AJM, Gries FA, Jervell JA. Guidelines for the diagnosis and outpatient management of diabetic peripheral neuropathy. *Diabet Med.* 1998;15:508–514.

36. Pirart J. Diabetes mellitus and its degenerative complications: a prospective study of 4,400 patients observed between 1947 and 1973. *Diabetes Metab.* 1977;3:97–107.

37. Vinik AI, Mehrabyan A. Understanding diabetic neuropathies. *Emerg Med.* 2004;5:39–44.

38. Vinik AI, Maser RE, Mitchell BD. et al. Diabetic autonomic neuropathy. *Diabetes Care.* 2003;26:1553–1579.

39. Boulton AJM, Malik RA, Arezzo JC. et al. Diabetic somatic neuropathies. *Diabetes Care.* 2004;27:1458–1486.

40. Argoff CE, Cole BE, Fishbain DA, et al. Diabetic peripheral neuropathic pain: clinical and quality-of-life issues. *Mayo Clin Proc.* 2006;81(4 suppl):S3–S11.

41. Sumner CJ, Sheth S, Griffin JW, et al. The spectrum of neuropathy in diabetes and impaired glucose tolerance. *Neurology.* 2003;60:108–111.

42. Singleton JR, Smith AG, Bromberg MB. Increased prevalence of impaired glucose tolerance in patients with painful sensory neuropathy. *Diabetes Care.* 2001;24:1448–1453.

43. Perkins BA, Greene DA, Bril V. Glycemic control is related to the morphological severity of diabetic sensorimotor polyneuropathy. *Diabetes Care.* 2001;24:748–752.

44. Tkac I, Bril V. Glycemic control is related to the electrophysiologic severity of diabetic peripheral sensorimotor polyneuropathy. *Diabetes Care.* 1998;21:1749–1752.

45. The Diabetes Control and Complications Trial Research Group. The effect of intensive diabetes therapy on the development and progression of neuropathy. *Ann Intern Med.* 1995;122:561–568.

46. Tesfaye S, Chaturvedi N, Eaton SEM. Vascular risk factors and diabetic neuropathy. *N Engl J Med.* 2005;352:341–350.

47. Vinik AI, Holland MT, Le Beau JM, et al. Diabetic neuropathies. *Diabetes Care.* 1992;15:1926–1975.

48. Raff MC, Asbury AK. Ischemic mononeuropathy and mononeuropathy multiplex in diabetes mellitus. *N Engl J Med.* 1968;279:17–21.

49. Vinik A, Mehrabyan A, Colen L, et al. Focal entrapment neuropathies in diabetes. *Diabetes Care.* 2004;27:1783–1788.

50. Malik RA. Focal and multifocal neuropathies. *Curr Diab Rep.* 2002;2:489–494.

51. American Diabetes Association. Clinical Practice Recommendations 2011. *Diabetes Care.* 2011;34(Suppl 1):S36.

52. Lavery LA, Higgins KR, Lanctot DR, et al. Home monitoring of foot skin temperatures to prevent ulceration. *Diabetes Care.* 2004;27:2642–2647.

53. Lavery LA, Higgins KR, Lanctot DR, et al. Preventing diabetic foot ulcer recurrence in high-risk patients: use of temperature monitoring as a self-assessment tool. *Diabetes Care.* 2007;30:14–20.

54. Arad Y, Fonseca V, Peters A. Beyond the monofilament for the insensate diabetic foot. *Diabetes Care.* 2011;34:1041–1046.

55. Pittenger GL, Ray M, Burcus NI, et al. Intraepidermal nerve fibers are indicators of small-fiber neuropathy in both diabetic and nondiabetic patients. *Diabetes Care.* 2004;27:1974–1979.

56. Shun CT, Chang YC, Wu HP, et al. Skin denervation in type 2 diabetes: correlations with diabetic duration and functional impairments. *Brain.* 2004;127:1593–1605.

57. Kennedy AJ, et al. Pathology and quantitation of cutaneous innervation. In: Dyck PJ, Thomas PK, eds. *Peripheral Neuropathy.* Philadelphia, PA: Elsevier Saunders; 2005:869–895.

58. http://www.aanem.org/Login.aspx?ReturnUrl=%2fPractice%2fCoding%2fFAQs%2fNerve-Conduction-Studies.aspx. Accessed December 5, 2011.

59. Perkins BA, Grewal J, Ng E, et al. Validation of a novel point-of-care nerve conduction device for the detection of diabetic sensorimotor polyneuropathy. *Diabetes Care.* 2006;29(9):2023–2027.

60. Kong X, Lesser EA, Gozani SN. Repeatability of nerve conduction measurements derived entirely by computer methods. *Biomed Eng Online.* 2009;8:33.

61. Berger A, Dukes EM, Oster G. Clinical characteristics and economic costs of patients with painful neuropathic disorders. *J Pain.* 2004;5:143–149.

62. Unger J. Obstacles surrounding the diagnosis and management of diabetic neuropathy. *The Pain Practitioner*. 2007;17:(3). 33–42.
63. Lee P, Chen R. Vitamin D as an analgesic for patients with type 2 diabetes and neuropathic pain. *Archive Intern Med*. 2008;168;(7):771–772.
64. Engelen W, Bouten A, De Leeuw I, et al. Are low magnesium levels in type 1 diabetes associated with electromyographical signs of polyneuropathy? *Magnet Res*. 2000;13:197–203.
65. Unger J. Diagnosis and management of diabetic peripheral neuropathic pain. *Female Patient Primary Care Edition*. 2005;30(8):27–30.
66. Begon S, Pickering G, Eschalier A. et al. Magnesium and MK-801 have a similar effect in two experimental models of neuropathic pain. *Brain Res*. 2000;887:436–439.
67. Veves A, et al. Endothelial cell dysfunction and the expression of nitric oxide synthase in diabetic neuropathy, vascular disease and foot ulcerations. *Diabetes*. 1998;47:457–463.
68. Jacobs AM. Abstracts of New Cardiovascular Horizons Meeting. 2008. L-methylfolate, methylcobalamin, and pyridoxal 5-phosphate reduces the symptoms of diabetic peripheral neuropaty. Oral presentations.
69. Hays L, Reid C, Doran M, et al. The use of methadone for the treatment of diabetic neuropathy. *Diabetes Care*. 2005;28(2):485–487.
70. Davis M, Walsh D. Methadone for relief of cancer pain: a review of pharmokinetics, pharmacodynamics. drug interactions and protocols of administration. *Support Care Cancer*. 2001;9:73–83.
71. Gilron I, Bailey JM, Dongsheng T, et al. Morphine, gabapentin or their combination for neuropathic pain. *New Engl J Med*. 2005;352:1324–1334.
72. Vinik AI, Erbas T. Recognizing and treating diabetic autonomic neuropathy. *Cleve Clin J Med*. 2001; 68:928–944.
73. O'Brian IA, McFadden JP, Corrall RJ. The influence of autonomic neuropathy on mortality in insulin-dependent diabetes. *Q J Med*. 1991;79:495–502.
74. Granberg B, Ejskjaer N, Peakman M, et al. Autoantibodies to autonomic nerves associated with cardiac and peripheral autonomic neuropathy. *Diabetes Care*. 2005;28:1959–1964.
75. Witte DR, Tesfaye S, Chaturvedi, et al. EURODIAB Prospective Complications Study Group. Risk factors for cardiac autonomic neuropathy in type 1 diabetes mellitus. *Diabetologia*. 2005;48:164–217.
76. Pop-Busui R, Low PA, Waberski BH, et al. DCCT/EDIC Research Group. Effects of prior intensive insulin therapy on cardiac autonomic nervous system function in type 1 diabetes mellitus: the Diabetes Control and Complications Trial/Epidemiology of Diabetes Interventions and Complications study (DCCT/EDIC). *Circulation*. 2009;119:2886–2893.
77. Gaede P, Vedel P, Parving HH, et al. Intensified multifactorial intervention in patients with type 2 diabetes mellitus and microalbuminuria: the Steno type 2 randomised study. *Lancet*. 1999;353:617–622.
78. Ziegler D, Gries FA, Muhlen H, et al. Prevalence and clinical correlates of cardiovascular autonomic and peripheral diabetic neuropathy in patients attending diabetes centers. The DiaCAN Multicenter Study Group. *Diabetes Metab*. 1993;19:143–151.
79. Nakano S, Uchida K, Kigoshi T, et al. Circadian rhythm of blood pressure in normotensive NIDDM subjects: its relationship to microvascular complications. *Diabetes Care*. 1991;14:707–711.
80. Parati G, Bilo G. Should 24-h ambulatory blood pressure monitoring be done in every patient with diabetes? *Diabetes Care*. 2009;32(Suppl 2):S298–S304.
81. Parati G, Bilo G, Mancia G. Prognostic and diagnostic value of ambulatory blood pressure monitoring. In: Oparial S, Weber MA, eds. *Hypertension: Companion to Brenner & Rector's The Kidney*. Philadelphia, PA: Elsevier Inc.; 2005:305–317.
82. Suzuki H, Kanno Y, Nakamoto H, et al. Decline of renal function is associated with proteinuria and systolic blood pressure in the morning in diabetic nephropathy. *Clin Exp Hypertens*. 2005;27:129–138.
83. Langer A, Freeman MR, Josse RG, et al. Detection of silent myocardial ischemia in diabetes mellitus. *Am J Cardiol*. 1991;67:1073–1078.
84. Solar NG, Bennet MA, Pentecost BI, et al. Myocardial infarction in diabetes. *Q J Med*. 1975;173:125–131.
85. Ikeda T, Matsuda K, Itoh H, et al. Plasma levels of brain and atrial natriuretic peptides elevate in proportion to left ventricular end-systolic wall stress in patients with aortic stenosis. *Am Heart J*. 1997;133(3):307–314.
86. Bhalla MA, Chiang A, Epshteyn VA, et al. Prognostic role of B-type natriuretic peptide levels in patients with type 2 diabetes mellitus. *J Am Coll Cardiol*. 2004;44(5):1047–1052.
87. Somaratne JB, Whalley GA, Bagg W, et al. Early detection and significance of structural cardiovascular abnormalities in patients with type 2 diabetes mellitus. *Expert Rev Cardiovasc Ther*. 2008;6(1): 109–125.

88. Vinik AI, Park TS, Stansberry KB, et al. Diabetic neuropathies. *Diabetologia.* 2000;43:957–973.

89. Hoeldtke RD, Israel BC. Treatment of orthostatic hypotension with octreotide. *J Clin Endocrinol Metab.* 1989;68:1051–1059.

90. Sheehy TW. Diabetic gustatory sweating. *Am J Gastroenterol.* 1991;86:15–17.

91. Tesfaye S, Boulton AJM, Dyck PJ, et al. Diabetic neuropathies: update on definitions, diagnostic criteria, estimation of severity and treatments. *Diabetes Care.* 2010;33(10):2285–2293.

92. Shaw JE, Abbott CA, Tindle K, et al. A randomized controlled trial of topical glycopyrrolate, the first specific treatment for diabetic gustatory sweating. *Diabetologia.* 1997;40:299–301.

93. Naumann M. Evidence-based medicine: botulinum toxin in focal hyperhidrosis. *J Neurol.* 2001; 248(Suppl 1):31–33.

94. Talley NJ. Diabetic gastropathy and prokinetics. *Am J Gastroenterol.* 2003;98:246–271.

95. Unger J, Marcus A. Insulin pump therapy: what you need to know. *Emerg Med.* 2002;34:24–33.

96. Hill SR, Fayyad AM, Jones GR. Diabetes mellitus and female lower urinary tract symptoms: a review. *Neurourol Urodyn.* 2008;27:362–367.

97. Unger J, Parkin C. Recognition, prevention and proactive management of hypoglycemia in patients with type 1 diabetes. *Postgraduate Medicine.* 2011;123(4):71–80.

98. UK Hypoglycaemia Study Group. Risk of hypoglycaemia in types 1 and 2 diabetes: effects of treatment modalities and their duration. *Diabetologia.* 2007;50(6):1140–1147.

99. Cryer PE, Davis SN, Shamoon H. Hypoglycemia in diabetes. *Diabetes Care.* 2003;26(6):1902–1912.

100. Cranston I, Lomas J, Maran A, et al. Restoration of hypoglyaemia awareness in patients with long-duration insulin dependent diabetes. *Lancet.* 1994;344(8918):283–287.

101. Burger AJ, Weinrauch LA, D'Elia JA, et al. Effect of glycemic control on heart rate variability in type 1 diabetic patients with cardiac autonomic neuropathy. *Am J Cardiol.* 1991;84:687–691.

102. Pfeifer MA, Schumer MP. Clinical trials of diabetic neuropathy: past, present, and future. *Diabetes.* 1995;l44:1355–1361.

103. NIH Consensus Conference. Impotence. *J Am Med Assoc.* 1993;270:83–90.

104. Bacon CG, Hu FB, Giovannucci E, et al. Association of type and duration of diabetes with erectile dysfunction in a large cohort of men. *Diabetes Care.* 2002;25(8):1458–1463.

105. Kalter-Leibovici O, Wainstein J, Ziv A, et al. Clinical, socioeconomic and lifestyle parameters associated with erectile dysfunction among diabetic men. *Diabetes Care.* 2005;28:1739–1744.

106. Montorsi P, Ravagnani PM, Galli S, et al. Common grounds for erectile dysfunction and coronary artery disease. *Curr Opin Urol.* 2004;14(6):361–365.

107. Urology Channel Web Site. Available at: http://www.urologychannel.com/erectiledysfunctiori/causes. shtml#dia. Accessed June 1, 2006.

108. Unger J. How to assess and treat erectile dysfunction. *Emerg Med.* 2004;36:28–37.

109. Cheitlin MD. Sexual activity and cardiovascular disease. *Am J Cardiol.* 2003;92:3M–8M.

110. Maddox PT, Saunders J, Chandrasekhar SS. Sudden hearing loss from PDE-5 inhibitors: a possible cellular stress etiology. *Laryngoscope.* 2009;119(8):1586–1589.

111. Cialis package insert. Indianapolis, IN: Eli Lilly and Company; 2010.

112. Gacci M, Eardley I, Giuliano F, et al. Critical analysis of the relationship between sexual dysfunctions and lower urinary tract symptoms due to benign prostatic hypertrophy. *Eur Urol.* 2011;60(4):809–825.

6

Prevention, Diagnosis, and Treatment of Microvascular Complications

PART 2 / DIABETIC NEPHROPATHY AND DIABETIC RETINOPATHY

I have figured out that if I drink water through a straw rather than gulp it from a large glass, I am better able to quench my thirst during these hot summer months in Southern California.

—*Eddie Hunter, kidney dialysis patient since 2009*

Diabetic Nephropathy

Introduction Diabetic nephropathy is characterized by proteinuria, hypertension, and progressive kidney failure. Thirty percent of patients with T1DM and 10% to 40% of patients with T2DM will eventually develop end-stage renal failure.[1] In patients with T2DM, the prevalence of diabetic nephropathy varies from 5% to 10% in Caucasian patients, 10% to 20% in African Americans, and nearly 60% in members of the Pima Indian tribe.[2] In 2008, the annual cost to society to support treatment of patients with end-stage renal disease (ESRD) was $38.45 billion.[3] The annual per patient cost of managing ESRD in the United States is approximately $64,000, with initial first year cost approaching $90,000.[3]

Primary care physicians (PCPs) should take a proactive stance in screening high-risk patients for the presence of chronic kidney disease (CKD). Once these individuals are identified, PCPs are well trained to provide interventional strategies designed to reverse or slow the progression of the disease. Confusion exists as to the most appropriate time to refer patients with diabetic nephropathy for renal consultation.[4] Demands for nephrology services across the United States are severely impacted by a shortage of specialist. In 2007, 6,891 nephrologists were listed as full-time equivalent clinicians.[5] Nephrology patients face a future clouded by limited specialty access. Even more worrisome is a glance into the future of the nephrology population. Although 235 nephrologists completed fellowship training in 2007, this number consistently falls approximately 200 trainees short of the projections required to manage the medical needs of renal patients in years to come. Interestingly, 30% of all currently practicing nephrologists are 55 years of age or older and may retire prior to the projected expansion of baby boomers into the ESRD market place. Currently, 13% of the U.S. population has clinical evidence of CKD.[6] Clearly, the burden of CKD detection and management will be shifting toward the primary care specialties where the patient-to-physician ratios are typically 1:1,100.[7]

Diabetes accounts for 38% of all ESRD in the United States. The mean A1C of patients initiating treatment for ESRD is 7.6%, suggesting that risk factors such as genetics, blood pressure (BP), smoking, obesity, and hyperlipidemia may be influential in determining both disease progression and outcomes.[8,9] Fortunately, diabetes-related ESRD has declined in all age groups by 3.9% per year from 1996 to 2006 as physicians become more aware of the importance of intensive metabolic management of glucose, BP, and hyperlipidemia.[10]

Diabetic dialysis patients and transplant recipients do have higher mortality and morbidity rates than their nondiabetic counterparts.[11] Microalbuminuria may substantially increase morbidity and mortality in diabetes patients.[12]

Patient awareness of CKD is extremely low. Less than 10% of 2,992 adult respondents in the 1994 to 2002 National Health and Nutrition Examination Survey (NHANES) who met criteria for CKD stage 1 to 3 answered yes to the question "Have you ever been told that you have weak or failing kidneys?" Only 42% of patients with CKD stage 4 were aware of their renal impairment.[13] Although PCPs are quick to obtain renal function labs on patients, few patients receive feedback on the interpretation of the results. Perhaps this adds further truth to the belief that PCP's familiarity with CKD is suboptimal.[14]

The early detection of diabetic nephropathy is dependent on measuring one's urinary albumin excretion (UAE) rate. UAE levels within microalbuminuric levels (30 to 299 mg per 24 hour or a spot urine albumin-to-creatinine ratio of 30 to 299 mg per g) identify patients at increased risk for development of overt diabetic nephropathy.[15] Kidneys damaged from diabetic nephropathy will experience a gradual decline in glomerular filtration rate (GFR). Over time, as more nephrons fail, CKD will progress and patient may eventually develop end-stage renal failure. Impaired renal function, as measured by GFR, may be present even in patients with a normal UAE rate. PCPs should feel confident assessing renal function studies in all patients with diabetes while providing appropriate initial and ongoing care to these individuals.

• Normal Renal Function

GFR is accepted as the best overall index of renal function and represents the total filtration rate of the functioning nephrons in the kidney. Chronic kidney disease is defined by the National Kidney Foundation as a decline in GFR to less than 60 mL per min per 1.73 m^2 for a minimum of 3 months.[16] Signs of kidney damage include proteinuria, but other markers such as persistent glomerulonephritis or structural damage from polycystic kidney disease may also be present.

Although serum creatinine can provide a rough index of GFR, used alone, the test may overestimate renal function by as much as 40%[16] (Fig. 6-1). Creatinine is produced at a fairly constant rate within muscle cells. However, the greater one's muscle mass, the greater will be the production of creatinine. Younger patients and African Americans have more muscle mass than older non-Hispanic white individuals. Men produce more creatinine than females. Because creatinine is filtered by the proximal tubules of the kidneys, any reduction in the number of nephrons (i.e., renal insufficiency—RI) will result in an elevation of serum creatinine. RI also will result in an increase in myocyte production, secretion, and clearance of creatinine.[17] Thus, validated GFR calculators must consider multiple factors including age, gender, serum creatinine, and race.[18]

A normal GFR ranges from 120 to 130 mL per min per 1.73 m^2. Normal kidney function is proportional to kidney size, which is determined by the body's surface area considered to be 1.73 m^2 for young adults. Thus, these units are included in the GFR formula. In healthy individuals, the GFR does not decrease to less than 90 mL per min per 1.73 m^2 until age 60. Early kidney disease is

Example: Serum Creatinine Does Not Accurately Reflect Renal Function

	70-year old, 100-kg non-Hispanic White Woman	25-year old, 100-kg African American Man
Serum Creatinine	1.5 mg/dL	1.5 mg/dL
GFR estimation by MDRD study equation	34 mL/min/1.73 m2	75 mL/min/1.73 m2

Figure 6-1 • Example: Serum Creatinine Does Not Accurately Reflect Renal Function. GFR is considered to be the best index of kidney function for both healthy and disease states. In this example, patients have the same weight and serum creatinine levels. They are of different races and their ages differ by 45 years. However, the calculation of their GFRs reveals substantial differences. The older woman has lost a significant number of nephrons, resulting in a diagnosis of advanced stage 3 CKD. The younger patient has evidence of CKD stage 2.
MDRD, Modification of Diet in Renal Disease.
(Reference: Shemesh O, Golbetz H, Kriss HP, et al. Limitations of creatinine as a filtration marker in glomerulopathic patients. *Kidney Int.* 1985;28(5):830–838.)

defined as having a GFR of 60 to 89 mL per min per 1.73 m² with proteinuria, suggesting that the kidneys have been exposed to some form of toxicity. CKD is diagnosed when one's GFR remains less than 60 mL per min per 1.73 m² for greater than 3 months.[19] Children reach adult values for mean GFR by approximately age 2 years.[20]

The Modification of Diet in Renal Disease (MDRD) equation is the preferred means by which GFR should be determined and may be accessed online.[21] The Cockroft-Gault equation is used to calculate medication dosing adjustments in patients with renal insufficiency.[22] Neither formula is validated for use during acute renal failure because a stable serum creatinine is required to ensure accuracy.

The MDRD has not been validated for patients with diabetic kidney disease, patients over age 70, or in those patients with normal renal function (GFR greater than 60 mL per min per 1.73 m²). The MDRD equation was developed from a study of 1,628 patients with impaired renal function, only 6% of whom had diabetes.[23] Both the MDRD equation and the Cockcroft-Gault formula tend to underestimate GFR in patients with T2DM who have microalbuminuria.[24] Despite the lack of precision and accuracy of the MDRD estimate, epidemiologic studies using the MDRD estimates of renal function have demonstrated a significant correlation between declining GFR trends with all-cause mortality and cardiovascular disease (CVD).[25,26]

The CKD-EPI equation may also be used to estimate GFR. Compared with the MDRD, CKD-EPI is more accurate at determining GFRs in patients with estimated GFR greater than 60 mL per min per 1.73 m².[27]

Internet and smartphone access to all GFR calculations are found in Table 6-1.

TABLE 6-1. Internet Sites for GFR and Renal Function Calculations

Renal Function Calculators	Site
CKD-EPI (GFR calculations >60 mL/min/1.73 m²)	http://www.nephromatic.com/egfr.php
Cockroft-Gault equation (calculates CC)	http://nephron.com/cgi-bin/CGSI.cgi
MDRD equation (calculates GFR)	www.kidney.org/professionals/tools
Smartphone app for all equations	http://www.freewarepocketpc.net/ppc-download-gfr-calc.html

TABLE 6-2. Screening Recommendations for Diabetic Nephropathy

T1DM	T2DM
• Assess UAE in all patients with diabetes duration >5 y.	• Assess annual UAE in all patients at time of diagnosis.
• Determine eGFR annually in all adults to stage the level of CKD if present.	• Determine eGFR annually in all adults to stage the level of CKD if present.

UAE, Urine albumin excretion; eGFR, estimated glomerular filtration rate, CKD, chronic kidney disease.
From American Diabetes Association. Clinical Practice Recommendations 2011. *Diabetes Care.* 2011;34(Suppl 1):S33.

• Importance of Screening for Diabetic Nephropathy

The American Diabetes Association (ADA) screening recommendations for nephropathy are displayed in Table 6-2. Both estimate glomerular filtration rate (eGFR), and UAE should be accessed annually in adult patients with T2DM. Once one is diagnosed with kidney damage (defined as having abnormalities on pathologic, urine, blood, or imaging tests) or a reduced eGFR for greater than or equal to 3 months, the GFR and UAE labs should be routinely evaluated to monitor disease progression.[28]

eGFR is the best measure of kidney function in both healthy and ill patients. The severity of RI is determined by the eGFR level shown in Figure 6-2. eGFR is calculated based upon the serum creatinine, as well as the patient's age, gender, and race. The GFR in patients with early stages of CKD due to diabetic nephropathy may be abnormally high due to hyperfiltration. Therefore, one must evaluate the presence of both UAE and eGFR to determine if kidney injury is present and, if so, what stage of CKD the patient is in.

Albuminuria may be determined with a spot urine test assessing the albumin-to-creatinine ratio. A result of less than 30 mg albumin per gram of creatinine is considered normal. Microalbuminuria is defined as 30 to 300 mg per g, whereas macroalbuminuria is diagnosed when one excretes greater than 300 m per g of albumin (Table 6-3).[28] Albuminuria is indicative of diabetic nephropathy, although other forms of CKD may occur in diabetic patients. One should note that the presence of albuminuria or other markers of renal damage are only necessary to diagnose CKD stages 1 and 2. Advanced CKD may be present without evidence of albuminuria.

Due to the intrasubject variability in UAE, at least two specimens, preferably first morning voids collected within a 3- to 6-month period, should be abnormal before diagnosing CKD. Stages 3 to

Both eGFR and Urine Albumin Excretion Predict Chronic Kidney Disease Progression

CKD Stage, eGFR (mL/min/1.73 m2)					
Normal > 90	**Stage 1** > 90 with kidney damage*	**Stage 2** 60-89 with kidney damage *	**Stage 3** 30-59	**Stage 4** 15-29	**Stage 5** < 15
	ICD-9: 581.1	ICD-9: 585.2	ICD-9: 585.3	ICD-9: 585.4	ICD-9: 585.5
	ICD-10: N18.1	ICD-10: N18.2	ICD-10: N18.3	ICD-10: N18.4	ICD-10: N18.5
CKD Progression					
Normal < 30 mg/g		Microalbuminuria 30-300 mg/g		Macroalbuminuria > 300 mg/g	

Figure 6-2 • Both eGFR and Urine Albumin Excretion Predict Chronic Kidney Disease Progression. (ICD-9 and ICD-10 coding provided courtesy of Reinhard Beel, rbeel@hotmail.com.)

TABLE 6-3. Clinical Definitions of Albuminuria

Category	Spot Collection: (Albumin/Creatinine Ratio) μg/mg Creatinine
Normal	<30
Premicroalbuminuria[a]	8–30
Microalbuminuria	30–300
Macroalbuminuria	>300

Note: A false-positive urine protein test may occur under the following circumstances: vigorous exercise within 24 hours of testing, preexisting fever or infection, presence of CHF, severe hypertension, or marked hyperglycemia. Once these conditions are identified and corrected, the urinary protein testing should be repeated. If the A:C ≥30 in two of three specimens within 3 months, the diagnosis of albuminuria is established.
[a]The presence of premicroalbuminuria can increase one's risk for developing hypertension.

5 CKD occurs in the absence of UAE in many patients with T2DM. Therefore, GFR should be used to stage, rather than screen, patients for CKD.

CKD increases cardiovascular (CV) risk including death. Figure 6-3 shows a graph relating GFR and albuminuria levels from 14,586 patients from the NHANES 1988 to 2000 dataset. The highest mortality rates are observed with macroalbuminuria (ACR greater than or equal to 300 mg per g) and a GFR less than 60 mL per min per 1.73 m². Such individuals are four times more likely to die from a CV event and three times more likely to die from any cause.[29] Lowest mortality rates are observed in patients with GFRs greater than or equal to 90 mL per min per 1.73 m² and without evidence of albuminuria.

Microalbuminuria is a marker of vascular disease, endothelial dysfunction, and all-cause mortality in the general population[30] (Fig. 6-4). Patients with microalbuminuria also have a greater chance of developing renal impairment over a 4-year follow-up period.[31]

Endothelial dysfunction may be defined as alterations in the normal properties of endothelium that are inappropriate for the preservation of organ function.[32] Under physiologic circumstances, the endothelium maintains homeostasis at the vascular wall. Normal healthy endothelium reduces vascular tone, regulates vascular permeability, limits platelet adhesion and aggregation, prevents activation of the coagulation cascade, and restricts leukocyte adhesion. One of the most potent mediators of endothelium function is nitric oxide (NO). NO acts as a potent vasodilator, inhibits inflammation, growth of vascular smooth muscle, and aggregation of platelets. Altered production and bioavailability of NO

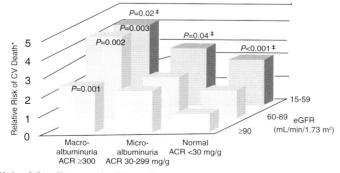

Risk of Cardiovascular Mortality In Relation To GFR and Albuminuria

Figure 6-3 • Risk of Cardiovascular Mortality in Relation to GFR and Albuminuria. The risk of CV mortality rises with each 10 mL per min per 1.73 m² decrease in estimated GFR, particularly when the GFR is less than 60 mL per min per 1.73 m². Below this level, the risk of CV mortality increased by 29% and all-cause mortality by 22% with each 10-point reduction in GFR. The risk of CV and all-cause death also increased with each doubling of albumin/creatinine ratio by 6.3%. (Adapted from Astor BC, Hallan SI, Miller ER III, et al. Glomerular filtration rate, albuminuria, and risk of cardiovascular and all-cause mortality in the U.S. population. *Am J Epidemiol.* 2008;167(10):1226–1234.)

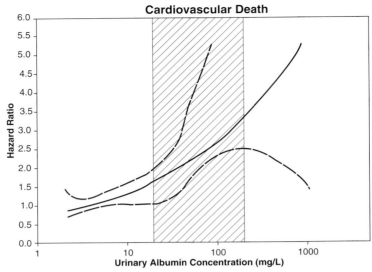

Figure 6-4 • **Urinary Albumin Excretion Predicts cardiovascular Mortality in the General Population.** Relationship between UAE and hazard ratio. The *dotted lines* represent 95% confidence limit and the *squared area* indicates the definition of microalbuminuria. (From Hillege HL, Fidler V, Diercks GF, et al. Urinary albumin excretion predicts cardiovascular and noncardiovascular mortality in general population. *Circulation.* 2002;106:1777–1782.)

are associated with endothelial dysfunction. NO production may be affected by diabetes, hypertension, aging, oxidative stress, genetic factors, and hyperlipidemia.[33] As endothelial cells become inflamed and dysfunctional due to alterations in NO production, vascular permeability is increased, allowing greater rates of transcapillary leakage of albumin systemically as well as through the glomeruli.[34]

Endothelial injury increases the release of renin, an enzyme produced primarily by the juxtaglomerular cells of the kidneys. Renin catalyzes the conversion of angiotensinogen into an inactive substance: angiotensin I (A-I) (Fig. 6-5). Angiotensin-converting enzyme (ACE) then converts A-I to the physiologically active angiotensin II (A-II), which causes potent vasoconstriction, aldosterone secretion, sympathetic activation, and hypertension.[35] ACE inhibitor drugs block the conversion of A-I to A-II. Angiotensin receptor blockers (ARBs) antagonize A-II-induced biologic actions, which include smooth muscle contractions, sympathetic pressor mechanisms, and aldosterone secretion.

Patients with both T1DM and T2DM who have microalbuminuria lose vasomotor control of their peripheral vessels.[36,37] Elevations of UAE are associated with vascular proinflammation. Higher levels of von Willebrand factor, tissue-type plasminogen activator (t-PA), and plasminogen activator inhibitor-1 (PAI-1) are found in patients with T2DM with microalbuminuria and surrogate markers of oxidative stress.[33] The resulting endothelial proinflammation and inflammation are shared metabolic consequences of hypertension and diabetes as mediated by factors such as oxidative stress. This may explain the heightened risk of CV mortality observed in all patients with microalbuminuria (Fig. 6-6).

• Chronic Kidney Disease and Cardiovascular Mortality

Patients with CKD stage 1 or 2 often have traditional Framingham CV risk factors such as diabetes, hypertension, dyslipidemia, obesity, tobacco use and advancing age. In more advanced CKD stages, the CV hazard ratio is accelerated due to the influence of nontraditional risk factors such as secondary hyperparathyroidism, anemia, oxidative stress, and vascular inflammation. Thus, proactive screening, recognition, and intensive management of renal insufficiency are required to prevent disease progression. Little can be done to reverse or delay diabetic nephropathy once the serum creatinine exceeds 2.5 mg/dL.

Increasing CV risk begins at the earliest stages of renal impairment and rises continuously as renal damage progresses toward ESRD (Fig. 6-7). There is a strong, continuous correlation between

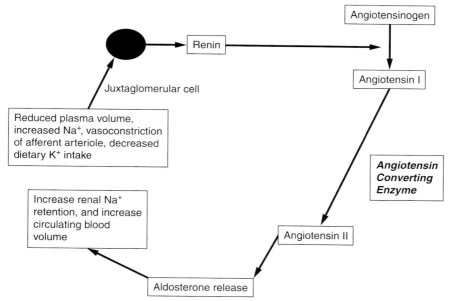

Figure 6-5 • The Renin-Angiotensin-Aldosterone System: Physiology and Pharmacology. Renin is released from juxtaglomerular cells acting as pressure and renal profusion sensors. A reduction in plasma volume is perceived by the juxtaglomerular cell as a threat to maintenance of BP homeostasis. Decreased dietary potassium (K^+) intake, increased plasma sodium (Na^+) levels, and sympathetic input from changes in posture also result in the renin release. Renin then catalyzes the conversion of angiotensinogen into angiotensin I (A-I). ACE converts inactive A-I into active angiotensin II (A-II). A-II results in vasoconstriction, sympathetic discharge, and hypertension. ARBs block the pharmacologic effects of A-II in the periphery: smooth muscle contraction, sympathetic discharge, and aldosterone secretion. Aldosterone secretion leads to sodium retention, an increase in circulation blood volume, and a rise in BP. (Adapted from Matsubara H. Pathophysiological role of angiotensin II receptor in cardiac and renal diseases. *Circ Res.* 1998;83:1182–1191.)

increased risk for CVD events and impaired renal function, which begins at the earliest stages of renal impairment and rises continuously to 20 to 30 times above the risk in the general population as renal damage progresses to ESRD.[38] The relative risk of mortality for patients in ESRD is 590% higher than patients in CKD stage 3.[25]

As shown in Figure 6-8, diabetic nephropathy significantly increases one's risk for congestive heart failure (CHF), atherosclerotic vascular disease, stroke, MI, peripheral vascular disease, and mortality.

As recommended by the American Heart Association, patients with diabetic nephropathy should be considered to have the "highest risk stratification" for subsequent cardiac events, even in early stages of CKD.[39] Any patient with early-stage CKD (eGFR greater than 60 mL per min per 1.73 m²) and demonstrated proteinuria should be treated as a coronary artery disease equivalent for purposes of risk stratification.[40]

• Predicting Risk of Chronic Kidney Disease Progression

CKD management is challenging due to the heterogeneity of the disease process, variability in rates of progression and high risk of CV mortality. Determining the probability of kidney failure may be useful for patient and provider communication, triage and management of nephrology referrals, and timing of dialysis access placement and living-related kidney transplant. eGFR is not a sufficient measure to predict progression toward ESRD.

Using a set of variables that are routinely measured in laboratories, disease progression may now be determined accurately within a primary care practice. The kidney risk equation provides

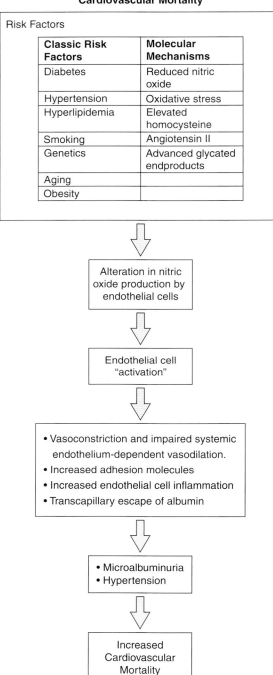

Figure 6-6 • Relationship between Microalbuminuria and Increased Cardiovascular Mortality.

the 2- and 5-year probability of progression to dialysis or transplantation for a patient with CKD stages 3 to 5.[41] Physicians will need to input the patient's age, sex, eGFR, urine albumin:creatinine ratio, calcium, phosphorus, albumin, and bicarbonate into an online formula available at: http://www.qxmd.com/calculate-online/nephrology/kidney-failure-risk-equation. A free app is also available at this web site for use on smartphones.

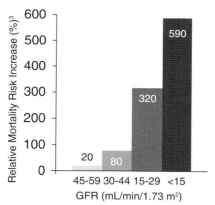

Figure 6-7 • **The Risk of All Cause Mortality Increases Sharply in Patients Having an eGFR Below 45 mL Per Minute Per 1.73 m².** In a registry study of over 1 million adult participants, patients with an eGFR less than 60 mL per min per 1.73 m² were found to have a dramatically increased risk of death from any cause, which increased in a nonlinear fashion with decreasing GFR. Patients with stage 3 CKD were subdivided into two categories. Those with eGFR between 45 and 59 mL per min per 1.73 m² had an increased rate of mortality of 20% compared to those patients with eGFR greater than 60 mL per min per 1.73 m². Patients in CKD stage 4 have a 320% greater risk of all cause mortality than those with GFR levels above 60 mL/min/1.73 m². Those patients with ESRD and a GFR < 15 mL/min/1.73 m² have a 590% increase in mortality. (Adapted from Go AS, Chertow GM, Fan D, et al. Chronic kidney disease and the risks of death, cardiovascular events, and hospitalization. *N Engl J Med.* 2004. 23;351(13):1296–305.)

• Specialty Referral Guidelines for Diabetic Nephropathy

Patients with CKD should be referred to a nephrologist for consultation and comanagement if a clinical action plan cannot be prepared, the appropriate evaluation cannot be performed, or the recommended treatment cannot be implemented. In most cases, patients with a GFR below 30 mL per min per 1.73 m² should be referred to a nephrologist.[15] Most patients will require either

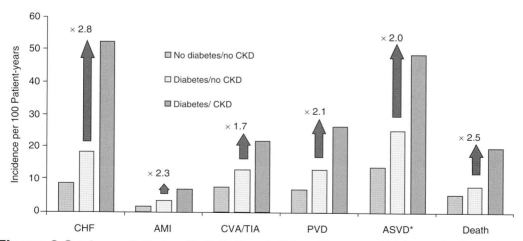

Figure 6-8 • **Among Patients with Both Chronic Kidney Disease and Diabetes, the Rate of Cardiovascular Events is More Than Twice the Rate Among Patients with Diabetes Alone.** Relative to healthy individuals, patients with CKD and diabetes have a 79% increased risk of CHF, a 41% increased risk of ASVD, and a 56% increased risk of death. These statistics are from a sample of the U.S. Medicare population from 1998 and 1999 (*n* = 1,091,201) who were divided according to diabetes and CKD status: no diabetes, no CKD (79.7%); diabetes, no CKD (16.5%); CKD, no diabetes (2.2%); and both CKD and diabetes (1.6%). (Adapted from Foley RN, Murray AM, Li S, et al. Chronic kidney disease and the risk for cardiovascular disease, renal replacement, and death in the United States Medicare population, 1998 to 1999. *J Am Soc Nephrol.* 2005;16(2):489–495.)

dialysis or renal transplantation once they progress into CKD stage 5. Unfortunately, few patients actually progress from CKD stage 4 to CKD stage 5. For patients with CKD stage 4 disease, death is twice as likely as progression to CKD stage 5.[42] Five percent to 20% of all patients in CKD stage 5 die annually.[43]

Renal biopsy should be considered in newly diagnosed patients with T1DM with proteinuria and a rapid decline in renal function. Because nephropathy and retinopathy so often coexist, patients with CKD *without* evidence of eye disease should also undergo a renal biopsy to determine if the kidney disease is related to diabetes or an unrelated disorder.[44] Diabetes causes unique changes in kidney structure. Classic glomerulosclerosis is characterized by increased glomerular basement membrane width, diffuse mesangial sclerosis, hyalinosis, microaneurysm, and hyaline arteriosclerosis.[45] Areas of extreme mesangial expansion called Kimmelstiel-Wilson nodules or nodular mesangial expansion are observed in 40% to 50% of patients developing proteinuria.[46] The indications for performing renal biopsies in patients with T2DM are unclear.

• Clinical Management of Diabetic Nephropathy

Treatment of patients with diabetic nephropathy includes the following: management of comorbid conditions, measures to slow loss of kidney function, measures to prevent and treat CVD, measures to prevent and treat complications of decreased kidney function, preparation for kidney failure and kidney replacement therapy, and replacement of kidney function by dialysis or transplantation if signs and symptoms of uremia are present.

Medications should be reviewed at all visits. Patients with stages 4 and 5 CKD should be questioned regarding the incidence of hypoglycemia. Dosage adjustments for medications such as dipeptidyl peptidase-4 (DPP-4) inhibitors (sitagliptin and saxagliptin), metformin, insulin, and sulfonylureas should be based on one's eGFR. The primary route of elimination for sulfonylureas is via the kidneys. Elderly, debilitated, and malnourished patients with renal or hepatic impairment are most at risk for developing severe hypoglycemia in association with the use of sulfonylureas. Renal patients should be prescribed with low doses of sulfonylureas or have the drug discontinued, especially when used in combination with insulin or other glucose-lowering agents.

The ADA recommends screening for complications related to CKD when the GFR is less than 60 mL per min per 1.73 m² (Table 6-4). Early vaccination against hepatitis B is indicated for patients likely to progress to ESRD.

The basis for prevention of diabetic nephropathy is treatment of known risk factors, including hypertension, hyperglycemia, anemia, and dyslipidemia. Lifestyle interventions should also be identified and enforced. Smoking cessation is a necessity. Patients who stop drinking alcohol may notice an improvement in their BP readings. Early recognition and management of secondary hyperparathyroidism and vitamin D deficiencies are within the realm of PCPs. Patients should be evaluated for possible coexisting obstructive sleep apnea and treated accordingly. In patients with moderate-to-severe obstructive sleep apnea, 3 months of continuous positive airway pressure (CPAP) therapy was found to lower BP, improve lipid profiles, and lower A1C by 0.2%.[47] Patients with advanced CKD should be identified as potential candidates for renal transplantation and referred to an appropriate transplant center.

Progression of CKD may best be halted by intensively targeting the following behavioral, pharmacologic, and nutritional therapies:

1. **Intensive glycemic control**

The DCCT demonstrated that intensively managing T1DM reduces the incidence of microalbuminuria by 39%.[48] "Graduates" from the intensively managed arm of the DCCT were able to reduce their incidence of microalbuminuria and hypertension by 40% even as their glycemic control deteriorated over time.[49] Patients with T2DM in the United Kingdom Prospective Diabetes Study (UKPDS) who were intensively managed demonstrated a 30% reduction in the development of microalbuminuria.[50] Thus, intensive treatment of glycemia targeting an A1C lower than 7% in most patients should be pursued as early as possible after the diagnosis of diabetes is made to prevent the development of microalbuminuria.

TABLE 6-4. American Diabetes Association Recommendations for Management of CKD in Diabetes

GFR (mL/min/1.73 m²)	Recommended Management
All patients with diabetes	• Yearly measurements of creatinine, UAE, potassium
45–60 (stage 3 CKD)[a]	• Refer to nephrologist if possibility for nondiabetic kidney disease exists (duration T1DM <10 y, albuminuria, abnormal renal ultrasound, treatment resistant hypertension, renal artery stenosis, rapid decline in eGFR) • Dose adjustments for all medications if needed • Biannual monitoring of eGFR • Annual monitoring of electrolytes, bicarbonate, hemoglobin, calcium, phosphorus, and iPTH for secondary hyperparathyroidism • Measure and treat vitamin D (25-hydroxyvitamin D_3 [25(OH)D_3]) levels • Consider dexa scan (bone density testing) • CDE or RD referral for dietary counseling
30-44 ("Advanced" stage 3 CKD)[a]	iPTH expansion: Intact parathyroid hormone • Monitor GFR every 3 months • Monitor electrolytes and bicarbonate annually • Screen hemoglobin, calcium, phosphorous, iPTH, and weight every 3–6 months • Adjust medication doses as needed per label
<30 (stage 4 CKD)[a]	Referral to nephrologist for comanagement of CKD

[a]Consider evaluating risk of renal disease progression: http://www.qxmd.com/calculate-online/nephrology/kidney-failure-risk-equation.
Adapted from American Diabetes Association. Clinical Practice Recommendations 2011. *Diabetes Care.* 2011;34 (Suppl 1):S35.

The glycemic targets of patients with renal insufficiency should be customized. Patients with CKD stages 1 and 2 may safely target A1C levels of 6.5-7% assuming they have no other significant contraindications for diabetes intensification. Because patients with advanced stage 3 through stage 5 CKD are at higher risk for cardiovascular events and hypoglycemia, targeting an A1C in the range of 7.5% appears to be prudent.[51]

2. Intensive management of hypertension

Both prospective and post hoc evidence indicates that systolic blood pressure (SBP) reduction to less than 130 mm Hg in nephropathic patients is associated with a decreased progression to ESRD.[52] In the Action in Diabetes and Vascular Disease Preterax and Diamicron MR Controlled Evaluation (ADVANCE) trial, a 21% reduction in the risk of new or worsening nephropathy was noted in patients as SBP was reduced to 110 mm Hg.[53]

Although the recommendation to lower BP to less than 130/80 mm Hg in diabetic and high-risk patients appears to have clear benefits in MOST patients, not all individuals appear to demonstrate improved outcomes with ambitious BP reduction. The ACCORD BP trial was a prospective randomized double-blind study that investigated whether therapy targeting normal SBP less than 120 mm Hg reduces CV event in high-risk patients with T2DM.[54] Despite the 14.2 mm Hg difference in SBP between the intensive and standard therapy groups, the rate of nonfatal MI, nonfatal stroke, or death from CV causes was identical. Intensive hypertensive therapy was associated with a lower rate of stroke, yet serious adverse events attributed to antihypertensive treatment occurred more frequently in the intensive therapy group than in the standard therapy group. Thus, as with glycemic targets, individualization of BP targets is warranted in all patients with diabetes.

TABLE 6-5. Treatment for Diabetic Nephropathy

Treatment Category	Recommended Treatment
T1DM or T2DM with micro- or macroalbuminuria	• ACE inhibitor or ARBs
T1DM with HTN and albuminuria	• ACE inhibitor delays progression of nephropathy
T2DM with HTN and microalbuminuria	• ACE inhibitor or ARBs delay the progression to macroalbuminuria
T2DM with HTN and macroalbuminuria and RI (serum creatinine > 1.5 mg/dL)	• ARBs delay the progression of nephropathy
T1DM or T2DM with microalbuminuria and *normal* BP	• ACE inhibitor or ARB[a]

[a]Gross JL, de Azevedo MJ, Silveiro SP, et al. Diabetic nephropathy: diagnosis, prevention and treatment. *Diabetes Care.* 2005;28(1):164–176.
ACE, angiotensin-converting enzyme inhibitors; ARB, angiotensin receptor blockers; RI, renal insufficiency; BP, blood pressure.
From American Diabetes Association. Clinical Practice Recommendations 2011. *Diabetes Care.* 2011;34(Suppl 1):S33.

Table 6-5 lists the treatment recommendations from the ADA diabetic nephropathy. Renoprotective effects of ACE inhibitors or ARBs appear to be independent of these agents' effect on BP lowering, possibly because of their ability to reduce intraglomerular pressure.[17] Both ACE inhibitors and ARBs decrease the risk of progression to macroalbuminuria by as much as 60% to 70%. Thus, these drugs are recommended as the first line pharmacologic treatment of microalbuminuria even in normotensive patients.[17] Patients with macroalbuminuria benefit from control of hypertension using either ACE or ARBs. Hypertension control in patients with macroalbuminuria from diabetic nephropathy slows decline in GFR independent of the BP-lowering effect.

Combination treatment with an ACE and an ARB does have additional renoprotective effects.[55] In a double-blind randomized two-period crossover trial of 8 weeks, an ARB, candesartan 16 mg daily, and placebo was added in random order to existing treatment to patients taking lisinopril 40 mg or captopril 150 mg per day. Addition of the dual blockade of the renin–angiotensin system (RAS) by the addition of candesartan resulted in a reduction in albuminuria as well as systolic and diastolic blood pressures. The changes in albuminuria did not correlate to changes in BP. Thus, the dual blockade of the RAS provided superior short-term renoprotection independent of systemic BP changes when compared with maximally recommended doses of ACE inhibitors in patients with T2DM and nephropathy.

Renin inhibition blocks the renin–angiotensin–aldosterone system (RAAS) at the first rate-limiting step of the cascade. Renin inhibition will decrease plasma renin activity and reduce levels of circulating A-I and A-II, resulting in a more efficient RAAS blockade. Combining a direct renin inhibitor (aliskiren) with an A-II receptor blocker (losartan) reduced albuminuria and renal dysfunction independent of baseline level of CKD in patients with T2DM, hypertension, and nephropathy.[56]

Critical renal artery stenosis (greater than 70%) occurs in approximately 17% of hypertensive T2DM patients and may be associated with hypertension and RI (ischemic nephropathy).[57] In these patients, the use of ACE inhibitors or ARBs could reduce transcapillary filtration pressure, leading to acute or chronic RI, especially if renal artery stenosis affects both kidneys or the sole functioning kidney. A rise in serum creatinine of higher than 50% after initiation suggests the presence of renal artery stenosis.[58] Other features of renal artery stenosis include renal impairment with minimal or absent proteinuria, absent or minimal diabetic retinopathy (DR), presence of macrovascular disease in other sites (coronary, carotid, and peripheral arteries), vascular bruits (especially femoral), and asymmetric kidney shrinkage on renal ultrasound.[57]

Although ACE inhibitors or ARBs are considered first-tier antihypertensive therapy in patients with diabetes, the choice of secondary agents requires treatment individualization. The National Kidney Foundation recommends adding either a thiazide diuretic or a long-acting CCB to the antihypertensive regimen if the BP target has not been achieved.[59] Using long-acting CCBs (verapamil HCl or diltiazem HCl) can help reduce proteinuria, whereas dihydropyridine calcium channel blocker (CCBs) have no such effect.[60]

β-blockers and CCBs are frequently used to control hypertension in patients with advanced CKD. Dihydropyridine CCBs (such as amlodipine and felodipine) are acceptable treatments provided they are used in combination with ACE inhibitors or ARBs.[61]

3. Dietary intervention

The ADA treatment recommendations for patients with diabetic nephropathy include dietary interventions for patients in both early and advanced stages of CKD.[62] A moderately low protein-restricted diet ($0.9 \, g \times kg^{-1} \times day^{-1}$) used in T1DM patients with progressive diabetic nephropathy reduced the risk of ESRD and death by 76% without affecting the decline in GFR.[63] Minimizing red meat and saturated fat consumption can reduce UAE by 46%.[64] Although protein and calorie restriction slows the progression of diabetic nephropathy in high-risk patients, more long-term studies are necessary to access the true benefits of nutritional therapy as being renoprotective.

4. Medication dosing adjustments

Most glucose-lowering agents undergo some renal clearance (glucophage, glimepiride, pioglitazone, exenatide, sitagliptin, saxagliptin, pramlintide, insulin, and glitinides). As a consequence, clearance may be slowed, resulting in higher blood levels of the drug and inducing hypoglycemia. Patients with advanced CKD stages 3 to 5 should periodically have their medications reviewed and doses adjusted based upon their CC. Drugs that require dosage adjustments include metformin, sulfonylureas, α-glucosidase inhibitors (AGIs), repaglinide, and insulin. Incretin-based therapies including exenatide and the DPP-4 inhibitors sitagliptin and saxagliptin require dosage reductions in persons with a CC of less than or equal to 50 mL per minute, whereas liraglutide and linagliptin require no adjustments.[65,66]

CKD increases one's risk for developing both acute hypoglycemia and hypoglycemia awareness autonomic failure as the renal clearance of both endogenous and exogenous insulin is reduced in patients with advanced CKD.[67] Insulin suppresses glucagon secretion, which in turn leads to impaired gluconeogenesis and hypoglycemia counterregulation.[68] One should consider reducing the total daily dose of insulin by 25% in hospitalized patients with GFR less than 45 mL per min per $1.73 \, m^2$ in order to minimize their risk of hypoglycemia.[69]

5. Management of anemia in patients with CKD

CKD is a known cause of anemia. Anemia is associated with lower exercise tolerance, poorer quality of life, left ventricular hypertrophy, and heart failure among patients with chronic RI.[70] Forty percent to 70% of patients beginning long-term hemodialysis in the United States have a history of CHF and left ventricular hypertrophy, both strong predictors of mortality.[71] This suggests that the harmful effects of anemia are progressive and reflective of the patient's declining GFR.

The anemia associated with diabetes is due to a reduction in erythropoietin production thought to be secondary to (a) renal denervation from diabetic neuropathy, (b) alterations in the structures within the renal cortex resulting in a reduced erythropoietin response to the hypoxic stimulus of anemia, and (c) a reduction in levels of androgen hormones that stimulate erythropoiesis.[72] Prior to the availability of recombinant human erythropoietin (rHuEPO, epoetin alfa), anemia was treated with iron supplements or blood transfusions. Both iron and erythropoietin are necessary for the formation of hemoglobin. Although epoetin therapy may improve outcomes in anemic patients with CKD and diabetic nephropathy, adverse events such as hypertension, seizures, hypercoagulation, hyperkalemia, and functional iron deficiency may occur.

In the United States, the available erythropoietic agents are epoetin alfa (Procrit, Epogen) and darbepoetin alfa (Aranesp), both of which are indicated for use in CKD whether or not patients are undergoing dialysis. Both drugs have similar efficacy and safety profiles in CKD, with pruritus occurring more frequently in patients using darbepoetin alfa.[73] Patients may safely transition between either erythropoietic agent.

Treatment of anemia with erythropoietin-stimulating agents (ESAs) can slow the progression of nephropathy while reducing the risk of heart disease and left ventricular hypertrophy.[74]

An assessment of the patient with CKD for anemia should include a hemoglobin and/or hematocrit, red blood cell (RBC) indices, reticulocyte count, iron parameters (serum iron, total iron-binding capacity, percent transferrin saturation, and serum ferritin), and a test for fecal occult blood. Normal values for hemoglobin are 12.0 to 16 g per dL for menstruating women and 13.5 to 17.5 g per dL for men and postmenopausal women. Mean normal hematocrit values are 36% to 46% for menstruating women and 41% to 53% for men and postmenopausal women.

The target hemoglobin range for patients with CKD has not been clearly determined. The use of epoetin alfa treatment for a median of 16 months in the CHOIR trial resulted in increased risk of death, myocardial infarction, hospitalization for CHF, and stroke in 17.5% of patients achieving hemoglobin targets of 13.5 g per dL and 13.5% of those patients treated to hemoglobin of 11.3 g per dL. The reasons for these findings are uncertain.[75] One might consider treating anemia to a range solely to avert the need for blood transfusions, targeting hemoglobin levels well below 12 g per dL. Rapid fluctuations in hemoglobin levels as well as normalization of anemia may increase the risk of adverse outcomes.[76]

An important aspect of management of anemia in patients with CKD is careful assessment of iron status to ensure that the transferrin saturation is between 20% and 50% while maintaining the ferritin level between 100 and 800 ng per mL. Serum transferrin saturation is an indicator of iron overload. Patients with serum transferrin saturations greater than 55% are at increased risk of all-cause mortality for reasons that are unclear.[77]

Ferritin levels in patients with a reduced GFR are an indicator of total iron storage but may also be a marker of systemic inflammation. Any acute loss of iron due to diet, malabsorption, and bleeding will result in a decline in ferritin levels. Serum iron is decreased in chronic anemia. Low ferritin levels will not likely respond to iron supplementation, whereas low serum iron should be treated with supplemental iron. Transferrin saturation, in combination with serum iron and ferritin levels, may be helpful in diagnosing functional iron deficiency, just as low serum ferritin level are used to diagnose iron deficiency anemia.[78] There is little correlation of iron measurements with stages of kidney disease.

The suggested dosing protocol for Epoetin alfa (Procrit) is listed in Table 6-6.

6. Aspirin use in patients with diabetic nephropathy

Patients with microalbuminuria or macroalbuminuria may be more aspirin resistant to the benefits of primary and secondary CV protection.[79] Therefore, patients with diabetic nephropathy may benefit from higher aspirin dosages (greater than 100 to 150 mg per day) with or without the combined use of antiplatelet agents such as clopidogrel.[80]

7. Management of hyperlipidemia

The goal for LDL cholesterol is lower than 100 mg per dL for diabetic patients in general and lower than 70 mg per dL for diabetic patients with CVD.[81] The effect of lipid reduction by antilipemic agents on progression of diabetic nephropathy is still unknown. So far, there have been no large trials analyzing whether the treatment of dyslipidemia could prevent the development of diabetic nephropathy or the decline of renal function. However, there is some evidence that lipid reduction by antilipemic agents might preserve GFR and decrease proteinuria in diabetic patients.[82] In the Heart Protection Study, 40-mg simvastatin reduced the rate of major vascular events and GFR decline in patients with diabetes, independent of cholesterol levels at baseline, by 25%.[83] A 56-week study in patients with combined hyperlipidemia and T2DM demonstrated no decline in GFR for patients taking either pitavastatin or atorvastatin.[84]

TABLE 6-6. Suggested Adult Dosing Protocols for Epoetin Alfa (Procrit)

- In an outpatient, nondialysis setting, subcutaneous injection is the preferred route of administration.
- Initial dose of 40,000 units given weekly. First recheck of Hgb should be 4 wk after initial injection.
- The baseline Hgb level is expected to increase in the rage of 0.7–2.5 g/dL in the 1st 4 wk.
- Reduce dose by 25% in 4 wk if Hgb exceeds a level needed to avoid transfusion or increases >1 g/dL in any 2-wk interval.
- Withhold dose if Hgb exceeds a level needed to avoid transfusion and restart at 25% below the previous dose when the Hgb approaches a level where transfusions are required.
- Increase dose by 60,000 units SC weekly if no increase in Hgb ≥ 1 g/dL is noted after 4 wk of therapy (in the absence of a RBC transfusion) to achieve and maintain the lowest Hgb needed to avoid the need for transfusion.
- Discontinue therapy if after 8 wk of therapy no increase in Hgb is noted or if transfusions are still required.

References:
National Kidney Foundation NDOQI Guidelines: http://www.kidney.org/professionals/kdoqi/guidelines_anemia/cpr31.htm. Accessed September 2, 2011.
Procrit prescribing information. Centocor Orthobiotech Products, L.P. Raritan, NJ, 2000.

8. Evaluation and management of secondary hyperparathyroidism in patients with diabetic nephropathy

Patients with CKD may develop secondary hyperparathyroidism, leading to renal osteodystrophy.[85] The pathophysiology of secondary hyperparathyroidism is shown in Figure 6-9. A decrease in GFR leads to renal retention of phosphate. Because the parathyroid glands are directly stimulated by elevated phosphate levels, hyperplasia of the glands occurs in response to hyperphosphatemia.

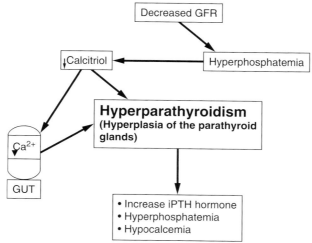

Figure 6-9 • **Pathophysiology of Secondary Hyperparathyroidism Associated with Chronic Kidney Disease.** Declining GFR leads to reduced phosphate excretion and hyperphosphatemia. The elevated phosphate levels directly stimulate PTH synthesis, resulting in glandular hyperplasia. Hyperphosphatemia also suppresses the activation of calcitriol by the kidneys. Low calcitriol directly enhances PTH secretion while reducing calcium absorption from the gut, leading to hypocalcemia and further increases in parathyroid production and secretion. Taken together, hyperphosphatemia, hypocalcemia, and reduced calcitriol synthesis all promote the production of PTH and parathyroid cell proliferation, resulting in secondary hyperparathyroidism.

As parathyroid hormone (PTH) levels rise, the absorption of calcitriol (vitamin D) is reduced, impairing the mobilization of calcium from bones. Calcitriol (1,25-dihydroxycholecalciferol) in a normal metabolic state would increase the absorption of both calcium and phosphate from the GI tract. Because calcitriol is a PTH suppressant, reduced absorption of calcitriol results in compensatory hyperparathyroidism. PTH levels will also rise independently in response to lower GI absorption of calcium from the gut. Patients with secondary hyperparathyroidism tend to have serum calcium levels that are either normal or marginally reduced despite an elevation intact parathyroid hormone levels (iPTH). Bone and joint pains may develop and slowly progress until the patient is bedridden. Clinically, patients may complain of pain that is usually vague and located in the lower back, hips, knees, and legs. Severe lower back pain occurs as a result of a collapsed vertebral body, and a spontaneous rib fracture can cause sharp chest pain. Joint pain may also occur as a result of periarticular deposition of hydroxyapatite crystals; this pain particularly occurs in marked hyperphosphatemia. Rarely, avascular necrosis of the femoral head may occur in association with renal osteodystrophy, causing pain and limping.

Secondary hyperparathyroidism may become evident during stage III CKD. All-cause mortality from CKD increases as patients develop hyperphosphatemia (PO_4 greater than 6.1 mg per dL), hypercalcemia (Ca greater than 10 mg per dL), and PTH (greater than 600 pg per mL), with hazard ratios of 1.18, 1.16, and 1.21, respectively.[86] The Kidney Disease Outcomes Quality Initiative (K/DOQI) recommends keeping PTH levels between 150 and 300 in order to minimize the risk of osteodystrophy and severe bone demineralization.[61]

The management of secondary hyperparathyroidism requires coordinated care between the PCP, nephrologist, dietitian and patient. Patients will require reduced phosphate diets, phosphate-binding drugs, calcimimetic agents, vitamin D derivatives, and possible surgical intervention.

Table 6-7 summarizes the screening and intervention strategies that should be standardized for all high-risk patients having CKD stages 3 to 5. Initially, one must optimize the levels of serum phosphorus and calcium within the recommended ranges based on the patient's CKD stage.

Patients with persistently elevated PTH levels should restrict their dietary intake of phosphate and be treated in, most cases, with a phosphate binder (aluminum hydroxide) and an active vitamin D analogue if their calcium levels are normal. Two vitamin D analogues are currently marketed in the United States: paricalcitol (e.g., Zemplar, Abbott Laboratories, Abbott Park, IL) and doxercalciferol (Hectorol, Genzyme Corp.). Patients receiving paricalcitol in one large randomized placebo controlled double-blind study demonstrated a 16% reduction in mortality than those subjects using calcitriol.[87] Serum levels of 25-hydroxyvitamin D (calcidiol) are decreased in many patients with advanced CKD. Supplementation with oral vitamin D_3 is recommended if levels fall to less than 30 ng per mL.[88]

The presence of extraskeletal calcification, calciphylaxis, debilitating bone disease, refractory pruritus, severe hypercalcemia, and PTH levels greater than 800 pg per mL are strong indications for parathyroidectomy in patients with secondary hyperparathyroidism.[89]

TABLE 6-7. Target Phosphorus, Calcium, and Parathyroid Hormone Levels for Patients with Chronic Kidney Disease (Stages 3–5)

CKD Stage	GFR (mL/min/1.73 m²)	Frequency of PTH Measurement	Frequency of Calcium and Phosphorus Measurement	Target PO_4 (mg/dL)	Target iPTH (pg/mL)
III	30–59	Annual	Annual	2.7–4.6	30–70
IV	15–29	Every 3 mo	Every 3 mo	2.7–4.6	70–110
V	<15 or on dialysis	Every 3 mo	Monthly	3.5–5.5	150–300

PTH, parathyroid hormone; CKD, chronic kidney disease; iPTH, intact parathyroid hormone; PO_4, serum phosphorus.
Adapted from National Kidney Foundation. K/DOQI clinical practice guidelines for bone metabolism and disease in chronic kidney disease. *Am J Kidney Dis.* 2003;42(4 Suppl 3):S1–S201.

9. Preparing a patient for dialysis

Still uncertain is whether patients with ESRD should initiate dialysis based upon the presence of uremic symptomatology or upon crossing a specific eGFR threshold. Observational studies published since 2002 suggest an association between early initiation of dialysis in patients with higher eGFRs and mortality rates.[90]

The IDEAL study enrolled patients above 18 years old with CC between 10 and 15 mL per min per 1.73 m².[91] Patients were randomized to two groups, named "early" and "late." The early group was planned to start dialysis when CC was 10 to 14 mL per min per 1.73 m² and the late group at 5 to 7 mL per min per 1.73 m². The study protocol allowed patients in either group to start dialysis based on clinical indications, regardless of CC, if that was deemed necessary by the patient's nephrologist. Mean follow-up was 3.5 years for over 800 patients in the study. No differences in mortality between the early and late groups were observed. Seventy-six percent of the patients in the late group started dialysis with CC greater than 7 mL per min per 1.73 m², the majority due to uremic symptoms. The late group started dialysis on average 6 months later than the early group.

PCPs may assist in preparing patients with ESRD for dialysis by adhering to the following principles:

1. Patients with advanced CKD should be prepared for dialysis, kidney transplant, or conservative care before their CKD becomes symptomatic.
2. Preparation for appropriate dialysis access should begin when the GFR is greater than 15 mL per min per 1.73 m².
3. Carefully observe patients for signs and symptoms of uremia (Table 6-8) when the GFR is less than mL per min per 1.73 m²
4. Dialysis should be considered in patients with a GFR of less than 15 mL per min per 1.73 m² based upon the presence of uremic signs and symptoms (Table 6-8), inability to control hydration status or BP, or a progressive deterioration in nutritional status. Most patients will require dialysis with a GFR in the range of 9 to 6 mL per min per 1.73 m².
5. The Cockcroft-Gault equation or reciprocal creatinine plots should not be used when the GFR is less than 30 mL per min per 1.73 m² to determine the need for dialysis. The MDRD-eGFR is useful in identifying CKD and estimating rate of progression but should not be used to determine the need for dialysis or to estimate renal function in stage 5 CKD (GFR less than 15 mL per min per 1.73 m²).
6. High-risk patients whose renal function is deteriorating greater than eGFR 4 mL per min per year require particularly close supervision. Where close supervision is not feasible and

TABLE 6-8. Signs and Symptoms of Uremia

System	Symptom or Sign
CNS	Drowsiness, fatigue, loss of concentration, personality changes, irritability, peripheral neuropathy, depression, loss of balance, slurred speech, seizures, coma
Muscular	Restless legs syndrome, cramping in legs
Skeletal	Bone pain, bone cysts, osteoporosis, fractures, calcium deposits in the skin and in the eyes that may cause redness and itching
Skin	Severe itching, pallor with a yellow tinge, subcutaneous calcium deposits may result in redness
Cardiac	CHF, pericardial rub, myocardial infarction, silent ischemia, arrhythmias
Pulmonary	Effusions, shortness of breath
Blood	Anemia, electrolyte imbalance, bruising, low testosterone

in patients whose uremic symptoms may be difficult to detect, a planned start to dialysis while still asymptomatic may be preferred. Supervision in a dedicated clinic for patients with advanced CKD is recommended.

10. Renal transplantation

Kidney transplantation is the treatment of choice for suitable patients with ESRD and should be discussed with individuals diagnosed with advanced CKD. In 2008, 382,343 Americans were receiving dialysis.[92] In that same year, 17,413 patients received kidney transplants, 65% from deceased donors and 35% from living donors.[93] The number of patients awaiting kidney transplants in September 2011 was 89,716.[94] Interestingly, the 10-year survival for a living donor transplant recipient is 76.6% compared with only 62.1% for a deceased donor.[93] Therefore, the living donor is the preferred method of transplantation in the United States.

Early referral to a transplant center will improve the chances of a patient receiving a preemptive transplant, especially those who have a potential living donor. However, patients who are referred for a living donor transplant are not guaranteed immediate transplantation.

In patients with T1DM with ESRD, early transplantation with a living donor followed by a pancreas-after-kidney transplantation is regarded as the best option.[95] A comprehensive medical, psychiatric, and surgical workup will be initiated and directed by the transplant center to which patients are referred.

Patients older than 60 years of age are at a greater risk of post-transplant infection and are more susceptible to immune-suppressive medication side effects. Appropriately evaluated and informed patients in their 70s may benefit in terms of life expectancy from transplantation. However, there are limited data on outcomes for assessing the benefits of renal transplantation for patients in their late 70s or early 80s. Considering the large number of patients on transplant waiting lists, elderly patients with ESRD should be encouraged to seek out a living donor.

• Reversing Advanced CKD with Bardoxolone Methyl, an Experimental Antioxidant Inflammation Modulator

Bardoxolone methyl is a novel antioxidant inflammation modulator that reduces the proinflammatory activity of the NF-κB pathway. Oxidative stress within the kidneys activates complication pathways leading to enlarged glomeruli, mesangial cell proliferation, thickened glomerular basement membranes, and glomerulosclerosis. This, in turn, will result in loss of kidney function as demonstrated by a persistent decline in eGFR. If redox homeostasis is restored and oxidative stress is minimized, inflammation within these structures is reduced and renal function may improve.[96]

Bardoxolone methyl was initially studied as an anticancer drug. In two phase 1 trials, bardoxolone methyl reduced serum creatinine levels with a corresponding improvement in eGFR. Improvements were more pronounced in a subset of patients with established CKD and were maintained over time in subjects who continued on bardoxolone methyl therapy for 5 months. Based on these observed effects and the well-described role of oxidative stress and inflammation in CKD, bardoxolone methyl was hypothesized to improve renal function in patients with T2DM and CKD.

In a multicenter, double-blind placebo-controlled phase 2b study, 227 patients with advanced CKD and T2DM were randomly assigned to receive either bardoxolone methyl in doses of 25 mg, 75 mg, or 150 mg daily or once daily placebo.[97] At 24 weeks, patients assigned to bardoxolone methyl experienced a mean increase in GFR of 10 mL per min per 1.73 m^2 versus no change in the placebo group. Approximately 60% of the patients assigned to bardoxolone methyl experience a reduction in the classification of the severity of their CKD after 24 weeks of treatment compared with only 17% of patients taking placebo. Thirteen percent of the placebo cohort experienced worsening of their CKD staging compared with only 4% of the bardoxolone methyl group. Significant reductions were also observed in other markers of kidney function, including uric acid, serum phosphorus, and BUN. The most common adverse event reported in the study in the bardoxolone methyl group was related to muscle spasm.

Bardoxolone methyl therefore appears to be an attractive agent for potentially reversing advanced kidney disease in select patients.

Diabetic Retinopathy

Introduction First, some good news! Considering the anticipated tripling of the number of people worldwide to develop T2DM by 2040, only 10% of at-risk patients are predicted to develop severe diabetic retinopathy (DR) over a 6-year observation period.[98] Primary care providers can reduce vision impairment by maintaining A1C levels at or near the recommended ADA targets, lowering fasting glucose levels and treating systolic hypertension in high-risk patients.

In the United States, the estimated prevalence of adult (age 40 years and older) DR and vision-threatening DR is 28.5% and 4.4%, respectively. DR is slightly more prevalent among men than women (31.6% vs. 25.7%). Non-Hispanic black individuals have a higher prevalence than non-Hispanic white patients of DR.[99] In the United States, DR remains the leading cause of blindness in adults ages 20 to 74.[100]

• Diabetic Retinopathy Classification

The American Academy of Ophthalmology has introduced a simplified rating scale to assess DR severity (Table 6-9). *Mild* refers to the presence of microaneurysms only. *Moderate* nonproliferative diabetic retinopathy (NPDR) is defined as the presence of microaneurysms and either hard exudates or blot hemorrhages, which are due to the deposition of lipoproteins and the exudation of RBCs from the retinal microaneurysms. *Severe* NPDR is characterized by a large number of retinal hemorrhages or the presence of cotton-wool exudates (microinfarcts within the nerve fiber layer of the retina) and the development of intraretinal microvascular abnormalities (collateral vessels) in the resulting ischemic areas of the retina. The progression of DR through these stages may be associated with leakage of fluids into the macular area that results in thickening (macular edema)

TABLE 6-9. International Clinical Diabetes Retinopathy Severity Scale

Proposed Disease Severity Level	Retinal Pathology	Retina Photo
No apparent retinopathy	No abnormalities	
Mild NPDR	Microaneurysms only	

(Continued)

TABLE 6-9. International Clinical Diabetes Retinopathy Severity Scale *(Continued)*

Proposed Disease Severity Level	Retinal Pathology	Retina Photo
Moderate NPDR	More than just microaneurysms but less than severe NPDR	
Severe NPDR	Any of the following: • >20 intraretinal hemorrhages in each of 4 quadrants • Definite venous beading in 2 or more quadrants • Prominent IRMA in 1 or more quadrants and no signs of proliferative retinopathy	
	One or both of the following: • Neovascularization • Vitreous or preretinal hemorrhage	

NPDR, nonproliferative diabetic retinopathy; IRMA, intraretinal microvascular abnormality.
Adapted from Gardner TW, Antonetti DA, Barber AJ, et al. Diabetic retinopathy: more than meets the eye. *Surv Ophthalmol.* 2002;(suppl):S253–S262, with permission.
Fundus photos courtesy of Jack Carlson, MD, Loma Linda, California.

and the gradual loss of visual acuity (VA). Proliferative diabetic retinopathy (PDR) is associated with the development of abnormal new retinal blood vessels that may bleed into the vitreous cavity and become fibrotic. The resulting traction on the macula leads to visual loss.

In the most destructive form of proliferative changes, diabetes may induce neovascularization beyond the posterior segment of the eye and into the anterior chamber angle. Here, the vessels block aqueous outflow and cause a dramatic rise in intraocular pressure. This devastating neovascular glaucoma (NVG) may result in total loss of the eye.

As with other microvascular complications of diabetes, the pathophysiology of DR appears to be multifactorial. Hyperglycemia results in increased adherence of white blood cells that traverse the tiny vascular channels of the retina. As the veins and arteries become obstructed, retinal blood flow is reduced, resulting in the abnormal vasculature appearance typically seen in patients with diabetes. Cotton-wool spots appear clinically when capillaries are completely occluded. As the leukocytes bind to the endothelium, inflammatory mediators are released that increase vascular permeability, producing hard exudates and edema.

As hyperglycemia damages more small vessels, hypoxemia develops within affected areas of the retina. In response to this ischemic state, the retinal endothelial cells release growth factors [vascular endothelial growth factor (VEGF)]. The proliferative stage of DR is then initiated as neovascularization attempts to restore blood flow to the ischemic areas of the retina. Unfortunately, these tiny, delicate, and fragile new vessels tend to leak and hemorrhage, resulting in sudden and profound vision loss. The fibrous tissue that accompanies neovascularization is difficult to treat, sprouting attachments between the internal surface of both the retina and the vitreous. Forces that result in traction to the fibrous tissue will result in hemorrhage with and without a retinal detachment.

Hyperglycemia has a direct effect on retinal cell death and subsequent retinal atrophy.[101] Retinal glial cells lose their ability to maintain the blood-retinal barrier in a hyperglycemic environment, resulting in vascular leakage and proliferation.[102]

Genetic factors also play an important role in DR pathogenesis. Genes are expressed in the presence of chronic hyperglycemia, which can lead to severe DR. Familial clustering of severe retinopathy has been observed in clinical trials.[103] Gene expression may occur independent of other risk factors for DR. Thus, genetic expression rather than the severity of hyperglycemia may be the most important risk factor for predicting likelihood of developing DR.

• Prevention of Diabetic Retinopathy

Once retinal damage has occurred, restoration of vision is often difficult and stabilization becomes the primary interventional strategy. Panretinal photocoagulation, focal macular laser therapy, and vitrectomy are the main arsenals in the treatment of established DR. Each treatment modality carries risks, such as loss of night vision, cataract progression, glaucoma, loss of accommodation, and infection. No intervention is available for ischemic maculopathy. Therefore, modification of identifiable risk factors at the earliest stage of diabetes is indicated to prevent and delay the onset of retinopathy.

Modifiable risk factors associated with DR include hyperglycemia, hypertension, hyperlipidemia, anemia, obstructive sleep apnea, and smoking. The DCCT and the UKPDS demonstrated the important role of diabetes intensification in reducing retinopathy. In the DCCT, patients who had no retinopathy at baseline and were treated intensively had a 76% reduction in risk of developing DR.[48] A subset of patients in the DCCT from both the intensively managed cohort and the conventional group had persistent A1C elevations of greater than 9% throughout the duration of the study. However, the conventional group had 2½ times as many patients who developed DR as the intensively managed patients despite having similar A1C levels.[103] The lower rate of DR in intensively managed patients is due to the minimization of glycemic variation and resulting oxidative stress that occurs with multiple daily injections of insulin when compared with using only twice-daily insulin.[104] T2DM patients in the UKPDS in the intensively managed cohort were able to reduce their A1C on average 1% when compared with conventionally managed patients. This 1% reduction in A1C was matched by a 25% reduction in microvascular complications (including fewer patients requiring photocoagulation for retinopathy).[105]

The Wisconsin Epidemiologic Study of Diabetic Retinopathy (WESDR) showed that progression to such end points as DR was lowest in patients having A1C values of 5.4% to 8.5% and highest in patients with A1Cs higher than 10.1%.[106] More than 70% of patients with A1C levels greater than 10% developed DR within 10 years.

As demonstrated by the EDIC study, early intervention and stabilization of blood glucose control result in a significant reduction in long-term risk of DR even if intensification deteriorates over time.[49] Therefore, targeting A1C levels to as close to normal (4.9% to 5.1%) as safely as possible appears to be appropriate to prevent progression to DR.

Normalization of BP also slows the progression of DR. In the UKPDS, the rate of progression of retinopathy was reduced by 34% and deterioration in VA by 47% when the mean BP was lowered to 144/82 mm Hg.[105] The WESDR showed that progression to DR was highest in patients with baseline hypertension at the time of their initial diagnosis.

Various trials have examined the possible benefits of ACE inhibitors on preventing and slowing the progression of DR in patients with and without hypertension. The EURODIAB Controlled Trial of Lisinopril in Insulin-Dependent Diabetes, for example, showed a 50% reduction in progression to retinopathy in those taking lisinopril.[107]

Like hypertension, hyperlipidemia may contribute to the progression of DR, yet, until recently, few studies have demonstrated the effect of lipid lowering on DR progression. Two major randomized trials, the Fenofibrate Intervention and Event Lowering in Diabetes (FIELD) and the ACCORD Eye trials, have firmly demonstrated that fenofibrate may play an important role in decreasing the progression of DR. In ACCORD Eye, fenofibrate (160 mg per day) with simvastatin resulted in a 40% reduction in the odds of retinopathy progressing over 4 years, compared with simvastatin alone. This occurred with an increase in HDL cholesterol and a decrease in the serum triglyceride level in the fenofibrate group as compared with the placebo group and was independent of glycemic control. The risk reduction in the ACCORD Eye trial in retinopathy progression was similar to that which was found in the FIELD study.[108,109] However, because this effect was not associated with a significant reduction in serum cholesterol levels, further trials are needed to better understand the mechanisms related to the positive effects of fenofibrate on DR. Perhaps fenofibrate may have effects on nonlipid pathways such as inflammation, endothelial function, and VEGFs. Several studies have demonstrated the correlation between hyperlipidemia and the accumulation of retinal and macular hard exudates, which are associated with visual impairment.

Anemia is also a risk factor for retinopathy and its treatment may help slow the progression of retinopathy.[110]

Two other risk factors that should not be overlooked in patients with diabetes are smoking and obstructive sleep apnea. Both are associated with worsening retinopathy and are amenable to treatment.[111] Both of these comorbid conditions are amenable to simple screening and interventions within the primary care setting.

• Screening Guidelines for Diabetic Retinopathy in Patients

DR must be detected and addressed early if the risk of visual loss is to be minimized. Current guidelines state that screening should begin in patients shortly after diagnosis of T2DM and 3 to 5 years after T1DM diagnosis; women with diabetes who are planning pregnancy should also have a comprehensive examination (Table 6-10). Researchers who retrospectively analyzed DCCT data, however, recommended starting annual eye examinations at the time of diagnosis for T1DM and T2DM, noting that this might identify patients at greatest risk for rapid progression of retinopathy. After the initial examination, annual follow-up is essential, even if no retinopathy is found. If retinopathy is discovered, the frequency of visits should be adjusted according to the severity of findings and need for treatment. Some physicians prefer to delay eye referral until a newly diagnosed patient with T2DM is stabilized. Delaying referral for 3 to 6 months as diabetes is intensively managed often will improve VA and retinal pathology. However, some patients who have had exposure to prolonged hyperglycemia may have significant retinal pathology and should be urgently referred for a comprehensive eye exam. Patients with poor glycemic control may initially develop a reversible deterioration in their VA once intensive management with insulin therapy is initiated. Frustration may mount as patients are informed that their "eyes are free of disease" yet they are unable to see clearly. Expensive glasses or contacts are prescribed, which will offer only temporary visual improvement as their A1C levels are lowered.

Despite these well-established guidelines, the rate of annual retinal screening examinations for patients with diabetes is low—ranging from 34% to 65%.[112] An ophthalmologist or optometrist fully trained in recognizing DR should provide these eye exams. Abnormal findings should result in

TABLE 6-10. Evidence Based Recommended Eye Examination Schedule For Patients With Diabetes

Diabetes Type	Recommended Initial Screening	Recommended Follow-up[a]
T1DM	• Adults and children aged 10 years or older should undergo a dilated, comprehensive eye exam by an ophthalmologist or optometrist within 5 years after date of diagnosis (Level of evidence: B) • Fundus photographs may serve as a screening tool for retinopathy but must be interpreted by a trained provider. Fundus photography should not be considered as a substitute for a comprehensive eye examination (Level of evidence: E)	• Annual comprehensive eye exams by an ophthalmologist or optometrist • If 1 or more eye exams are considered as being "normal" patients may opt for comprehensive evaluations every 2-3 years • More frequent examinations are required if one has evidence of progressive retinopathy (Level of evidence: B)
T2DM	• Patients should have a comprehensive eye exam by an ophthalmologist or optometrist soon after being diagnosed (Level of evidence: B)	• Recommendations for follow-up are comparable with those of patients with T1DM (Level of evidence: B)
Pregnancy	• A comprehensive eye examination should be performed in all women with preexisting diabetes who are contemplating pregnancy or who become pregnant so that the risk of progressive DR may be determined. (Level of evidence: B)	• No DR to mild or moderate NPDR every 3 months • Severe NPDR every 1-3 months • Comprehensive follow-up should continue for 1 year postpartum (Level of evidence: B)

[a]Abnormal findings may warrant more frequent follow-up.
DR, diabetic retinopathy; NPDR, nonproliferative diabetic retinopathy.
From Gardner TW, Antonetti DA, Barber AJ, et al. Diabetic retinopathy: more than meets the eye. *Surv Ophthalmol.* 2002;(suppl):S253–S262, with permission.

either prompt treatment or timely referral for the management of DR. Any patient with persistent visual complaints should be referred more frequently.

Communication between the eye care team and the PCP is essential. Results of the eye examinations should be a part of the patient's permanent medical record. The PCP should provide the eye care specialist with the patient's current A1C and BP values.

• Treatment of Diabetic Retinopathy

The use of aspirin and anticoagulant drugs is safe for patients with DR and does not increase the risk of vitreous hemorrhage. The Early Treatment of Diabetic Retinopathy Study (ETDRS) found that the cumulative incidence of new vitreous hemorrhage was similar in patients taking either aspirin (650 mg per day) or placebo over a 4-year period.[113]

Consensus based on the available evidence is that achievement of recommended targets for A1C and BP ameliorate but do not eliminate the risk of DR, suggesting the need to target other potential risk factors that may be implicated in the pathogenesis of DR. Other vital therapeutic targets are considered for potential benefit in the treatment and prevention of DR. Futuristic interventions include the use of intravitreal injection of VEGF inhibitors, such as ranibizumab and pegaptanib. Ranibizumab has shown extensive trial data of benefit in diabetic macular edema.[114] Bevacizumab, currently unlicensed for ocular use, showed improved outcomes in patients with macular edema compared with laser therapy in the smaller BOLT study.[115] Other trials of new medical therapies have focused on blockade of the protein kinase C pathway (ruboxistaurin) showing an effect with reduction of laser treatment and visual loss in patients with diabetes with maculopathy, such that this agent has an approvable letter from the U.S. FDA while further trial data are being completed.[116]

Ranibizumab (RBZ), an anti-VEGF antibody fragment designed for intraocular use in DR, has been found in clinical trials to lead to rapid and sustained improvement in both vision and retinal anatomy. The drug also reduces progression of DR and improves patient-reported function.[117,118] The use of RBZ resulted in patients being able to correctly identify greater than 15 letters on the Snellen equivalent chart versus laser rescue patients who received placebo injections. Of the placebo randomized patients, 72% required laser rescue versus only 33% of the RBZ patients over 24 months.

Patients with PDR have elevated levels of insulin-like growth factor 1 (IGF-1) in their serum and vitreous.[119] The IGF-1 induces retinal neovascularization through the hormonal activation of VEGF. Two studies ($n = 585$) evaluated the efficacy of monthly doses of a long-acting IGF-1 inhibitor (octreotide, sandostatin) on limiting the progression of preexisting DR, reducing the time to development of macular edema and the loss of VA.[120] Although octreotide did not reduce the incidence of macular edema, the IGF-1 inhibitor did limit the clinically relevant progression of DR.

Although laser photocoagulation is the standard treatment for diabetic macular edema associated with DR, vision improvement after treatment is uncommon. Therefore, the use of RBZ may represent an important therapeutic advance by improving vision and reducing the severity of DR in patients with coexisting macular edema.

• Effects of Diabetes on Other Ocular Tissues

Although diabetes is a well-known risk factor for visual impairment in adults, hyperglycemia can affect a wide spectrum of ocular structures. Being generally more susceptible to infection, diabetic patients are more at risk of developing blepharitis and orbital cellulitis. Recurrent hordeola and blepharitis may be an early sign of diabetes in naive patients secondary to *Staphylococcus epidermis*.[121] Patients with diabetes are prone to developing bacterial conjunctivitis, which may result in squamous metaplasia. This may account for the higher incidence of dry eye syndrome observed in the diabetic population. Severity of dry eye syndrome is related to worsening of glycemic control. Dry eyes also tend to become worse following panretinal photocoagulation.[121] An increased deposition of advanced glycation end products within the lacrimal ducts may also impair tear production, resulting in dry eye syndrome when diabetes is poorly controlled.[122]

Corneal sensitivity is enhanced in diabetes which increases the risk of dry eyes, corneal trauma, and neurotrophic corneal ulcers.[123] The corneal epithelial barrier, which protects the eye against common infections, is weakened in diabetes patients. A rise in A1C has been shown to correlate with a greater frequency of severe infections such as fungal keratitis.[124] Chronic hyperglycemia may result in corneal thickening. PCPs should assure that patients who wish to undergo laser *in situ* keratomileusis (LASIK) procedures have well-controlled diabetes in advance of the procedure. Halkiadakis and associates examined the outcome of LASIK in 24 tightly controlled diabetic patients. None of these patients displayed any significant epithelial complications, and all ended up with a postoperative VA of 20/20. The foregoing notwithstanding, 28% of these individuals ultimately required enhancements compared with 10% of nondiabetic patients.[125] Proliferative retinopathy is considered a contraindication for LASIK.[126]

Contact lenses may be worn safely by patients with diabetes without experiencing an increase likelihood of infection or corneal ulceration.[127]

Patients with poorly controlled diabetes will often experience a transient change in VA associated with improvement in glycemic control. Most patients complain of hyperopia (farsightedness). These visual changes appear to be related to alterations in the lens as well as accommodation and should normalize within 6 to 8 weeks.[128]

The Framingham Eye Study reported as much as a fourfold increase in the prevalence of cataracts in diabetic patients younger than 65 years of age, and up to a twofold increase in patients over 65 years of age.[129,130] A 1% increase in HbA1c increased the risk of cataracts by 15% in patients with diabetes.[131] Cataracts tend to develop earlier and progress more rapidly in diabetic patients, often necessitating surgical intervention at an earlier age. Surgery in patients with cataracts may be necessary in order to evaluate retinal health in patients with significant cataracts and poorly controlled diabetes.

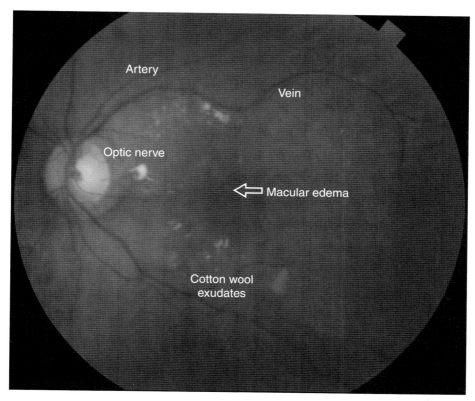

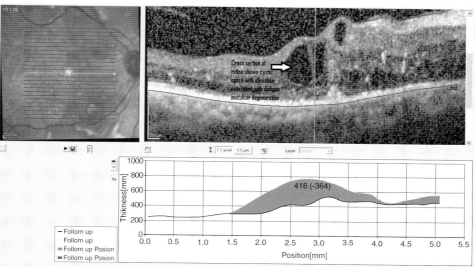

Figure 6-10 • Diabetic Retinopathy and Macular Edema. A. Sixty-two-year-old newly diagnosed T2DM patient with DR (cotton wool exudates) and macular edema on screening retinal photography. **B.** OCT demonstrates classic cystic formation within the retina consistent with macular edema. (Photos courtesy of Anshul Varshney, MD.)

Diabetic macular edema is among the leading causes of persistent, severe vision loss in patients with DR. A patient is said to have clinically significant macular edema if:

- Retinal thickening is located at or within 500 μm (1/3 DD) from the center of the macula
- Hard exudates are found within 500 μm of the center of the macula if associated with thickening of the adjacent retina
- Zones of retinal thickening 1 DD in size are present, at least a part of which are within 1 DD of the center of the macula[121] (Fig. 6-10A).

Optical coherence tomography (OCT) facilitates the detection of clinically significant macular edema and also allows for the assessment of the effects of vitreous traction on macular changes[132] (Fig. 6-10B).

The hypercoagulable state of hypertensive patients with diabetes appears to increase their risk of developing retinal vein and artery occlusions.[133] Symptoms would include sudden blurred or loss of vision in all or portions of one's field of vision.

Macrovascular disease may have a direct impact on the eyes. Carotid occlusive disease may result in ocular ischemic syndrome, the signs of which include gradual or sudden loss of vision, amaurosis fugax, NVG, and retinal hemorrhages. NVG is a complication of PDR that is thought to develop as a result of VEGF-induced neovascularization of the iris and angle; the newly formed blood vessels and fibrous tissue block aqueous outflow from the anterior chamber.[134] Proper detection and diagnosis of carotid occlusive disease are important, as visual prognosis tends to be poor, especially when iris neovascularization is present. Treatment with panretinal photocoagulation, trabeculectomy, and carotid reconstruction has little or no effect on visual outcome.[135]

Individuals with uncontrolled diabetes develop a variety of ocular pathologies that affect nearly all tissues in the eye. While the more well-known complications are sight-threatening retinopathy, macular edema, and cataract, it is important to be aware of the effects of this disease on the other ocular tissues, which can also result in compromised visual function. Recent advancements in the treatment of some of these complications, such as the use of VEGF inhibitors and intravitreal steroid injections, have improved the visual outcome in patients. The most important approach to the prevention of ocular complications in diabetic patients remains to be the maintenance of ambitious metabolic control.

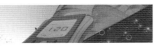

SUMMARY

Although chronic kidney disease and diabetic retinopathy are two of the most dreaded complications associated with diabetes, awareness of either disorder among both patients and physicians is marginal. Primary care physicians are quick to test for renal dysfunction, yet provide limited feedback to patients with evidence of chronic kidney disease. Few nephrologists would expect PCPs to manage patients with end-stage renal failure. However, the role of the PCP is to first identify patients who have early stages of CKD and then provide evidence-based guidance on how the disease progression may be slowed or even reversed. Patients should be informed that targeted intervention requires improvement in glycemic control, normalization of blood pressure, reversal of microalbuminuria, improvement in lipids, weight management, smoking cessation, use of ACE inhibitors or ARBs, and reversal of anemia. Published guidelines provide providers with not only targeted intervention strategies, but when specialty consultation should be obtained.

Fortunately, the risk of visual loss due to diabetes is in decline among Americans. Nevertheless, clinicians must remain vigilant by encouraging all patients to have comprehensive eye examinations preformed by qualified practitioners. Clinicians should also remember that diabetes may affect ocular structures beside the retina, such as the macula, lens, and cornea. Patients are prone to dry eyes as well as transient changes in visual acuity.

REFERENCES

1. National Kidney Foundation: http://www.kidney.org/atoz/content/diabetes.cfm. August 29, 20111.
2. Cowie CC, Port FK, Wolfe RA, et al. Disparities in incidence of diabetic end-stage renal disease according to race and type of diabetes. *N Engl J Med.* 1989;321:1074–1079.
3. Kidney and Urologic diseases statistics for the United States. kidney.niddk.nih.gov/KUDiseases/pubs/kustats/KU_Diseases_Stats_508.pdf -08-24-2011 Accessed August 29, 2011.
4. De Coster C, McLaughlin K, Noseworthy TW. Criteria for referring patients with renal disease for nephrology consultation: a review of the literature. *J Nephrol.* 2010;23(04):399–407.
5. Rosenberg ME. Adult nephrology fellowship training in the United States: trends and issues. *J Am Soc Nephrol.* 2007;18:1027–1033.
6. Coresh J, Selvin E, Stevens LA, et al. Prevalence of chronic kidney disease in the United States. *JAMA.* 2007;298:2038–2047.
7. United States Government Accountability Office. Testimony before the Committee on Health, Education, Labor, and Pensions, U.S. Senate. Primary Care Professionals. Recent supply trends, projections, and valuation of services. February 12, 2008. http://www.gao.gov/new.items/d08472t.pdf. Accessed February 15, 2011.
8. USRDS 2009 Annual Data Report. Volume 3: Reference Tables on ESRD in the United States. Bethesda, MD: NIH, NIDDK; 2009:453–468. http://www.usrds.org/2009/ref/B_Ref_09.PDF. Accessed August 29, 2011.
9. USRDS 2009 Annual Data Report. Volume 3: Reference Tables on ESRD in the United States. Bethesda, MD: NIH, NIDDK; 2009:241–248: http://www.usrds.org/2009/pdf/V2_03_09.PDF. Accessed August 29, 2011.
10. Burrows NR, Li Y, Geiss LS. Incidence of treatment for end-stage renal disease among individuals with diabetes continues to decline. *Diabetes Care.* 2010;33(1):73–77.
11. Muntner P, He J, Hamm L, et al. Renal insufficiency and subsequent death resulting from cardiovascular disease in the United States. *J Am Soc Nephrol.* 2002;13:745–753.
12. Garg JP, Bakris GL. Microalbuminuria: marker of vascular dysfunction, risk factor for cardiovascular disease. *Vasc Med.* 2002;7:35–43.
13. Plantiga LC, Boulware LE, Coresh J. Patient awareness of chronic kidney disease: trends and predictors. *Arch Intern Med.* 2008;168:2268–2275.
14. Israni RK, Shea JA, Joffe MM, et al. Physician characteristics and knowledge of CKD management. *Am J Kidney Dis.* 2009;54:238–247.
15. National Kidney Foundation: K/DOQI clinical practice guidelines for chronic kidney disease: evaluation, classification, and stratification. *Am J Kidney Dis.* 2002;39:S1–S266.
16. Shemesh O, Golbetz H, Kriss HP, et al. Limitations of creatinine as a filtration marker in glomerulopathic patients. *Kidney Int.* 1985;28 (5):830–838.
17. Gross JL, de Azevedo MJ. Diabetic nephropathy: diagnosis, prevention, and treatment. *Diabetes Care.* 2005;28(1):164–176.
18. Miller WG. Estimating glomerular filtration rate. *Clin Chem Lab Med.* 2009;47:1017–1019.
19. Fink JC, Burdick RA, Kurth SJ, et al. Significance of serum creatinine values in new end-stage renal disease patients. *Am J Kidney Dis.* 1999;34:694–701.
20. Atiyeh BA, Dabbagh SS, Gruskin AB: Evaluation of renal function during childhood. *Pediatr Rev.* 1996;17:175–179.
21. National Kidney Foundation. Modification of Diet in Renal Disease study calculator. Available at www.kidney.org/professionals/tools. Accessed December 15, 2011.
22. http://nephron.com/cgi-bin/CGSI.cgi. Accessed December 15, 2011.
23. Levey AS, Bosch JP, Lewis JB, et al. A more accurate method to estimate glomerular filtration rate from serum creatinine: a new prediction equation: Modification of Diet in Renal Disease Study Group. *Ann Intern Med.* 1999;130:461–470.
24. Rossing P, Rossing K, Gaede P, et al. Monitoring kidney function in type 2 diabetic patients with incipient and overt diabetic nephropathy. *Diabetes Care*;2006:29(5):1024–1030.
25. Go AS, Chertow GM, Fan D, et al. Chronic kidney disease and the risks of death, cardiovascular events, and hospitalization. *N Engl J Med.* 2004;351:1296–1305.
26. Anavekar NS, McMurray JJ, Velazquez EJ, et al. Relation between renal dysfunction and cardiovascular outcomes after myocardial infarction. *N Engl J Med.* 2004;351:1285–1295.
27. Levey AS, Stevens LA, Schmid CH, et al. A new equation to estimate glomerular filtration rate. *Ann Intern Med.* 2009;150(9):604–612.
28. National Kidney Foundation. KDOQI Clinical Practice Guidelines and Clinical Practice Recommendations for Diabetes and Chronic Kidney Disease. *Am J Kidney Dis.* 2007;49(Suppl 2):S1–S179.

29. Astor BC, Hallan SI, Miller ER III, et al. Glomerular filtration rate, albuminuria, and risk of cardiovascular and all-cause mortality in the U.S. population. *Am J Epidemiol.* 2008;167(10):1226–1234.

30. Hillege HL, Fidler V, Diercks GF, et al. Urinary albumin excretion predicts cardiovascular and noncardiovascular mortality in general population. *Circulation.* 2002;106:1777–1782.

31. Verhave JC, Gansevoort RT, Hillege HL, et al. An elevated urinary albumin excretion predicts de novo development of renal function impairment in the general population. *Kidney Int Suppl.* 2004;92:S18–S21.

32. Stehouwer CD. Endothelial dysfunction in diabetic nephropathy: state of the art and potential significance for non-diabetic renal disease. *Nephrol Dial Transplant.* 2004;19:778–781.

33. Ochodnicky P, Henning RH, van Dokkum RPE, et al. Microalbuminuria and endothelial dysfunction: emerging targets for primary prevention of end-organ damage. *J Cardiovasc Pharmacol.* 2006;47:S151–S162.

34. Jensen JS, Borch-Johnsen K, Jensen G, et al. Microalbuminuria reflects a generalized transvascular albumin leakiness in clinically healthy subjects. *Clin Sci (London).* 1995;88:629–633.

35. Fliser D, Buchholz K, Haller H. Antiinflammatory effects of angiotensin II subtype 1 receptor blockade in hypertensive patients with microinflammation. *Circulation.* 2004;110:1103–1107.

36. Zenere BM, Arcaro G, Saggiani F, et al. Noninvasive detection of functional alterations of the arterial wall in IDDM patients with and without microalbuminuria. *Diabetes Care.* 1995;18:975–982.

37. Yu Y, Suo L, Yu H, et al. Insulin resistance and endothelial dysfunction in type 2 diabetes patients with or without microalbuminuria. *Diabetes Res Clin Pract.* 2004;65:95–104.

38. Berl T, Henrich W. Kidney-heart interactions: epidemiology, pathogenesis, and treatment. *Clin J Am Soc Nephrol.* 2006;1:8–18.

39. Sarnak M, Levey A, Schoolwerth A, et al. Kidney disease as a risk factor for development of cardiovascular disease: a statement from the American Heart Association Councils on Kidney in Cardiovascular Disease, High Blood Pressure Research, Clinical Cardiology, and Epidemiology and Prevention. *Circulation.* 2003;108:2154–2169.

40. Whaley-Connel A, Chaudhary K, Misra M, et al. A case for early screening for diabetic kidney disease. *Cardiorenal Med.* 2011;1(4):235–242.

41. Tangri N, Stevens LA, Griffith J, et al. A predictive model for progression of chronic kidney disease to kidney failure. *JAMA.* 2011;305(15):1553–1559.

42. Kinchen KS, Sadler J, Fink N, et al. The timing of specialist evaluation in chronic kidney disease and mortality. *Ann Intern Med.* 2002;137:479–486.

43. Mohanram A, Toto RD. Outcome studies in diabetic nephropathy. *Semin Nephrol.* 2003;23:255–271.

44. Serra A, Romero R, Bayes B, et al. Is there a need for changes in renal biopsy criteria in proteinuria in type 2 diabetes? *Diabetes Res Clin Pract.* 2002;58:149–153.

45. Mauer SM, Steffes MW, Brown DM. The kidney in diabetes. *Am J Med.* 1981;70:603–612.

46. Kimmelstiel P, Wilson C. Intercapillary lesions in the glomeruli of kidney. *Am J Pathol.* 1936;12:83–97.

47. Sharma SK, Agrawal S, Damodaran D, et al. CPAP for the metabolic syndrome in patients with obstructive sleep apnea. *N Engl J Med.* 2011;365(24):2277–2286.

48. Diabetes Control and Complications Trial Research Group. The effect of intensive treatment of diabetes on the development and progression of long-term complications in insulin-dependent diabetes mellitus. *N Engl J Med.* 1993;329:977–986.

49. The Diabetes Control and Complications Trial/Epidemiology of Diabetes Interventions and Complications Research Group. Retinopathy and nephropathy in patients with type 1 diabetes four years after a trial of intensive therapy. *N Engl J Med.* 2000;342:381–389.

50. Adler AI, Stevens RJ, Manley SE, et al. Development and progression of nephropathy in type 2 diabetes: the United Kingdom Prospective Diabetes Study (UKPDS 64). *Kidney Int.* 2003;63:225–232.

51. Schernthaner G, Ritz E, Schernthaner GH. Strict glycaemic control in diabetic patients with CKD or ESRD: beneficial or deadly? *Nephrol Dial Transplant.* 2010;25:2044–2047.

52. Mancia G, Laurent S, Agabiti-Rosei E, et al. Reappraisal of European guidelines on hypertension management: a European Society of Hypertension Task Force Document. *J Hypertens.* 2009;27:2121–2158.

53. The ADVANCE Collaborative Group. Intensive blood glucose control and vascular outcomes in patients with type 2 diabetes. *N Engl J Med.* 2008;358:2560–2572.

54. Cushman WC, Evans GW, Byington RP, et al. Effects of intensive blood-pressure control in type 2 diabetes mellitus. *N Engl J Med.* 2010;362:1575–1585.

55. Rossing K, Jacobsen P, Pietrasek L. Renoprotective effects of adding angiotensin II receptor blocker to maximal recommended doses of ACE inhibitor in diabetic nephropathy: a randomized double-blind crossover trial. *Diabetes Care.* 2003;26:2268–2274.

56. Persson F, Lewis JB, Lewis EJ, et al. Impact of baseline renal function on the efficacy and safety of aliskiren added to losartan in patients with type 2 diabetes and nephropathy. *Diabetes Care.* 2010;33(11):2304–2309.

57. Nicholls AJ. The impact of atherosclerotic renovascular disease on diabetic renal failure. *Diabet Med.* 2002;19:889–894.

58. Caramori ML, Fioretto P, Mauer M. The need for early predictors of diabetic nephropathy risk: is albumin excretion rate sufficient? *Diabetes.* 2000;49:1399–1408.

59. Bakris GL, Williams M, Dworkin L, et al., for the National Kidney Foundation Hypertension and Diabetes Executive Committee Working Group. Preserving renal function in adults with hypertension and diabetes: a consensus approach. *Am J Kidney Dis.* 2000;36:646–661.

60. Tuomilehto J, Rastenyte D, Birkenhäger W, et al. Effects of calcium-channel blockade in older patients with diabetes and systolic hypertension. *N Engl J Med.* 1999;340:677–684.

61. National Kidney Foundation. K/DOQI clinical practice guidelines for bone metabolism and disease in chronic kidney disease. *Am J Kidney Dis.* 2003;42(4 Suppl 3):S1-S201.

62. American Diabetes Association. Clinical Practice Recommendations 2011. *Diabetes Care.* 2011;34 (Suppl 1):S33.

63. Hansen HP, Tauber-Lassen E, Jensen BR, et al. Effect of dietary protein restriction on prognosis in patients with diabetic nephropathy. *Kidney Int.* 2002;62:220–228.

64. Gross JL, Zelmanovitz T, Moulin CC, et al. Effect of a chicken-based diet on renal function and lipid profile in patients with type 2 diabetes: a randomized crossover trial. *Diabetes Care.* 2002;25:645–651.

65. Davidson JA, Brett J, Falahati A, et al. Mild renal impairment has no effect on the efficacy and safety of liraglutide. *Endocrine Pract.* 2011;17(3):345–355.

66. Sloan L, Newman J, Sauce C, et al. Safety and efficacy of linagliptin in type 2 diabetes patients with severe renal impairment. American Diabetes Association. 71st Scientific Sessions. San Diego, CA. June 24–28, 2011. 413-PP.

67. Unger J, Parkin C. Recognition, prevention and proactive management of hypoglycemia in patients with type 1 diabetes. *Postgrad Med.* 2011;123(4):71–80.

68. Cryer PE. Glucose counterrefgulation in man. *Diabetes.* 1981;30:261–264.

69. Zander J, Raghu P, Hong L, et al. Initial insulin doses should be decreased in hospitalized patients with renal insufficiency and type 2 diabetes. American Diabetes Association. 71st Scientific Sessions. 2011. San Diego, CA. June 24–28. 1081 p.

70. Foley RN, Parfrey PS, Kent GM, et al. Long-term evolution of cardiomyopathy in dialysis patients. *Kidney Int.* 1998;54:1720–1725.

71. The USRDS Dialysis Morbidity and Mortality Study: wave 2: United States Renal Data System. *Am J Kidney Dis.* 1997;30(Suppl 1):S67–S85.

72. Bosman DR, Winkler AS, Marsden JT, et al. Anemia with erythropoietin deficiency occurs early in diabetic nephropathy. *Diabetes Care.* 2001;24:495–499.

73. Vanrenterghem Y, Barany P, Mann JF, et al. Randomized trial of darbepoetin alfa for treatment of renal anemia at a reduced dose frequency compared with rHuEPO in dialysis patients. *Kidney Int.* 2002;62:2167–2175.

74. Macdougall IC. How to improve survival in pre-dialysis patients. *Nephron.* 2000;85(Suppl 1):15–22.

75. Unger EF, Thompson AM, Blank MJ, et al. Erythropoesis-stimulating agents-time for reevaluation. *N Engl J Med.* 2010;362(3):189–192.

76. FDA briefing information for the joint meeting of the Cardiovascular and Renal Drugs Advisory Committee and the Drug Safety and Risk Management Committee. Rockville, MD: Food and Drug Administration, 2007. Accessed September 2, 2011 at http://www.fda.gov/ohrms/dockets/ac/07/briefing/2007-431b1-01-FDA-PDF.

77. Mainous AG, Gill JM, Carek PJ. Elevated Serum transferrin saturation and mortality. *Ann Fam Med.* 2004;2(2):133–138.

78. Sunder-Plassman G, Horl W. Erythropoietin and iron. *Clin Nephrol.* 1997;47:141–157.

79. Sacco M, Pellegrini F, Roncaglioni MC, et al. Primary prevention of cardiovascular events with low-dose aspirin and vitamin E in type 2 diabetic patients: results of the Primary Prevention Project (PPP) trial. *Diabetes Care.* 2003;26:3264–3272.

80. Watala C, Golanski J, Pluta J, et al. Reduced sensitivity of platelets from type 2 diabetic patients to acetylsalicylic acid (aspirin): its relation to metabolic control. *Thromb Res.* 2004;113:101–113.

81. Grundy SM, Cleeman JI, Merz CN, et al. Implications of recent clinical trials for the National Cholesterol Education Program Adult Treatment Panel III guidelines. *Circulation.* 2004;110:227–239.

82. Fried LF, Orchard TJ, Kasiske BL. Effect of lipid reduction on the progression of renal disease: a meta-analysis. *Kidney Int.* 2001;59:260–269.

83. Collins R, Armitage J, Parish S, et al. MRC/BHF Heart Protection Study of cholesterol-lowering with simvastatin in 5963 people with diabetes: a randomised placebo-controlled trial. *Lancet.* 2003;361:2005–2016.

84. Sponseller CA, Gumprecht J, Zhu B, et al. Long-term effects of pitavastatin on renal function in patients with type 2 diabetes and combined dyslipidemia and in non-diabetic patients with primary hyperlipidemia or mixed dyslipidemia and ≥ 2 risk factors for CHD. American Diabetes Association. 71st Scientific Sessions. San Diego, CA. June 24–28, 2011. p. 1085.

85. Sherrard DJ, Hercz G, Pei Y. The spectrum of bone disease in end-stage renal failure: an evolving disorder. *Kidney Int.* 2003;43:436–442.

86. Tentori F, Blayney MJ, Albert JM, et al. Mortality risk for dialysis patients with different levels of serum calcium, phosphorus and PTH: the Dialysis Outcomes and Practice Patterns Study (DOPPS). *Sm J Kidney Dis.* 2008;52:519–530.

87. Teng M, Wolf M, Lowrie E, et al. Survival of patients undergoing hemodialysis with paricalcitol or calcitriol therapy. *N Engl J Med.* 2003;349:446–456.

88. Kidney Disease: Improving Global Outcomes (KDIGO) CKD–MBD Work Group. KDIGO clinical practice guideline for the diagnosis, evaluation, prevention, and treatment of chronic kidney disease–mineral and bone disorder (CKD–MBD). Kidney Int. 2009;76(Suppl 113):S31.

89. Kostakis A, Vaiopoulos G, Kostantopoulos K, et al. Parathyroidectomy in the treatment of secondary hyperparathyroidism in chronic renal failure. *Int Surg.* 1997;82:85–86.

90. Tattersall J, Dekker F, Heimburger O, et al. When to start dialysis. *Nephrol Dial Transplant.* 2011;26(7):2082–2086.

91. Cooper BA, Branley P, Bulfone L, et al. A randomized, controlled trial of early versus late initiation of dialysis. *N Engl J Med.* 2010;363:609–619.

92. Centers for Disease Control and Prevention (CDC). National chronic kidney disease fact sheet: general information and national estimates on chronic kidney disease in the United States, 2010. Atlanta, GA: U.S. Department of Health and Human Services (HHS), CDC, 2010.

93. National Kidney and Urologic Disease Information Clearinghouse. http://kidney.niddk.nih.gov/kudiseases/pubs/kustats/#3. Accessed September 3, 2011.

94. OPTN: Organ Procurement and Transplantation Network website: www.optn.transplant.hrsa.gov. Accessed September 3, 2011.

95. Bunnapradist S, Danovitch GM. Evaluation of adult kidney transplantation candidates. American Journal of Kidney Diseases 2007;50(5):890–898.

96. Pergola PE, Krauth M, Huff JW, et al. Effect of bardoxolone methyl on kidney function in patients with T2D and stage 3b-4 CKD. *Am J Nephrol* 2011;33:469–476.

97. Pergola PE, Raskin P, Toto RD, et al. Bardoxolone methyl and kidney function in CKD and type 2 diabetes. *N Engl J Med.* 2011;365:327–336.

98. Zavrelova H, Hoekstra T, Alssema M, et al. Progression and regression: distinct patterns of diabetic retinopathy in patients with type 2 diabetes treated in the Diabetes Care System West-Friesland, the Netherlands. *Diabetes Care.* 2011;34:867–872.

99. Zhang X, Saaddine JB, Chou CF, et al. Prevalence of diabetic retinopathy in the United States, 2005–2008. *JAMA.* 2010;304(6):649–656.

100. Centers for Disease Control and Prevention. Blindness caused by diabetes—Massachusetts 1987–1994. *MMWR Morb Mortal Wkly Rep.* 1996;45:937–941.

101. Gardner TW, Antonetti DA, Barber AJ, et al. Diabetic retinopathy: more than meets the eye. *Surv Ophthalmol.* 2002;(Suppl):S253–S262.

102. The Diabetes Control and Complications Research Group. Clustering of long-term complications in families with diabetes in the diabetes control and complications trial. *Diabetes.* 1996;46:1829–1839.

103. The Diabetes Control and Complications Trial Research Group. The relationship of glycemic exposure (HbA1c) to the risk of development and progression of retinopathy in the Diabetes Control and Complications Trial. *Diabetes.* 1995;44:968–983.

104. Brownlee M, Hirsch IB. Glycemic variability: a hemoglobin A1C-independent risk factor for diabetic complications. *JAMA.* 2006;295:1707–1708.

105. UK Prospective Diabetes Study Group. Tight blood pressure control and risk of macrovascular and microvascular complications in type 2 diabetes: UKPDS 38. *BMJ.* 1998;317:703–713.

106. Klein R, Klein BE, Moss SE, et al. The Wisconsin Epidemiologic Study of Diabetic Retinopathy: XVII. The 14-year incidence and progression of diabetic retinopathy and associated risk factors in type 1 diabetes. *Ophthalmology.* 1998;105:1801–1815.

107. van Hecke MV, Dekker JM, Stehouwer CDA, et al. Diabetic retinopathy is associated with mortality and cardiovascular disease incidence. The EURODIAB Prospective Complications Study. *Diabetes Care.* 2005;28:1383–1389.

108. Chew EY, Ambrosius WT, Davis MD, et al. ACCORD Study Group; ACCORD Eye Study Group. Effects of medical therapies on retinopathy progression in type 2 diabetes. *N Engl J Med.* 2010; 363:233–244).

109. Keech A, Simes RJ, Barter P, et al. FIELD Study Investigators. Effects of long-term fenofibrate therapy on cardiovascular events in 9795 people with type 2 diabetes mellitus (the FIELD study): randomized controlled trial. *Lancet.* 2005;366(9500):1849–1861.

110. Sinclair SH, DelVecchio C, Levin A. Treatment of anemia in the diabetic patient with retinopathy and kidney disease. *Am J Ophthalmol.* 2003;135:740–743.

111. Resnick HE, Redline S, Shahar E, et al. Diabetes and sleep disturbances. Findings from the Sleep Heart Health Study. *Diabetes Care.* 2003;26:702–709.

112. Ciulla TA, Amador AG, Zinman B. Diabetic retinopathy and diabetic macular edema: pathophysiology, screening, and novel therapies. *Diabetes Care.* 2003;26:2653–2664.

113. The ETDRS Research Group: Impaired color vision associated with diabetic retinopathy. Early Treatment Diabetic Retinopathy Study (ETDRS Report No. 15). *Am J Ophthalmol.* 1999;128:612–617.

114. Elman MJ, Aiello LP, Beck RW, et al. Randomized trial evaluating ranibizumab plus prompt or deferred laser or triamcinolone plus prompt laser for diabetic macular oedema. *Ophthalmology* 2010;117: 1064–1077.

115. Michaelides M, Kaines A, Hamilton RD, et al. A prospective, randomised trial of intravitreal bevacizumab or laser therapy in the management of diabetic macular oedema (BOLT study) 12 month data; report 2. *Ophthalmology.* 2010;117:1078–1086.

116. The PKC-DRS Study Group. The effect of ruboxistaurin on visual loss in patients with moderately severe to very severe non-proliferative diabetic retinopathy: initial results of the protein kinase C beta inhibitor retinopathy study (PKC-DRS) multicentre randomised clinical trial. *Diabetes.* 2005;54:2188–2197.

117. A Study of Ranibizumab Injection in Subjects With Clinically Significant Macular Edema With Center Involvement Secondary to Diabetes Mellitus (RISE). NCT00473330. http://www.clinicaltrials.gov/ct2/show/NCT00473330?term=NCT00473330&rank=1. Accessed September 16, 2011.

118. A Study of Ranibizumab Injection in Subjects With Clinically Significant Macular Edema With Center Involvement Secondary to Diabetes Mellitus (RIDE). http://www.clinicaltrials.gov/ct2/show/NCT00473382?term=NCT00473382&rank=1. Accessed September 16, 2011.

119. Diabetic retinopathy—diagnostic and treatment novelties. Symposium. Program and abstracts of the American Diabetes Association 66th Scientific Sessions; June 9–13, 2006, Washington, DC.

120. Grant M. Treating diabetic retinopathy with IGF-1 antagonists. Diabetic retinopathy—diagnostic and treatment novelties. Symposium. Program and abstracts of the American Diabetes Association 66th Scientific Sessions; June 9–13, 2006, Washington, DC.

121. Skarbez K, Priestly Y, Hoepf M, et al. Comprehensive review of the effects of diabetes on ocular health. *Expert Rev Ophthalmol.* 2010;5(4):557–577.

122. Alves M, Calegari VC, Cunha DA, et al. Increased expression of advanced glycation end-products and their receptor, and activation of nuclear factor κ-B in lacrimal glands of diabetic rats. *Diabetologia* 2005;48:2675–2681.

123. Mishima S. The effects of the denervation and stimulation of the sympathetic and the trigeminal nerve on the mitotic rate of the corneal epithelium in the rabbit. *Jpn J Ophthalmol.* 1957;1:65–73.

124. Goebbels M, Spitznas M, Oldendoerp J. Impairment of corneal epithelial barrier function in diabetics. *Graefes Arch Clin Exp Ophthalmol.* 1989;227:142–144.

125. Halkiadakis I, Belfair N, Gimbel HV. Laser *in situ* keratomileusis in patients with diabetes. *J Cataract Refract Surg.* 2005;31:1895–1898.

126. Ghanbari H, Ahmadieh H. Aggravation of proliferative diabetic retinopathy after laser *in situ* keratomileusis. J. *Cataract Refract Surg.* 2003;29:2232–2233.

127. March W, Long B, Hofmann W, et al. Safety of contact lenses in patients with diabetes. *Diabetes Technol Ther.* 2004;6(1):49–52.

128. Wiemer NGM, Dubbelman M, Kostense PJ, et al. The influence of chronic diabetes mellitus on the thickness and the shape of the anterior and posterior surface of the cornea. *Cornea* 2007;26(10):1165–1170.

129. Klein BE, Klein R, Moss SE. Prevalence of cataract in a population-based study of persons with diabetes mellitus. *Ophthalmology* 1985;92:1191–1196.

130. Ederer F, Hiler R, Taylor HR. Senile lens changes and diabetes in two population studies. *Am J Ophthalmol.* 1981;91:381–395.

131. Klein BEK, Klein R, Lee KE. Diabetes, cardiovascular disease, selected cardiovascular disease risk factors, and the 5-year incidence of age-related cataract and the progression of lens opacities: the Beaver Dam Eye Study. *Am J Ophthalmol.* 1998;126:782–790.

132. Koleva-Georgieva D, Sivkova N. Assessment of serous macular detachment in eyes with diabetic macular edema by use of spectral domain optical coherence tomography. *Graefes Arch Clin Exp Ophthalmol.* 2009;247:1461–1469.
133. Klein R, Klein BE, Moss SE, et al. The epidemiology of retinal vein occlusion: the Beaver Dam Eye Study. *Trans Am Ophthalmol Soc.* 2000;98:133–143.
134. Brown GC, Magargal LE, Schachat A, et al. Neovascular glaucoma: etiologic considerations. *Ophthalmology.* 1984;91:315–320.
135. Ino-ue M, Azumi A, Kajiura-Tsukahara Y, et al. Ocular ischemic syndrome in diabetic patients. *Jpn J Ophthalmol.* 1999;43:31–35.

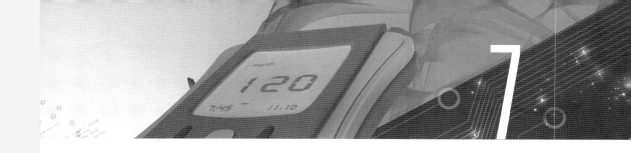

Exploring the Association between Diabetes and Cardiovascular Disease

Stop thinking in terms of limitations and start
thinking in terms of possibilities.
—*Terry Josephson, 20th/21st-century*
motivational author

Introduction   Diabetes is considered a cardiovascular (CV) risk equivalent disease. In 1998, Haffner et al. reported that Finnish patients with T2DM have a risk for future major coronary events similar to that of patients with previous myocardial infarction (MI).[1] Other studies have shown that coronary mortality at the time of acute myocardial infarction (AMI) is essentially doubled in patients with diabetes compared with those without diabetes.[2,3] Moreover, the mortality rates for patients with diabetes who survive an initial MI are doubled for subsequent events when compared to patients who are euglycemic.[4]

Due to the high risk of both primary events and mortality following onset of coronary heart disease (CHD), intensive prevention of atherosclerosis in all patients with diabetes appears to be a reasonable objective.[5]

Adult Treatment Panel III (ATP III) defines CHD risk equivalent as the likelihood of developing a major coronary event (myocardial infarct + coronary death) within 10 years of greater than 20%.At current retail drug prices, when 10-year risk for hard CHD events (MI + CHD death) ranges from 10% to 20% per year, statins carry an acceptable cost-effectiveness according to a cost analysis by ATP III.[5]

Eighty percent of diabetes-related mortality is attributable to the three major forms of macrovascular complications, which include CHD, stroke, and peripheral arterial disease (PAD).[6] Table 7-1 shows the predictors of CV mortality in patients with diabetes, and Table 7-2 displays the features commonly associated with CHD and diabetes.

Roughly 85% of acute strokes are atherothrombotic, and the rest are hemorrhagic (10% primary intracerebral hemorrhage and 5% subarachnoid hemorrhage). The risk of atherothrombotic stroke is two- to threefold higher in patients with diabetes, while the rates of hemorrhagic stroke and transient ischemic attacks (TIAs) are similar to those of the nondiabetic population.[7]

Predictors of increased mortality among stroke patients with diabetes include (a) severity of hyperglycemia on admission, (b) infarct of the middle cerebral artery, (c) advanced age, (d) presence

TABLE 7-1. Predictors of CV Mortality in Patients with T1DM and T2DM

T1DM	T2DM
Overt nephropathy	Presence of CAD
Hypertension	Overt proteinuria
Age	Hemoglobin A1C
Smoking	Hypertension
Microalbuminuria	
Autonomic cardiac neuropathy	

Adapted from Donnelly R, Emslie-Smith AM, Gardner ID, et al. ABC of arterial and venous disease: vascular complications of diabetes. *BMJ.* 2000;320:1062–1066.

of atrial fibrillation, (e) history of congestive heart failure, (f) chronic kidney disease (CKD), and (g) a low Glasgow coma score. Renal failure is a rare cause of death in acute stroke, yet suggests the presence of significant vascular disease. Stroke patients with diabetes also require longer hospital stays when compared to euglycemic individuals. This will inevitably translate into higher overall cost. The longer length of stay might possibly be caused by the difficulties in controlling the blood glucose during the hospital stay.[8,9]

Pathogenesis of Macrovascular Compromise in Patients with Diabetes

Vascular disease and endothelial dysfunction are accelerated in diabetes due to the multiple metabolic anomalies associated with hyperglycemia (Fig. 7-1). Damaged endothelial cells produce lower levels of nitric oxide (NO), thereby inhibiting vasodilation. Vascular smooth-muscle proliferation in association with higher circulating levels of plasminogen activator inhibitor-1 (PAI-1) leads to a state of hypercoagulation, increased thrombosis, and progressive atherogenesis. Inflammation within the endovascular environment is accelerated in the presence of hypertension, dyslipidemia, cigarette smoking, and direct endothelial cell damage from cytokines such as tumor necrosis factor (TNF) and C-reactive protein (CRP).

TABLE 7-2. Features of CHD in Diabetic Patients

Atherosclerosis	AMI	Revascularization
• Prevalence of fatal and nonfatal CHD events 2–20 times higher than for nondiabetics of similar age	• In-hospital and 6-mo mortality double that in nondiabetics	• 5-y survival rates after coronary artery bypass graft or percutaneous coronary angioplasty lower than for nondiabetics
• Protective effect of female gender is lost.	• Complications (e.g., arrhythmias, heart failure, death) more common	• 5-y survival better after coronary artery bypass graft than percutaneous coronary angioplasty because of higher restenosis rates
• Plaque rupture leading to unstable angina and MI is more common.	• Reperfusion rates after thrombolysis are similar to those of nondiabetics, but reocclusion and reinfarction rates are higher.	
• Higher incidence of diffuse, multivessel disease	• Mortality reduced by insulin glucose infusion immediately after MI	
• Superimposed thrombosis more likely		

Adapted from Donnelly R, Emslie-Smith AM, Gardner ID, et al. ABC of arterial and venous disease: vascular complications of diabetes. *BMJ.* 2000;320:1062–1066.

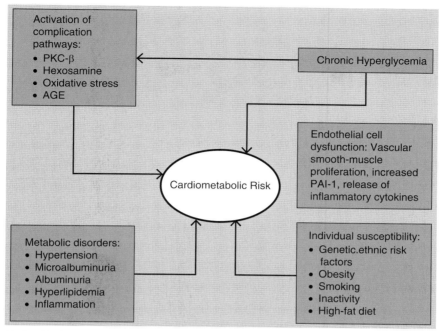

Figure 7-1 • Pathogenesis of CV Complications in Patients with Diabetes. Multiple acquired and genetic risk factors favor progression to CVD in patients with diabetes. All of these components with the exception of genetics and ethnicity are modifiable risk factors. Chronic hyperglycemia increases one's glycemic burden favoring progression toward heart disease, stroke, and peripheral vascular disease. (AGE, advanced glycosylated end products; PKC, protein kinase-C.)

Glucose can react extracellularly in nonenzymatic reactions. One pathologic mechanism shared with microvascular complications involves the glycosylation of protein within arterial wall matrix in a process that induces cross-linking of collagen within the vessel wall, reducing compliance. Direct glycation of low-density lipoprotein cholesterol (LDL-C) prolongs the half-life of these atherogenic lipoproteins, further increasing CV risk. Activation of the protein kinase C (PKC)-β pathway in association with the oxidative stress induced by glycemic variability increases risk of cardiomyopathy.[10,11] Glycemic variability and oxidative stress appear to be the cornerstone for both microvascular and macrovascular pathogenesis.[12]

Why are some tissues (such as neurons or endothelial cells) prone to develop complications, whereas others (digestive cells) appear to be immune to the effects of prolonged exposure to hyperglycemia? The answer may lie in a cell's ability to assimilate the amount of glucose required as an energy source, before pumping any excess glucose to the outside of the cell. Neurons, nephrons, retinal cells, and endothelial cells are inefficient interstitial transporters of glucose. As glucose levels rise above 180 mg per dL in these "at risk cells," reactive oxygen species (ROS) form within their mitochondria electron transport chain, triggering a cascade of events leading to microvascular and macrovascular disease.[13] The "downstream" targets of ROS formation include increased activity of PKC, activation of nuclear factor (NF)-κB, collagen synthesis, and cell death.[14] Exposure to blood glucose levels above 180 mg per dL for just 4 hours can cause the downstream effects of ROS to persist for up to 7 days, even if the blood glucose levels are quickly normalized.[15] One can easily understand the biologic link between the extremely high incidence of cardiovascular disease (CVD) and hyperglycemia as shown in Figure 7-2.

CV risk is increased in individuals who have glucose abnormalities that are considered as being below the diagnostic threshold level for diabetes.[16] The A1C levels of 10,232 patients were assessed from 1995 to 1997. CVD events and mortality rates were subsequently assessed through 2003. As shown in Figure 7-3, the risk for CVD and mortality increased continuously across the A1C distribution.

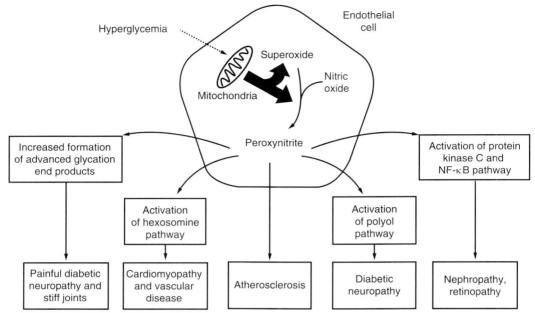

Figure 7-2 • **Hyperglycemia Activates Pathways within Endothelial Cells Leading to Multiple Long-term Complications.** The action of endothelium-derived vasodilators (e.g., NO and prostacyclin) has been associated with antiatherogenic mechanisms, whereas endothelium-derived vasoconstrictors (e.g., endothelin-1 and thromboxane) promote atherosclerosis. NO keeps the endothelial cells free of adhesion molecules and regulates vascular tone. Peroxynitrate (an NO derivative) is formed when NO interacts with oxidative forces (superoxide) within the endothelial cells. Perioxynitrate inhibits the endothelial cell's mitochondrial electron transport system leading to endothelial dysfunction and the transcription of endothelial-derived cytokines that induce pathways responsible for microvascular and macrovascular complications. (From Unger J. Reducing oxidative stress in patients with type 2 diabetes mellitus: a primary care call to action. *Insulin.* 2008;3:176–184.)

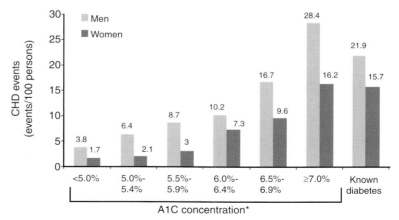

Figure 7-3 • **A1C Is Predictive of CHD Event Rates.** The risk for CVD and total mortality associated with A1C concentrations increased continuously through the sample distribution. Most of the events in the sample occurred in persons with moderately elevated A1C concentrations. A1C levels greater than or equal to 7% infer the highest risk in this study population. (Adapted from Khaw KT, Wareham N, Bingham S, et al. Association of hemoglobin A1C with cardiovascular disease and mortality in adults: the European prospective investigation into cancer in Norfolk. *Ann Intern Med.* 2004;141(6):413–420.)

TABLE 7-3. Relative Risk Reduction of CHD Events in UKPDS and 10-Year UKPDS Follow-up Suggesting Importance of Intensive Intervention

Treatment Group	Reduction in MI (1997)	Reduction in MI (2007)	Reduction in All-cause Mortality (1997)	Reduction in All-cause Mortality (2007)
Sulfonylurea/ Insulin	16% $p = 0.052^a$	15% $p = 0.01$	6% $p = 0.44^a$	13% $p = 0.007$
Metformin	39% $p = 0.01^a$	33% $p = 0.005$	36% $p = 0.011$	27% $p = 0.002$

Reductions in MI and all-cause mortality rates, which had not been statistically significant in the original trial, became significant for the intensively treated participants during the long-term follow-up study.
$^a p$ value not statistically significant.
From Holman RR, Paul SK, Bethel MA, et al. Long-term follow-up of intensive glucose control in type 2 diabetes. *N Engl J Med.* 2008;359:1577–1589.

As with microvascular disease, improvement in glycemic control can significantly lower the risk of macrovascular complications. The UK Prospective Diabetes Study (UKPDS) demonstrated that each 1% reduction in A1C was associated with a corresponding 14% reduction in the risk of MIs.[17] There was no A1C threshold that targeted the optimal macrovascular risk reduction. Thus, lowering the A1C as close to normal as possible is certainly a desirable target.

The 10-year UKPDS follow-up observed a "legacy effect" of intensive glucose therapy suggesting continued vascular benefits despite loss of glycemic differences from conventional treatment.[18] Reductions in MI and all-cause mortality, which had not been statistically significant in the original trial, became significant for the intensively treated participants during the post-trial period (Table 7-3). Thus, the UKPDS follow-up supports initiation of intensive glucose therapy as early as possible for patients with T2DM.

Patients with T1DM who were intensively managed on average for 6.5 years in the Diabetes Control and Complications Trial (DCCT) and then followed for 17 years once the study concluded had a significantly lower rate of CV events than those patients treated with conventional therapy (Fig. 7-4).[19] Intensive insulin management in T1DM patients reduced the risk of nonfatal MI, stroke, or death from CVD by 57% and the risk of any CVD event by 42% compared with conventionally treated DCCT patients. Associated with the prolonged improvement in the A1C, intensively managed patients had lower A1C levels as well as lower incidences of microalbuminuria and albuminuria, both of which are associated with CVD. Other studies have demonstrated that intensive therapy reduced the progression of atherosclerosis, measured by carotid intima–media thickness (CIMT), as well as the prevalence of coronary artery calcification.[20,21] The mechanisms responsible for the improvement in outcomes and for the prolonged effects on early intervention remain uncertain. Some investigators feel that "metabolic memory" results in long-term beneficial effects on macrovascular risk reduction in intensively managed patients with T1DM. Regardless of the protective mechanism associated with improved glycemic control, the risk reduction achieved by initiating intensive therapy in T1DM patients as soon as the diagnosis is made is compelling. Risk reduction achieved with other proven interventions such as lowering cholesterol and BP is far less than those attained by intensively managing patients with diabetes.

Risk reduction for macrovascular disease involves targeting treatment at each one of the metabolic abnormalities that coexist with hyperglycemia.[22]

Determining Cardiovascular Risk Assessment in Patients with Diabetes

The use of a mathematical model to predict the likelihood of developing long-term diabetes-associated complications would help the physician target specific treatment targets, which should lower the

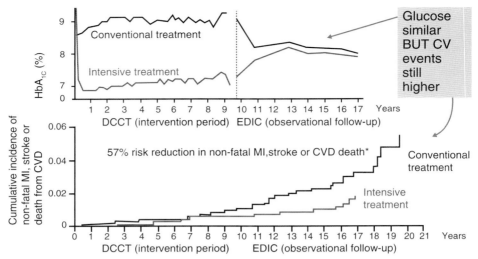

Figure 7-4 • Long-term Effects of Intensive Management of T1DM Patients on CV Outcomes.
Patients who were intensively managed during the DCCT demonstrated a 57% reduction in nonfatal MI, stroke, and CV-related deaths during the 10-year follow-up study (EDIC). (Adapted from The Diabetes Control and Complications Trial/Epidemiology of Diabetes Interventions and Complications (DCCT/EDIC) Study Group. Intensive diabetes treatment and cardiovascular disease in patients with type 1 diabetes. *N Engl J Med.* 2005;353:2643–2653.)

risk. In addition, global risk assessment models could be useful in educating patients regarding the importance of fine-tuning metabolic therapy or maintaining adherence to a prescribed treatment plan. Risk factor assessment may target two different populations. Patients who have already suffered a diabetes-related complication, such as a stroke or AMI, should be evaluated to determine which interventions may be prescribed to prevent the occurrence of a secondary event. Primary prevention strategies are used to delay or avoid an initial event from occurring in high-risk patients such as AMI, stroke, acute coronary syndrome (ACS) (angina), and lower extremity amputation due to PAD.

The major and independent risk factors for CHD are cigarette smoking of any amount, elevated BP, elevated serum total cholesterol and LDL-C, low serum high-density lipoprotein cholesterol (HDL-C), diabetes mellitus, and advancing age (Table 7-4). Preventive efforts should target each major risk factor. Any major risk factor, if left untreated for many years, has the potential to produce CHD. Nonetheless, an assessment of total (global) risk based on the summation of all major risk factors can be clinically useful for three purposes: (a) identification of high-risk patients who deserve immediate attention and intervention, (b) motivation of patients to adhere to risk-reduction therapies, and (c) modification of intensity of risk-reduction efforts based on the total risk estimate.

The Framingham Risk Score (FRS) incorporates well-established risk factors such as age, sex, smoking history, blood pressure (BP), total serum cholesterol, HDL-C, and blood glucose (or history of diabetes) into a risk calculation model.[23] However, Framingham tends to underestimate the true 10-year CV risk associated with having T2DM.[24] The initial Framingham cohort included a low baseline prevalence of patients with diabetes while omitting any reference to triglycerides (TGs), an important determinant in CV risk for patients with T2DM.[25] This leads to wide confidence intervals in the overall predicted risk. A wide confidence interval implies that more data should be collected before conclusions may be made in regard to defining specific risk within a given cohort.

The modified FRS (Fig. 7-5) addresses short- and long-term CV risks in adults with existing CHD. Patients characterized as being "high risk" are predicted to have at least a 2% to 3% yearly likelihood of having a significant cardiac event.[26] The American College of Cardiology recommends aggressive risk reduction for all patients with diabetes as displayed in Table 7-5 as these individuals have CHD risk equivalent disease.[27]

Disease risk factors can be defined as measurable biologic characteristics of an individual that precede a well-defined outcome of a disease (such as myocardial infarct), predict that outcome, and

TABLE 7-4. Risk Factors for CVD

Major Risk Factors	Predisposing Risk Factors		
Smoking	Obesity[a]		
Hypertension	**BMI categories**		
Elevated LDL-C, low HDL-C	• 18.5–24.9 kg/m^2		Normal
Diabetes	• 25–29 kg/m^2		Overweight
Advancing age	• >30.0 kg/m^2		Obesity
	Abdominal obesity (defined as a waist circumference >40 inches in men and 35 inches in women)		
	Physical inactivity[a]		
	Family history of premature CHD		
	Ethnic characteristics		
	Psychosocial factors[b]		
	Elevated serum TGs		
	Small LDL-C particles		
	Elevated serum homocysteine[c]		
	Elevated serum LP(a)		
	Prothrombotic factors (e.g., fibrinogen, PAI-1)		
	Inflammatory markers (e.g., CRP)		

[a]These risk factors are defined as major risk factors by the AHA.
LDL-C, low-density lipoprotein cholesterol; HDL-C, high-density lipoprotein cholesterol; BMI, body mass index; PAI-1, plasminogen activator inhibitor-1; CRP, C-reactive protein.

are directly related to the pathogenic pathway. In contrast, nontraditional biomarkers are biologic indicators of a disease process that are involved in the development of the disease, which may or may not be causal.[28] Risk factors identify asymptomatic individuals who have a greater chance of developing a disease compared with the general population. A clinically useful biomarker should meet both of the following criteria: (1) evidence from prospective studies either cohort or randomized trials across a broad range of populations demonstrating independent prediction of vascular events with reclassification of risk based upon the inclusion of that biomarker and (2) therapies that modify a given biomarker should be available that would otherwise not be used in the at-risk population. A biomarker that is not useful in predicting disease causality is not considered a risk factor, yet may still elucidate vital information related to disease progression. Biomarkers may also be useful in drug development and measuring therapeutic outcomes. Table 7-6 lists several novel biomarkers related to inflammation, oxidative stress, and insulin resistance.

The U.S. Preventive Services Task Force (USPSTF) has stated that the use of "high-sensitivity C-reactive protein (hs-CRP), ankle-brachial index (ABI), leukocyte count, fasting blood glucose level, periodontal disease, CIMT, coronary artery calcification score on electron-beam computed tomography (EBCT), homocysteine level, and lipoprotein(a) [Lp(a)] level are insufficient to screen asymptomatic patients with no history of CHD for primary prevention."[29] To be fair, the USPSTF recommendation statement clearly says that the critical gap in the evidence for screening with nontraditional risk factors is the lack of information on subsequent reductions in risk for CHD events in persons identified by the new risk factors.

The Centers for Disease Control and Prevention (CDC) and the American Heart Association (AHA) released a joint statement in 2003 on the use of hs-CRP in assessing CHD risk.[30] Their recommendations include the following:

a. hs-CRP is the CHD inflammatory marker of choice for clinical practice.
b. Patients with an intermediate (10% to 20%) risk of CHD may benefit from measurement of hs-CRP for evaluation and therapy decisions (this would include all patients with diabetes).
c. hs-CRP may be useful for estimating prognosis in patients with CHD (including death and recurrent events).

Step 1

Age		
Years	LDL Pts	Chol Pts
30-34	-1	[-1]
35-39	0	[0]
40-44	1	[1]
45-49	2	[2]
50-54	3	[3]
55-59	4	[4]
60-64	5	[5]
65-69	6	[6]
70-74	7	[7]

Step 2

LDL - C		
(mg/dL)	(mmol/L)	LDL Pts
<100	<2.59	-3
100-129	2.60-3.36	0
130-159	3.37-4.14	0
160-190	4.15-4.92	1
≥190	≥4.92	2

Cholesterol		
(mg/dL)	(mmol/L)	Chol Pts
<160	<4.14	[-3]
160-199	4.15-5.17	[0]
200-239	5.18-6.21	[1]
240-279	6.22-7.24	[2]
≥280	≥7.25	[3]

Step 3

HDL - C			
(mg/dL)	(mmol/L)	LDL Pts	Chol Pts
<35	<0.90	2	[2]
35-44	0.91-1.16	1	[1]
45-49	1.17-1.29	0	[0]
50-59	1.30-1.55	0	[0]
≥60	≥1.56	-1	[-2]

Step 4

Blood Pressure					
Systolic (mm Hg)	Diastolic (mm Hg)				
	<80	80-84	85-89	90-99	≥100
<120	0 [0] Pts				
120-129		0 [0] Pts			
130-139			1 [1] Pts		
140-159				2 [2] Pts	
≥160					3 [3] Pts

Note: When systolic and diastolic pressures provide different estimates for point scores, use the higher number

Step 5

Diabetes		
	LDL Pts	Chol Pts
No	0	[0]
Yes	2	[2]

Step 6

Smoker		
	LDL Pts	Chol Pts
No	0	[0]
Yes	2	[2]

(sum from steps 1-6)

Step 7

Adding up the points	
Age	_____
LDL-C or Chol	_____
HDL-C	_____
Blood Pressure	_____
Diabetes	_____
Smoker	_____
Point total	_____

(determine CHD risk from point total)

Step 8

CHD Risk			
LDL Pts Total	10 Yr CHD Risk	Chol Pts Total	10 Yr CHD Risk
<-3	1%		
-2	2%		
-1	2%	[<-1]	[2%]
0	3%	[0]	[3%]
1	4%	[1]	[3%]
2	4%	[2]	[4%]
3	6%	[3]	[5%]
4	7%	[4]	[7%]
5	9%	[5]	[8%]
6	11%	[6]	[10%]
7	14%	[7]	[13%]
8	18%	[8]	[16%]
9	22%	[9]	[20%]
10	27%	[10]	[25%]
11	33%	[11]	[31%]
12	40%	[12]	[37%]
13	47%	[13]	[45%]
≥14	≥56%	[≥14]	[≥53%]

(compare to average person your age)

Step 9

Comparative Risk			
Age (years)	Average 10 Yr CHD Risk	Average 10 Yr Hard* CHD Risk	Low** 10 Yr CHD Risk
30-34	3%	1%	2%
35-39	5%	4%	3%
40-44	7%	4%	4%
45-49	11%	8%	4%
50-54	14%	10%	6%
55-59	16%	13%	7%
60-64	21%	20%	9%
65-69	25%	22%	11%
70-74	30%	25%	14%

Key	
Color	Relative Risk
green	Very Low
white	Low
yellow	Moderate
rose	High
red	Very high

* Hard CHD events exclude angina pectoris

** Low risk was calculated for a person the same age, optimal blood pressure, LDL-C 100-129 mg/dL or cholesterol 160-199 mg/dL, HDL-C 45 mg/dL for men or 55 mg/dL for women, non-smoker, no diabetes

Risk estimates were derived from the experience of the Framingham Heart Study, a predominantly Caucasion population in Massachusetts, USA

Figure 7-5 • Framingham Modified Risk Score Calculations. Online calculator available at: http://www. mdcalc.com/framingham-cardiac-risk-score. Note: *The modified FRS is validated for patients ages 35 to 74.*

TABLE 7-5. Interpretation and Treatment Intensification Based on Modified FRSs

Low Risk (~35% of patients)	Low-risk Framingham Risk Score and no major CHD risk factors; minimal risk estimate	Provide reassurance and retest in about 5 y
Intermediate Risk (~40% of patients)	≥1 major abnormal risk factor or positive family history of CHD; global risk estimate: 0.6%–2%/y	Patients may benefit from noninvasive testing for further risk assessment
High Risk (~25% of patients)	Established CHD or atherosclerotic disease (PAD, CAD, atherosclerotic cardiovascular disease (ASCVD), TIA, or stroke); T2DM or multiple CHD risk factors; hard CHD risk: >20% in 10 y	Candidates for intensive risk factor intervention without further risk factor assessment to determine treatment goals

From Greenland P, Smith SC Jr, Grundy SM. Improving coronary heart disease risk assessment in asymptomatic people: role of traditional risk factors and noninvasive cardiovascular tests. *Circulation.* 2001;104(15):1863–1867.

Hyperglycemia is associated with a rise in hs-CRP. Hypertensive patients with T2DM have the highest plasma levels of hs-CRP suggesting that these individuals have an active and on-going inflammatory process perhaps predisposing them to CVD.[31] In 2008, the JUPITER trial was published that showed that statin use (rosuvastatin) in healthy men aged greater than 50 and in healthy women aged greater than 60 with an LDL-C of less than 130 mg per dL and an hs-CRP greater than 2 mg per L decreased the incidence of a first MI by 48% and stroke by 55%.[32] The best primary prevention CV outcomes occurred in patients who attained an LDL-C of less than 70 mg per dL and an hs-CRP of less than 1 mg per L with rosuvastatin.[33] In general, hs-CRP levels may be reduced with the use of statins, β-blockers, or aspirin by 20% to 30%.[34,35]

A 15-year longitudinal observational study demonstrated that plasma vitamin D levels less than 13.9 nmol per L in patients with T2DM place them at increased risk for all-cause mortality including deaths from CVD.[36] Vitamin D appears to mitigate vascular inflammation by affecting foam cell (macrophages which ingest oxidized LDL) formation and signaling in individuals who do not have diabetes.[37]

Several risk engines are useful in assessing the likelihood of developing heart disease and strokes. The UKPDS Risk Engine (available for downloading at: http://www.dtu.ox.ac.uk/index.html7maindoc=/riskengine/download.html) provides risk estimates and 95% confidence intervals in patients with T2DM not known to have heart disease. A patient's risk for heart disease and stroke can be calculated for any given duration of T2DM based on current age, sex, ethnicity, smoking status, presence or absence of atrial fibrillation, and levels of A1C, systolic BP, total cholesterol, and HDL-C.

One of the most detailed and patient-friendly global risk engines, Diabetes PHD (Personal Health Decisions), can be accessed as a link through the American Diabetes Association (ADA) Web site (https://www.diabetes.org/phd/profile/start.jsp). Diabetes PHD can be used to explore the effects of a wide variety of health-care interventions (both behavioral and pharmacologic) on the 30-year risk of developing a heart attack, stroke, kidney disease, lower extremity amputation, and DR. Information that needs to be uploaded into the site includes a detailed health history (MI, stroke, angina, bypass surgery, angioplasty, heart failure, retinopathy, albuminuria, CKD or ESRD, diabetic neuropathy, neuropathic ulcer), age, ethnicity, sex, height, weight, lipid levels, smoking history, BP reading, dates of last eye exam, frequency and intensity of exercise, frequency of office visits, A1C, foot exam, presence and level of proteinuria, list of medications, length of time patient has used aspirin, family history of diabetes and/or CVD, and a list of all current medications related to managing diabetes, hypertension, and hyperlipidemia. Diabetes PHD, as powered by a health modeling program known as Archimedes, then calculates the patient's risk of developing microvascular and macrovascular

TABLE 7-6. Novel Biomarkers Used in the Assessment of Patients with Diabetes

Biomarker	Comment
Leptin	One of the adipose tissue's adipokines (bioactive proteins). In animal models, leptin levels are higher with higher fat mass. Leptin theoretically acts as a regulator to decrease appetite in the presence of obesity and to increase energy expenditure. Obese people may be "leptin resistant." Subcutaneous injections of leptin restores normal appetite and reduces fat mass in children.
Adiponectin	Adipose-specific hormone that has anti-inflammatory and insulin-sensitizing properties. Protective vs. obesity. PPAR drugs, such as thiazolidinediones act, in part, by increasing circulating levels of adiponectin. Metabolic surgery also increases adiponectin levels.
Plasma 8-isoprostanes and F2 α-isoprostanes	Markers of oxidative stress. Higher levels indicate greater risk of endothelial cell dysfunction. Unfortunately, oxidative stress is not measured clinically in adults or children. Experimental measurements of oxidative stress have not been shown to predict future risk of CV events in observational studies. No interventional trials altering oxidative stress have affected CV event rates.
CRP	A downstream marker of inflammation that has multiple effects including complement binding, augmentation of expression of adhesions molecules, and decreased expression of the vasodilator endothelial NO synthase. CRP may also stimulate the expression of the thrombotic factor, PAI-1 and induce oxidative stress. Adipocytes release IL-6 and TNF-α that stimulate the liver to produce CRP. Obesity and CRP levels are positively correlated. CRP levels are independent predictors of stroke and MI.[a] Weight loss and reducing saturated fat intake reduce CRP levels in children.
Vitamin D	Plasma levels of vitamin D (25-hydroxyvitamin D3) <13.9 nmol/L are predictive of CV mortality independent of conventional risk factors including glycemic control and independent of one's history of CKD.[b]

[a]Ridker PM, Danielson E, Fonseca FAH, et al. JUPITER Trial Study Group. Reduction in C-reactive protein and LDL cholesterol and cardiovascular event rates after initiation of rosuvastatin: a prospective study of the JUPITER trial. *Lancet.* 2009;373(9670):1175–1182.
[b]Joergensen C, Gall MA, Schmedes A, et al. Vitamin D levels and mortality in type 2 diabetes. *Diabetes Care.* 2010;33:2238–2243.

complications over the next 30 years. Patients can explore the effects various treatment interventions (both pharmacologic and behavioral) will have on predicted microvascular and macrovascular outcomes using this web site. An updated version of Diabetes PHD is currently being developed by the ADA.

Targeting Optimal Metabolic Control in Patients with T2DM

Data from the UKPDS suggested that improved glycemic control reduced the risk of CVD and deaths as well as all-cause mortality.[38] However, three recently published large, randomized, controlled trials (ADVANCE, ACCORD, and VADT) found no evidence that intensive glycemic control had a major effect on CV outcomes (Table 7-7).[39–41]

ACCORD identified an increased risk for death from CV causes and total mortality associated with intensive glucose control, thereby providing little guidance on how to manage metabolic control in high-risk patients with type T2DM. The lessons learned from these landmark studies are listed in Table 7-8.

TABLE 7-7. Summary of ACCORD, ADVANCE, and VADT Clinical Trial Data

Study	Demographics	Goal of Study	Primary End Point	Secondary End Points	Results	Interpretation
VADT	1,791 veterans. Median A1C >75%. Mean age 60.4 y. 40% of subjects had history of a CV event.	Reduce A1C <1.5% in the intensive-therapy group compared with the standard-therapy group Median follow-up 5.6 y Modifiable risk factors were treated identically in the 2 groups	Time from randomization to 1st occurrence of MI, stroke, death from CV event, CHF; surgery for vascular disease, inoperable coronary disease, amputation for ischemic gangrene	Progression to sensory neuropathy, albuminuria, and retinopathy	No differences noted in primary outcomes No differences in secondary outcomes Intensive therapy doubled the frequency of severe hypoglycemia (2.3 vs. 1.1%/y) Median weight gain of 6.8 kg in intensive group	Glucose control has no impact on CV outcomes
ACCORD	10,251 patients. Median A1C 8.1%. 38% of women and 35% of men had a previous CV event 4,733 patients were randomly assigned to receive intensive BP therapy (systolic target <120 mm Hg) vs. standard BP therapy (systolic target <140 mm Hg)	Intensive therapy targeted an A1C <6% vs. standard therapy targeting A1C to 7%–7.9%	Nonfatal MI, nonfatal stroke, death from CV causes	Death from any cause	At 1 year, the stable median A1C was 6.4% in intensive group and 7.5% in standard group. 257 patients in the intensive group died vs. 203 in the conventional cohort. This led to a discontinuation of intensive therapy after a mean of 3.5 years of follow-up.	Intensive control may reduce risk of MIs, but favors an increased risk of death

(Continued)

TABLE 7-7. Summary of ACCORD, ADVANCE, and VADT Clinical Trial Data (Continued)

Study	Demographics	Goal of Study	Primary End Point	Secondary End Points	Results	Interpretation
	5,518 patients were randomly assigned to receive either fenofibrate or placebo while maintaining good control of LDL-C with simvastatin				3 times more frequent annual episodes of severe hypoglycemia in intensive group vs. conventional group (4.6 vs. 1.5%). 27.8% of intensive group gained >10 kg vs. only 14.1% of conventional group. Median weight gain of intensive group was 3.5 kg. No differences in progression toward cardiac autonomic neuropathy between the 2 groups	
ADVANCE	11,140 patients. Median A1C = 7.2%.32% had history of prior macrovascular disease. 3% had macroalbuminuria and 7% had retinopathy	Intensive glucose control using gliclazide plus other drugs as required to achieve an A1C ≤6.5% vs. standard glucose control BP was controlled with either perindopril + indapamide or matching placebo Median 5 y follow-up	Death from CV causes nonfatal MI or stroke. New or worsening macroalbuminuria, doubling of serum creatinine to at least 2.26 mg/dL needed for renal replacement, death due to renal disease. Development of retinopathy (proliferative retinopathy, macular edema or diabetes-related blindness or the use of retinal photocoagulation therapy	Deaths from any cause, death from CV causes, coronary revascularization, TIA, CHF, worsening of New York Heart Association class of CHF, new or worsening nephropathy, new or worsening retinopathy, development of microalbuminuria, new or worsening neuropathy, decline in cognitive function, hospitalization for more than 24 h, hypoglycemic events	No reduction in macrovascular events with intensive therapy. 21% reduction in nephropathy, 5% reduction in retinopathy (not significant) 3 time greater annual incidence of severe hypoglycemia in intensive cohort vs. conventional group (1.8 vs. 0.6%). Median weight gain of intensive group was 0.7 kg	Intensive glucose control has no impact on CV risk reduction but may slightly improve progression of nephropathy

Data from Action to Control Cardiovascular Risk in Diabetes Study Group. Effects of intensive glucose lowering in type 2 diabetes. *N Engl J Med.* 2008;358:2545–2559; Group AC, Patel A, MacMahon S, et al.; ADVANCE Collaborative Group. Intensive blood glucose control and vascular outcomes in patients with type 2 diabetes. *N Engl J Med.* 2008;358:2560–2572; Duckworth W, Abraira C, Moritz T, et al.; VADT Investigators. Glucose control and vascular complications in veterans with type 2 diabetes. *N Engl J Med.* 2009;360:129–139.

Based upon the studies mentioned above, health-care providers should focus their efforts on combining elements of lifestyle modification, glycemic control, which minimizes hypoglycemia and weight gain, BP reduction, and optimal lipid lowering to reduce macrovascular complications in patients with T2DM.

Macrovascular Complications in Patients with T1DM

Although less studied than in patients with T2DM, macrovascular complications can impact those individuals with T1DM at a younger age (less than 40 years), be more diffuse, have a greater accelerated course to end-stage outcomes than observed in the general population. The Pittsburgh Epidemiology of Diabetes Complications study demonstrated that both men and women had similarly increased risk of premature coronary artery disease (CAD), although risk factors, such as renal impairment appeared to be gender specific.[42] As with T2DM, risk factors for macrovascular complications in T1DM include hypertension, smoking and dyslipidemia, insulin resistance, African American race, and disease duration.[43,44]

Genetic variation may play a major role in predicting which patients may be predisposed to CHD. In the Pittsburgh EDC study, patients who carried the haptoglobin (Hp)2-2 genotype had a twofold greater risk of CHD than those expressing the Hp1-1. A major limitation for the management of CHD in T1DM is the lack of a validated risk engine for this patient population. Therefore, genetic studies may prove valuable in future risk assessment in patients with T1DM.[45]

Long-term follow-up of the intensively treated patients in the DCCT suggest that treatment to A1C targets less than 7% in the years soon after the diagnosis of the disease is associated with reduction in macrovascular risk.[19] The establishment of "metabolic memory," appears to warrant treating hyperglycemia as soon as possible, for as long as possible, as low as possible, as safely as possible, and as rationally as possible in all patients with diabetes.[46]

Reducing Macrovascular Risk in Patients with Diabetes

• Targeting Hypertension in Diabetes Patients

BP reduction in patients with diabetes improves long-term outcomes. The HOT study reported a 51% reduction in cardiac events in the diabetes subpopulation ($n = 1,501$) who were able to intensively reduce their diastolic BP to lower than 80 mm Hg.[47] Likewise, the UKPDS reported significant reductions in all diabetes-related endpoints, deaths, stroke, and microvascular complications when the BP in diabetic subjects was intensively lowered to 144/82 mm Hg versus 154/87 mm Hg.[17]

Hypertension must be treated vigorously in all patients with diabetes to limit and/or prevent the progression of both macrovascular and microvascular complications. The BP target for a patient without evidence of microalbuminuria is less than 130/80 mm Hg.[48] Patients with isolated systolic hypertension (systolic BP greater than 180 mm Hg) should be treated to a target of 160 mm Hg initially and then to 140 mm Hg if the treatment is well tolerated.[49] The treatment of hypertension for patients with CKD is addressed in Chapter 6.

As a general rule, reductions in systolic or diastolic BP of 5% to 10% occur with most single antihypertensive agents. Therefore, more than one drug is often needed to treat patients with diabetes and hypertension to target. Often the addition of a small or moderate dose of a second drug offers better control with fewer side effects than using full doses of the first agent of choice.

Dietary and lifestyle management of hypertension may be effective at lowering BP in some individuals. Weight reduction of 1 kg independent of sodium restriction can reduce mean arterial pressure by 1 mm Hg.[50] Sodium restriction has not been tested in controlled trials enrolling patients

TABLE 7-8. Lessons Learned from ACCORD, ADVANCE, and VADT (Implications for Clinical Practice)

- Patients with recently recognized diabetes and no prior CVD history should have metabolic targets directed toward normal or near-normal levels.

- In patients with established T2DM (≥8–10 y duration) and recognized CVD, glycemic control targets should be carefully scrutinized and individualized. Normalizing glucose levels in such patients does NOT reduce the risk of further CVD events or mortality

- Aggressive glucose titration to A1C targets <6.5% were associated with a threefold increased risk of severe hypoglycemia

- Intensive glycemic therapy is likely to result in weight gain. Weight gain in ACCORD averaged 6 lb. 20% of ACCORD subjects gained >10 kg.

- Medications (including insulin) that are weight neutral or favor weight loss are preferred agents for patients with diabetes

- Intensive glycemic control appears to reduce the risk of nephropathy progression

- In order to achieve and maintain A1C targets of <6.5% in patients with advanced T2DM of long duration, multiple medications are required

- Patients with heart disease, hypoglycemic unawareness, advanced neuropathy, reduced life expectancy, advanced age, or those who live alone and may be unable to manage a hypoglycemic event should have a target A1C of ≥7.5%

- Hypoglycemia risk was greatest for those who attempted to achieve targeted control but did not succeed. This suggests a relationship between hypoglycemia, glycemic variability, and weight gain.

- For patients who died during ACCORD, no glucose was recorded at the time of death

- Safety and efficacy of medications trump cost (per American Association of Clinical Endocrinologists)

- Physicians should aggressively manage hyperglycemia during the earliest phases of diabetes in order to minimize microvascular and macrovascular complications

- These studies did NOT address strategies for lowering A1C in low-risk patients with T2DM (those without CVD)

- Appropriate management of diabetes requires interpretation and treatment of glycemia, BP, lipids, and the patient's hypercoagulation state. Lifestyle interventions such as smoking cessation and promoting physical activity and weight loss remain the foundations of diabetes care.

From Gaede P, Lund-Andersen H, Parvig HH, et al. Effect of a multifactorial intervention on mortality in type 2 diabetes. *N Engl J Med.* 2008;358 (6):580–591.

with diabetes. However, a reduction of 2 to 4 g of sodium per day can reduce systolic BP by 5 mm Hg and diastolic BP by as much as 2 to 3 mm Hg. Excessive use of sodium (3 to 5 g per day) may nullify the positive BP lowering effects of angiotensin converting enzyme (ACE) inhibitors.[51] Walking 30 to 45 minutes daily while stopping smoking and alcohol consumption will likely improve hypertension.

The treatment for hypertension as recommended by the ADA is summarized in Table 7-9.

• Ambulatory Blood Pressure Monitoring for Patients with Diabetes

Ambulatory blood pressure monitoring (ABPM) should be considered as a means of assessing hypertensive treatment in patients with diabetes. Ambulatory monitoring provides information regarding the true, or mean, BP level, the diurnal rhythm of BP, and the BP variability.[52] ABPM has had limited use in the United States outside of clinical trials over the past decade, while becoming

TABLE 7-9. Management of Hypertension in Patients with Diabetes

Screening and Diagnosis	Goals	Treatment
• Measure BP at each visit • A BP ≥130/≥80 mm Hg on 2 separate days confirms the diagnosis of hypertension	• Target BP <130/80 for most patients	• Patients with a SBP of 130–139 mm Hg or a DBP of 80–89 mm Hg may receive a lifestyle intervention trial for 3 mo. If targets are not met, pharmacotherapy should be initiated • Lifestyle interventions of choice include weight loss, DASH diet (sodium reduction, increasing potassium intake, increased physical activity, and moderation of alcohol intake) (www.dashdiet.org). • Pharmacotherapy should be initiated in patients with SBP ≥140 mm Hg or DBP ≥90 mm Hg at diagnosis • ACE inhibitors or ARBs are the preferred drug. If one class is not tolerated, switch to the other. • A thiazide diuretic may be added to those with a GFR ≥30 mL/min/1.73 m² • A loop diuretic should be used for those with a eGFR <30 mL/min/1.73 m² • Multiple medications may be necessary to control BP in patients with diabetes • Monitor serum potassium levels in patients using ACE inhibitors and ARBS

ACE, angiotensin converting enzyme inhibitors; ARBs, angiotensin receptor blockers; eGFR, estimated glomerular filtration rate; SBP, systolic blood pressure; DBP, diastolic blood pressure; DASH, Dietary Approaches to Stop Hypertension; BP, blood pressure.
Adapted from American Diabetes Association. Standards of Medical Care. *Diabetes Care.* 2012;35(suppl 1):S29.

the standard of care for monitoring BP in Europe and Asia. Patients wear the BP cuff on one arm and a recorder on their belt for 24 hours. The data can be downloaded by a physician or through a web site portal. Several disease state patterns are easily discernible using ABPM as shown in Figure 7-6.

The typical circadian variation in BP for the majority of hypertensive patients follows a nadir occurring during the nighttime hours and a surge observed as the individual arises. Patients who demonstrate persistently elevated BP while sleeping are classified as "nondippers." Others develop a morning "surge" between the hours of 6:00 AM and noon, which follows nocturnal dipping of BP. Surge patients typically exhibit nocturnal BPs that are greater than 20% lower than diurnal pressures.[53] A healthy individual may have a surge that normalizes within a few hours of awakening. The morning surge is due to increases in cortisol release by the adrenal glands as well as activation of the renin–angiotensin–aldosterone system.[54]

The morning surge is an independent risk factor for MI and stroke. The risk of CV events may be related to an increase in platelet aggregation, hematocrit, and fibrinogen levels, which create a thrombogenic environment. The Framingham Heart Study suggests that the risk of sudden cardiac death is 70% higher during the periods between 7:00 AM and 9:00 AM compared with other times of the day.[55] For every 10 mm Hg rise in morning systolic BP, the risk of stroke increases by 22%.[55] Alcohol consumption, smoking, obesity, advancing age, and uncontrolled hypertension tend to exacerbate the morning surge.

For patients suspected of having a morning surge, the Omron 10 series BP monitor system (http://www.omronhealthcare.com/products/10-series-plus/) allows accurate digital tracking of both evening and morning BP readings. BP readings for 8 weeks may be reviewed at an office visit. The device costs $110.

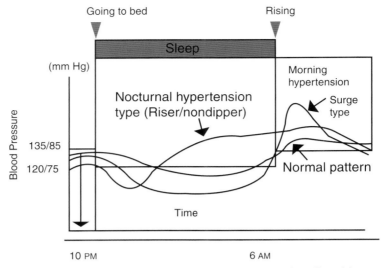

Figure 7-6 • Circadian BP Variability. Nocturnal hypertension (riser/nondipper) is associated with essential hypertension, diabetes, congestive heart failure, sleep apnea, and orthostatic hypertension. Surge-type hypertension increases one's risk for left ventricular hypertrophy, prolonged QTc interval, stroke, and myocardial infarct. (Adapted from Kario K. Time for focus on morning hypertension: pitfall of current antihypertensive medication. *Am J Hypertens.* 2005;18:149–151 with permission.)

Comprehensive Assessment and Management of Hyperlipidemia and Atherosclerosis in Patients with Diabetes

Lipid abnormalities that accelerate atherosclerosis and increase CHD risk are more common in patients with T2DM than in nondiabetic subjects. Combined with central obesity, dyslipidemia has become a major cause of morbidity and mortality in T2DM.

• Atherosclerosis Pathogenesis

The word "atherosclerosis" is of Greek origin and means focal accumulation of lipid [i.e., athere (gruel)] and thickening of arterial intima [i.e., sclerosis (hardening)]. Atherosclerosis affects large and medium-sized arteries and is characterized by endothelial dysfunction, vascular inflammation, and the accumulation of lipid, calcium, and cellular debris within the intima of the vessel wall. The resulting disruption of normal intima anatomy results in plaque formation, vascular remodeling, acute and chronic luminal obstruction, alterations of blood flow, and target organ hypoxemia.[56] The end result of the reduced oxygen flow to a given target organ could result in stroke, myocardial infarct, loss of vision, PAD, hypertension, and neuropathy. Plaque within coronary vessels may rupture, resulting in ACS and AMI. Fifty percent of AMIs are the direct result of plaque rupture from vulnerable plaques and 50% are secondary to vascular occlusion from stable plaque.[57] The vulnerable plaque consists of a large lipid core, inflammatory cells, and a thin, fibrous cap subject to biomechanical stress leading to rupture. Most vulnerable plaque cannot be identified (Fig. 7-7). Primary prevention should target plaque rupture and reversal of atherosclerosis with appropriate pharmacologic intervention.

The coronary artery consists of an inner monolayer of endothelial cells, which line the lumen, known as the intima. The media separates the intima from the adventitia, which consists of fibroblasts, smooth muscle cells (SMCs), and a complex matrix consisting of collagen and proteoglycans.

The endothelium provides a nonthrombogenic surface through which blood may freely flow. Endothelium cells also serve as a potent vasodilator (via the secretion of endothelium-derived relaxing factor) and inhibit platelet aggregation. Fibrin clots are also lysed by the endothelium via

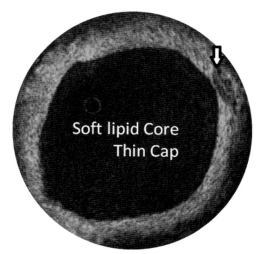

Figure 7-7 • Prelude to Sudden Death from Plaque Rupture. An optical coherence tomography (OCT) scan was performed on this 48-year-old patient with atypical chest pain and angiographically minimal coronary artery disease on catheterization. A thin fibrous plaque (*arrow*) lying adjacent to a soft lipid core places this patient at high risk for plaque rupture and sudden death. (OCT courtesy of Robert Chilton, DO.)

the production and secretion of plasminogen, von Willebrand factor, and plasminogen activator inhibitor type 1 (PAI-1). The endothelium secretes cytokines and adhesion molecules such as vascular cell adhesion molecule-1 and platelet-derived growth factor, which may have a role in vasoconstriction. The endothelium regulates vascular tone, platelet activation, monocyte adhesion and inflammation, thrombus generation, lipid metabolism, cellular growth, and vascular remodeling.[58]

Atherosclerotic plaques (or atheromas), which may require 10 to 15 years for full development, characteristically develop in regions of branching and marked curvature at areas of geometric irregularity and where blood undergoes sudden changes in velocity and direction of flow. Decreased shear stress and turbulence may promote atherogenesis (the deposition of plaque within the intima) at these important sites within the coronary arteries, the major branches of the thoracic and abdominal aorta, and the large conduit vessels of the lower extremities[59] (Figs. 7-8 and 7-9).

The primary trigger of atherogenesis is LDL cholesterol. LDL-C binds to receptors located on the endothelial surface after which the lipoproteins become internalized and accrue within the subendothelial space. The atherogenic LDL particles stimulate the endothelial host cells to produce cytokines that recruit monocytes allowing for LDL to become oxidized within the intimal space. The oxidized LDL is subsequently picked up by scavenger receptors on macrophages that transform into "foam cells." The inflammatory process progresses as endothelial cells produce leukocyte adhesion molecules [i.e., cytokines and growth factors that regulate SMC proliferation, collagen degradation, and thrombosis (e.g., vascular cell adhesion molecule-1, intercellular cell adhesion molecule-1)].[60]

Oxidized LDL inhibits NO synthase activity and increasing ROS generation reducing endothelial-dependent vasodilation. Oxidative stress has been recognized as the most significant contributor to atherosclerosis by causing LDL oxidation and increasing NO breakdown. Over time, SMCs proliferate from the media into the intima to become advanced atherosclerotic lesions.[61]

The earliest pathologic lesion of atherosclerosis is the fatty streak, which is observed in the aorta and coronary arteries of most individuals by age 20 years. The fatty streak is the result of focal accumulation of serum lipoproteins within the intima of the vessel wall. The fatty streak may progress to form a fibrous plaque, the result of progressive lipid accumulation and the migration

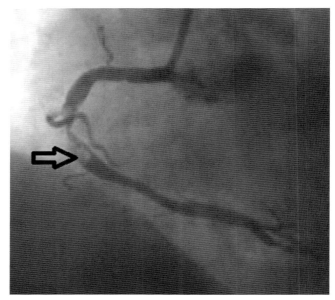

Figure 7-8 • Acute Coronary Syndrome. A 42-year-old woman with T2DM presents to the ED complaining of chest tightness, shortness of breath, and "anxiety" of 2 days duration. During her subsequent heart catheterization, she was found to have right coronary artery thrombus in the middle of the RCA (*arrow*). (Photograph courtesy of Robert Chilton, DO.)

and proliferation of SMCs. The SMCs are responsible for the deposition of extracellular connective tissue matrix and form a fibrous cap that overlies a core of lipid-laden foam cells, extracellular lipid, and necrotic cellular debris. Growth of the fibrous plaque results in vascular remodeling, progressive luminal narrowing, blood-flow abnormalities, and compromised oxygen supply to the target organ.[59] Luminal stenosis may occur only when the plaque occupies more than 40% of the area bounded by the internal elastic lamina.[62]

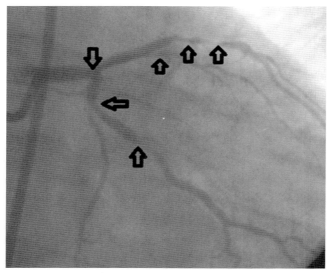

Figure 7-9 • Advanced CAD. A 43-year-old woman with T2DM and unstable angina. This angiogram shows multiple areas of advanced atherosclerosis (*arrows*) involving the distal left main, left anterior descending (LAD), and circumflex arteries. (Photograph courtesy of Robert Chilton, DO.)

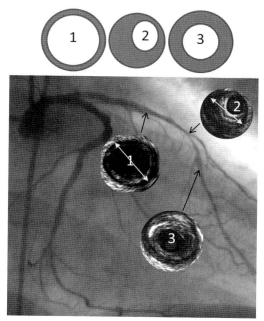

Figure 7-10 • Negative and Positive Vascular Remodeling. A 48-year-old patient with poorly controlled T1DM of 15 years duration. Prior to beginning an exercise program, the patient was referred to a cardiologist for an exercise stress test that revealed prolonged ST-T depression during the recovery stage. His coronary angiogram demonstrates narrowing of the LAD coronary artery and corresponding intravascular ultrasound (IVUS) findings of negative remodeling and advanced atherosclerosis. IVUS of the proximal vessel (*1*) shows little evidence of atherosclerosis. The midportion of the LAD (*2*) has a high-grade stenosis. The distal portion of the LAD (*3*) has moderate atherosclerosis. This finding illustrates negative remodeling of the coronary artery in a patient with T1DM. (Photograph courtesy of Robert Chilton, DO.)

As endothelial injury and inflammation progress, plaque may remodel. Positive remodeling is an outward compensatory remodeling in which the arterial wall bulges outward and the lumen remains uncompromised (Fig. 7-10). Such positively remodeled lesions thus form the bulk of the vulnerable plaques, grow for years, and are more prone to result in plaque rupture and ACS than stable angina, as documented by intravascular ultrasonography (IVUS) studies.

Many of the plaques with initial positive remodeling eventually progress to the negative remodeling stage, causing narrowing of the vascular lumen. Such plaques usually lead to the development of stable angina. They are also vulnerable to plaque rupture and thrombosis and dissection (Fig. 7-11). Plaque rupture is the etiology of AMI and sudden death. Most atheromas resulting in ACS are less than 50% occlusive and do not usually result in ACS or an MI.[63] Plaque ruptures occur secondary to a weakness of the fibrous cap allowing contact between the highly thrombogenic lipid core and the blood (Fig. 7-7).

• Dyslipidemia in T2DM

The dyslipidemia of T2DM is characterized by a number of abnormalities fueled by insulin resistance and predating the onset of clinically apparent hyperglycemia by years. Dyslipidemia consists of increased levels of TG-rich lipoproteins [very low-density lipoprotein (VLDL), intermediate-density lipoprotein and remnant particles], low levels of HDL-C, as well as increased levels of small, dense LDL particles. (Fig. 7-12).

Indirect LDL-C measurement underestimates the influence of LDL in atherogenesis; the LDL particle is heterogeneous, its size being smaller and its cholesterol content lower in states of obesity,

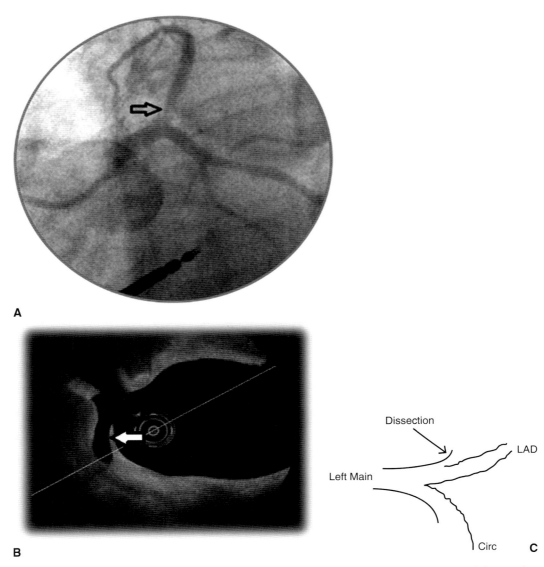

Figure 7-11 • LAD Artery Dissection. A 38-year-old man presents with sudden onset of chest pain. At catheterization **(A)**, the patient was found to have dissection of ostium of the LAD. The diagnosis was confirmed with OCT **(B)**. The anatomic location of dissection is shown in **C**. (Photographs courtesy of Robert Chilton, DO.)

insulin resistance, and T2DM.[64] Patients with T2DM tend to demonstrate increased particle size of VLDL and decreased sizes of both LDL-C and HDL-C. However, the cholesterol content in large LDL-C is *increased* while the cholesterol content in small LDL-C is *decreased* in patients with insulin resistance and T2DM. Yet the calculated LDL-C is unchanged despite patients having an increased LDL-particle number (Fig. 7-13).

Ninety-seven percent of adults with diabetes have at least one lipid abnormality, with the primary characteristic being elevated TGs and low HDL-C levels.[65] In patients with diabetes, the LDL-C is usually not significantly different from what is seen in nondiabetic patients. Yet, patients with T2DM typically have a smaller, denser LDL particle, which increases lipoprotein atherogenicity even if the absolute concentration of the LDL-C is not elevated.[66]

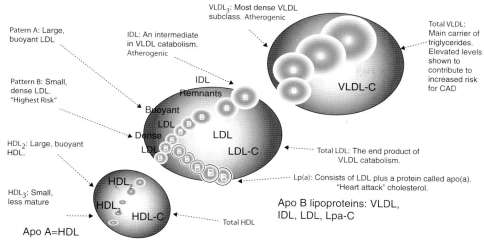

Figure 7-12 • Components of Lipoproteins. LDL cholesterol is divided into four subtypes based upon particle diameter size. Large LDL (greater than or equal to 26 nm), medium LDL II (25.5 to 26 nm), small LDL III (24.2 to 25.6 nm), and very small LDL IV (less than or equal to 24.2 nm). (VLDL, very low-density lipoproteins; HDL-C, high-density lipoprotein cholesterol; IDL, intermediate-density lipoprotein; TG, triglyceride; Apo, apolipoprotein A or B.)

• Lipoprotein Production and Packaging

Overview of Lipoprotein Structure and Function

Cholesterol is a natural steroid retaining multiple critical physiologic functions such as stabilization of cell membranes and interacting with membrane-bound enzymes.

Lipoprotein particles are comprised of cholesterol esters, free cholesterol, protein, phospholipids, and TGs in different percentages. These lipoproteins are involved in systemic cholesterol delivery to and removal from peripheral cells. (The addition of the protein component to the cholesterol allows the lipoprotein to become water soluble and easily transportable throughout the body.) Cholesterol is produced primarily by the liver, or provided as a source of dietary saturated fat absorbed through the small intestine. All cells have the capacity to synthesize cholesterol de novo, but only hepatocytes are able to catabolize the steroid. While an excess of cholesterol is pathogenic, this crucial sterol is a key component of the steroidal hormones (e.g., estrogen, testosterone, aldosterone, cortisol) and an essential part of human development, growth, and reproduction.

Lipoproteins are complex molecules (Fig. 7-14) that are hydrophobic (nonpolar) on one end and have a hydrophilic (polar) region on the opposite end. A lipoprotein particle is generally composed of a hydrophobic lipid core primarily containing triacylglycerol (TG) and cholesteryl ester (CE). A lipoprotein plasma membrane surrounds the core. The relative amounts of lipid and protein contained in these particles determine lipoprotein particle density.[67]

Five major lipoprotein classes have been characteristically defined by particle density and electrophoretic mobility (Table 7-10 and Fig. 7-13). The protein component increases the relative density of a given particle compared to the lipid component. As such, denser lipoprotein families have a higher protein:lipid ratio compared to the less dense lipoproteins, which have more cholesterol and TG composition.

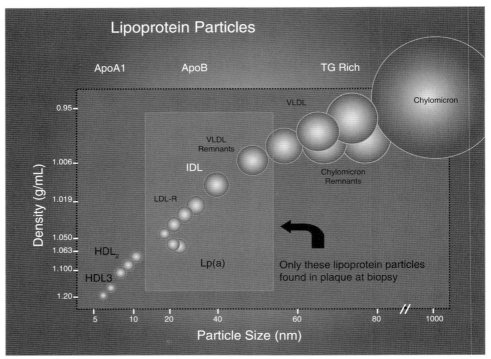

Figure 7-13 • Lipoprotein subfractions represent a continuum of particles that vary in size and density. The largest lipoproteins are TG-rich IDL, VLDL, and chylomicrons. Technologies that sort lipoproteins by particle size (NMR and GGE) cannot separate IDL and Lp(a) from LDL-R because these particles have overlapping size. However, the particles do differ in density allowing ultracentrifugation as the best means to separate LDL into its three components. Total LDL is comprised of Lp(a), IDL and real LDL or R-LDL-R. R-LDL is defined as total LDL-C minus Lp(a)-C minus IDL-C. Each subcomponent, has a different inheritance, requires different therapies, and confers a different risk. For example, both Lp(a) and IDL are more atherogenic than LDL itself. Lp(a) doubles CV risk. However, when small dense LDL is elevated in partnership with Lp(a) risk increases 25-fold. Lp(a) can only be measured with advanced lipid testing. Dense, small LDL is called Pattern B and increases risk 4×. Intermediately dense LDL is called Pattern A/B and doubles risk. HDL2 is the most protective HDL subfractions. HDL3 may be mildly protective to inert. A patient may have a normal HDL-C but low protective HDL2. Atherogenic remnant lipoproteins, including IDL and VLDL 3 (small/dense) are elevated in T2DM and metabolic syndrome.

• Standard versus Advanced Lipid Testing for Patients at High Risk for CHD

Lipoproteins vary in size and density and are designated as LDL, HDL, and VLDL. Standard laboratory-reported LDL concentration (via gel electrophoresis) represents a measurement of not just one lipoprotein, but a spectrum of LDL particles ranging in size and density as shown in Figure 7-13. Standard lipid testing does not provide enough data to provide clinicians with an accurate assessment of one's true CV risk profile. Standard lipid testing may actually underestimate the number of one's atherogenic lipoprotein particles including the residual remnants that are present in the plasma (Fig. 7-15).

Advanced lipid testing may provide a more sophisticated measurement of the components of LDL-C, HDL-C, very low-density lipoprotein cholesterol (VLDL-C), non-HDL-C, and other emerging risk factors. The types of advanced lipid tests that are currently available are listed in Table 7-11. The "Berkeley" test measures HDL and LDL size as a distribution of five subclasses (HDL 2a, 2b, 3a, 3b, and 3c) and seven subclasses (LDL I, IIa, IIb, IIa, IIb, Iva, and IVb). The HDL2b subclass best reflects the efficacy of the reverse cholesterol transport system and cholesterol clearance by the liver.

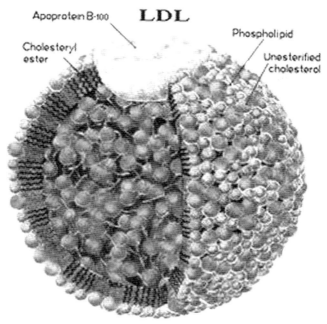

Figure 7-14 • Structure of a Lipoprotein Molecule. Each lipoprotein's (VLDL, IDL, LDL, HDL) internal core contains a specific quantity of cholesterol, TGs, free cholesterol, and cholesterol esters. Apolipoproteins bind to lipid surfaces. Attachment of the apolipoprotein to a lipid surface allows the phospholipid to become water soluble for simple transportation through the blood and lymphatic systems. Apolipoproteins also serve as receptor ligands allowing lipids to attach to tissues and become oxidized.

Low levels of HDL2b are correlated with a two- to threefold increase in CV risk and have been used to predict the progression of coronary atherosclerosis and disease severity. Both apoB and ulta-apoB are only measured per request of the physician.

The Nuclear Magnetic Resonance (NMR) LipoProfile Test provides direct measure of the number of LDL particles and includes a standard lipid panel. Very high risk is inferred when the LDL particle is greater than 2,000 nmol per L. Optimal LDL particle is less than 1,000 nmol per L.[68]

Vertical Auto Profile (VAP) tests report the relative distribution of cholesterol content of all lipoproteins and subfractions including 22 components of cholesterol, half of which would be missed with standard lipid testing. VAP testing may be performed in nonfasting patients, measure LDL directly, and report all lipoproteins and apolipoproteins considered necessary by the ADA and the American College of Cardiology.[68]

Candidates for advanced lipid profiling would include patients with established atherosclerosis, a history of MI, stroke, or TIA, coronary artery bypass grafting, stent placement, arterectomy, angina, ACS, and T2DM. Patients with a premature family history of atherosclerosis or those with at least two of five National Cholesterol Education Program (NCEP) risk factors should also be tested.[68] The five major NCEP risk factors other than elevated LDL-C include smoking, hypertension (BP 140/90 mm Hg or on antihypertensive medication), HDL-C less than 40 mg per dL, family history of premature CHD (CHD in male first-degree relative less than 55 years; CHD in female first-degree relative less than 65 years), or advanced age (men 45 years; women 55 years). In ATP III, an HDL-C 60 mg per dL counts as a "negative" risk factor; its presence removes one risk factor from the total count.[69]

A patient's LDL profile can be further classified into two distinct patterns (A and B) based on average particle diameter or the LDL particle subtype with the highest concentration. Pattern A denotes larger average particle diameter (20.6 to 23 nm), whereas pattern B denotes smaller average particle diameter (18 to 20.5 nm).[68] Patterns A and B patients also differ in other components of the lipid panel, as noted in Table 7-12.

TABLE 7-10. Major Classes of Lipoproteins[a]

Lipoprotein Class	Subclasses	Composition	Apolipoproteins	Comment
Chylomicrons	None	100% TGs	apoB-48	Atherogenic Treatment targets carbohydrate reduction Pharmacotherapy options include omega-3 acid ethyl esters (lovaza) and/or fenofibric acid (Trilipix, fibricor, fenoglide, lofibra, antra, lipofen) The use of fenofibrate in patients with T2DM (FIELD Study) reduces the need for laser treatment for diabetic retinopathy, although the mechanism appears to be independent of the drug's lipid-lowering effect. Fenofibrate does NOT lower risk of stroke or MI (ACCORD).
VLDL (Very low-density lipoproteins)	VLDL 1 and 2 VLDL3 remnant	90% TGs 10% cholesterol	apoB-100 apoE	Main carrier of TGs. Elevated levels shown to contribute to increased risk for CVD. Treatment includes alcohol cessation and carbohydrate reduction Pharmacologic interventions: fenofibric acids, ethyl ester acids or nicotinic acids (Niaspan) VLDL remnants (VLDL3) are atherogenic
IDL (Intermediate density lipoproteins)	I and II	50% TGs 50% cholesterol	apoB-100 apo E	IDL is an intermediate of VLDL catabolism Highly atherogenic, but persists in circulation for a very short time Treat with behavioral interventions similar to that of VLDL Pharmacologic treatment with fenofibric acids, ethyl ester acids, or nicotinic acids
LDL (Low density lipoproteins)	LDL 1 + 2 = buoyant LDL 4 + 3 = small dense	90% cholesterol rich 10% TG	apoB-100	End product of VLDL catabolism LDL has the highest "residence time" within the plasma of all lipoproteins and is also the most abundant lipoprotein. This enhances its atherogenic potential. Oxidized LDLs and small dense LDL subclasses are highly atherogenic Behavioral treatment targets include reducing dietary saturated fat intake Pharmacotherapy includes the use of statins, ezetimide, and/or nicotinic acid

| HDL (High density lipoproteins) | 2a 2b 3a 3b 3c | Composition varies with increasing size of HDL subclass | apoA-I, but particles may have multiple other apolipoproteins | HDL2b subclass is considered the most atheroprotective Low levels of HDL2b can increase CV risk 2–3 fold Nicotinic acid can raise HDL |

[a]Nomenclature for subcomponents of lipoproteins has not be standardized. Some tests have been validated by individual laboratories only and have not been approved for use by the FDA. Data from Gofman JW, Delalla O, Glazier, et al. The serum lipoprotein transport system in health, metabolic disorders, atherosclerosis and coronary heart disease. *Journal of Clinical Lipidology.* 2007;1(2):104–141; Cobble M, Sellers J. Advanced lipid testing. A better alternative for cardiovascular risk prediction. *Practical Diabetology.* 2010; Keech AC, Mitchell P, Summanen PA. Effect of fenofibrate on the need for laser treatment for diabetic retinopathy (FIELD study): a randomized controlled trial. *Lancet.* 2007;370:1687–1697; Action to Control Cardiovascular Risk in Diabetes Study Group. Effects of intensive glucose lowering in type 2 diabetes. *N Engl J Med.* 2008;358:2545–2559.

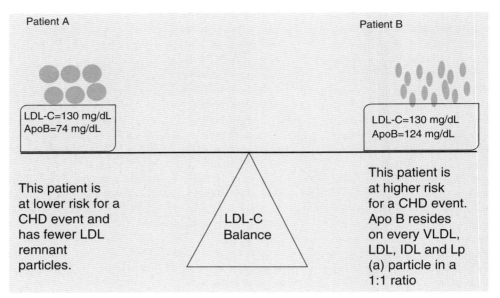

Patient A

LDL-C=130 mg/dL
ApoB=74 mg/dL

This patient is
at lower risk for a
CHD event and
has fewer LDL
remnant
particles.

LDL-C
Balance

Patient B

LDL-C=130 mg/dL
ApoB=124 mg/dL

This patient is
at higher risk
for a CHD event.
Apo B resides
on every VLDL,
LDL, IDL and Lp
(a) particle in a
1:1 ratio

Figure 7-15 • Standard Lipid Testing Underestimates Atherogenic Lipoprotein Particle Numbers. Individuals with predominantly small dense LDL particles **(right)** have a greater atherosclerotic risk than those with large buoyant LDL. Apo B resides in a 1:1 ratio on all atherogenic lipoproteins. Patient A (*pattern A*) has large, buoyant LDL particles and a lower plasma level of apo B compared with Patient B (*pattern B*) whose plasma lipoprotein level is considered to be highly atherogenic, although their LDL-C levels are equivalent.

Lower-density lipoproteins (LDL) are rich in TGs, resulting in an increased atherogenic potential within the endothelium. HDLs are comprised primarily of protein, making them less atherogenic than LDL phospholipids. Atherogenesis is also enhanced by the duration of exposure each lipoprotein spends within the circulation. For example, VLDL-C residence times are much greater than HDL-C (Table 7-13).

The standard lipid panel uses the Friedewald formula to mathematically estimate the LDL-C as noted in Figure 7-16. Although used universally, the measurement is inaccurate when the patient is NOT fasting and has a TG level greater than 200 mg per dL or an LDL-C less than 100 mg per dL. For patients who do not smoke, have normal glucose tolerance, normal body weight, and no CV risk factors, the Friedewald formula may be adequate. High-risk patients warrant direct measuring of their atherogenic remnant phenotype, particle number, pattern, and density. Advanced lipid testing allows clinicians to customize lipid risk management strategies for patients with diabetes.

 TABLE 7-11. Advanced Lipid Testing

Common Name of Lipid Test	Methodology	Manufacturer
Berkeley	HDL and LDL subclass distribution by gradient gel electrophoresis	Berkeley Heart Lab, Inc. http://www.bhlinc.com/
NMR LipoProfile Test	Nuclear magnetic resonance	LipoScience, Inc. http://www.theparticletest.com/home-heathcare.html
VAP Test	High-speed ultracentrifugation	Atherotech Diagnostics Lab http://www.atherotech.com/

TABLE 7-12. Atherogenic Pattern A versus Pattern B

Pattern A	Pattern B
Large buoyant LDL	Small dense LDL
Normal TG	Increased postprandial TGs
Normal HDL	Decreased HDL
Lower CVD risk	Increased CVD risk

CVD, cardiovascular disease; HDL, high-density lipoprotein; LDL, low-density lipoprotein.
From Hoffman TK, tucker MA, Parker DL. Emerging risk factors and risk markers for cardiovascular disease: looking beyond NCEP ATP III. *Formulary.* 2009;44:237–247.

• Apolipoproteins, Lipoproteins, and Other Lipid Components

Apolipoproteins

The protein component located on the surface of a lipoprotein is known as an apolipoprotein (ALP). ALPs transport cholesterol within the plasma, provide structural stability for each associated lipoprotein complex, and facilitate uptake of the lipoprotein and enzymatic action within target cells.

HDL-C contains apolipoproteins A1 and AII (ApoA). ApoA is the protein that promotes cholesterol efflux from the tissues back to the liver for excretion. Thus, Apo A is a "good form" of ALP that assists in reverse cholesterol transport.

ApoB resides on all non-HDL lipoproteins in a uniform 1:1 relationship. Every VLDL, LDL, IDL, and Lp(a) particle has one, and only one, ApoB.[70] ApoB subtypes include apoB-100 and apoB-48.[71]

 TABLE 7-13. Size Matters: Why Are Small Dense LDLs More Atherogenic Than Large Buoyant LDLs?

- Small dense LDL independently increases CVD risk threefold even with "normal" LDL-C concentration.
- There is a 2-fold greater rate of arteriographic progression in untreated CVD patients with elevated small dense LDLs, while appropriate treatment to lower small dense LDLs results in significant arteriographic benefit.
- Small dense LDL residence time in the plasma is longer than large buoyant LDL.
- Small dense LDL gains easier entry into arterial walls, allowing for oxidation and initiation of atherosclerosis.
- Small dense LDL binds to interstitial glycosaminoglycans, increasing rate of atherogenesis.
- Small dense LDLs have decreased affinity for LDL receptors.
- LDL subfractions have different susceptibility to oxidative stress, a factor contributing to atherogenesis.
- Large buoyant LDL particles are more resistant and small dense LDL particles are more susceptible to oxidation within arterial walls.

Data from Superko HR. What can we learn about dense low density lipoprotein and lipoprotein particles from clinical trials? *Curr Opin Lipidol.* 1996;7(6):363–368; Austin MA, Edwards KL. Small, dense low density lipoproteins, the insulin resistance syndrome and noninsulin-dependent diabetes. *Curr Opin Lipidol.* 1996;7(3):167–171; Galeano NF, Al-Haideri M, Keyserman F, et al. Small dense low density lipoprotein has increased affinity for LDL receptor-independent cell surface binding sites: a potential mechanism for increased atherogenicity. *J Lipid Res.* 1998;39(6):1263–1273; Tribble DL, Rizzo M, Chait A, et al. Susceptibility and reduced antioxidant content of metabolic precursors of small, dense low-density lipoproteins. *Am J Med.* 2001;1;110(2):103–110; Stampfer MJ, Krauss RM, Ma J, et al. A prospective study of triglyceride level, low-density lipoprotein particle diameter, and risk of myocardial infarction. *JAMA.* 1996;276(11):882–888; Zambon A, Brown BG, Deeb SS, et al. Hepatic lipase as a focal point for the development and treatment of coronary artery disease. *J Investig Med.* 2001;49(1):112–128.

- LDL = Total Cholesterol - HDL - 1/5 Triglycerides, but only if the serum triglyceride is 400 mg/dL or less

- Person A has directly calculated total cholesterol of 300mg/dL , HDL of 50 mg/dL, and TGs of 125mg/dL

  LDL= 300-50- 125/5 (=25); LDL= 225 mg/dL

- Person B has the same total cholesterol and HDL as A, but his TGs are 250 mg/dL

  LDL=300-50-250/5 (=50); LDL= 200.

(Reference: Friedewald WT, Levy RI, Fredrickson DS. Estimation of the concentration of low-density lipoprotein cholesterol in plasma, without use of the preparative centrifuge. *Clin Chem.* 1972; 18:499–50)

Figure 7-16 • Friedewald Formula "Optical Illusion" Effect for LDL Calculation. (From Friedewald WT, Levy RI, Fredrickson DS. Estimation of the concentration of low-density lipoprotein cholesterol in plasma, without use of the preparative centrifuge. *Clin Chem.* 1972;18:499–450.)

ApoB provides a more accurate indication of the number of circulating atherogenic non-HDL-C particles than simply calculating the LDL-C plasma concentration (see Fig. 7-15). ApoB levels are directly measured unlike the commonly reported Friedewald calculation of LDL-C (Fig. 7-16). Higher levels of plasma ApoB may signify increased coronary disease risk, even when LDL-C is not in the high-risk range.[72] Therefore, for comprehensive cardiac risk assessment, one must measure the plasma ApoB in addition to the LDL-C concentration to determine the actual number of atherogenic VLDL, IDL, Lp(a), and LDL particles.[73]

TG levels above 400 mg per dL falsely elevate apo B because of influx of apoB containing chylomicrons and VLDLs. Ultracentrifugation removes the influence of the chylomicrons and VLDLs allowing accurate reporting of apoB in patients with hypertriglyceridemia.

Small, dense LDL particles confer a three- to sevenfold increased risk of CVD compared with that of large buoyant LDL particles.[74] The sdLDL particles are more easily delivered to the endothelial wall where they become trapped, oxidized, and inflamed. One could picture the sdLDL particles as being golf balls and the large buoyant LDLs as beach balls. If your best friend were to throw golf balls at your head all morning, there is a very good chance that you would be knocked unconscious by day's end. If your friend were to throw beach balls at you, not much would happen except that you would probably become bored after two hours and suggest playing a different game to pass the time of day. Beach ball size LDL particles do not get trapped within the arterial walls and, as such, do not cause atherosclerosis. The golf ball size LDLs do become trapped and inflamed and cause considerable damage (Fig. 7-17).

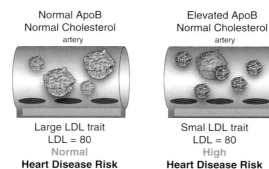

Normal ApoB
Normal Cholesterol
artery

Elevated ApoB
Normal Cholesterol
artery

Large LDL trait
LDL = 80
Normal
Heart Disease Risk

Smal LDL trait
LDL = 80
High
Heart Disease Risk

Figure 7-17 • The large, buoyant LDL **(left)** would have difficulty adhering to damaged arterial walls. The small, dense LDL particles (*right*) can easily access damaged arterial walls. In patients with similar LDL concentrations, if one patient has more small dense LDL particles, that patient will have higher ApoB levels and greater atherogenic risk.

HDL-C

HDL-C is the smallest of the lipoprotein particles and contains the highest proportion of protein (apo A-I and apo A-II) to cholesterol. Known as the reverse cholesterol transporter, HDL ferries cholesterol to the liver, adrenal glands, ovaries, or testes via the cholesteryl ester transfer protein (CETP) pathway. The delivery of HDL-C to steroidogenic organs is important for the synthesis of steroid hormones. Cholesterol delivered to the liver is excreted into the bile, and then into the intestines, following conversion into bile acids.[75]

HDL particles consist of several heterogenous subgroups that differ in density, size, and lipid composition. Thus, not all HDL particles offer equal protection against atherogenesis.[76] HDL subclasses vary in their ability to extract cholesterol from target sites. The HDL2b subclass reflects the best efficacy of the reverse cholesterol transport system and cholesterol clearance by the liver. Low levels of HDL2b are correlated with a two- to threefold increase in CVD risk and have been used to predict the progression of coronary atherosclerosis and disease severity.[77]

Low HDL-C is often associated with elevated TGs, excess body weight, physical inactivity, cigarette smoking, very high carbohydrate intake, insulin resistance, T2DM, and certain drugs (i.e., β-blockers, anabolic steroids, progestins). Low HDL-C substantially increases CHD risk at all levels of LDL-C.[78]

Triglycerides

TGs are fats consisting of three fatty acids covalently bonded to a glycerol molecule. TGs are either synthesized by the liver or derived from dietary sources. Transportation through the circulation occurs through chylomicrons, VLDLs, and IDLs.

TGs packaged within lipoproteins must be converted to fatty acids for storage uptake into tissues (adipocytes and muscle cells). The conversion of dietary fat to TGs occurs within the enterocytes cells lining the intestines where they form chylomicrons that enter the plasma via the thoracic duct. Once in the bloodstream, TGs provide an energy source for glycolysis (a metabolic pathway responsible for the production of ATP). TGs may be produced de novo in the liver and packaged as VLDL.[79]

Significant elevations of TG may be secondary to obesity (insulin resistance and T2DM), renal failure, alcoholism, and genetic mutations that affect the production of lipoprotein lipase, apo CIII, and apo E. Central obesity paired with insulin resistance is probably a major factor contributing to the dyslipidemia associated with T2DM.[80] Certain medications are also associated with treatment of emergent hypertriglyceridemia:

- Estrogens
- Testosterone
- Thiazide diuretics
- Alcohol
- Glucocorticosteroids
- β-blockers
- Antipsychotics
- Cyclosporines
- Valproic acid
- Isotretinoin
- Tacrolimus
- Protease inhibitors

The independent impact of elevated TG on CHD has yet to be definitively proven. Whether hypertriglyceridemia causes CHD or is merely a marker for other lipoprotein abnormalities that cause premature CHD is also controversial.[81] Nevertheless, the evidence that elevated TG is independently associated with an increased risk for CHD is clearly growing.[82] Plasma TG levels show a strong relationship with impaired LV relaxation, an early marker of diastolic dysfunction. The accumulation of lipids within myocytes appears to potentiate the LV diastolic dysfunction.[83] In 1998, Austin et al.

investigated the relationship between TG levels and CHD risk in a meta-analysis of 17 prospective studies that included 46,413 men and 10,864 women. Their findings suggested that for every 89 mg per dL increase in TG levels a corresponding increase of 36% was seen in the risk of CV events in men, and a 76% increased risk in women.[84]

TGs are routinely and variably elevated after eating. Significant postprandial hypertriglyceridemia has been shown to be a specific marker for the presence of CHD. Certain postprandial lipid levels and resultant TG-rich chylomicron and lipoprotein remnants are thought to drive early atherogenesis. These remnants diminish endothelial function, promote the generation of atherogenic small dense LDL particles, and are correlated with prothrombotic and proinflammatory biomarkers, such as PAI-1 and CRP.[85]

Hypertriglyceridemia is an independent risk factor for nontraumatic lower extremity amputations in patients with diabetes.[86] Patients with TG levels greater than 500 mg per dL have a hazard ratio of 1.65 for lower extremity amputation compared with a cohort having TG levels of 150 to 199 mg per dL and a hazard ratio of 1.10.

Non-HDL-Cholesterol

Non-HDL-C, in contrast to LDL-C, includes the cholesterol carried within every highly atherogenic TG-rich lipoprotein. All the lipoprotein particles included in the non-HDL-C calculation carry apo B on their surface. Not surprisingly, non-HDL-C is regarded as a better correlate of apo B levels than LDL-C in patients with both normotriglyceridemia and hypertriglyceridemia.[87] Because the meta-analysis by Austin suggests that TG levels are strongly and independently related to CHD risk, calculating all TG-rich "remnant particles" provides the clinician with another option for evaluating the likelihood of developing a CHD event.

Non-HDL-C is strongly related to CV risk among persons of various ages, among both sexes, in patients with and without diabetes, and among persons with and without documented CVD. Non-HDL-C predicts atherosclerosis progression after as little as 2 years of follow-up, and CV events and mortality over follow-up periods as short as 5 years and as long as 24 years. Because LDL-C and non-HDL-C levels are strongly correlated, direct comparison of the prognostic value of the LDL-C level and non-HDL-C level is difficult. Available data suggest that non-HDL-C is as good as or better than LDL-C in predicting CV risk.[88-93] Furthermore, currently available lipid-lowering agents can substantially reduce non-HDL-C levels and these reductions correlate with reductions in subsequent CV morbidity and mortality.

The calculation of the non-HDL-C is made simply by subtracting the HDL-C level from the patient's total cholesterol. For example, if the total cholesterol is 200 mg per dL and the HDL-C is 30 mg per dL, the non-HDL-C is 170 mg per dL. In general, the non-HDL-C should be less than 30 mg per dL higher than the patient's acceptable LDL-C level. All patients with diabetes should have a targeted LDL-C of less than 100 mg per dL.[48]

Only a few clinical trials have reported non-HDL-C levels and changes in non-HDL-C level in relation to physiologic outcomes or clinical events and mortality. The 4S study randomized 4,444 patients with CHD, serum cholesterol level of 213 to 310 mg per dL, and TG levels less than 220 mg per dL to simvastatin or placebo for 5.4 years. In this cohort of patients, each 1% decrease in levels of non-HDL-C and LDL cholesterol with simvastatin therapy resulted in a 1.7% reduction in events.[94]

ADA Recommendations for Screening and Managing Patients with Hyperlipidemia

The recommendations for screening and targeted treatment goals for patients with hyperlipidemia are shown in Table 7-14. Current guidelines for CHD management in diabetes are based on the premise that most patients with diabetes are at high risk for CV event. When diabetes exists in patients with established coronary disease, absolute risk for future events is very high. Performing a

TABLE 7-14. Screening and Managing Lipid Disorders in Patients with Diabetes

Screening	Treatment Recommendations	Primary Lipid Targets	Alternative Targets
• Annual fasting lipid panel	• Lifestyle modification focusing on reducing saturated fat, transfat, and cholesterol intake. Increase omega-3 fatty acids, fiber, and plant sterols	*LDL-C* • With CVD risk <70 mg/dL • Without CVD risk<100 mg/dL • 30%–40% reduction from *baseline* is an alternative treatment target	For statin-treated patients in whom the LDL-C goal would be <70 mg/dL, the non-HDL-C target should be <100 mg/dL and Apo B should be measured and treated to <80 mg/dL.
	• Weight loss if *indicated* • Increased physical activity	*TG* • <150 mg/dL *HDL-C* >50 mg/dL (women) <40 mg/dL (men)	For statin-treated patients with an LDL-C goal of <100 mg/dL the non-HDL-C target should be <130 mg/dL and the Apo B should be measured and treated to <90 mg/dL
	• Statin[a] therapy for all *patients* with diabetes (with overt CVD who are over age 40 or who have 1 or more CV risk factors) regardless of baseline lipid levels • Consider statins if age <40 without overt *CVD* if LDL >100 mg/dL or if patient has multiple risk factors		

[a]Statins are contraindicated in pregnancy.
From the American Diabetes Association. Standards of medical care. *Diabetes Care.* 2012;35(suppl 1):S30–S32.

customized global risk assessment, such as those mentioned in this chapter, is useful for prescribing appropriate interventions for each patient based upon age, lifestyle, coexisting medical conditions, family history, traditional risk factors, and emergent risk factors.

Lifestyle intervention must target weight reduction in patients with diabetes. Weight reduction in obese persons will reduce all of the CHD risk factors associated with T2DM and improve chronic hyperglycemia. Moderate weight loss (e.g., 7% to 10% of body weight in 1 year) is often attainable, whereas efforts to achieve ideal body weight in short periods of time usually fail. Even if no weight reduction can be achieved, weight maintenance is certainly preferable to weight gain. A patient over age 50 who gains no weight over the course of 5 years by exercising 5 days each week has actually lost the equivalent of 2.5 lb, as most patients over the age of 50 can expect to gain 0.5 lb per year. Diets low in carbohydrate (and therefore high in fat) may be associated with greater weight loss in the short term but have not been demonstrated to result in greater weight loss after 1 year than diets with more balanced proportions of fats and carbohydrates.[95]

In the first year of the Look AHEAD trial, a study evaluating the effectiveness of intentional weight loss using individual and group therapy versus standardized diabetes support and education, intensively managed patients lost an average of 8.6% from their baseline weight. Intensively managed patients also demonstrated a 21% improvement in CV fitness.[96] Additionally, 42% achieved the ADA goal for LDL-C, 66% for BP, and 71% for A1C, all significantly greater than at baseline and comparable to individuals with a BMI less than 40 kg per m[2]. Thus, intensive behavioral intervention even in severely obese patients will achieve positive metabolic outcomes during the first 12 months.

To improve glycemic control, assist with weight maintenance, and reduce the risk of CHD, at least 150 minutes of moderate-intensity aerobic physical activity per week or at least 90 minutes of vigorous aerobic exercise per week is recommended.[48] Encourage patients with diabetes to perform 30 to 60 minutes of moderate-intensity aerobic activity such as brisk walking on most (preferably all) days of the week, supplemented by an increase in daily lifestyle activities (e.g., walking breaks during the workday, gardening, and household work). For long-term maintenance of major weight loss, a larger amount of exercise (a minimum of 7 hours of moderate or vigorous aerobic physical activity per week) is helpful.

Prior to beginning a program of physical activity that is more vigorous than brisk walking, people with diabetes should be assessed for conditions that might contraindicate certain types of exercise or predispose to injury (e.g., severe autonomic neuropathy, severe peripheral neuropathy, preproliferative or proliferative retinopathy). Unfortunately, no randomized trials or large cohort studies have evaluated the utility of exercise stress testing specifically in people with diabetes. Moreover, even if cardiac stress imaging is performed and interpreted as "normal," one may not be able to guarantee a patient's low CV risk status.[97] The low predictive value of a negative stress test in those with diabetes confirms the need to treat risk factors for atherosclerosis intensively regardless of the results of exercise testing and indicates that patients with diabetes require close follow-up, with a lower threshold for proceeding to angiography than patients without diabetes. Yet those patients with diabetes who are unable to exercise are at the greatest risk of developing a "hard" macrovascular event! Therefore, performing a gaited exercise test on a patient prior to initiation of strenuous physical activity becomes a customizable decision based upon need assessment.

The typical lipid phenotype in a patient with T2DM includes elevated TGs, low HDL-C, and mildly elevated LDL-C. The LDL-C particles are small and dense, carrying less cholesterol per particle. Apo B levels are elevated as are non-HDL-C reflecting a greater number of small, dense LDL-C atherogenic particles. Although an elevated LDL-C level generally is not recognized as the major lipid abnormality in patients with T2DM, clinical trials amply demonstrate that LDL-C lowering with drugs will reduce risk for major coronary events regardless of diabetes status.[98]

Elevated LDL-C is identified as the primary target of lipid-lowering therapy by both the ADA and the AHA. The focus on LDL-C is supported by results of controlled clinical trials demonstrating the safety and efficacy of targeting LDL-C reduction in patients with diabetes.

The MRC/BHC Heart Protection Study and the Collaborative Atorvastatin Diabetes Study (CARDS) included large numbers of patients over age 40 with either T1DM or T2DM, having at least 1 CV risk factor, but no known history of a primary CV event. Subjects were randomized to receive simvastatin 40 mg per day in the Heart Protection Study and atorvastatin 10 mg per day in CARDS, which produced, respectively, a 33% and 40% reduction in LDL-C and a 31% and 37% reduction in combined CV end points.[99,100]

The ADA recognizes serum TGs as a surrogate for atherogenic TG-rich lipoprotein remnants (VLDL and IDL) and a secondary target of lipid-lowering therapy once the goal of LDL-C is attained. The ADA recommends targeting the TG level to less than 150 mg per dL.[48]

The ADA specifies therapeutic goals for HDL-C (greater than 40 mg per dL, with consideration of a higher target of greater than 50 mg per dL in women).[48] The most effective available drug for raising HDL-C levels is nicotinic acid (niacin). Niacin (in doses less than or equal to 2.5 g per day) alone or in combination with statins may raise fasting glucose 4% to 5% and A1C less than or equal to 0.3%. These elevations in glycemic control appear to be transient, reversible, and amenable to adjustments in oral hypoglycemic regimens without having to discontinue the use of niacin. On a population basis, significant reductions in incidences of CV events and the degree of atherosclerotic progression associated with long-term niacin (or niacin-statin) therapy in patients with diabetic dyslipidemia outweigh the typically mild effects of this therapy on glycemic regulation.[101]

• Antiplatelet Therapy

Aspirin is widely regarded as the most cost-effective intervention to reduce CHD in the general population and in patients with diabetes. The Early Treatment of Diabetic Retinopathy Study is the

TABLE 7-15. Antiplatelet Therapy Recommendations for Patients with Diabetes

- Aspirin therapy (75–162 mg/d) should be recommended as a primary prevention strategy in those with diabetes at increased CV risk, including those who are >40 y of age or who have additional risk factors (family history of CHD, hypertension, smoking, dyslipidemia, or albuminuria)

- People with aspirin allergy, bleeding tendency, existing anticoagulant therapy, recent gastrointestinal bleeding, and clinically active hepatic disease are not candidates for aspirin therapy. Other antiplatelet agents may be a reasonable alternative for patients at high risk.

- Aspirin therapy should not be recommended for patients under the age of 21 y because of the increased risk of Reye syndrome

From Buse JB, Ginsberg HN, Bakris GL, et al. Primary prevention of cardiovascular disease in patients with diabetes mellitus: A scientific statement from the American Heart Association and the American Diabetes Association. *Circulation.* 2007;115:114–126.

only large randomized, controlled trial of aspirin in people with diabetes, but included people with and without CHD.[102] For the overall population in this study, the relative risk among aspirin-treated patients was 0.91 for death and 0.83 for fatal and nonfatal MI. Because aspirin may cause bleeding in low CV risk patients, the use of the drug for primary prevention should be limited as shown in Table 7-15.

• Aleglitazar

Aleglitazar is a novel, balanced dual peroxisome proliferator-activated receptor (PPAR)α/γ agonist designed to optimize lipid and glycemic benefits and minimize PPAR-related adverse effects. The drug is being studied in phase 3 clinical trials (ClinicalTrials.gov identifier: NCT01042769).[103]

PPARα and PPARγ agonists target genes relevant to atherosclerosis and inflammation while also benefiting metabolic parameters in patients with diabetes. Fibrates activate PPARα receptors, whereas thiazolidinediones work as insulin receptors through their expression of PPARγ.

Several dual PPARα/γ agonists have been clinically developed. However, the emergence of toxic effects in clinical trials has resulted in their failure to progress beyond phase 3 development. Tesaglitazar was discontinued due to indications that the drug could cause renal impairment. Muraglitazar was linked with CV safety issues.[104]

Aleglitazar was designed to optimize glycemic and lipid benefits while minimizing potential adverse events including weight gain and edema. Aleglitazar has greater affinity for both PPAR receptors unlike tesalitazar and muraglitazar. The overall toxicity profile from nonclinical safety studies with aleglitazar was consistent with that of pioglitazone.

Table 7-16 differentiates the effects of PPARα and PPARγ activation.

During the 16-week phase 2 SYNCHRONY study, aleglitazar reduced baseline A1C fasting plasma glucose, and all lipid parameters in a dose-dependent manner versus placebo. A 10% reduction from baseline LDL-C was observed with aleglitazar 150 μg. By comparison, pioglitazone increases LDL-C by 2% to 16%. Aleglitazar 150 μg also demonstrated statistically significant improvement in reducing TG and apo B versus placebo and pioglitazone. The increase in HDL-C was 25 mg per dL for aleglitazar 150 μg versus 4 mg per dL for placebo and 16 mg per dL for pioglitazone 45 mg.[105] The significant improvement in lipids and glycemic endpoints coupled with the favorable safety profile represent promising data for aleglitazar.

TABLE 7-16. Balanced Pharmacologic Activation of PPARα and PPARγ Receptors

PPAR Receptor	Drug Responsible for Activation	Pharmacologic Response to Receptor Activation
PPARα	Fibrates	• Lower TGs • Raise HDL-C • Reverse atherosclerosis • Reverse vascular inflammation • Decrease cytokines, chemokines, cholesterol efflux, and adhesion molecules
PPARγ	Thiazolidinediones	• Improve insulin sensitivity in fat, liver, and skeletal muscles • Improve plasma glucose • Decrease inflammation • Decrease atherosclerosis

Prevention of Cardiovascular Disease in Patients with T1DM

The relative risk of CHD in patients with T1DM compared with age-matched euglycemic individuals is dramatically increased in both men and women. The risk factors for CHD in T1DM are similar to those with T2DM. However, glycemic control does *not* predict progression.[42,106] Interventions that are beneficial for reducing CHD risk in T2DM are equally effective for patients with T1DM.[107] Epidemiologic studies suggest that addressing traditional risk factors including albuminuria, markers of inflammation and customized metabolic targets including A1C, lipids, and BP have a synergistic effect on reducing CHD risk in patients with T1DM.[108]

Utility of Carotid Intima–Media Thickness Measurements as a Surrogate Marker of Cardiovascular Disease in Patients with Diabetes

Ultrasonographic assessment of CIMT is used as a surrogate marker of CHD in people with diabetes. CIMT allows physicians to identify patients with subclinical atherosclerosis affording the initiation of preventative therapies to minimize one's chances of developing a primary CV event. CIMT may also be used to track and monitor therapeutic interventions over time for patients with atherosclerosis.

CIMT is determined using a B-mode high-resolution vascular ultrasound transducer and represents the area of tissue beginning at the edge of the artery lumen and ending at the boundary between the media and the adventitia (Fig. 7-18). CIMT increases with age (0.015 mm per year) and varies between sex and race as shown in Table 7-17. When risk is assessed using percentiles, a CIMT greater than the 75th percentile is considered high risk.

Carotid artery intima–media thickness increases are most significant (0.017 to 0.026 mm per year) in patients with a history of CAD. Patients with diabetes and inflammatory disorders, such as rheumatoid arthritis, also experience a more rapid increase in CIMT thickness due to accelerated rates of atherosclerosis.[109–111]

A study evaluating CIMT and plaque in 118 young patients, ages 36 to 59 years, with 1 CV risk factor (family history of premature CVD, smoking, hyperlipidemia, or hypertension), determined that 97% of patients had a Framingham annualized CV event rate risk score of less than 1%. However, 34% of these subjects demonstrate the appearance of carotid plaque, whereas 13% had a high-risk CIMT greater than the 75th percentile.[112] Therefore, a gap may exist in some individuals who

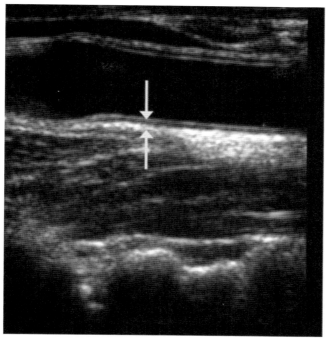

Figure 7-18 • **Carotid Artery Intima–Media Thickness Measurement.** The double-line pattern between the two echogenic lines representing the lumen–intima interface and the media–adventitia interface represents the intima media. CIMT in healthy middle-aged adults measure 0.6 to 0.7 mm. Greater than 1.20 mm is considered abnormal. The appearance of plaque within the carotid artery is suggestive of atherosclerosis. (From Jacoby DS, Mohler IE, Rader DJ. Noninvasive atherosclerosis imaging for predicting cardiovascular events and assessing therapeutic interventions. *Curr Atheroscler Rep.* 2004;6(1):20–26 with permission.)

appear to be at low risk based on Framingham scores, yet may have evidence of early atherosclerotic disease. CIMT may be useful in detecting subclinical atherosclerosis in these young adults.

The presence and type of carotid plaque (soft, heterogenous, mixed, fully calcified) should also be reported when performing CIMT. Plaque is an independent risk factor for CHD increasing one's probability of having a MI or stroke.[113] Internal carotid artery plaque that exceeds 1.5 mm in thickness doubles CV risk over 8 years (when compared to patients having no plaque).[114]

Multiple drug classes have been demonstrated to have a positive effect on CIMT. Many antihypertensive drugs [calcium channel blockers, α- and β-blockers, ACE inhibitors, diuretics, and angiotensin receptor blockers (ARBs)] induce regression of CIMT after 6 to 52 months of treatment.[115] Niacin in combination with statin therapy has an insignificant effect on CIMT progression after 1 year. However, during the open-label extension phase of the same study, (ARBITER 3), patients who switched from placebo to extended-release niacin experienced a significant regression of CIMT versus placebo over 24 months.[116]

Long-term treatment with statins have demonstrated a favorable effect on CIMT. In the Measuring Effects on Intima–Medial Thickness: An Evaluation of Rosuvastatin (METEOR) study, patients with low risk (less than or equal to one risk factor or greater than or equal to two risk factors and a FRS of less than 10% annualized CV event rate) but with mild hyperlipidemia and subclinical atherosclerosis based on CIMT were treated with rosuvastatin or placebo for 2 years.[117] Atherosclerosis progression was significantly reduced with rosuvastatin compared with placebo (–0.0014 mm per year and 0.0131 mm per year, respectively; $p < 0.001$). As a result of this trial, rosuvastatin has a label indication for slowing the progression of atherosclerosis.

Other drugs that slow the progression of CIMT include pioglitazone[118] and rosiglitazone.[119]

TABLE 7-17. Mean Far Wall Common Carotid CIMT Values and 75th Percentiles

Age (years)	25	30	35	40	45	55	65
Black Women							
Mean value, 0.78 mm	0.67	0.71	0.76	0.81	0.58	0.67	0.75
75th percentile	0.72	0.78	0.83	0.89	0.64	0.75	0.85
Black Men							
Mean value, 0.78 mm	0.73	0.78	0.83	0.87	0.64	0.73	0.86
75th percentile	0.71	0.82	0.92	1.02	0.72	0.83	0.99
White Women							
Mean value, 0.78 mm	0.63	0.67	0.70	0.73	0.55	0.64	0.73
75th percentile	0.70	0.73	0.76	0.79	0.61	0.71	0.81
White Men							
Mean value, 0.78 mm	0.69	0.73	0.77	0.81	0.62	0.71	0.80
75th percentile	0.83	0.85	0.87	0.88	0.70	0.80	0.93

From Howard G, Sharrett AR, Heiss G, et al. Carotid artery intimal-medial thickness distribution in general populations as evaluated by B-mode ultrasound. ARIC Investigators. *Stroke.* 1993;24(9):1297–1304.

Patients regardless of age with risk factors such as prediabetes, diabetes, tobacco use, hyperlipidemia, or family history of CAD could benefit from a CIMT evaluation. CIMT should be performed annually if the study is abnormal and every 2 to 5 years if the results are normal.[120] Specific guidelines addressing candidates for CIMT testing, testing intervals, and a standardized protocol for performing the evaluation are forthcoming from the Society of Atherosclerosis Imaging and Prevention (SAIP).

Primary Care and Primary Prevention of CHD

Most primary care physicians are trained to prevent the acute events associated with chronic diseases with the use of screening tests, vaccines, or medications that improve outcomes. While attempting to prevent CHD in high-risk patients, such as those with diabetes, we must be able to micromanage hyperglycemia, prevent hypoglycemia, reduce hypertension, and treat hyperlipidemia to the recommended individual targets. One public health model predicted that every 10% increase in hypertension treatment will prevent 14,000 deaths, while every 10% increase in treatment of elevated LDL-C with statin use or initiation of aspirin prophylaxis would lead to 8,000 prevented deaths/year in patients less than 80 years of age. These simple interventions using generic medications (ACE inhibitors, statins, and aspirin) could save 25,000 to 40,000 lives per year for those who are less than 65 years old.[121] Simply stated, early intervention with metformin, coupled with primary prevention using medications costing on average less than $20 per month may have a huge impact on minimizing CHD morbidity and mortality in the United States.

Primary prevention refers to prevention of coronary disease before clinical heart disease is evident, a diagnosis is made, or an event has occurred in a patient with multiple risk factors. Patients who have already experienced a primary CV event may be offered secondary prevention with the hope of delaying or reversing disease progression. The most important aspect of primary prevention involves patient participation. Behavioral intervention measures that are applied over a prolonged "incubation period" such as proper nutrition, practicing sound sleep hygiene, and participating in a regular exercise program can delay disease progression.

Once medications are prescribed to minimize CV risk, physicians must be cognizant of patient nonadherence. In clinical trials, patient adherence rates to medication regimens range from 43% to

TABLE 7-18. The "Top 5" Goals for Successful Diabetes Management

1. Understand your metabolic targets (A1C, lipids, and BP).

2. Know how to successfully achieve these metabolic targets (via behavioral and pharmacologic intervention).

3. Stop smoking (if patient does not smoke, move to goal no. 4).

4. Be adherent to your treatment plan. If, by chance, you become uncomfortable with any of the components of the plan, discuss your concerns with your health-care provider.

5. Obtain your medical care from a knowledgeable and caring physician who understands your individual needs and will help guide you toward successful treatment rather than steer you into a path of failure.

Goals provided by Bill Polonsky, CDE, PhD, Director, Diabetes Behavioral Institute. San Diego, CA.

78%. Yet, in clinical practice, the adherence rates are much lower. Patients with CHD and stroke fail to fill their prescriptions within 1 week after discharge 23% of the time due to simple refusal to use the medications, lack of understanding, polypharmacy, fear of side effects, cultural issues, or cost.[122]

Patients are not the only ones to blame for lack of effort toward prevention of CHD and all-cause mortality. Only 29% of patients with a prior history of CHD are taking statins upon hospital discharge.[123]

A survey of PCPs concluded that only one-third considered evidence-based guidelines important in achieving optimum patient management.[124] Less than 50% of PCPs in this survey felt confident providing nutritional counseling to patients with hyperlipidemia despite the fact that dietary intervention is the foundation of management for diabetes, hyperlipidemia, and primary prevention of CHD. PCPs significantly underestimate CAD risk, are often unaware of published disease state guidelines, and are inclined to not utilize risk engines.[122]

Thus, the responsibilities for disease prevention lie with both the patient and the treating physician. Because patients do not "feel" the benefits of statins, aspirin, ACE inhibitors, or even some glucose-lowering agents, our job as educators is to explain that we are treating our bodies as if we are funding our retirement account. Appropriate and timely interventions (both behavioral and pharmacologic) at the earliest stages of metabolic dysfunction will often result in improved outcomes. Medical costs will be minimized by simply exercising, stopping smoking, reducing one's weight, and using aspirin prophylaxis when indicated.[122]

Finally, how can we effectively and efficiently treat our patient's multiple risk factors? A treatment-naive patient just informed that he has diabetes will simply "freak out" thinking that within weeks he will likely lose his eye, a kidney, and a foot as his Aunt Leslie did 30 years ago. Patients need not fear the diagnosis of diabetes as being a death sentence considering all of the medications and technology we have at our disposal. In order to successfully self-manage diabetes, one must understand and adhere to the top five goals listed in Table 7-18.

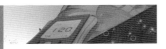

SUMMARY

Because diabetes is considered a cardiovascular risk-equivalent disease, intensive primary prevention of atherosclerosis in patients with abnormal glucose tolerance appears to be a reasonable objective. Glycemic variability, oxidative stress, and prolongation of one's glycemic burden (elevation of A1C) all contribute to cardiovascular pathogenesis. Once a patient has had a primary cardiovascular event, his or her risk of all-cause mortality actually increases if one targets A1C levels < 7 %. However, for the vast majority of patients who have few, if any co-existing disorders or comorbidities, clinicians should attempt to reduce the A1C as low and safely as possible, for as long as possible, as rationally as possible and as soon as possible. The UKPDS 10-year follow-up and the DCCT/EDIC studies both support evidence demonstrating the induction of "metabolic memory" or a "legacy effect" for patients who are intensively managed soon after being diagnosed with diabetes. Thus, intensification of glycemic control will likely result in continued vascular benefits despite loss of glycemic differences from conventional treatment over time.

Atherosclerosis and cardiovascular disease are characterized by a number of abnormalities fueled by insulin resistance. Ninety-seven percent of adults with T2DM have at least one lipid abnormality with the primary phenotype being elevated triglycerides and reduced levels of HDL-C. Advanced lipid testing may provide a more sophisticated measurement of the components of LDL-C, HDL-C, VLDL-C, non-HDL-C and other emerging risk factors. Candidates for advanced lipid profiling would include patients with established atherosclerosis, a history of myocardial infarction, stroke or transient ischemic attack, coronary artery bypass grafting, stent placement, arterecotomy, angina, acute coronary syndrome, and T2DM. Patients with a premature family history of atherosclerosis or those with at least two of five NCEP risk factors should also be tested.

Surrogate markers of cardiovascular disease such as CIMT measurements allow clinicians the opportunity to track and monitor the efficacy of therapeutic interventions over time in hopes of reducing one's cardiovascular risk.

Unfortunately, PCPs significantly underestimate coronary artery disease risk, are often unaware of published disease state guidelines and are inclined to not utilize risk engines. The responsibilities for primary prevention of heart disease lies with both the patient and the treating clinician. Appropriate and timely interventions (both behavioral and pharmacologic) at the earliest stages of metabolic dysfunction will often result in improved outcomes.

REFERENCES

1. Haffner SM, Lehto S, Ronemaa T, et al. Mortality from coronary heart disease in subjects with type 2 diabetes and in nondiabetic subjects with and without prior myocardial infarction. *N Engl J Med.* 1998;339:229–234.
2. Herlitz J, Karlson BW, Edrardsson N, et al. Prognosis in diabetics with chest pain or other symptoms suggestive of acute myocardial infarction. *Cardiology.* 1992;80:237–245.
3. Miettinen H, Lehto S, Salomaa V, et al.; the FINMONICA Myocardial Infarction Register Study Group. Impact of diabetes on mortality after the first myocardial infarction. *Diabetes Care.* 1998;21:69–75.
4. Gustafsson I, Hildebrandt P, Seibaek M, et al.; the TRACE Study Group: Long-term prognosis of diabetic patients with myocardial infarction: relation to antidiabetic treatment regimen. *Eur Heart J.* 2000;21:1937–1943.
5. National Cholesterol Education Program (NCEP) Expert Panel on Detection, Evaluation, and Treatment of High Blood Cholesterol in Adults (Adult Treatment Panel III): Third Report of the National Cholesterol Education Program (NCEP) Expert Panel on Detection, Evaluation, and Treatment of High Blood Cholesterol in Adults (Adult Treatment Panel III) final report. *Circulation.* 2002;106:3143–3421.

6. Laakso M. Epidemiology of diabetic dyslipidemia. *Diabetes Rev*. 1995;3:408–422.

7. Donnelly R, Emslie-Smith AM, Gardner ID, et al. ABC of arterial and venous disease: vascular complications of diabetes. *BMJ*. 2000;320:1062–1066

8. Hamidon BB, Raymond AA. The impact of diabetes mellitus on in-hospital stroke mortality. *J Postgrad Med*. 2003;49(4):307–310.

9. Arboix A, Rivas A, Garcia-Eroles L, et al. Cerebral infarction in diabetes: clinical pattern, stroke subtypes, and predictors of in-hospital mortality. *BMC Neurol*. 2005;5(9). doi:10.1186/1471-2377-5-9.

10. Henry RR. Preventing cardiovascular complications of type 2 diabetes: focus on lipid management. *Clin Diabetes*. 2001;19:113–120.

11. Wakasaki H, Koya D, Schuen FJ, et al. Targeted overexpression of protein kinase C isoform in myocardium causes cardiomyopathy. *Proc Natl ACVD U S A*. 1997;94:9320–9325.

12. Brownlee M, Hirsch IB. Glycemic variability: a hemoglobin A1C-independent risk factor for diabetic complications. *JAMA*. 2006;295:1707–1708.

13. Monnier L, Mas E, Ginet C, et al. Activation of oxidative stress by acute glucose fluctuations compared with sustained chronic hyperglycemia in patients with type 2 diabetes. *JAMA*. 2006;295:1681–1687.

14. Hirsch IB, Brownlee M. Should minimal blood glucose variability become the gold standard of glycemic control? *J Diabetes Complications*. 2005;19:178–181.

15. Brownlee M. Biochemistry and molecular cell biology of diabetic complications. *Nature*. 2001;414:813–820.

16. Khaw KT, Wareham N, Bingham S, et al. Association of hemoglobin A1c with cardiovascular disease and mortality in adults: the European prospective investigation into cancer in Norfolk. *Ann Intern Med*. 2004;141(6):413–420.

17. UK Prospective Diabetes Study (UKPDS) Group. Intensive blood-glucose control with sulphonylureas or insulin compared with conventional treatment and risk of complications in patients with type 2 diabetes (UKPDS 33). *Lancet*. 1998;352:837–853.

18. Holman RR, Paul SK, Bethel MA, et al. Long-term follow-up of intensive glucose control in type 2 diabetes. *N Engl J Med*. 2008;359:1577–1589.

19. Diabetes Control and Complications Trial/Epidemiology of Diabetes Interventions and Complications (DCCT/EDIC) Study Group. Intensive diabetes treatment and cardiovascular disease in patients with type 1 diabetes. *N Engl J Med*. 2005;353:2643–2653.

20. Diabetes Control and Complications Trial/Epidemiology of Diabetes Interventions and Complications Research Group. Intensive diabetes therapy and carotid intima-media thickness in type 1 diabetes mellitus. *N Engl J Med*. 2003;348:2294–2903.

21. Cleary P, Orchard T, Zinman B, et al. Coronary calcification in the Diabetes Control and Complications Trial/Epidemiology of Diabetes Interventions and Complications (DCCT/EDIC) cohort. *Diabetes*. 2003;52(suppl 2):A152–A152.

22. Gaude P, Vedel P, Larsen N, et al. Multifactorial interventions and cardiovascular disease in patients with type 2 diabetes. *N Engl J Med*. 2003;348:383–393.

23. Grundy SM, Pasternak R, Greenland P, et al. Assessment of Cardiovascular Risk by Use of Multiple-Risk-Factor Assessment Equations: A Statement for Healthcare Professionals From the American Heart Association and the American College of Cardiology. *Circulation*. 1999;100(13):1481–1492.

24. Coleman RL, Stevens RJ, Retnakaran R, et al. Framingham, SCORE, and DECODE risk equations do not provide reliable cardiovascular risk estimates in type 2 diabetes. *Diabetes Care*. 2007;30(5):1292–1293.

25. Yeo WW, Yeo KR. Predicting CHD risk in patients with diabetes mellitus. *Diabet Med*. 2001;18:341–344.

26. Jacobson TA, Griffiths GG, Varas C, et al. Impact of evidence-based "clinical judgment" on the number of American adults requiring lipid-lowering therapy based on updated NHANES III data. National Health and Nutrition Examination Survey. *Arch Intern Med*. 2008;160(9):1361–1369.

27. Smith SC, Allen J, Blair SN, et al. AHA/ACC guidelines for secondary prevention for patients with coronary and other atherosclerotic vascular disease: 2006 update: endorsed by the National Heart, Lung, and Blood Institute. *Circulation*. 2006;113(19):2363–2372.

28. Vasan RS. Biomarkers of cardiovascular disease: molecular basis and practical considerations. *Circulation*. 2006;113:2335–2362.

29. Helfand M, Buckley DI, Freeman M, et al. Emerging risk factors for coronary heart disease: a summary of systematic reviews conducted for the U.S. Preventive Services Task Force. *Ann Intern Med*. 2009;151:496–507.

30. Pearson TA, Mensah GA, Alexander RW, et al; Centers for Disease Control and Prevention; American Heart Association. Markers of inflammation and cardiovascular disease: application to clinical public

health practice: a statement for healthcare professionals from the Centers for Disease Control and Prevention and the American Heart Association. *Circulation*. 2003;107(3):499–511.

31. Luciana ML, das GC M, Anna LS, et al. High sensitivity C-reactive protein in subjects with type 2 diabetes mellitus and/or high blood pressure. *J Arg Bras Endocrinol Meta*. 2007;51:6–10.

32. Ridker PM, Danielson E, Fonseca FAH, et al. Rosuvastatin to prevent vascular events in men and women with elevated C-reactive protein. *N Engl J Med*. 2008;359(21):2195–2207.

33. Ridker PM, Danielson E, Fonseca FAH, et al. JUPITER Trial Study Group. Reduction in C-reactive protein and LDL cholesterol and cardiovascular event rates after initiation of rosuvastatin: a prospective study of the JUPITER trial. *Lancet*. 2009;373(9670):1175–1182.

34. Mora S, Musunuru K, Blumenthal RS. The clinical utility of high-sensitivity reactive protein in cardiovascular disease and the potential implication of JUPITER on current practice guidelines. *Clin Chem*. 2009;55:219–228.

35. Jenkins NP, Keevil BG, Hutchinson IV, et al. Beta-blockers are associated with lower C-reactive protein concentrations in patients with coronary artery disease. *Am J Med*. 2002;112:269–274.

36. Joergensen C, Gall MA, Schmedes A, et al. Vitamin D levels and mortality in type 2 diabetes. *Diabetes Care*. 2010;33:2238–2243.

37. Oh J, Weng S, Felton SK, et al. 1,25(OH)2 vitamin D inhibits foam cell formation and suppresses macrophage cholesterol uptake in patients with type 2 diabetes mellitus. *Circulation*. 2009;120:687–698.

38. UK Prospective Diabetes Study (UKPDS) Group. Effect of intensive blood-glucose control with metformin on complications in overweight patients with type 2 diabetes (UKPDS 34). *Lancet*. 1998;352:854–865.

39. Action to Control Cardiovascular Risk in Diabetes Study Group. Effects of intensive glucose lowering in type 2 diabetes. *N Engl J Med*. 2008;358:2545–2559.

40. Group AC, Patel A, MacMahon S, et al.; ADVANCE Collaborative Group. Intensive blood glucose control and vascular outcomes in patients with type 2 diabetes. *N Engl J Med*. 2008;358:2560–2572.

41. Duckworth W, Abraira C, Moritz T, et al.; VADT Investigators. Glucose control and vascular complications in veterans with type 2 diabetes. *N Engl J Med*. 2009;360:129–139.

42. Orchard TJ, Olson JC, Erbey JR, et al. Insulin resistance-related factors, but not glycemia, predict coronary artery disease in type 1 diabetes: 10-year follow-up data from the Pittsburgh Epidemiology of Diabetes Complications Study. *Diabetes Care*. 2003;26(5):1374–1379.

43. Forrest KYZ, Becker DJ, Kuller LH, et al. Are predictors of coronary heart disease and lower extremity arterial disease in type 1 diabetes the same? A prospective study. *Atherosclerosis*. 2000;148:159–169.

44. Roy MS, Peng B, Roy A. Risk factors for coronary disease and stroke in previously hospitalized African-Americans with type 1 diabetes: a 6-year follow-up. *Diabet Med*. 2007;24(12):1361–1368.

45. Costacou T, Ferrell RE, Orchard TJ. Haptoglobin genotype and renal disease progression in type 1 diabetes. *Diabetes*. 2008;57:1702–1706.

46. Unger J, Parkin CG. Type 2 diabetes: an expanded view of pathophysiology and therapy. *Postgrad Med*. 2010;122(3):145–157.

47. Hansson L, Zanchetti A, Carruthers SG, et al. Effects of intensive blood-pressure lowering and low-dose aspirin in patients with hypertension: principal results of the Hypertension Optimal Treatment (HOT) randomised trial. *Lancet*. 1998;351:1755–1762.

48. American Diabetes Association. Standards of medical care in diabetes—2012. *Diabetes Care*. 2012;35(suppl 1):S11–S63.

49. Chobanian AV, Bakris GL, Black HR, et al. The Seventh Report of the Joint National Committee on Prevention, Detection, Evaluation, and Treatment of High Blood Pressure: the JNC 7 report. *JAMA*. 2003;289:2560–2572.

50. Staessen J, Fagard R, Lijnen P, et al. Body weight, sodium intake and blood pressure. *J Hyperten* 1989;7(suppl 1):S19–S23.

51. Cutler JA, Fohnann D, Allender PS. Randomized trials of sodium reduction: an overview. *Am J Clin Nutr*. 1997;65(suppl 2):643S–651S.

52. Meyers MG, Tobe SW, McKay DW, et al. New algorithm for the diagnosis of hypertension. *Am J Hypertens*. 2005;18:1369–1374.

53. Kario K, Schwartz JE, Gerin W, et al. Psychological and physical stress-induced cardiovascular reactivity and diurnal blood pressure variation in women with different work shifs. *Hypertens Res*. 2002;25:543–551.

54. Naito Y, Tsujino T, Fujioka, et al. Augmented diurnal variations of the cardiac renin-angiotensin system in hypertensive rats. *Hypertension*. 2002;40:827–833.

55. Kario K, Shimada K, Pickering TG. Clinical implications of morning blood pressure surge in hypertension. *J Cardiovasc Pharmaocol*. 2003;42(S1):S87–S91.

56. Ross R, Fuster V. The pathogenesis of atherosclerosis. In: Ross R, Fuster V, Topol EJ, eds. *Atherosclerosis and Coronary Artery Disease*. Philadelphia: Lippincott-Raven; 1996;441–462.

57. Stary HC, Chandler AB, Dinsmore RE, et al. A definition of advanced type of atherosclerotic lesions and a histological classification of atherosclerosis: a report from the committee on vascular lesions of the Council on Arteriosclerosis, American Heart Association. *Circulation*. 1995;92(5):1355–1374.

58. Michiels C. J. Endothelial cell functions. *Cell Physiol*. 2003;196(3):430–443.

59. Weissber PL. Atherogenesis: current understanding of the causes of atheroma. *Heart*. 2000;83:247–225.

60. Orasanu G, Plutzky J. The pathologic continuum of diabetic vascular disease. *J Am Coll Cardiol*. 2009;53(5 suppl):S35–S42.

61. Simionescu A, Schulte JB, Fercana G, et al. Inflammation in cardiovascular tissue engineering: the challenge to a promise: a mini review. *Int J Inflam*. 2011;2011:958247. Epub 2011 Jul 9.

62. Kolodgie FD, Gold HK, Burke AP, et al. Intraplaque hemorrhage and progression of coronary atheroma. *N Engl J Med*. 2003;349(24):2316–2325.

63. O'Rourke RA, Brundage BH, Froelicher VF, et al. American College of Cardiology/American Heart Association Expert Consensus Document on electron-beam computed tomography for the diagnosis and prognosis of coronary artery disease. *J Am Coll Cardiol*. 2000;36(1):326–340.

64. Garvey WT, Kwon S, Zheng D, et al. Effect of insulin resistance and type 2 diabetes on lipoprotein subclass particle size and concentration determined by nuclear magnetic resonance. *Diabetes*. 2003;52:453–462.

65. Fagot-Campagna A, Rolka DB, Beckles GL, et al. Prevalence of lipid abnormalities, awareness, and treatment in U.S. adults with diabetes. Abstract 318. *Diabetes*. 2000;49(suppl 1).

66. Grundy SM. Small LDL, atherogenic dyslipidemia, and the metabolic syndrome [editorial]. *Circulation*. 1997;95:1–4.

67. Superko HR. The atherogenic lipoprotein profile. *Sci Med*. 1997;4(5):36–45.

68. Cobble M, Sellers J. Advanced lipid testing: a better alternative for cardiovascular risk prediction. *Practical Diabetology*. 2010;September/October:22–26.

69. ATP III Guidelines At-A-Glance. Quick Desk Reference. http://www.nhlbi.nih.gov/guidelines/cholesterol/atglance.pdf. Accessed 3/24/12.

70. Elovson J, Chatterton JE, Bell GT, et al. Plasma very low density lipoproteins contain a single molecule of apolipoprotein B. *J Lipid Res*. 1988;29(11):1461–1473.

71. Contois JH, McConnell JP, Sethi AA, et al. Apolipoprotein B and cardiovascular disease risk: a position statement from the AACC Lipoproteins and Vascular Disease Division Working Group on Best Practices. The Fats of Life 2008;XXII(3):5.

72. Thompson A, Danesh J. Associations between apolipoprotein B, apolipoprotein AI, the apolipoprotein B/AI ratio and coronary heart disease: a literature-based meta-analysis of prospective studies. *J Intern Med*. 2006;259(5):481–492.

73. Tian L, Fu M. The relationship between high density lipoprotein subclass profile and apolipoptrotein concentrations. *J Endocrinol Invest*. 2011;34(6):461–472.

74. Rizzo M, Berneis K. Who needs to care about small, dense low-density lipoproteins? *Int J Clin Pract*. 2007;61(11):1949–1956.

75. Barter P, Gotto AM, LaRosa J, et al. HDL cholesterol, very low levels of LDL cholesterol and cardiovascular events. *N Engl J Med*. 2007;357(13):1301–1310.

76. Ueda M, Sethi AA, Freeman LA, et al. High density lipoproteins: overview and update on new findings from diagnostics to therapeutics. *J Clin Ligand Assay*. 2005;28:216–232.

77. Zeljokovic A, Vekic J, Spasojevic-Kalmanovska V, et al. LDL and HDL subclasses in acute ischemic stroke: prediction of risk and short-term mortality. *Atherosclerosis*. 2010;210(2):548–554.

78. Kannel WB. Status of risk factors and their consideration in antihypertensive therapy. *Am J Cardiol*. 1987;23;59(2):80A–90A.

79. Kolovou GD, Anagnostopoulou KK, Kostakou PM, et al. Primary and secondary hypertriglyceridaemia. *Curr Drug Targets*. 2009;10(4):336–343.

80. Despres JP, Lemieux I. Abdominal obesity and metabolic syndrome. *Nature*. 2006;444:881–887.

81. Bansal S, Buring JE, Rifai N, et al. Fasting compared with nonfasting triglycerides and risk of cardiovascular events in women. *JAMA*. 2007;298(3):309–316.

82. Nordestgaard BG, Benn M, Schnohr P, et al. Nonfasting triglycerides and risk of myocardial infarction, ischemic heart disease, and death in men and women. *JAMA*. 2007;18;298(3):299–308.

83. Pacold I, Ackerman L, Johnson B, et al. The effects of acute hypertriglyceridemia and high levels of free fatty acids on left ventricular function. *Am Heart J.* 1985;110(4):836–840.

84. Austin MA, Hokanson JE, Ewards KL. Hypertriglyceridemia as a cardiovascular risk factor. *Am J Cardiol.* 1998;81(4, suppl 1):7B–12B.

85. Zilversmit DB. Atherogenesis: a postprandial phenomenon. *Circulation.* 1979;60(3):473–850.

86. Callaghan BC, Feldman E, Liu J, et al. Triglycerides and amputation risk in patients with diabetes ten-year follow-up in the DISTANCE study. *Diabetes Care.* 2011;34(3):635–640.

87. Sniderman AD, St-Pierre AC, Cantin B, et al. Concordance/discordance between plasma apolipoprotein B levels and the cholesterol indexes of atherosclerotic risk. *Am J Cardiol.* 2003;91:1173–117.

88. Keys A, Karvonen MJ, Punsar S, et al. HDL serum cholesterol and 24-year mortality of men in Finland. *Int J Epidemiol.* 1984;13:428–435.

89. Pocock SJ, Shaper AG, Phillips AN, et al. High density lipoprotein cholesterol is not a major risk factor for ischaemic heart disease in British men. *BMJ.* 1986;292:515–519.

90. Cui Y, Blumenthal RS, Flaws JA, et al. Non-high-density lipoprotein cholesterol level as a predictor of cardiovascular disease mortality. *Arch Intern Med.* 2001;161:1413–1419.

91. Lu W, Resnick HE, Jablonski KA, et al. Non-HDL cholesterol as a predictor of cardiovascular disease in type 2 diabetes. *Diabetes Care.* 2003;26:16–23.

92. Frost PH, Davis BR, Burlando AJ, et al. Serum lipids and incidence of coronary heart disease. *Circulation.* 1996;94:2381–238.

93. Von Muehlen D, Langer RD, Barrett-Connor E. Sex and time differences in the associations of non-high-density lipoprotein cholesterol versus other lipid and lipoprotein factors in the prediction of cardiovascular death: the Rancho Bernardo Study. *Am J Cardiol.* 2003;91:1311–1315.

94. Pedersen TR, Olsson AG, Faergeman O, et al. Lipoprotein changes and reduction in the incidence of major coronary heart disase events in the Scandinavian Simvastatin Survival Study (4S). *Circulation.* 1998;97:1453–1460.

95. Foster GD, Wyatt HR, Hill JO, et al. A randomized trial of a low-carbohydrate diet for obesity. *N Engl J Med.* 2003;348:2082–2090.

96. The Look AHEAD Research Group. Reduction in weight and cardiovascular disease risk factors in individuals with type 2 diabetes reduction in weight and one-year results of the Look AHEAD trial. *Diabetes Care.* 2007;30:1374–1383.

97. Kamalesh M, Feigenbaum H, Sawada S. Challenge of identifying patients with diabetes mellitus who are at low risk for coronary events by use of cardiac stress imaging. *Am Heart J.* 2004;147:561–563.

98. Baigent C, Keech A, Kearney PM, et al. Cholesterol Treatment Trialists' (CTT) Collaborators. Efficacy and safety of cholesterol lowering treatment: prospective meta-analysis of data from 90,056 participants in 14 randomised trials of statins. *Lancet.* 2005;366:1267–1278.

99. Collaborative Group. MRC/BHF Heart Protection Study of cholesterol lowering with simvastatin in 5963 people with diabetes: a randomised placebo-controlled trial. *Lancet.* 2003;361:2005–2016.

100. Colhoun HM, Betteridge DJ, Durrington PN, et al. CARDS Investigators. Primary prevention of cardiovascular disease with atorvastatin in type 2 diabetes in the Collaborative Atorvastatin Diabetes Study (CARDS): multicentre randomised placebo-controlled trial. *Lancet.* 2004;364:685–696.

101. Goldberg RB, Jacobson TA. Effects of niacin on glucose control in patients with dyslipidemia. *Mayo Clin Proc.* 2008;83(4):470–478.

102. ETDRS Investigators. Aspirin effects on mortality and morbidity in patients with diabetes mellitus: Early Treatment Diabetic Retinopathy Study report 14. *JAMA.* 1992;268:1292–1300.

103. ClinicalTrials.gov identifier: NCT01042769. http://www.clinicaltrials.gov/ct2/show/NCT01042769?term=Aleglitazar&rank=6. Accessed 3/25/12.

104. Nissen SE, Wolski K, Topol EJ. Effect of muraglitazar on death and major adverse cardiovascular events in patients with type 2 diabetes mellitus. *JAMA.* 2005;294:2581–2586.

105. Henry RR, Lincoff AM, Mudaliar S, et al. Effect of the dual peroxisome proliferator–activated receptor-α/γ agonist aleglitazar on risk of cardiovascular disease in patients with type 2 diabetes (SYNCHRONY): a phase II, randomized, dose-ranging study. *Lancet.* 2009;374:126–135.

106. Laing SP, Swerdlow AJ, Slater SD, et al. Mortality from heart disease in a cohort of 23,000 patients with insulin-treated diabetes. *Diabetologia.* 2003;46:760–765.

107. Buse JB, Ginsberg HN, Bakris GL, et al. Primary prevention of cardiovascular disease in patients with diabetes mellitus: a scientific statement from the American Heart Association and the American Diabetes Association. *Circulation*. 2007;115:114–126.

108. Wajchenberg BL, Feitosa AC, Rassi N, et al. Glycemia and cardiovascular disease in type 1 diabetes mellitus. *Endocr Pract*. 2008;14(7):912–923.

109. Botts ML, Evans GW, Riley WA, et al. Carotid intima-media thickness measurements in intervention studies: design options, progression rates, and sample size considerations: a point of view. *Stroke*. 2003;34(12):2985–2994.

110. Rabago RR, Gomez-Diaz RA, Tanus HJ, et al. Carotid intima-media thickness in pediatric type 1 diabetic patients. *Diabetes Care*. 2007;30(10):2599–2602.

111. Del Rincon I, O'Leary DH, Freeman GL, et al. Acceleration of atherosclerosis during the course of rheumatoid arthritis. *Atherosclerosis*. 2007;195(2):354–360.

112. Lester SJ, Eleid MF, Khandheria BK, et al. Carotid intima-media thickness and coronary artery calcium score as indications of subclinical atherosclerosis. *Mayo Clin Proc*. 2009;84(3):229–233.

113. Hunt KJ, Sharrett AR, Chambless LE, et al. Acoustic shadowing on B-mode ultrasound of the carotid artery predicts CHD. *Ultrasound Med Biol*. 2001;27(3):357–365.

114. Polak JF, Pencina MJ, Pencin KM, et al. Carotid-wall intima–media thickness and cardiovascular events. *N Engl J Med*. 2011;365:213–221.

115. Riccioni G. the effect of antihypertensive drugs on carotid intimia media thickness: an up-to-date review. *Curr Med Chem*. 2009;16(8):988–996.

116. Taylor AJ, Lee HJ, Sullenberger LE. The effect of 24 months of combination statin and extended-release niacin on carotid intima-media thickness: ARBITER 3. *Curr Med Opin*. 2006;22(11):2243–2250.

117. Crouse JR, Raichlen JS, Riley WA, et al. Effect of rosuvastatin on progression of carotid intima-media thickness in low-risk individuals with subclinical atherosclerosis: the METEOR Trial. *JAMA*. 2007;297(12):1344–1353.

118. Mazzone T, Meyer PM, Feinstein SB, et al. Effect of pioglitazone compared with glimepiride on carotid intima-media thickness in type 2 diabetes: a randomized trial. *JAMA*. 2006;296(21):2572–2581.

119. Lonn EM, Gerstein HC, Sheridan P, et al. Effect of ramipril and rosiglitazone on carotid intima-media thickness in people with impaired glucose tolerance or impaired fasting glucose: STARR (STudy of Atherosclerosis with Ramipril and Rosiglitazone). *J Am Coll Cardiol*. 2009;53(22):2028–2035.

120. Cobble M, Bale B. Carotid intima-media thickness: knowledge and application to everyday practice. *Postgrad Med*. 2010;122(1):7–15.

121. Farley TA, Dalal MA, Mostashari F, et al. Deaths preventable in the U.S. by improvements in the use of clinical preventive services. *Am J Prev Med*. 2010;38:684–685.

122. Kones R. Is prevention a fantasy, or the future of medicine? Status of prevention performance. *Ther Adv Cardiovasc Dis*. 2011;5(1):61–81.

123. Sachdeva A, Cannon DP, Deedwania PC, et al. Lipid levels in patients hospitalized with coronary artery disease. An analysis of 136,905 hospitalizations in Get With The Guidelines. *Am Heart J*. 2009;157:111–117.

124. Hajjar I, Kotchen TA. Trends in prevalence, awareness, treatment, and control of hypertension in the United States 1988–2000. *JAMA*. 2003;290:199–206.

8

Comanaging Disorders Commonly Associated with Diabetes

Expecting the world to treat you fairly
because you are a good person is a little like
expecting the bull not to attack you because
you are a vegetarian.
—*Dennis Wholey, 20th/21st-century self-help
author and journalist*

Diabetes is associated with a number of chronic disease states often seen within the primary care setting, such as peripheral arterial disease (PAD), pulmonary disorders, Parkinson disease (PD), cancer, sleep disorders, and hearing loss. The pathogenic pathways shared between diabetes and these associated disorders often involve expression of oxidative stress, inflammation, and increased insulin resistance. Recognition of the cause-and-effect relationship may afford primary care physicians a window of opportunity to screen high-risk patients for these important disorders. Conversely, if these ailments are undiagnosed or managed inappropriately, they may adversely affect glycemic control.

- Patients with *PAD* are at risk for critical leg ischemia and amputation as well as coronary artery disease.
- Chronic hyperglycemia and hyperlipidemia can induce inflammation of the blood–brain barrier leading to *PD* in susceptible individuals.
- Patients with *asthma and chronic obstructive pulmonary disease (COPD)* are twice as likely to develop diabetes than age-matched controls. The true challenge for PCPs is to train those patients requiring glucocorticoids how to skillfully manage their gycemic variability.
- Patients with diabetes have a higher incidence of all forms of *cancer* and significantly greater rates of all-cause mortality once diagnosed with a malignancy. Coordination of care between the PCP, oncologist, and other specialists is therefore of utmost importance for these patients.
- The neuroendocrine axis of *sleep* becomes dysfunctional after just one night of insomnia or sleep deprivation. Chronic sleep disorders can increase insulin resistance, promote weight gain, and favor progression of normal glucose tolerance to clinical diabetes.
- With nearly 60% of all patients at risk for developing *hearing loss* between ages 50 and 60 years, periodic audiometric screening for diabetes patients may be appropriate.

Practicing clinicians should find the scientific correlates discussed in this chapter to be intriguing and intellectually challenging. Some of the teleologic links between hyperglycemia and other chronic disease states are unknown even among diabetes specialists. Whereas a PCP may screen a newly diagnosed patient with Parkinson disease for diabetes, the specialist would likely begin managing a patient's PD by referral, years after the diabetes control has begun to deteriorate. Thus, PCPs have an opportunity to screen, prevent and optimize diabetes care in patients with commonly observed associated disorders.

Peripheral Arterial Disease

The prevalence of PAD in the United States is 5 million persons, or 14.5% of the general population greater than 70 years of age.[1] However, the prevalence of PAD is approximately threefold greater in patients with diabetes and more often seen in a younger cohort of individuals (greater than age 50) when compared to age-matched controls.[2] Contributing risk factors for PAD include duration of diabetes, age of the patient, hyperlipidemia, body mass index (BMI), smoking history, atrial fibrillation, stroke, renal insufficiency, and a history of coronary artery bypass grafting.[3]

Clinical Presentation and Pathogenesis

PAD manifests as insufficient tissue perfusion caused by areas of atherosclerosis, which may be acutely exacerbated by embolic or thrombotic disease. The Arterial Disease Detection, Awareness, and Treatment in Primary Care (PARTNERS) study screened asymptomatic patients in 350 primary care offices within the United States for PAD. Patients eligible for screening [using ankle brachial index (ABI) testing] included those aged ≥70 years, or persons aged 50 to 69 years with a history of cigarette smoking or diabetes. PAD was detected in 29% of the 7,000 patients screened.[4] Fewer than 10% of patients with PAD had classic symptoms of exercise-induced claudication. The vast majority of patients experienced "atypical symptoms." Moreover, only 49% of physicians correlated patient symptomatology as being representative of PAD prior to screening.

During exercise, blood flow cannot maximally increase through muscles oxygenated via proximally occluded arteries. When the metabolic demands of the muscle exceed blood flow, claudication ensues. Patients also experience a longer recovery period for claudication to ease, during which time normal blood flow resumes within the affected muscle. Aortoiliac disease (Fig. 8-1) manifests as pain in the thighs and buttocks, whereas femoral–popliteal PAD presents as calf pain. Symptoms of PAD are precipitated by walking a predictable distance and are relieved by rest.

PAD is characterized as being either acute or chronic, each with different etiologies (Table 8-1). Acute ischemia most often results from an embolus originating from the heart (secondary to valvular insufficiency or atrial fibrillation). Alternatively, the origin of an embolism can be debris from an atherosclerotic plaque in the aorta or a large peripheral vessel such as the superficial femoral artery. The embolic occlusion most commonly occurs at the arterial bifurcation points of the aorta, iliac, femoral, or popliteal artery. Patients experience a sudden onset of lower extremity pain initially in the feet and toes, which progresses proximally within a short time. The symptoms may be partially and temporarily relieved by placing the extremity in a dependent position. In chronic disease, symptoms are less severe because collateral circulation around the occluded vessel is well developed, minimizing the pain of exercise-induced ischemia.

Patients with chronic PAD will typically relate their onset of pain to a particular walking distance (e.g., 1 block claudication). Claudication due to PAD is reproducible within the same muscle group that has obstructed arterial flow. The pain stops within 2 to 5 minutes of initiating rest. Chronic arterial occlusive disease may be difficult to diagnose prospectively because many patients have atypical claudicatory symptoms. Screening patients at risk for PAD using a Doppler ABI may allow physicians the opportunity to identify patients with PAD and initiate a proactive approach to slow disease progression.[5] More importantly, these patients are at higher risk for cardiovascular ischemic events and mortality. Identifying patients with PAD will allow the timely initiation of statins and antiplatelet agents.

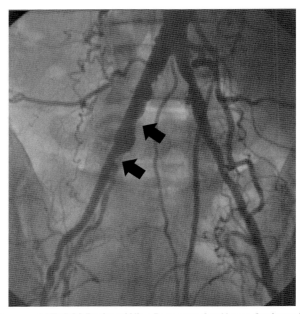

Figure 8-1 • **A 56-year-old T2DM Patient Who Presents for Heart Catheterization Due to Medical Failure of Antianginal Drugs.** Prior to heart catheterization, the patient was noted by the nurse to have poor leg pulses. This patient has significant right-sided aortofemoral disease (*arrows*) secondary to severe atherosclerosis. (Photograph courtesy of Robert Chilton, DO.)

 TABLE 8-1. Differentiation of Acute and Chronic Peripheral Arterial Disease

	Acute Ischemia	Chronic Ischemia
Risk factors	Valvular heart disease, atrial fibrillation History of cardiac catheterization, hypertension, diabetes, smoking, family history of CVD, hyperlipidemia	Atherosclerosis, diabetes, smoking, BMI, hypertension, hyperlipidemia
Etiology	Embolic	Occlusive mural thrombus
Historical clues	No prior history of intermittent claudication Known source of embolic etiology	History of intermittent claudication History of coronary heart disease
Clinical signs	Limb is pale and pulseless Paresthesias develop followed by paralysis	May be asymptomatic or symptoms may be atypical Pain with ambulation; subsides with rest Hair loss Brittle nails Dry, scaly, atrophic skin Dependent rubor Pallor with leg elevation after 1 min at 60 degrees (normal color should return in 10–15 sec; longer than 40 sec indicates severe ischemia) Ischemic tissue ulceration (punched-out, painful, with little bleeding), gangrene Absent or diminished femoral or pedal pulses Arterial bruits

(Continued)

TABLE 8-1. Differentiation of Acute and Chronic Peripheral Arterial Disease *(Continued)*

	Acute Ischemia	Chronic Ischemia
Pain trigger	Acute embolic etiology or in situ plaque thrombosis	Intermittent claudication, characterized by cramping, tightness, or tired sensation induced by exercise Pain location in buttock, hip, thigh, calf, foot Distance to claudication is consistent Pain does *not* occur with standing and is relieved by cessation of activity
Appearance	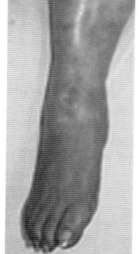Fixed, mottled, cyanotic limb	Ischemic, necrotic toes, with multiple erythematous granulating lesions on dorsum of foot (Note, most patients have no visual findings on examination)
Diagnostic workup	Arteriography	ABI for screening Magnetic resonance angiography for imaging large and small vessels
Treatment	Anticoagulation Thrombolytic therapy Surgical intervention Embolectomy Percutaneous angioplasty	Improved walking distance and ABI have been attributed to smoking cessation Walk 45–60 min daily. Walk until claudication occurs. Rest until pain subsides, then resume exercise. Customize the metabolic management of patient's disease state. Control diabetes, lipids, and blood pressure Cilostazol (Pletal) 50–100 mg b.i.d Percutaneous angioplasty followed by surgical intervention Stenting

Adapted from Cronenwett JL, Warner KG, Zelenock GB, et al. Intermittent claudication: current results of nonoperative management. *Arch Surg.* 1984;119(4):430–436; Couch NP. On the arterial consequences of smoking. *J Vasc Surg.* 1986;3(5):807–812; Conen D, Everett BM, Kurth T, et al. Smoking, smoking status, and risk for symptomatic peripheral artery disease in women: a cohort study. *Ann Intern Med.* 2011;154(11):719–726; Rowe VL, Lee W, Weaver FA, et al. Patterns of treatment for peripheral arterial disease in the United States: 1996-2005. *J Vasc Surg.* 2009;49(4):910–917; Krajewski LP, Olin J. Atherosclerosis of the aorta and the lower extremities. In: Young JR, Graor RA, Olin J, Bartholomew JR, eds. *Peripheral Vascular Diseases.* Chicago, IL: Mosby Year Book; 1991:18.

Screening Patients for PAD

PAD predicts future all-cause mortality. A recently published observational study of 6,292 patients suggested that patients with diabetes and hypertension [but no prior history of cardiovascular disease (CVD)] who had a normal resting ABI had a 41.2% 10-year mortality rate if their *postexercise* ABI was less than 0.85. Therefore, ABI screening, especially if performed after an exercise session, may be a powerful predictor of all-cause mortality in high-risk patients.[6]

Why should an abnormal postexercise ABI be predictive of all-cause mortality? At baseline, a healthy person may have a higher measured ankle pressure than arm pressure. When exercise begins, no change in measured blood pressure occurs in the healthy extremity as there is little or no evidence of atherosclerosis that would narrow the vessels. In the atherosclerotic limb, each stenotic segment acts to reduce the pressure head experienced by distal muscle groups. Correspondingly, at rest, the measured blood pressure at the ankle is less than that of a healthy person. Once physical activity starts, there is increased demand for blood flow by the exercised muscles. The narrowed vessels are unable to accommodate the increase in blood flow required, and distal pressure is further reduced.

The phenomenon of increased blood flow causing decreased pressure distally to an area of stenosis is based on Poiseuille's law (Fig. 8-2). In the 19th century, this French physician performed numerous experiments using liquid and cylindric tubes. He observed that flow rate of liquid through a tube is proportional to the radius of the cylindrical tube raised to the fourth power and inversely proportional to the length of the tube and the liquid viscosity. Thus, the radius of the blood vessels is the most important factor in determining the blood flow rate. If the radius of a peripheral vessel (or coronary artery) is decreased by 50%, the blood flow through that vessel will decrease 16-fold.

In 2011, the American College of Cardiology Foundation and the American Heart Association Task Force published updated guidelines for the management of patients with PAD.[7] Patients with diabetes should be screened for PAD based on their recommendations shown in Table 8-2.

Performing the Ankle Brachial Index Test

ABI testing is a simple, painless procedure that may be performed within the primary care office (Fig. 8-3). Initial equipment costs are approximately $2,300 to $6,000. The procedure is reimbursable by private payers and Medicare under CPT Code 93922. ABI pressures must be measured using

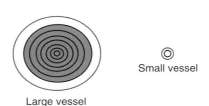

Large vessel

Small vessel

Figure 8-2 • **Poiseuille's Law.** The relationship between conductance and diameter can be explained by considering the "layers" of blood in a vessel. Per Poiseuille's law, the velocity is derived by integrating the velocities of all concentric rings of flowing blood and multiplying them by the areas of the rings. A small vessel has a large proportion of blood in contact with the walls. A larger vessel has fewer layers of blood in contact with the walls. The radius of a given vessel is the most influential factor of blood flow through that artery. Blood flowing through a large artery meets with very little resistance. However, if the radius of the artery is narrowed, resistance is raised to the fourth power and additive when two or more occlusive lesions are located sequentially within the same artery. (Modified from Sutera SP, Skalak R. The history of Poiseuille's law. *Ann Rev Fluid Mech.* 1993;25:1–19.)

TABLE 8-2. Recommendations for Performing ABI Screening for Detecting Peripheral Arterial Disease in Patients with Diabetes

- A resting ABI should be used to establish the diagnosis of PAD in high-risk patients. The ABI is calculated as the ratio of systolic blood pressure at the ankle to the arm.

- High-risk patients include those with exertional claudication, nonhealing wounds, age ≥65 y, or those age ≥50 y with a history of smoking or diabetes.

- Normal ABI values are defined as 1.00–1.40.

- Borderline ABI values are defined as 0.91–0.99.

- Abnormal ABI values are defined as ≤ 0.90

Adapted from Rooke TW, Hirsch AT, Misra S, et al. 2011 ACCF/AHA focused update of the guideline for the management of patients with peripheral artery disease (Updating the 2005 Guideline). A report of the American College of Cardiology Foundation/American Heart Association Task Force on Practice Guidelines. *Circulation.* 2011;124:00–00. DOI: 10.1161/CIR.0b013e31822e80c3.

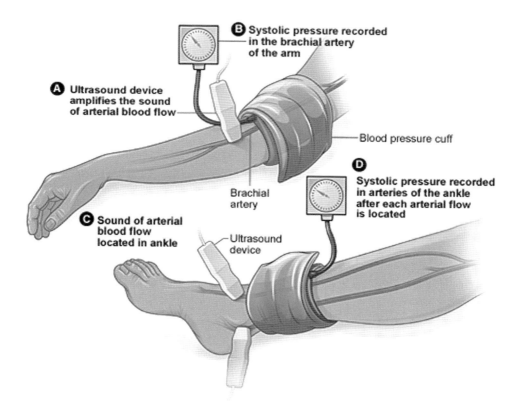

Figure 8-3 • Ankle Brachial Index Examination. A blood pressure cuff is applied to the patient's arm and inflated. A Doppler ultrasound placed at the radial artery is used to record the first sound as the cuff is deflated. The cuff is then applied to the other arm and the procedure is repeated. The highest of the two arm blood pressures is accepted as the "baseline" upper extremity reading. The cuff is then applied to the midcalf on one leg and inflated. The Doppler ultrasound is placed at the dorsalis pedis (DP) and the posterior tibial (PT) arteries to record the first sound as the cuff is deflated. The cuff is then placed on the opposite leg, and the procedure is repeated. The highest ankle pressure for each leg is used as the lower extremity "baseline" reading. The ratio of each ankle to brachial pressure is determined by dividing the ankle by the highest brachial pressure. An equal ratio implies no blockage of blood flow into the lower extremities. If the ratio of blood flow into the ankles is less than 0.9, PAD is likely to exist. A ratio of less than 0.8 correlates with symptomatic exercise induced claudication. Patients with a ratio of less than 0.4 are likely to experience pain at rest in their legs. Severe, limb-threatening PAD is diagnosed when the ratio is less than 0.25.

both the posterior tibial (PT) and the dorsalis pedis (DP) arteries. To calculate the ABI for each leg, simply use the higher of the DP or PT pressures divided by the higher of the brachial pressures from the arms. Prior to billing under CPT code 93922, discuss which ICD-9 codes are covered by each insurer for the procedure. Testing requires less than 10 minutes and may be performed by a medical assistant. The computerized interpretation printout provides a hard copy for the patient's medical record. If the ABI does not provide a hard copy of the results, the evaluation is considered to be part of the E/M service and is not separately reportable.

ABI measurements may actually be misleading in patients with diabetes because the presence of medial calcinosis renders the arteries incompressible. False elevations in ABI readings will result in suprasystolic ankle pressures (ABI > 1.3). Patients suspected of having a false elevation in their ABI readings should be referred to an accredited vascular lab where measurements of digital arterial systolic pressure (toe pressure), transcutaneous oxygen tension, and/or pulse volume recordings may be performed.[8]

◼ Management of Patients with PAD

Patients with typical symptoms of intermittent claudication represent fewer than 20% of patients with objective evidence of PAD.[9] Patients with lifestyle-interfering claudication and evidence of aortoiliac disease should undergo primary stenting as the initial therapy. Proximal atherosclerotic disease does not respond well to exercise and medical therapy. The long-term patency rates for conservative care approach those of surgical interventions without the associated morbidity, prolonged hospital stays, and recovery time.[9]

Those with disease below the inguinal ligament should undergo a trial of medical therapy consisting of a walking program and cilostazol (Pletal) 50 to 100 mg b.i.d (assuming no history of heart failure). Cilostazol has been shown to improve walking distance in patients with stable intermittent claudication in eight large randomized placebo-controlled, double-blind trials of 12 to 24 weeks.[10] If the patient does not respond to a 4-month trial of conservative management, a revascularization procedure should be considered. Nevertheless, patients with claudication progress to limb loss at a low rate of approximately 5% per year. Therefore, revascularization is best reserved for patients with favorable anatomy who fail conservative therapy and have lifestyle or vocational limiting symptoms. The therapeutic goals for such patients are symptom relief, increased walking distance, and improved functionality and quality of life.

Patients with critical limb ischemia (CLI) (rest pain, nonhealing ulcers, or gangrene) have more extensive disease than patients with intermittent claudication. As such, these individuals require a more urgent revascularization approach for limb salvation. Patients with diabetes and CLI have multilevel disease involving arteries below the knee in addition to small-vessel (microvascular) disease that may not improve even with revascularization. Patients with diabetes who smoke and present with CLI are 10 times more likely to require a nontraumatic lower extremity amputation than age-matched controls.[9] More than half of all lower extremity amputations occur in patients greater than 80 years of age. The clinical outcome for patients presenting with CLI is grim. Within 3 months of presentation, 12% will require an amputation and 9% will die.[9]

The 1-year all-cause mortality rate for patients with CLI is 22%. The Bypass versus Angioplasty in Severe Ischaemia of the Leg trial compared an initial strategy of angioplasty with vascular surgery in 452 patients with CLI.[11] The primary outcome was time to amputation or death (amputation-free survival) over 6 months. There was no statistical difference between the groups for quality of life outcomes. For the first year of follow-up, costs associated with a surgery-first strategy were higher than for angioplasty. Thus, percutaneous intervention first strategy appears to be the intervention of choice for patients who are candidates for either surgery or percutaneous angioplasty. Aortoiliac and aortofemoral bypass procedures are associated with 74% and 95% 5-year patency rates, respectively, which are comparable, yet not superior to percutaneous therapies.[12,13]

Patients with aortoiliac disease are being managed with percutaneous kissing-balloon-expandable stents designed to scaffold the lumen and prevent embolization rather than simply employing balloon angioplasty.[14]

Medical therapy, percutaneous angioplasty, and surgery have been compared in several trials in symptomatic patients with femoral–popliteal disease. While angioplasty may provide for a better short-term improvement in claudication, the benefits of exercise are not only longer lasting but also multifactorial and should always be the initial treatment recommendation in these patients.[15], Revascularization procedures (either angioplasty or surgery) offer significant advantages compared with medical therapy for improvement in walking distance.[16]

Peripheral artery stents may be recommended as salvage therapy for patients with femoral, popliteal, and tibial PAD who have failed angioplasty (residual diameter stenosis greater than 50% or flow-limiting dissection).[17] Stents may also be feasible for long or heavily calcified lesions.

Below-knee angioplasty is reserved for patients with CLI or those individuals with severe claudication due to extensive multilevel disease. Limb-salvage rates at 2 to 5 years are 80% to 90% with modern endovascular techniques.[9] Success is determined by relief of rest pain, healing rate of ulcers, and avoidance of limb loss.

Newer therapies for the minimally invasive endovascular treatment of claudication and CLI include rotational and orbital atherectomy for which there are no long-term or comparative results. Short-term results have been promising, but these technologies may be more expensive than conventional therapies. At this time, surgery still provides the best long-term patency and limb salvage results when compared to all other modalities. Alternatively, surgical revascularization is associated with higher morbidity and mortality rates than endovascular therapies. Which modality to choose for a particular patient depends upon the pattern and extent of arterial disease, indications for the procedure, coexisting complications, and the projected life span of the patient. Clinical trials are currently assessing the safety and efficacy of minimally invasive drug-eluting stents as well as balloon and biodegradable stents. These devices may provide better long-term patencies and improved limb salvation outcomes while lessening the morbidity associated with surgical revascularization.

A summary of the current recommendations for medical and surgical interventions related to PAD is displayed in Table 8-3.

Parkinson Disease

The risk of PD is approximately 40% greater among patients who have had diabetes for longer than 10 years compared with euglycemic individuals.[18] Common pathogenic processes such as chronic inflammation or oxidative stress may first lead to diabetes and then, years later, to a higher risk of PD. Diabetes may also predispose patients to insulin dysregulation and subsequent neurodegeneration. Insulin receptors are expressed in the substantia nigra. The two major neuropathic findings in patients with PD are loss of pigmented dopaminergic neurons in the substantia nigra and the presence of Lewy bodies. Approximately 70% of dopaminergic neurons are lost before the motor signs of PD emerge. Although Lewy bodies are not specific to PD, their presence within the substantia nigra is believed to represent the presymptomatic phase of the disorder.[19]

Patients with PD demonstrate decreased stimulation of dopamine within the basal ganglia.[20] In animal models, reduced dopamine levels are observed in the insulin-resistant state and normalize as rodents become insulin sensitive.[21] Consistent with these observations in animals, administration of bromocriptine (a sympatholytic D2-dopamine agonist) improves glycemic control in patients with T2DM.[22]

Hyperglycemia, which contributes to endothelial dysfunction, may also favor neurodegeneration as supported by the association between PD incidence and diabetes duration.[23] Insulin acts as a growth factor in the brain and reduces oxidative stress, whereas insulin resistance decreases the transport of insulin into the brain.[24] The densely concentrated insulin receptors located in the

TABLE 8-3. Management of Patients with Peripheral Arterial Disease

Management Modality	Recommendations
Smoking cessation	• Patients who smoke or former smokers should be asked about status of tobacco use at every visit • Counsel patients on smoking cessation at every visit • Unless contraindicated, pharmacologic interventions may include varenicline, bupropion, and nicotine replacement therapy
Antiplatelet therapy	• Antiplatelet therapy can be useful to reduce the risk of MI, stroke, or vascular death in asymptomatic individuals with an ABI ≤0.90 • Aspirin 75–325 mg/d is recommended as safe and effective therapy to reduce the risk of MI, stroke, or vascular death in patients with symptomatic PAD, CLI, prior lower extremity revascularization, or prior amputation for lower extremity ischemia • Clopidogrel 75 mg/d is an effective alternative antiplatelet therapy to aspirin to reduce the risk of MI, ischemic stroke, or vascular death in patients with symptomatic PAD, CLI, prior lower extremity revascularization, or prior amputation for lower extremity ischemia • The combination of aspirin + clopidogrel may be considered to reduce the risk of CV events in patients with symptomatic atherosclerotic PAD • Warfarin is of no benefit and is potentially harmful when used in patients with PAD due to an increased risk of major bleeding
Critical limb ischemia: Endovascular and open surgical limb salvage	• Patients with combined inflow and outflow disease with CLI should have inflow lesions addressed initially • For patients with combined inflow and outflow disease in whom symptoms of CLI or infection persist after inflow revascularization, an outflow revascularization procedure should be performed • Balloon angioplasty is reasonable to perform for patients with limb-threatening lower extremity ischemia and an estimated life expectancy of ≤2 y to improve distal blood flow • For patients with limb-threatening ischemia and an estimated life expectancy of ≥2 y, bypass surgery is reasonable to perform as the initial treatment to improve distal blood flow

Adapted from Rooke TW, Hirsch AT, Misra S, et al. 2011 ACCF/AHA focused update of the guideline for the management of patients with peripheral artery disease (Updating the 2005 Guideline). A report of the American College of Cardiology Foundation/American Heart Association Task Force on Practice Guidelines. *Circulation.* 2011;124:00–00. DOI: 10.1161/CIR.0b013e31822e80c3.

substantia nigra appear to play a role in the expression of central dopamine concentrations, which is deficient in PD.[25]

T2DM and hyperlipidemia may induce a chronic inflammatory pathway, leading to destruction of both pancreatic islet β-cells and dopaminergic neurons in the substantia nigra. The brain is considered an immunologically privileged organ, free from immune attack due to the protection afforded by the blood–brain barrier. However, with aging and under conditions of chronic inflammation, the blood–brain barrier becomes breached and more permeable. Consequently, proinflammatory factor, reactive oxygen species, and neurotoxins may cross the blood–brain barrier and induce neurodegeneration. Both central and peripheral inflammation appears to be dysregulated in patients with PD.[26]

Although the direct relationship between PD and diabetes is unclear, patients with PD should certainly be screened for diabetes and lipid disorders. What is uncertain is whether improving one's hyperglycemia or other metabolic abnormalities will influence outcomes for patients who are afflicted with both disorders.

Anectodotal observations suggest that some patients with advanced PD and symptoms such as dysphagia and bradykinesia and diabetes may experience temporary improvement with exenatide and exanatide LAR. However, additional clinical trials must be performed prior to advocating the preferential use of any antidiabetes drug in patients with PD.

COPD, Asthma, and Glucocorticoid-induced Hyperglycemia

In a prospective cohort study involving 100,000 women, subjects with COPD had a statistically significant increased risk of developing T2DM.[27] Inflammatory markers that are increased in patients with T2DM have been observed to be up-regulated in patients with COPD, suggesting that inflammation may be a common link. Elevated levels of CRP, IL-6, and TNF-α are linked to the development of insulin resistance in T2DM, supporting a role for inflammation in the pathogenesis of diabetes.[27] In addition, patients with COPD tend to minimize their exercise capacity, leading to an increase in adipose tissue mass and a subsequent rise in systemic markers of inflammation. The link between systemic inflammation may be persistent even when weight loss is not apparent.[28]

A population-based retrospective database study comparing medical records of 2,392 patients with asthma with those of 4,784 age-matched controls suggested that the incidence rate for diabetes was 188.6 per 100,000 versus 134 per 100,000 within the control group. Patients with asthma are twice as likely to have coexisting diabetes.[29] The hazard ratio for CVD in this study was 1.48 ($p = 0.0349$) indicating that a diagnosis of asthma increases one's probability of developing both diabetes and heart disease. The authors of the study suggest that inflammatory, environmental, and genetic mechanisms may be implicated as mediators for all three disease states.

Youths with dual diagnoses of T1DM and asthma have a higher mean A1C than those with diabetes alone (7.77% vs. 7.49%; $p = 0.034$). Younger patients treated with leukotriene modifiers, either as monotherapy or in combination with rescue or other inhaled medications, had the best glycemic control. A total of 72% of these patients were considered as having "good control" among all groups of medication users. Those patients who were receiving no drug therapy for asthma had the highest A1Cs in the study.[30] The suggestion is that specific asthma medications may both decrease systemic inflammation and have a positive effect on long-term glycemic control.

Effect of Glucocorticoids on Glycemic Control

Patients with diabetes and coexisting COPD or asthma may require glucocorticoids during periods of acute exacerbations. Other patients, such as those with rheumatoid arthritis, are often prescribed maintenance doses of steroids. Glucocorticoids are not only the most common cause of drug-induced diabetes, they also are likely to induce severe postprandial hyperglycemia in patients with preexisting diabetes.

Glucocorticoids induce a state of insulin resistance rather than decrease insulin production. In euglycemic subjects, the liver decreases its glucose output in response to insulin. However, glucocorticoids decrease the liver's sensitivity to insulin, thereby increasing hepatic glucose output.[31] Steroids also inhibit glucose uptake in muscle and fat, reducing insulin sensitivity as much as 60% in healthy volunteers due to a postreceptor defect.[32] The peak effect of prednisone on glycemic excursions occurs between 4 and 6 hours after dosing and persists for up to 16 hours.

Prednisone does not affect fasting plasma glucose levels if given once daily in the morning at doses of ≤30 mg. Short-term medium-dose prednisone (20 mg per day for 3 days induces postprandial hyperglycemia in T2DM and in patients with prediabetes from midday to midnight due to suppression of insulin secretion followed by decreased insulin action that dissipates overnight.[33] Insulin requirements may double, depending on the glucocorticoid dose. For patients with T1DM taking prednisone 60 mg daily for 3 days, mean blood glucose levels increased 30 mg per dL and persisted for 24 hours after the drug was discontinued. Insulin doses increased on average 69% for patients with T1DM using prednisone for just 3 days.[34]

Targeted Glycemic Management for Patients with Diabetes Using Glucocorticoids

The random or 1 to 2 hour postprandial glycemic target for patients treated with chronic or acute steroid therapy is less than 220 mg per dL. Patients with T2DM should have their doses of OADs titrated to minimize these postprandial excursions as shown in Table 8-4.

Glucose levels exceeding 300 mg per dL result in symptomatic hyperglycemia (e.g., fatigue, polyuria, polydipsia) as well as activation of oxidative stress pathways favoring vascular inflammation. Patients managing asthma or autoimmune disorders with chronic steroids will either need to initiate insulin therapy or adjust their prescribed dose of insulin based on postprandial glycemic excursions.

Patients who had been using only basal insulin and have not experienced a significant increase in fasting glucose levels should minimize postprandial excursions by initiating a rapid-acting

TABLE 8-4. Therapeutic Options to Optimize Glycemic Control for Patients Using Glucocorticoids

	Random or 1–2 Postprandial Glucose 140–220 mg/dL	Random or 1–2 Postprandial Glucose 220–300 mg/dL	Random or 1–2 Postprandial Glucose >300 mg/dL
Suggested Therapeutic Options	• Metformin 850–100 mg b.i.d with food • DPP-4 inhibitor • GLP-1 agonist • Meglitinides (longer-acting forms of sulfonylureas may not be suitable if the fasting plasma glucose is normal)	Metformin + sulfonylurea Metformin + DPP-4 Metformin + meglintinide Metformin + GLP-1 agonist	Insulin

DPP-4, Dipeptidyl peptidase-4 inhibitor, GLP-1, Glucagon-like peptide agonist.
Adapted from Lansang MC. Glucocorticoid-induced diabetes and adrenal suppression: how to detect and manage them. *Cleve Clin J Med.* 2011;78 (11) 748–756.

analogue (lispro, glulisine, or aspart) at each meal. The dose of the rapid-acting insulin is calculated as 0.1 U per kg per meal. Thus, a 100-kg person would require 10 U of insulin injected 15 minutes prior to eating. Due to the increased insulin resistance caused by the use of prednisone, consider increasing the baseline dose of prandial insulin by 10% to 20% targeting a 2-hour postmeal glucose value of less than 180 mg per dL. Patients who also experience a rise in fasting glucose levels while on steroids can increase their basal insulin dose by 1 U each night until their fasting levels are less than 110 mg per dL.

Patients who are insulin naive and require chronic glucocorticoid therapy may also be placed on a mixed insulin analogue (bi-aspart 70/30, lispro mix 50/50, and lispro mix 75/25). The initial dose may be calculated as 0.3 U per kg per day. For example, a 100-kg patient with T2DM who has been taking a DPP-4 inhibitor plus metformin should add 30 U of a mixed insulin analogue once daily at lunch if postprandial glucose values consistently exceed 300 mg per dL. Dose titrations should be made every 2 to 3 days until the patient has achieved the 2-hour postmeal glucose target of less than 180 mg per dL.

Frequent paired glucose testing should be suggested for all diabetes patients using acute or chronic steroid regimens. Glucose values are monitored fasting, as well as before and 2 hours after each meal. Normal 2-hour postprandial excursions should not exceed 50 mg per dL from baseline. For example, if the prelunch glucose level is 125 mg per dL, the 2-hour postprandial glucose value should be less than 175 mg per dL. Patterns suggestive of extreme postprandial or fasting glycemic excursions would require adjustments in insulin dosing.

While tapering off steroids, glucose levels will also need to be assessed. Within 24 hours of reducing the prednisone dose to less than 7.5 mg per day, patients may be at risk of developing iatrogenic hypoglycemia unless insulin dosing is downtitrated.

▌ Cancer

The association between diabetes and cancer was first reported in the 1960s.[35] Accumulating evidence from case control and observational studies advocates an association between T2DM and cancer at multiple sites. The American Cancer Society Cancer Prevention Study II reported that, irrespective of BMI, adults with diabetes had a mortality risk from breast, colon, pancreatic, and liver cancers in excess of those without diabetes.[36,37] Patients with diabetes have a 2-fold increased risk for developing cancers of the liver, pancreas, and endometrium, and a 1.2- to 1.5-fold likelihood of developing cancers of the colon, rectum, breast, and bladder (Fig. 8-4). Other cancers, such as those arising from the lung, do not appear to be associated with diabetes.[35] The data on renal cell carcinoma, and non-Hodgkin lymphoma are inconclusive. Interestingly, few studies have explored the associated risks between T1DM and cancer. Only prostate cancer appears to have a lower risk in patients with T2DM. Although circulating testosterone levels have not been associated with prostate cancer, men with T2DM are generally noted to have reduced total and free plasma testosterone concentrations. The presence of diabetes also appears to increase the risk of all-cause mortality in patients with cancer.[38]

In 2007, 26 million Americans were estimated to be living with diabetes, whereas 12 million patients were receiving treatments for cancer.[39] Approximately 25% of people living in the developed world succumb to cancer.[40] Most patients present to their PCP with disease-state–specific symptoms. The PCP has the formidable task of determining if the individual has a benign or malignant disorder. PCPs are more experienced in diagnosing what is *not* cancer than counseling patients as to what metabolic, genetic, or lifestyle behaviors might adversely affect one's future cancer risk. Assuming that primary care is the setting in which cancer is most often diagnosed, or at least suspected, the PCP should be at the forefront of performing routine presymptomatic oncologic risk assessments in patients regardless of their glycemic status. High-risk patients should be screened for cancer according to the evidence-based guidelines shown in Table 1-6 of the Introduction chapter. One should also assess each patient's family

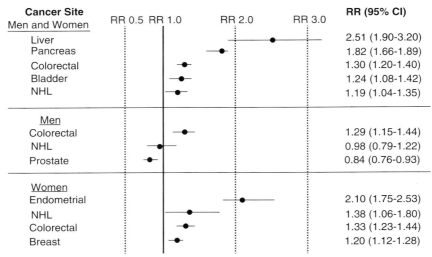

Figure 8-4 • Results of a Meta-analysis of Cohort and Case-controlled Studies Examining Cancer Risk at Specific Sites in Patients with Diabetes. The *dots* represent relative risk and the *bars* represent 95% confidence intervals (CI). NHL, non-Hodgkin lymphoma. (Modified from Gallagher EJ, Fierz Y, Ferguson RD, et al. The pathway from diabetes and obesity to cancer, on the route to targeted therapy. *Endocrine Pract.* 2010;16(5):864–873.)

history and modifiable risk factors (smoking, obesity, and alcohol use). Clinicians should be willing to comanage a cancer patient's metabolic disorders in consultation with oncologic and surgical specialists.

Relationship between Obesity, Diet, Physical Activity, Diabetes, and Cancer

Overweight individuals (BMI ≥ 30 kg per m²) have a higher cancer risk compared with those individuals having normal BMIs (18.5 to less than 25 kg per m²). The cancers most consistently associated with obesity are breast, colon, endometrium, pancreas, esophagus, gallbladder, kidney, liver, and prostate.[35] Unfortunately, the positive benefits of intentional weight loss on reducing one's risk of cancer are less certain. The Nurses' Health Study did demonstrate a statistically significant inverse association between weight loss and postmenopausal breast cancer.[41] The role of bariatric surgery in reducing cancer occurrence and mortality has not been established through prospective trials.

Diets that are low in red and processed meats but high in vegetables, fruits, and whole grains are associated with a lower cancer risk. Adding fiber to meals will protect against T2DM and improve insulin sensitivity.[42,43] Physical activity may prevent colon, breast, and endometrial cancers while improving metabolic outcomes in patients with T2DM.[35,44]

The relationship between diabetes and cancer occurrence has preventive, behavioral, and therapeutic implications as outlined in Table 8-5. Clearly, lower levels of adiposity, healthy diets, and regular physical activity are associated with reduced risk of both T2DM and several common types of cancer. However, these risk factors are interrelated, making the individual contribution of each component difficult to assess. Little is known about how modifiable lifestyle factors actually influence the prognosis of cancer patients. Still, one could speculate as to which biologic mechanisms in patients with diabetes may influence the neoplastic process.

TABLE 8-5. Implied Pathogenic Associations between T2DM and Cancer

Speculated Associations That May Increase Cancer Risk among Patients with Diabetes	Clinical Implications
Insulin is produced by the pancreatic β-cells and then transported via the portal vein to the liver. In cases of severe insulin resistance, more endogenous insulin is produced, increasing the exposure of the liver and pancreas to insulin receptor binding	Obesity increases insulin resistance. Weight reduction may be useful in reducing insulin resistance.
Insulin resistance increases steatosis and nonalcoholic fatty liver disease. This could increase the risk of liver cancer	Identify and treat patients with insulin resistance and steatosis. Lifestyle intervention is certainly appropriate. Also, screen patients for sleep apnea.
Smoking and obesity have been implicated as risk factors in pancreatic cancer	Among individuals with a history of diabetes for >5 y, the relative risk of developing pancreatic cancer is ~50% lower than for patients in whom the disease history is shorter. Patients with newly diagnosed T2DM should be counseled to stop smoking. Weight loss should be encouraged.
Dietary influences	Diets low in red and processed meats and high in vegetables, fruits, and whole grains are associated with a lower cancer risk. The addition of high fiber to meals will protect against T2DM and improve insulin sensitivity.
Physical inactivity	30 min of moderate-intensity exercise, such as walking at least 5 d a week, reduces risk of diabetes progression in patients with prediabetes.
Alcohol increases the risk of cancers of the mouth, pharynx, esophagus, liver, colon, and female breast. Excess alcohol consumption also increases risk of developing diabetes in both men and women	Address alcohol consumption. Refer for counseling if necessary.
IGF-1, and IGF-2 signaling through the insulin receptor and IGF-1 receptor can induce tumorigenesis by up-regulating the insulin receptor and IGF-1 receptor signaling pathways.	Disrupting these receptors or blocking their activity in animal models prevents tumor growth and metastasis by inhibiting downstream signaling.
Chronic hyperglycemia favors tumor growth via glycolysis	Uncertain as to whether improvement in glycemic control will reduce incidence of tumors or slow tumor growth
Inflammatory cytokines enhance cancer cell proliferation while suppressing host anti-tumor immunity.	Obesity and sleep apnea may trigger the release of inflammatory cytokines in patients with diabetes. Uncertain whether behavioral therapy or CPAP may mitigate cancer risk.

Adapted from Canonici A, Steelant W, Rigot V, et al. Insulin-like growth factor-I receptor, E-CVDherin and alpha v integrin form a dynamic complex under the control of alpha-catenin. *Int J Cancer*. 2008;122:572–582; Huxley R, Mansary-Moghaddam A, Berrington de Gonzalez A. Type-II diabetes and pancreatic cancer: a meta analysis of 36 studies. *Br J Cancer*. 2005;92:2076–2083; Kastorini CM, Panagiotakos DB. Dietary patterns and prevention of type 2 diabetes: from research to clinical practice; a systematic review. *Curr Diabetes Rev*. 2009;5:221–227; Kushi LH, Byers T, Doyle C, et al. American Cancer Society 2006 Nutrition and Physical Activity Guidelines Advisory Committee. American Cancer Society guidelines on nutrition and physical activity for cancer prevention: reducing the risk of cancer with healthy food choices and physical activity. *CA Cancer J Clin*. 2006;56:254–281.

Molecular Biology of the Insulin Growth Factor-1 Receptor

Insulin growth factor-1 (IGF-1) is a polypeptide hormone similar in molecular structure to insulin. The IGF-1 receptor (IGF-1R) mediates the effects of IGF-1 at the sites of target tissues throughout the body (Fig. 8-5). The IGF-1R and insulin receptors share 60% homology. Once activated by a ligand, postreceptor signaling occurs within the targeted tissue, which could affect tumorigenesis. IGF-1R has been implicated in breast, prostate, and lung cancers.[45] Increased levels of the IGF-IR are expressed in the majority of primary and metastatic prostate cancer tumor cells.[46]

Insulin is produced by the pancreatic β-cells, whereas IGF-1 is synthesized primarily in the liver in response to the growth hormone action. Insulin increases the expression of growth hormone receptors while enhancing postreceptor signaling. Thus, hyperinsulinemia may lead to increased production of IGF-1. IGF-1 plays an important role in childhood growth and continues to have anabolic effects in adults. Selective receptor activation of either IGF-1 or insulin may activate either metabolic or mitogenic effects as shown in Figure 8-6.

Does a biologic link between IGF-1 and cancer actually exist? In a cohort of men older than 50 years from the Rancho Bernardo Study, a significant association was found between IGF-1 levels and cancer mortality. Those men with an IGF-1 concentration greater than 100 ng per mL had an adjusted risk of cancer mortality of 1.82 compared with men whose IGF-1 concentration was less than 100 ng per mL.[47] Further observational studies involving persons with diabetes have reported that those treated with insulin or insulin secretagogues have an increased risk of developing cancer compared with those taking metformin. Whether these results are because secretagogues and insulin confer an increased risk, or whether metformin has a protective effect is unclear.[48] Inhaled insulin was suggested to carry an increased risk of lung cancer, although large studies were never performed to investigate this possible association before it was withdrawn from the market. In light of the epidemiologic data, the association of diabetes and obesity with the increased risk of developing cancer appears to possibly be through hyperinsulinemia and/or increased IGF-1 levels.

Elevated fasting serum insulin levels are also associated with an increase in all-cause cancer mortality in both sexes suggesting a link between cancer, diabetes, and mortality rates.[49]

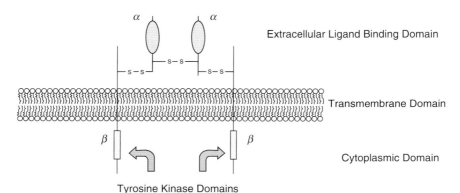

Figure 8-5 • IGF-1R Structure and Function. The IGF-1R consists of two subunits. The α chain, located extracellularly, has a 60% homology between IGF-1 and the insulin receptor. Once the receptor is activated by ligand binding, the α chain induces tyrosine autophosphorylation of the β chains, triggering a cascade of intracellular signaling events that promote cell survival and proliferation. IGF-1 binds to either the IGF-1 receptor or the insulin receptor. The IGF-IR binds IGF-1 at significantly higher affinity than the insulin receptor. Compared to insulin, IGF-1 activates the insulin receptor at 1/10th the potency of insulin. (Modified from Butler AA, Yakar S, Gewolb IH, et al. Insulin-like growth factor-I receptor signal transduction: at the interface between physiology and cell biology. *Comp Biochem Physiol B Biochem Mol Biol.* 1999;121(1):19–26.)

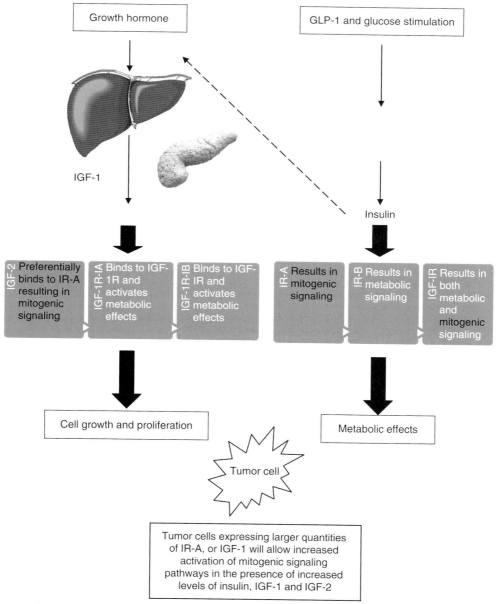

Figure 8-6 • Differentiation of IGF-1 and Insulin Receptor-binding Activity. Insulin is produced in response to glucose stimulation and GLP-1 release from the L-cells of the small intestines. The production of IGF-1 in the liver is mediated primarily by growth hormone. Insulin increases the expression of growth hormone receptors, thereby increasing growth hormone concentration in the plasma. Insulin signals primarily through insulin receptors, while IGF-1 activates the IGF-1R. Insulin receptor activation results *primarily* in changes in metabolism, whereas expression of the IGF-IR receptor results in cellular growth and proliferation. IGF-1 activation can cause relocation of transmembrane glycoproteins (integrins) to the edge of migrating cells, which enhance cancer metastasis. (Modified from Gallagher EJ, Fierz Y, Ferguson RD, et al. The pathway from diabetes and obesity to cancer, on the route to targeted therapy. *Endocrine Pract.* 2010;16(5):864–873.)

IGF-1 activation can cause relocation of transmembrane glycoproteins (integrins) to the edge of migrating cells, which enhance cancer metastasis.[50] In summary, increased insulin and IGF-1 receptor activation favors tumorigenesis. Blocking or inhibiting postreceptor signaling of the IGF-1 receptors may prevent tumor growth and metastasis.[50]

Relationship between Hyperglycemia and Tumor Growth

Hyperglycemia may directly influence cancer growth and metastasis. Many cancers are dependent upon glycolysis for energy; a metabolic pathway which is dependent upon large quantities of glucose for activation. Many tumors, therefore, become glucose dependent for growth and metastasis.[51] Positron emission tomography (PET) scanning detects pairs of gamma rays emitted indirectly by a positron-emitting tracer injected into the body. The biologically active molecule chosen for PET scanning is fluorodeoxyglucose, a glucose analogue, which accumulates in tissues of heightened metabolic activity depending on regional glucose uptake, such as rapidly growing malignant tumors.[52] (See Fig. 8-7) Whether hyperglycemia directly stimulates tumor growth or secondarily stimulates hyperinsulinemia is uncertain. Perhaps each cell type may have different modulating factors, which predispose to tumor progression.

Cytokines are molecular mediators of cellular injury. The presence of inflammatory cytokines has, in general, reflected the severity of disease and predicted future outcomes. Cytokines such as PAI-1 and IL-6 are elevated in both lean and obese patients with diabetes.[53] PA1-1 is linked to poor outcome in breast cancer patients.[54] The inflammatory cytokine, IL-6, is known to enhance cancer cell proliferation and suppress host antitumor immunity.[55]

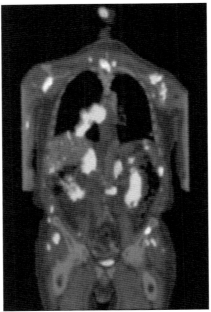

Figure 8-7 • A PET/CT Scan of a 64-year-old Man with a 12-year History of T1DM and Metastatic Lung Cancer. An intravenous injection of radioactive glucose (fluorodeoxyglucose) is administered to the patient. Cancer cells are highly metabolic and rapidly synthesize the radioactive glucose at primary and metastatic sites. This patient was found to have multiple metastases to the shoulders, pelvis, abdominal lymph nodes, and right adrenal gland. The primary tumor is seen in the right hilum. (Photo courtesy of Jeff Unger, MD.)

Practical Therapeutic Strategies That May Minimize Cancer Risk in Patients with T2DM

Therapeutic interventions for patients with T2DM should be directed toward safe and efficacious glycemic control while minimizing one's potential risk of developing cancer. No specific drug has been endorsed as being the "preferred antihyperglycemic agent" in high-risk cancer patients. Nevertheless, primary care physicians should be familiar with the defined risks and benefits each therapeutic options has in relation to minimizing cancer risk in patients with T2DM.

• Metformin

A prospective study following patients using metformin for 9.6 years found that cancer mortality was reduced by approximately 50% versus patients not taking metformin at baseline (Fig. 8-8).[56] The benefits of metformin related to cancer mortality appear to be dose related. The hazard ratio for cancer mortality decreased 42% for every 1 g increase in metformin dose. Patients with T2DM who were not taking metformin demonstrated an increased cancer mortality ratio compared with that of the general population, whereas the use of metformin inferred a mortality risk equal to that of the general population. In laboratory studies, metformin has been shown to inhibit cell proliferation, reduce colony formation, and cause partial cell cycle arrest in cancer cell lines.[57]

Controversy notwithstanding a meta-analysis of 2,126 abstracts, 55 publications, and 12 randomized controlled trials failed to support the hypothesis that metformin lowers cancer risk.[58] However, few would argue that metformin remains the foundation of drug therapy for patients with T2DM. Further research is needed to establish whether metformin is a definite beneficial causal factor in reducing the risk of cancer mortality.

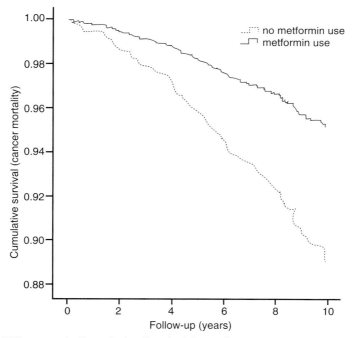

Figure 8-8 • Differences in Cumulative Survival Curve for 10-year Cancer Mortality for Patients Using Metformin versus Not Using Metformin. In patients with T2DM, after a median follow-up time of 9.6 years, metformin use at baseline was associated with a 50% reduction in cancer-related mortality. The mortality of patients taking metformin was comparable with that of the general population. (Modified from Landman GWE, Kleefstra N, Van Hateren KJJ, et al. Metformin associated with lower cancer mortality in type 2 diabetes. ZODIAC-16. *Diabetes Care.* 2010.33:322–326.)

• Pioglitazone

Bladder cancer occurs in 20 per 100,000 persons per year in the United States with the risk being higher in patients with diabetes.[59] (FDA Drug Safety Podcast: http://www.fda.gov/Drugs/DrugSafety/DrugSafetyPodcasts/ucm226749.htm; accessed on January 5, 2012). Risk factors for bladder cancer include cigarette smoking, urinary tract infections, occupational exposure to aromatic amines and polycyclic aromatic hydrocarbons, and the use of certain drugs (e.g., cyclophosphamide, glucocorticosteroids).[60] Genetic factors also play an important role in determining bladder cancer risk. Mutations in several genes (*FGFR3*, *RB1*, *HRAS*, *TP53*, and *TSC1*) affect one's ability to completely and safely metabolize certain drugs or environmental chemicals. This increases one's sensitivity and exposure mitogenic agents such as nicotine and other chemicals. Bladder cancer is not an inherited disease. Yet, some individuals may be carriers of genetic variants for certain alleles similar to BRCA2 genes, which increase one's odds ratio of developing breast, pancreas, and ovarian cancer. Inheritance of the "wimp SNPs" are likely to reduce one's ability to detoxify carcinogens within the bladder, minimize localized control of cell death and maintenance of bladder cell DNA integrity.[61]

Reports recorded between 2004 and 2009 in the FDA Adverse Event Reporting System (AERS) related to bladder cancer in patients with diabetes were recently analyzed and published.[62] Ninety-three reports of bladder cancer were retrieved corresponding to 138 drug-reaction pairs. Pioglitazone was noted to increase the risk of bladder cancer in patients exposed to the drug for over 2 years.

A link between pioglitazone and bladder cancer first appeared in preclinical studies and was initially reported on the U.S. pioglitazone label in 1999. Although animal models suggested that the association may be a rat-specific phenomenon, the large PROactive (PROspective pioglitAzone Clinical Trial In macroVascular Events) study demonstrated 14 cases of bladder cancers in the pioglitazone arm (0.5%) versus 6 in the placebo arm (0.2%).[63] In September 2010, the FDA mandated that Takeda conduct a 10-year observational study to address the possible risk of bladder cancer in humans exposed to pioglitazone.[64]

On June 13, 2011, the FDA stated that "patients who have used the highest dose of pioglitazone (45 mg) for more than 1 year should be aware of the association between bladder cancer and high dose pioglitazone therapy."[65] The directive noted that patients using pioglitazone for more than 1 year showed a 40% higher risk of bladder cancer. However, a review of the 5-year interim results of an ongoing, 10-year epidemiologic study described in FDA's September 2010 ongoing safety review showed that there was no overall increased risk of bladder cancer with pioglitazone. Consequently, the FDA recommended that no patient with urinary bladder cancer or a prior history of such a malignancy be started or maintained on pioglitazone without a thorough evaluation and informed consent provided by the treating physician. Continuation of pioglitazone therapy in patients without bladder cancer is a matter for individual consideration by patients and physicians, according to the FDA.

• Sulfonylureas

A small number of observational studies found a higher risk of cancer or cancer death among individuals with diabetes treated with sulfonylureas compared with those treated with metformin or other diabetes medications.[35] Most of these studies had very few cancer cases among users of sulfonylureas, and therefore power was limited to examine associations with specific cancer sites. Studies regarding dose, duration, and persistence of use are limited.

An observational-cohort study evaluating 33,000 diabetic women treated with a single oral agent at the Cleveland Clinic from 1998 to 2006 determined that the cancer risk for sulfonylurea-exposed patients was 18% greater than for metformin use.[66]

• Incretin Therapies

Incretin-based therapies initially received approval for marketing in 2005. No impact on human cancer incidence has been observed with either the GLP-1 analogues or DPP-4 inhibitors. Preclinical trials in rodents exposed to supraphysiolic doses of liraglutide for 2 years produced C-cell adenomas in 20% of rats and 50% of mice. A subsequent study using high-dose liraglutide treatment for up to 87 weeks did not produce any signs of C-cell hyperplasia in nonhuman primates. Liraglutide did not increase calcitonin levels (a serologic marker of C-cell dysfunction) or the incidence of C-cell hyperplasia in human phase III clinical trials.[67]

GLP-1 receptors are expressed in C cells of normal rat and mice thyroids. Their density is markedly increased in rat C-cell hyperplasia, but is present in all rat medullary thyroid cancers. No GLP-1 or GIP receptors are detected in *normal* human thyroids. Whereas only 27% of all human medullary thyroid carcinomas (MTC) express GLP-1 receptors, 89% express GIP receptors in high density.[68] Because liraglutide binds to and activates the expression of GLP-1 receptors, any patients at risk for developing MTC should NOT be treated with liraglutide.[69] The risk should also be noted for patients with multiple endocrine neoplasia type 2, a constellation of pathologic conditions including MTC, primary hyperparathyroidism, and/or pheochromocytoma.[70]

MTC is a rare tumor originating in the parafollicular C-cells of the thyroid gland. Approximately 1,000 cases of MTC are reported annually, typically in patients aged 50 to 60.[71] Nearly 25% of MTC cases have a genetic predisposition due to mutations in the rearranged during transfection (RET) protooncogene encoded on chromosome 10. Asymptomatic patients who screen positive for the RET mutation should consider undergoing a prophylactic total thyroidectomy.[71] Calcitonin, a hormone secreted by thyroid C cells, is used as a biomarker for the detection of MTC. Normal calcitonin levels are less than 10 pg per mL, whereas levels exceeding 100 pg per mL are highly predictive of MTC.[72] In clinical trials, the rise in calcitonin levels for patients treated with liraglutide is similar to those subjects treated with placebo.[73]

Exenatide, liraglutide, and DPP-4 inhibitors increased β-cell proliferation in animal studies, and in one small study of a transgenic rodent model, the DPP-4 inhibitor sitagliptin was demonstrated to increase pancreatic ductal hyperplasia.[74] The clinical significance of this finding is unclear.

When prescribed to appropriate patients, the incretin class of drugs appears to offer improvement in glycemic control, weight neutrality or weight loss, and an uncertain, yet probably minimal increase in mitogenic potential.

• Insulin

Concern has arisen relating a possible link between hyperinsulinemia and cancer risk. Insulin binds to IGF-1 receptors as well as to insulin receptors as noted above. The affinity of a given insulin analogue for an IGF-1 receptor may influence mitogenic potential. Insulin receptors are also located on tumor cell surfaces as well as on targeted metabolic organ. Direct activation of the insulin receptors on cancer cells may influence their neoplastic behavior.[75,76]

In 2009, a series of widely publicized European-based epidemiologic analyses examined a possible association between cancer occurrence and the use of insulin glargine.[77–80] These studies were inconclusive and probably misleading in their interpretation of the data. Limitations among some or all of these studies included payer restrictions for insulin usage, inability to adjust for confounders such as BMI, lack of data on specific dosing regimens, limited use of glargine in Europe, resulting in small cohorts, and sparse outcomes among exposed patients, industry sponsorship, and relatively short follow-up time (1 to 3 years for cohort studies and 4 to 6 years for case-control or prospective studies).

A U.S.-based cohort study of 81,681 patients (mean age 77 years) followed for a mean of 23.1 months from 2003 to 2008 evaluated the potential risk of cancer for individuals treated with glargine versus other insulin preparations. Twenty-one percent of patients used glargine, 61% non-glargine insulin, and 18% were managed with mixed insulin. This study found no associations between glargine at any dose and increased cancer risk.[81]

Data from the ACCORD trial was assessed to determine a possible association between any insulin preparation and increased cancer risk over 5 years. Of the 10,251 patients randomized in ACCORD, insulin glargine or neutral protamine Hagedorn (NPH) was used in 79% of the intensively managed cohort and in 61% of the standardized group. Exposure to *any* insulin was not associated with an increased risk of cancer-related outcomes.[82]

Randomized clinical trial data from an open-label 5-year trial of insulin glargine versus NPH insulin did not find evidence of excess cancer risk in the insulin glargine arm among the 1,000 subjects randomized. Only 57 cancer cases developed within the glargine cohort compared with arm 62 cases in the NPH arm.[83]

The ongoing randomized ORIGIN trial (glargine vs. placebo in patients with impaired fasting glucose or newly diagnosed T2DM) is much larger; 12,000 patients randomized and followed for 6 to 7 years.[84] However, this trial is powered for cardiovascular outcomes and may not provide definitive evidence regarding cancer incidence in this high-risk population.

In summary, the currently marketed insulin preparations do not appear to be associated with an increased risk of cancer. However, any patient who is insulin resistant and obese is already at a higher risk of developing cancer. Therefore, one should look toward environmental and lifestyle factors as being the most common factors linking diabetes to cancer risk.

• Sodium–Glucose Transporter-2 Inhibitors

Of the new classes of oral agents that are currently in clinical development, those that induce renal glucosuria by targeting the renal sodium–glucose transporter-2 (SGLT2) appear to hold promise. Recent studies have shown that dapagliflozin added to metformin produced superior glycemic control versus metformin and placebo. However, faint signals of bladder and breast cancers were observed in the drug-treated cohort,[85] and in early 2012, the FDA requested additional data to evaluate the drug's benefit-risk profile.[86]

The observations of increased cancer frequency in the dapagliflozin treatment cohort is worrisome, because some patients may have actually had cancer prior to enrollment in the clinical trial, although SGLT2 is not expressed in either bladder or breast tissue.[87] Some may argue that the short duration of registry trials for dapagliflozin limits the likelihood that patients could have developed cancer as a direct result of using this agent. Dapagliflozin is the first drug in the SGLT2 class to undergo FDA review and as such will be open to careful safety scrutiny by the agency.

Canagliflozin, another SGLT-2 inhibitor is currently in phase 3b clinical trials. Unlike dapagliflozin, cancer occurrence has not been reported in any patients receiving this investigational drug.

▌ Does Diabetes Influence Mortality Rates in Cancer Patients?

Both from an acute and chronic disease state perspective, patients with diabetes are at a distinct disadvantage after being diagnosed with cancer and vice versa.

Preexisting diabetes is associated with a twofold increased risk of acute postoperative mortality across all cancer types.[88] Mortality risk appears to be heightened due to sepsis, perioperative hyperglycemia, and postoperative myocardial infarction. Therefore, oncologists, surgeons, primary care physicians, and the patients themselves must work together to optimize perioperative care for these high-risk patients.

Patients diagnosed with cancer who have preexisting diabetes have a more rapid advancement to all-cause mortality compared to cancer patients without diabetes.[38] Patients with endometrial, breast, and colon cancers are at highest risk for mortality.

Glycemic variability observed in cancer patients with glucocorticoid-induced diabetes has also been shown to impact all-cause mortality. A retrospective cohort study evaluated 66,062 blood glucose measurements obtained from 1,175 patients who underwent allogeneic hematopoietic stem cell (HSC) transplantation between 2000 and 2005.[89] HSC transplantation is a procedure in which progenitor cells capable of reconstituting normal bone marrow function are administered to a patient. The procedure is performed to eliminate a bone marrow infiltrative process, such as leukemia, or to correct a congenital immunodeficiency disorder.[90] HSC transplant patients are known to have substantial rates of nonrelapse mortality, implying that they are extremely ill at the time they receive their transplant. Not all HSC transplant patients have diabetes. However, the introduction of high-dose steroids as antirejection drugs tends to cause a treatment-emergent secondary form of diabetes. Steroid-dependent patients with hyperglycemia are placed on insulin and must monitor their blood glucose values throughout the day. Hammer et al. determined that the transplanted patients with the greatest daily glycemic variability in their blood glucose values ("malglycemia") had a 15-fold increased risk of nonrelapse mortality within 200 days of their transplant when compared with patients having the least variability ($p < 0.0001$). Thus, severe fluctuations in glycemic control on a daily basis may be more predictive of mortality in extremely ill patients with coexisting diabetes and cancer than simply having chronic hyperglycemia alone while undergoing chemotherapy.

From a clinical perspective, patients with diabetes and cancer must minimize their exposure to hyperglycemia, hypoglycemia, and glycemic variability ("malglycemia"). Hyperglycemia impairs immune function by affecting granulocyte formation, increasing the expression of proinflammatory cytokines, and inhibiting antibody production.[91]

Severe sepsis is complicated by the frequent occurrence of hypoglycemia. Hospitalizations are prolonged by episodes of severe hypoglycemia. Allograft patients appear to have a poor tolerance to glucose values less than 89 mg per dL.[89]

Malglycemia is associated with heightened morbidity and mortality most often secondary to infection. Glycemic variability is also an indicator of endogenous insulin deficiency. Patients will require higher doses of exogenous insulin, which would make them more susceptible to iatrogenic treatment-emergent hypoglycemia. Wide diurnal glycemic variability will also activate oxidative stress pathways leading to an increased state of vascular and neurologic inflammation.[92]

Summary of Strategic Comanagement of Patients with Diabetes and Cancer

Because of the heightened risk of cancer in patients with T2DM, primary care physicians should be vigilant in screening patients as per the recommended guidelines published by the American Cancer Society (Table 1-6, Chapter 1). The mounting evidence linking obesity, insulin resistance, and reduced physical activity with cancer suggests that a proactive approach to promoting healthy lifestyle choices should begin sooner, rather than later in one's life. Therapeutic choices should be based on improving glycemic control, minimizing glycemic variability, and limiting one's exposure to agents that may predispose an individual to cancer risk.

Table 8-6 summarizes the clinical implications of the associations between diabetes and cancer.

Sleep Disorders

• Relationship between Sleep and Diabetes

Sleep deprivation is a common condition in modern society. U.S. adults are sleeping on average only 6.8 hours per night, which is 1.5 hours less than we did a century ago.[93] Nearly 30% of adults report sleeping less than 6 hours per night, leading some to suggest we live in a sleep-deprived society.[94] Factors responsible for this change include increases in longer workdays/commuting time, an increase in shift and night work opportunities, and the advent of television, radio, and the Internet.

Physiologic data suggest that short-term partial sleep restriction results in striking alterations in metabolic and endocrine function such as carbohydrate tolerance (i.e., for any given plasma glucose level, the β-cells must increase insulin production in order to maintain euglycemia), insulin resistance, increased sympathetic tone, and elevated cortisol concentrations, obesity, and memory loss. These findings suggest that long-term sleep curtailment may predispose high-risk individuals

TABLE 8-6. Screening, Preventing, and Managing Cancer Risk in Patients with Diabetes in Primary Care

- T2DM is associated with an increased risk of liver, pancreas, endometrium, colon, rectum, and breast cancers. Screen ambitiously for early detection and prevention

- The association between diabetes and some cancers is strongest with aging, obesity, poor dietary habits, and reduced physical activity.

- Hyperinsulinemia, hyperglycemia, and inflammation increase cancer risk

- Healthy lifestyle choices, including low-fat diets, increased physical activity, and weight management may improve outcomes for both diabetes care and cancer mortality

- Evidence-based cancer screening recommendations for all patients regardless of their metabolic status may be found in Table 1-6, Chapter 1.

- Preferred drugs that appear to minimize cancer risk include metformin, DPP-4 inhibitors, GLP-1 agonists, and metformin. Sulfonylureas, pioglitazone, and dapagliflozin may increase cancer risk, in some patients. However, a direct link between cancers and specific drug therapies has not been proven.

- Patients with cancer should have their diabetes and metabolic control optimized prior to undergoing any operative intervention in order to minimize perioperative risk of sepsis or myocardial infarction. Communication between the oncologist, surgeon, and primary care physician is likely to reduce postoperative risk for perioperative cancer patients with coexisting diabetes.

- Bone marrow transplant patients who have steroid-induced diabetes should minimize their glycemic variability and avoid hypoglycemia, both of which can negatively impact all-cause mortality.

to overt clinical diabetes, impair glucose metabolism in patients afflicted with diabetes, and increase cardiovascular mortality.[95]

Darukhanavala et al. studied sleep pathophysiology over 13 days in 47 healthy volunteers who had a parental history of T2DM.[96] Individuals who slept on average between 4.5 and 6 hours per night felt more daytime fatigue than those who slept more than 6 hours per night. The short duration sleepers were found to be considerably more insulin resistant and had higher circulating serum insulin levels, allowing them to maintain normal glucose tolerance during the study period.

Wrist actigraphy is a means by which one measures sleep characteristics, such as exact times when one lies down, falls asleep, awakens, or experiences sleep fragmentation. Data obtained from actigraphy may be stored for months allowing researchers to observe specific sleep patterns of individuals and compare them to metabolic assessments of insulin resistance.[97] Several small observational studies using actigraphy suggest that both short- and long-duration sleepers have developed defective glucose metabolism favoring hyperglycemia over time.[98]

Insomnia has several variations as defined within clinical trial inclusion criteria. Patients with insomnia may complain of (a) inability to fall asleep within 30 minutes of going to bed more than three times per week, (b) waking up after falling asleep more than three times per week, and (c) reduced average sleep efficiency (sleep duration divided by time in bed obtained from actigraphy data of less than 80%). Insomnia patients with coexisting diabetes demonstrate a 23% higher fasting glucose level and a 48% higher fasting insulin level than subjects who have normal sleep patterns.[99] From a clinical perspective, a patient with well-controlled diabetes who has no insomnia would typically awaken with a fasting blood glucose of ≤ 140 mg per dL. A similar patient with a sleep disorder who takes any form of pharmacotherapy for hyperglycemia might awaken daily with elevated fasting glucose levels.

Sleep-restricted patients with T1DM who sleep for less than 4.5 hours in a single night experience a 14% to 21% reduction in insulin-stimulated peripheral glucose uptake.[100] Thus, chronic sleep deprivation in patients with T1DM is likely to result in insulin resistance and an increase in basal insulin dosing.

Sleep deprivation may also be used to predict the onset of clinical diabetes. A cohort of men from the Massachusetts Male Aging Study without diabetes at baseline (1987 to 1989) was followed until 2004 for the development of diabetes.[101] Average number of hours of sleep per night was grouped into the following categories: 5, 6, 7, 8, and 8 hours. Incidence rates and relative risks were calculated for the development of diabetes in each sleep duration category. Those reporting 7 hours of sleep per night served as the reference group. Men reporting either 5 to 6 hours of sleep per night or more than 8 hours of sleep per night were at a two- to threefold increased risk of developing T2DM.[95] These elevated risks were independent of age, hypertension, smoking status, self-rated health status, and education.

Can sleep disturbance be considered an independent risk factor for the development of T2DM? In a meta-analysis study of sleep literature, Cappuccio et al.[102] concluded that there is an "unambiguous increased risk of developing T2DM at either end of the distribution of sleep duration and with qualitative disturbances of sleep." Subjects averaging less than 5 to 6 hours per night of sleep have a 28% chance of developing T2DM, whereas those with difficulty maintaining sleep have an 84% likelihood of developing the disorder.

• Neuroendocrine Pathways of Sleep Dysfunction

Sleep disorders potentiate insulin resistance and promote the development of diabetes by disrupting the delicate balance between two food-intake–regulating hormones: leptin and ghrelin. Leptin is released by adipocytes and provides information about energy status to hypothalamic regulatory centers. In humans, circulating leptin levels rapidly decrease or increase in response to acute caloric shortage or surplus. Elevated plasma leptin levels *minimize* hunger and vice versa. Ghrelin is produced predominantly by the stomach. In contrast to leptin, elevation in plasma ghrelin *stimulates* appetite (Fig. 8-9).[103,104]

In a small randomized, 2-period, 2-condition crossover clinical study involving 12 healthy men, 2 days of sleep restriction, and 2 days of sleep extension under controlled conditions of caloric intake and physical activity, short sleep duration decreased leptin (−8%) and increased ghrelin levels (+18%).[105] Sleep restriction increased hunger by 24% and appetite by 23%, favoring foods with high carbohydrate content. Thus, sleep deprivation, sleep fragmentation, and insomnia appear to create a hormonal imbalance that dysregulates satiety in favor of hunger, weight gain, and insulin resistance.

The neuroendocrine and metabolic status of sleep has been studied in patients with T1DM in a laboratory environment during which euglycemic conditions were maintained. Concentrations of epinephrine, cortisol, growth hormone, and adrenocorticotropic hormone were elevated during sleep, suggesting a tendency favoring hyperglycemia and neuroendocrine stress. Serum leptin levels were similar to those of age- and BMI-matched controls.[106]

• Obstructive Sleep Apnea

Obstructive sleep apnea (OSA) syndrome is characterized by the recurrent collapse of the pharyngeal airway during sleep, which generally requires arousal to reestablish airway patency and resume breathing. Thus, the patient suffers from both sleep fragmentation (frequent arousal) and the recurrent hypoxemia and hypercapnia (accumulation of carbon dioxide) resulting from the respiratory pause. Sleep apnea patients experience decreased neurocognitive function (sleepiness, mood changes), cardiovascular complications (systemic and pulmonary hypertension, cor pulmonale, arrhythmias, myocardial infarction, and stroke), and ultimately death in severe cases. Associated symptoms include snoring, dry mouth, headaches, heartburn, nocturia, daytime fatigue, restless legs syndrome (which could be confused with the pain of diabetic peripheral neuropathy), depression, memory loss, and loss of productivity. Sleep apnea is a major risk factor for motor vehicle accidents.[107]

The prevalence of OSA among obese patients has been reported to exceed 30%, reaching as high as 50% to 98% in the morbidly obese population.[108] Sleep apnea worsens with weight gain and improves with weight loss. Current estimates reveal that 93% of women and 82% of men with moderate to severe sleep apnea remain undiagnosed.[109]

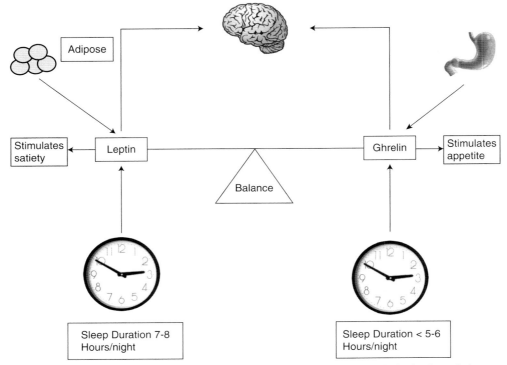

Figure 8-9 • Leptin is produced by adipose cells and acts on receptors within the hypothalamus to inhibit appetite by counteracting the potent feeding stimulation of neuropeptide Y (secreted by the gut and hypothalamus). In obese patients with sleep apnea, leptin levels are increased, yet patients are unable to lose weight corresponding with a state of "leptin resistance." Correction of sleep apnea with continuous positive airway pressure (CPAP) reverses leptin resistance. Ghrelin is produced primarily by P/D1 cells within the fundus of the stomach as well as in the epsilon cells of the pancreas. Once secreted, ghrelin increases adipose cell mass while activating receptors in the arcuate nucleus of the hypothalamus. Neuropeptide Y is expressed and appetite will increase. Ghrelin also activates other hedonic pathways that reinforce aspects of natural rewards such as food, addictive drugs, and alcohol. Patients with sleep fragmentation, insomnia, or sleep apnea or those with a history of chronic sleep deprivation (less than 5 hours per night) tend to favor the release of ghrelin over leptin. This will increase adiposity, elevated fasting blood glucose levels, insulin resistance, and a predilection for diabetes. (Taheri S, Lin L, Austin D, et al. Short sleep duration is association with reduced leptin, elevated ghrelin, and increased body mass index. *PLOS Med.* 2004;1(3):e62. 10.1371/journal.pmed.0010062.)

The clinical features, which are suggestive of obstructive sleep apnea are shown in Figure 8-10A. Although the diagnosis of sleep apnea must be confirmed by overnight polysomnography, PCPs may screen for the disorder using a device known as ApneaLink (Fig. 8-10A,B).

The ApneaLink (manufactured by ResMed Corporation) is a portable, battery-powered single-channel screening device that uses a simple nasal cannula to record a patient's breathing while asleep. The downloaded data are then summarized in a simple report that also predicts the likelihood (risk indicator) of a patient testing positive for OSA on a detailed sleep study. ApneaLink studies are useful screening tools for patients who are experiencing a rise in their A1C due to elevations in fasting glucose levels. Some centers require patients to be screened for OSA prior to undergoing metabolic (bariatric) surgery. Patients may also believe that their CPAP devices are no longer needed if they have lost some weight. ApneaLinks can be useful to determine if weight loss has, in fact, reversed the patient's apnea, hypoxia, and snoring episodes.

The sensitivity of the ApneaLink is 100% and specificity is 87.5% when the patient's apnea-hypopnea index is ≥10.[110] The ApneaLink does not discriminate obstructive from central sleep apnea because the signal is based only on airflow and there is no recording of respiratory effort. Patients

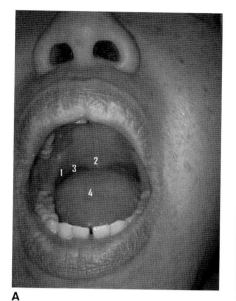
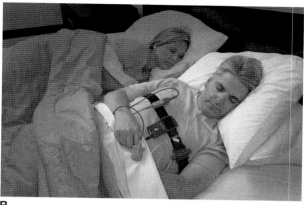

A   **B**

Figure 8-10 • (A) shows the anatomic abnormalities of the oropharynx associated with increased risk of obstructive sleep apnea: (*1*) lateral narrowing of the posterior pharynx defined by the presence of bands of tissue impinging into the observable posterior pharyngeal space, (*2*) uvular enlargement of greater than 1.5 cm in length or more than 1.0 cm in width, (*3*) low-lying soft palate defined as more than one third of the uvula extending below the level of the last molar in the mandible, and (*4*) macroglossia suggested when the tongue lies above the level of the last molar. **B.** A patient using the ApneaLink device for sleep apnea screening. (Schellenberg JB, Maislin G, Schwab RJ. Physical findings and the risk for obstructive sleep apnea: the importance of oropharyngeal structures. *Am J Respir Crit Care Med.* 2000;162:740–748; Photograph 8-10A courtesy of Jeff Unger, MD. Photograph 8-10B courtesy of ResMed, used with permission.)

who sleep on their sides while wearing the device rather than on their backs may demonstrate a false negative reading. In fact, during a patient's actual sleep study, technicians will work to keep patients sleeping on their backs during the diagnostic and titration portion of the evaluation. Table 8-7 lists the appropriate CPT and ICD codes for the ApneaLink device. An ApneaLink Plus with oximetry is a four-channel device that can be used to screen and/or diagnose patients with OSA, central apneas, and mixed apneas and to identify patients with a Cheyne-Stokes respiration pattern.

OSA is associated with sleep fragmentation, daytime sleepiness, and loss of insulin sensitivity. Babu et al. reported that 83 days on CPAP resulted in significant reduction of glucose levels as well as A1C, with a significant correlation between CPAP treatment and reduction in A1C.[111] Leptin levels are often paradoxically elevated in patients with OSA. One could speculate that obese patients with sleep apnea are resistant to the appetite-suppressing effects of leptin. The use of CPAP decreases

TABLE 8-7. CPT and ICD-9 Codes for ApneaLink Usage

Device	Description	Suggested ICD-9 Code	Suggested CPT Code
ApneaLink with oximetry	Three-channel type IV home sleep test, which measures flow, pulse, oxygen saturation	780.79 (fatigue) 327.26 (sleep related hypoventilation) 278.03 (obesity/hypoventilation) 327.23 (OSA)	G0400 (Medicare) 95806 (Commercial payers)

leptin levels and appears to reverse leptin resistance.[112] Levels of the appetite-stimulating hormone, ghrelin, are also increased in patients with OSA. The serum levels of ghrelin decline after only 2 days of CPAP.[113]

• Nocturnal Hypoglycemia Unawareness

A primary concern and complication of patients with T1DM is nocturnal hypoglycemia. Patients with T1DM may experience prolonged episodes of hypoglycemia while at rest (Fig. 8-11). The effects of rapid induction of short-term (less than 1 hour) hypoglycemia in T1DM patients and normal controls were evaluated in a recent clinical trial.[114] As these otherwise healthy subjects entered their second stage of sleep, an insulin infusion was initiated that lowered their blood glucose levels to 40 mg per dL. Once the nadir of the glycemia was attained, the insulin infusion was discontinued and the glucose levels were normalized. Neurocognitive testing was performed prior to bedtime as well as in the morning upon rising following hypoglycemia induction.

Hypoglycemia was found to adversely affect both mood and memory functions in patients with T1DM and normal controls. Some authors believe that repetitive episodes of nocturnal hypoglycemia may result in deterioration of memory and cognitive functioning over time.[115]

• Dead-in-Bed Syndrome

Tattersall first described the dead-in-bed syndrome in 1991 by illustrating 22 cases of unexplained death in young patients with T1DM. In each case, the patient was found dead in the morning in their undisturbed bed.[116] All patients were in good health on the day before the night of their death. Autopsies failed to find any anatomic cause for the deaths of these patients. Dead-in-bed syndrome is estimated to be responsible for 6% of deaths in patients with T1DM younger than age 40 years.[116] The syndrome has been found to be associated with the onset of severe nocturnal hypoglycemia in patients with hypoglycemia awareness autonomic failure (HAAF)[117] (Fig. 8-12).

Patients with diabetes have impaired counterregulation to hypoglycemia while asleep.[118] This impairment makes patients more susceptible to both hypoglycemia and hypoglycemia unawareness. Both epinephrine and norepinephrine concentrations (an index of central sympathetic activation) are reduced. Other indexes of central sympathetic activity such as heart rate, blood pressure, and peripheral vascular resistance are also reduced during the deeper stages of non-REM sleep in patients with diabetes. Impaired defenses against hypoglycemia during sleep may contribute to the vicious

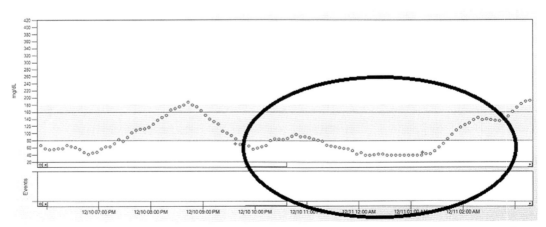

Figure 8-11 • A 35-year-old Patient with 12-year History of T1DM. The patient wears an insulin pump and a continuous glucose monitoring system (CGMS). The sensor data demonstrate a period of prolonged nocturnal hypoglycemia extending from 11:00 PM until 2:00 AM. (Case courtesy of Jeff Unger, MD.)

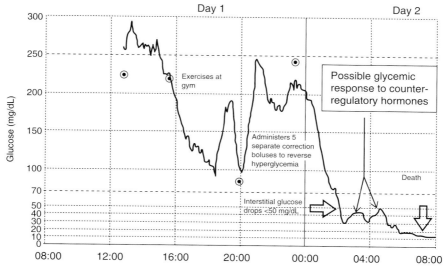

Figure 8-12 • Death of a Patient with T1DM Due to Severe Nocturnal Hypoglycemia. A 23-year-old man with a prior history of severe hypoglycemia resulting in seizure activity. The patient is wearing an insulin pump and a continuous glucose sensor. The interstitial glucose (ISG) tracing on the evening prior to his death shows readings above 250 mg per dL from 1:00 PM to 3:00 PM. After dinner the patient went to the gym. The drop in glucose level corresponds with his intense exercise session. He performed a self-glucose calibration at 8 PM, which correlated with the ISG level. He apparently consumed a snack at 8 PM and noted his ISG had risen to 250 mg per dL. In an attempt to correct the elevated reading, he administered 5 separate boluses of insulin totaling 7.35 U from 9:30 PM to midnight as noted from his insulin pump download. After he went to bed, his ISG dropped precipitously below 50 mg per dL by 2:00 AM. Between 3:00 AM and 4:30 AM, the ISG demonstrates a slight rise on two occasions as his body attempts an emergency counterregulatory reversal of the severe hypoglycemia. The patient was found dead in bed at 9:00 AM. The vitreous humor glucose level was only 25 mg per dL, consistent with death due to severe hypoglycemia. (Adapted and reprinted from Tanenberg RJ, Newton CA, Drake AJ. Confirmation of hypoglycemia in the "Dead-in-Bed" syndrome as captured by a retrospective continuous glucose monitoring system. *Endocr Pract.* 2010;16:244–248, with permission.)

cycle of impaired counterregulation when patients are either awake or asleep. Thus, both asymptomatic and symptomatic episodes of nocturnal hypoglycemia have potential serious consequences for patients with diabetes.

In summary, the complex hormonal pathways linking obesity, insulin resistance, diabetes, and sleep disorders in patients with T2DM suggest a need to screen and aggressively manage high-risk patients. Primary care physicians may be able to reduce cardiovascular risk, restore metabolic integrity, and improve one's quality of life by recognizing these related disorders. Patients with T1DM are not immune from the effects of poor sleep hygiene. Individuals who sleep less than 6 hours per night or longer than 8 hours are likely to experience resistance to peripheral glucose disposal resulting in elevated diurnal glucose levels. Stress hormones that are elevated while sleeping also favor a hyperglycemia state. One could attempt to mitigate the nocturnal rise in glucose levels by compensatory bolusing at dinnertime, increasing nocturnal basal insulin dosing or changing one's overnight pump basal insulin parameters. However, without appropriate blood glucose monitoring, nocturnal hypoglycemia could be induced. Patients with T1DM lack appropriate counterregulatory mechanisms to acutely reverse nocturnal hypoglycemia. Therefore, hypoglycemia unawareness during sleep is likely to be prolonged, recurrent, and responsible for inducing cognitive and memory impairment in some patients.

Sleep may be defined as a "natural periodic state of rest for the mind and body." However, in patients with diabetes, sleep may become a timebomb ticking its way toward leptin resistance, obesity, fatigue, neuroendocrine stress, HAAF, memory loss, hypertension, motor vehicle accidents, stroke, heart attacks, and sudden death. Some might argue that sleep should be avoided altogether. An informed physician should discuss the metabolic relationships that are shared between sleep disorders and diabetes with their patients. Those individuals who clearly have poor sleep hygiene or who are at risk for having sleep disorders should be carefully monitored, evaluated, and treated.

• Hearing Loss

Hearing impairment affects nearly two-thirds of all adults with diabetes.[119] Diabetes-related hearing loss is a progressive, sensorineural impairment affecting audiometric thresholds between 500 and 8,000 Hz.[119] Age-related hearing loss (presbycusis) typically begins in the higher frequencies and progresses to the middle and lower frequencies as people age. Patients with diabetes may exhibit both mid- and high-frequency progressive hearing loss associated with aging. Figure 8-13 shows the audiogram changes expected with aging versus the audiogram pattern of a patient with diabetes-related hearing loss.

Hearing impairment is most commonly diagnosed in patients with diabetes aged 56 to 57 years.[120] Diabetes-related hearing loss is more prevalent among non-Hispanic whites and male subjects possibly due to the contribution of chronic noise exposure at work or recreational noise exposure.[120] Interestingly, hearing loss affects the right ear more than the left in patients with diabetes.[121]

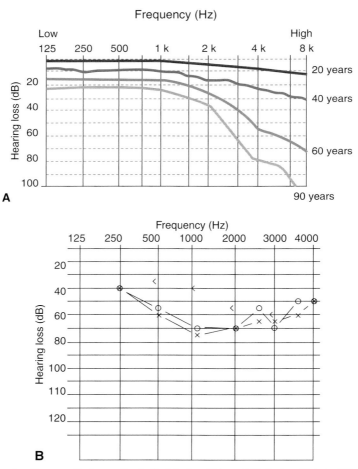

Figure 8-13 • Audiogram Patterns Typical of Aging (A) and Diabetes-Related Hearing Loss (B).
Mid-frequency hearing loss (also referred to as a "cookie bite audiogram pattern") differentiates patients with diabetes from those with sensorineural hearing loss due to aging. (Audiogram courtesy of Richard Borello and Baseline Hearing Aid Center, Upland, CA).

TABLE 8-8. Associated Risk Factors for Hearing Loss in Patients with Diabetes

- HDL-C < 40 mg/dL
- Symptoms of peripheral neuropathy
- Advancing age
- Non-Hispanic white males
- Lower income
- History of coronary artery disease
- Patients report overall poor health

Adapted from Bainbridge KE, Hoffman HJ, Cowie CC. Risk factors for hearing impairment among U.S. adults with diabetes. National Health and Nutrition Examination Survey 1999–2004. *Diabetes Care.* 2011;34:1540–1545.

The estimated cost to an individual for hearing impairment is $43,000. Hearing aids account for only 11% of this cost. The remainder of the costs is attributed to lost productivity and job retraining. Cost per person is closely related to the age of the individual at the time they become hearing impaired with younger patients incurring the greatest lifetime expenses.[122]

Interestingly, neither the duration of diabetes nor the level of glycemic control as measured by A1C is predictive of hearing loss. Table 8-8 lists the risk factors that are strongly associated with progressive, sensorineural hearing loss in adult patients with diabetes.

One possible cause of hearing loss in diabetes involves mechanistic basilar membrane thickening similar to that observed in patients with other microvascular complications (nephropathy and retinopathy). Vascular inflammation was observed in proximity to the cochlear capillaries as well as in the internal auditory artery and the stria vascularis among autopsied people who had diabetes but not in people without diabetes.[123] Atrophy of the spiral ganglion and demyelination of the eighth cranial nerve among autopsied diabetic patients suggest a neurologic etiology to diabetes-related hearing impairment.[124] Regardless of whether the primary lesion is angiopathic or neuropathic, hyperglycemia may contribute via mechanisms related to oxidative stress or deposition of advanced glycosylated end products within the structures of the auditory system.

Although no expert guidelines or recommendations have been published suggesting appropriate timing or mechanism by which patients should be screened for hearing loss, timely recognition of this coexisting disorder may improve hearing and quality of life.[125] The Hearing Handicap Inventory for the Elderly-Screening Version may be downloaded and completed by patients waiting to see the physician for their routine office visit (http://www.anvita.info/wiki/Hearing_Handicap_Inventory_In_The_Elderly_Screening_Version). An audiometer may also be used for screening purposes. (Pure tone, air only screen test CPT code: 92551.)

Some patients may benefit from referral to an audiologist or an otolaryngologist, although the majority of individuals with diabetes and hearing loss may only require protective devices to minimize their risk of further auditory injury. Patients with evidence of a perforated tympanic membrane, those with evidence of severe infection with persistent drainage, those with significant and acute-onset unilateral or asymmetric hearing loss, as well as those with rapidly declining hearing loss of uncertain etiology warrant further evaluation.

Hearing loss commonly occurs with both T1DM and T2DM. Patients who lose hearing experience functional decline, depression, and social isolation. Those individuals with sensory neuropathy and visual disorders may have a higher risk of falls.[126] Primary care physicians may be the first, and in some cases, the only health-care professionals to assess patients with both diabetes and hearing loss. Patients who have evidence of mid-frequency hearing loss should be educated regarding hearing protection. Audiology referral may be necessary in patients with rapidly declining or acute-onset loss of hearing.

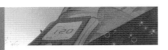

SUMMARY

Primary care physicians manage patients with multiple disorders and chronic diseases many of which have a direct physiologic and teleologic association with diabetes. If a clinician diagnoses a patients as having obstructive sleep apnea, not only is a prescription for behavioral modification and CPAP advisable, but one must further investigate if that individual may have insulin resistance, abnormal glucose tolerance, PCOS, and even a higher risk for cancer. Similarly patients with PAD are at higher risk of stroke and CAD, whereas patients with Parkinson disease tend to have a higher prevalence of diabetes. The epidemiology of associated disorders within the field of diabetes requires that clinicians take a careful history and perform a comprehensive physical evaluation on all of their patients. Simply determining that a patient has elevated morning glucose values is insufficient, especially if clinical evidence demonstrates weight gain and increasing fatigue. Medications that are prescribed to treat the fasting hyperglycemia may not be necessary if the primary cause of the patient's insulin resistance is a dysfunction in the neuroendocrine axis of sleep.

With diabetes being an independent risk factor for several forms of cancers, prescribers must be vigilant regarding use of medications that not only minimize weight gain, but also reduce one's likelihood of developing cancer. Patients should be informed about the risks and benefits of using all medications to treat hyperglycemia. Those patients who have both cancer and diabetes should pursue optimal glycemic control in order to minimize glycemic variability, which has been shown to increase mortality rates.

Although guidelines for evaluating auditory function in patients with diabetes have not been published, clinicians should not hesitate to perform an audiogram on individuals with T2DM as nearly 66% have hearing impairment. Neither the duration of diabetes nor the level of glycemic control as measured by A1C are predictive of hearing loss.

REFERENCES

1. Selvin E, Erlinger TP. Prevalence of and risk factors for peripheral arterial disease in the United States: results from the National Health and Nutrition Examination Survey, 1999–2000. *Circulation.* 2004;110:738–774.
2. Bembi V, Singh S, Singh P, et al. Prevalence of peripheral artery disease in a cohort of diabetic patients. *South Med J.* 2006;99(6):564–569.
3. Badheka AO, Rathod AD, Bharadawaj AS, et al. Outcomes and risk prediction model for peripheral arterial disease in patients with stable coronary artery disease. *Angiology.* 2011;62(6):473–479.
4. Hirsch AT, Criqui MH, Treat-Jacobson D, et al. Peripheral arterial disease detection, awareness, and treatment in primary care. *JAMA.* 2001;286:1317–132.
5. Gey DC, Lesho EP, Manngold J. Management of peripheral arterial disease. *Am Fam Physician.* 2004;69(3):525–532.
6. Sheikh MA, Bhatt DL, Li J, et al. Usefulness of postexercise ankle-brachial index to predict all cause mortality. *Am J Cardiol.* 2011;107(5):778–782.
7. Rooke TW, Hirsch AT, Misra S, et al. 2011 ACCF/AHA focused update of the guideline for the management of patients with peripheral artery disease (Updating the 2005 Guideline). A report of the American College of Cardiology Foundation/American Heart Association Task Force on Practice Guidelines. Circulation. *Circulation.* 2011;124:00-00. DOI: 10.1161/CIR.0b013e31822e80c3).
8. Boulton AJM, Armstrong DG, Albert SF, et al. Comprehensive foot examination and risk assessment: a report of the Task Force of the Foot Care Interest Group of the American Diabetes Association, with endorsement by the American Association of Clinical Endocrinologists. *Diabetes Care.* 2008;31(8): 1679–1685.
9. White CJ, Gray WA. Endovascular therapies for peripheral arterial disease: an evidence-based review. *Circulation.* 2007;116:2203–2215.

10. Pletal package insert. Otsuka Pharmaceutical Co. Ltd. Tokushima, Japan. May 2007.

11. Adam DJ, Beard JD, Clevelant D, et al. Bypass versus angioplasty in severe ischaemia of the leg (BASIL): multicenter, randomized controlled trial. *Lancet*. 2005;366:1925–1934.

12. Johnston K. Balloon angioplasty: predictive factors for long-term success. *Semin Vasc Surg*. 1989;3:117–122.

13. Murphy TP, Ariaratnam NS, Carney WI Jr, et al. Aortoiliac insufficiency: long-term experience with stent placement for treatment. *Radiology*. 2004;231:243–249.

14. Scheinert D, Schroder M, Balzer JO, et al. Stent-supported reconstruction of the aortoiliac bifurcation with the kissing balloon technique. *Circulation*. 1999;100(suppl II):II-295–II-300.

15. de Vries SO, Visser K, de Vries JA, et al. Intermittent claudication: cost-effectiveness of revascularization versus exercise therapy. *Radiology*. 2002;222:25–36.

16. Hunink MG, Wong JB, Donaldson MC, et al. Revascularization for femoropopliteal disease: a decision and cost-effectiveness analysis. *JAMA*. 1995;274:165–171.

17. Schillinger M, Sabeti S, Loewe C, et al. Balloon angioplasty versus implantation of nitinol stents in the superficial femoral artery. *N Engl J Med*. 2006;354(18):1879–1888.

18. Xu Q, Park Y, Huang X, et al. Diabetes and risk of Parkinson disease. *Diabetes Care*. 2011;34:910–915.

19. Kordower JH, Chu Y, Hauser RA, et al. Lewy body-like pathology in long-term embryonic nigral transplants in Parkinson disease. *Nat Med*. 2008;14(5):504–506.

20. Grimes DA, Lang AE. Treatment of early Parkinson disease. *Can J Neurol Sci*. 1999;26(suppl 2):S39–S44.

21. Luo S, Meier AH, Cincott AH. Bromocriptine reduces obesity, glucose intolerance and extracellular monoamine metabolite levels in the ventromedial hypothalamus of Syrian hamsters. *Neuroendocrinology*. 1998;68:1–10.

22. Pijl H, Ohashi S, Matsuda M, et al. Bromocriptine: a novel approach to the treatment of type 2 diabetes. *Diabetes Care*. 2000;23:1154–1161.

23. Rönnemaa E, Zethelius B, Sundelöf J, et al. Glucose metabolism and the risk of Alzheimer's disease and dementia: a population-based 12 year follow-up study in 71-year-old men. *Diabetologia*. 2009;52:1504–1510.

24. Craft S, Watson GS. Insulin and neurodegenerative disease: shared and specific mechanisms. *Lancet Neurol*. 2004;3:169–178.

25. Cardoso S, Correia S, Santos RX, et al. Insulin is a two-edged knife on the brain. *J Alzheimers Dis*. 2009;18:483–507.

26. Lu M, Hu G. Targeting metabolic inflammation in Parkinson disease: implications for prospective therapeutic strategies. *Clin Exp Pharmacol Physiol*. November 29, 2011. DOI: 10.1111/j.1440-1681.2011.

27. Rana JS, Mittleman MA, Sheikh J, et al. Chronic obstructive pulmonary disease, asthma, and risk of type 2 diabetes in women. *Diabetes Care*. 2004;27(10):2478–2484.

28. Eid AA, Ionescu AA, Nixon LS, et al. Inflammatory response and body composition in chronic obstructive pulmonary disease. *Am J Respir Crit Care Med*. 2001;164:1414–1418.

29. Yun H, et al. Asthma and proinflammatory conditions: a population-based retrospective matched cohort study. *American Academy Allergy Asthma and Immunology Meeting*. San Francisco, CA. March 21–24, 2011. Abstracts 293.

30. Black MH, Anderson A, Bell RA, et al. Prevalence of asthma and its association with glycemic control among youth with diabetes. *Pediatrics*. 2011;128(4):e839–e847.

31. Rizza RA, Mandarino LJ, Gerich JE. Cortisol-induced insulin resistance in man: impaired suppression of glucose production and stimulation of glucose utilization due to a postreceptor detect of insulin action. *J Clin Endocrinol Metab* 1982;54:131–138.

32. Lansang MC. Glucocorticoid-induced diabetes and adrenal suppression: how to detect and manage them. *Cleve Clin J Med*. 2011;78 (11) 748–756

33. Yuen KC, McDaniel PA, Riddle MC. Twenty-four hour profiles of plasma glucose, insulin, C-peptide and free fatty acid in subjects with varying degrees of glucose tolerance following short-term medium-dose prednisone (20 mg/day) treatment: evidence for differing effects on insulin secretion and action. *Clin Endocrinol*. October 4, 2011. DOI: 10.1111/j.1365-2265.2011.04242.x. [Epub ahead of print]).

34. Bevier WC, Zisser HC, Jovanovic L, et al. Use of continuous glucose monitoring to estimate insulin requirements in patients with type 1 diabetes mellitus during a short course of prednisone. *J Diabetes Sci Technol*. 2008;2:578–583.

35. Giovannucci E, Harlan DM, Archer MC, et al. Diabetes and cancer: a consensus report. *Diabetes Care*. 2010;33:1674–1685.

36. Campbell PT, Newton CC, Dehal AN, et al. Impact of body mass index on survival after colorectal cancer diagnosis: the Cancer Prevention Study-II Nutrition Cohort. *J Clin Oncol*. 2012;30(1):42–52.

37. Dehal AN, Newton CC, Jacobs EJ, et al. Impact of diabetes mellitus and insulin use on survival after colorectal cancer diagnosis: the Cancer Prevention Study-II Nutrition Cohort. *J Clin Oncol*. 2012;30(1):53–59.

38. Barone BB, Yeh HC, Snyder CF, et al. Long-term all-cause mortality in cancer patients with preexisting diabetes mellitus: a systematic review and meta-analysis. *JAMA*. 2008;300:2754–2764.
39. Li C, Ballus L, Ford ES, et al. Association between diagnosed diabetes and self-reported cancer among U.S. adults. *Diabetes Care*. 2011;34:1356–1368.
40. Hamilton W. Cancer diagnosis in primary care. *Br J Gen Pract*. 2010;60(571):121–128.
41. Eliassen AH, Colditz GA, Rosner B, et al. Adult weight change and risk of postmenopausal breast cancer. *JAMA*. 2006;296:193–201.
42. Kastorini CM, Panagiotakos DB. Dietary patterns and prevention of type 2 diabetes: from research to clinical practice: a systematic review. *Curr Diabetes Rev*. 2009;5:221–227.
43. Kushi LH, Byers T, Doyle C, et al. American Cancer Society 2006 Nutrition and Physical Activity Guidelines Advisory Committee. American Cancer Society guidelines on nutrition and physical activity for cancer prevention: reducing the risk of cancer with healthy food choices and physical activity. *CA Cancer J Clin*. 2006;56:254–281.
44. Physical Activity Guidelines Advisory Committee Report. 2008. Washington, DC. U.S. Department of Health and Human Services. Available from http://www.health.gov/paguidelines/committeereport.asp. Accessed September 14, 2011.
45. Jones HE, Goddard L, Gee JM, et al. Insulin-like growth factor-I receptor signaling and acquired resistance to gefitinib (ZD1839; Iressa) in human breast and prostate cancer cells. *Endocr Relat Cancer*. 2004;11(4):793–814.
46. Hellawell GO, Turner GD, Davies DR, et al. Expression of the type 1 insulin-like growth factor receptor is up-regulated in primary prostate cancer and commonly persists in metastatic disease. *Cancer Res*. 2002;62(10):2942–2950.
47. Major JM, Laughlin GA, Kritz-Silverstein D, et al. Insulin-like growth factor-I and cancer mortality in older men. *J Clin Endocrinol Metab*. 2010;95:1054–1059.
48. Bowker SL, Majumdar SR, Veugelers P, et al. Increased cancer-related mortality for patients with type 2 diabetes who use sulfonylureas or insulin. *Diabetes Care*. 2006;29:254–258.
49. Simon D, Lange C, Charles M-A, et al. Fasting serum insulin as a predictive marker for cancer mortality in a healthy population—The Telecom Study. American Diabetes Association. *71st Scientific Sessions*. San Diego, CA. June 24–28, 2011,1306-p.
50. Canonici A, Steelant W, Rigot V, et al. Insulin-like growth factor-I receptor, E-CVDherin and alpha v integrin form a dynamic complex under the control of alpha-catenin. *Int J Cancer*. 2008;122:572–582.
51. Vander Heiden MG, Cantley LC, Thompson CB. Understanding the Warburg effect: the metabolic requirements of cell proliferation. *Science*. 2009;324:1029–1033.
52. Phelps ME. *PET: Physics, Instrumentation, and Scanners*. New York, NY: Springer; 2006;8–10. ISBN: 0387349464.
53. Roytblat L, Rachinsky M, Fisher A, et al. Raised interleukin-6 levels in obese patients. *Obesity Res*. 2000;8. 673–675.
54. Ulisse S, Baldini E, Sorrenti S, et al. The urokinase plasminogen activator system: a target for anticancer therapy. *Curr Cancer Drug Targets*. 2009;9:32–71.
55. Yu H, Pardoll D, Jove R. STATs in cancer inflammation and immunity: a leading role for STAT3. *Nat Rev Cancer*. 2009;9:798–809.
56. Landman GWE, Kleefstra N, Van Hateren KJJ, et al. Metformin associated with lower cancer mortality in type 2 diabetes. ZODIAC-16. *Diabetes Care*. 2010;33:322–326.
57. Alimova IN, Liu B, Fan Z, et al. Metformin inhibits breast cancer cell growth, colony formation and induces cell cycle arrest in vitro. *Cell Cycle*. 2009;8:909–915.
58. Metformin Trial Lists' Collaboration Group. American Diabetes Association. *71st Scientific Sessions*. San Diego, CA. June 24–28, 2011;950-p.
59. FDA Drug Safety Podcast: http://www.fda.gov/Drugs/DrugSafety/DrugSafetyPodcasts/ucm226749.htm. Accessed January 5, 2012.
60. Dietrich K, Schned A, Fortuny J, et al. Glucocorticoid therapy and risk of bladder cancer. *Br J Cancer*. 2009;101:1316–1320.
61. Golka K, Selinski S, Lehmann ML, et al. Genetic variants in urinary bladder cancer: collective power of the "wimp SNPs." *Arch Toxicol*. 2011;85(6):539–554.
62. Piccinni C, Motola D, Marchesini G, et al. Assessing the association of pioglitazone use and bladder cancer through drug adverse event reporting. *Diabetes Care*. 2011;34(6):1369–1371.
63. Dormandy J, Bhattacharya M, van Troostenburg de Bruyn AR. Safety and tolerability of pioglitazone in high-risk patients with type 2 diabetes: an overview of data from PROactive. *Drug Saf*. 2009;32:187–202.

64. U.S. Food and Drug Administration. FDA drug safety communication: ongoing safety review of actos (pioglitazone) and potential increased risk of bladder cancer after two years exposure [Internet], 2010. Silver Spring, MD, U.S. Food and Drug Administration. Available from http://www.fda.gov/Drugs/DrugSafety/ucm226214.htm. Accessed June 11, 2011.

65. http://www.fda.gov/Drugs/DrugSafety/ucm259150.htm Accessed June 15, 2011.

66. Sun G, Wells B, Zimmerman R, et al. Increased cancer risk with sulfonylurea vs metformin in women with diabetes: an observational cohort study. American Diabetes Association. *71st Scientific Sessions*. San Diego, CA. June 24–28, 2011;-p. 1350.

67. Croom KF, McCormack PL. Liraglutide. A review of its use in type 2 diabetes mellitus. *Drugs*. 2009;69(14):1985–2004.

68. Waser B, Beetschen K, Pellegata NS. Incretin receptors in non-neoplastic and thyroid C cells in rodents and humans: relevance for incretin-based diabetes therapy. *Neuroendocrinology*. 2011;94(4):291–301.

69. Victoza Risk evaluation and mitigation strategy. Novo Nordisk. Princeton, NJ. http://www.victozapro.com/rems-program.aspx. Accessed September 16, 2011.

70. Carling T. Multiple endocrine neoplasia syndrome: genetic basis for clinical management. *Curr Opin Oncol*. 2005;17(1):7–12.

71. Kloos RT, Eng C, Evans DB, et al. Medullary thyroid cancer: management guidelines of the American Thyroid Association. *Thyroid*. 2009;19(6):565–612.

72. Costante G, Meringolo D, Durante C, et al. Predictive value of serum calcitonin levels for preoperative diagnosis of medullary thyroid carcinoma in a cohort of 5817 consecutive patients with thyroid nodules. *J Clin Endocrinol Metab*. 2007;92:450–455.

73. Parks M, Rosebraugh C. Weighing the risks and benefits of liraglutide: The FDA's review of a new antidiabetic therapy. *N Engl J Med*. 2010;362:774–777.

74. Butler PC. Insulin glargine controversy: a tribute to the editorial team at Diabetologia. *Diabetes*. 2009;58:2427–2428.

75. Cox ME, Gleave ME, Zakikhani M, et al. Insulin receptor expression by human prostate cancers. *Prostate*. 2009;69:33–40.

76. Law JH, Habibi G, Hu K, et al. Phosphorylated insulin-like growth factor-i/insulin receptor is present in all breast cancer subtypes and is related to poor survival. *Cancer Res*. 2008;68:10238–10246.

77. Currie CJ, Poole CD, Gale EA. The influence of glucose-lowering therapies on cancer risk in type 2 diabetes. *Diabetologia*. 2009;52:1766–1777.

78. Jonasson JM, Ljung R, Talback M, et al. Insulin glargine use and short-term incidence of malignancies: a population based follow-up study in Sweden. *Diabetologia*. 2009;52:1745–1754.

79. Colhoun HM, SDRN Epidemiology Group. Use of insulin glargine and cancer incidence in Scotland: a study from the Scottish Diabetes Research Network Epidemiology Group. *Diabetologia*. 2009;52:1755–1765.

80. Hemkens LG, Grouven U, Bender R, et al. Risk of malignancies in patients with diabetes treated with human insulin or insulin analogues: a cohort study. *Diabetologia*. 2009;52:1732–1744.

81. Morden NE, Liu SK, Smith J, et al. Further exploration of the relationship between insulin glargine and incident cancer: a retrospective cohort study of older Medicare patients. *Diabetes Care*. 2011;34:1965–1971.

82. Hamaty M, Miller MI, Gerstein HC, et al. American Diabetes Association. *71st Scientific Sessions*. San Diego, CA. June 24–28, 2011;366-OR.

83. Rosenstock J, Fonseca V, McGill JB, et al. Similar risk of malignancy with insulin glargine and neutral protamine Hagedorn (NPH) insulin in patients with type 2 diabetes: findings from a 5 year randomised, open-label study. *Diabetologia*. 2009;52:1971–1973.

84. The ORIGIN Trial-Outcome Reduction With Initial Glargine Intervention-[registered clinical trial], 2009. Clinical trial reg. no. NCT00069784, clinicaltrials-.gov. Accessed September 15, 2011.

85. Bailey CJ, Gross JL, Yadav MJ, et al. Long-term efficacy of dapagliflozin as add-on to metformin (MET) in T2DM inadequately controlled with MET alone. American Diabetes Association. *71st Scientific Sessions*. San Diego, CA. June 24–8, 2011;988–P.

86. http://www.medpagetoday.com/Endocrinology/Diabetes/30747. Accessed February 24, 2012.

87. Chao EC, Henry RR. SGLT2 inhibition: a novel strategy for diabetes treatment. *Nat Rev Drug Discov*. 2010;9(7):551–559.

88. Barone BB, Yeh HC, Snyder CF, et al. Postoperative mortality in cancer patients with preexisting diabetes: systematic review and meta-analysis. *Diabetes Care*. 2010;33:931–939.

89. Hammer MJ, Casper C, Gooley TA, et al. The contribution of malglycemia to mortality among allogeneic hematopoietic cell transplant recipients. *Biol Blood Marrow Transplant*. 2009;15(3):344–351.

90. Cutler C, Antin JH. Peripheral blood stem cells for allogeneic transplantation: a review. *Stem Cells.* 2001;19(2):108–117.

91. Butler SO, Btaiche IF, Alaniz C. Relationship between hyperglycemia and infection in critically ill patients. *Pharmacotherapy.* 2005;25:963–976.

92. Brownlee M. The pathobiology of diabetic complications: a unifying mechanism. *Diabetes.* 2005;54:1615–1625.

93. Webb WB, Agnew HW. Are we chronically sleep deprived? *Bull Psychonomic Soc.* 1975;6:47.

94. Bonnet MH, Arand DL. We are chronically sleep deprived. *Sleep.* 1995;18:908–911.

95. Yaggi HK, Araujo AB, McKinlay JB. Sleep duration as a risk factor for the development of type 2 diabetes. *Diabetes Care.* 2006;29:657–661.

96. Darukhanavala A, Booth JN, Bromley L, et al. Changes in insulin secretion and action in adults with familial risk for type 2 diabetes who curtail their sleep. *Diabetes Care.* Published Ahead of Print. August 11, 2011. DOI:10.2337/dcii-0777.

97. Pollak CP, Tryon WW, Nagaraja H, et al. How accurately does wrist actigraphy identify states of sleep and wakefulness? *Sleep.* 2001;24(8):957–965.

98. Trento M, Broglio F, Riganti F, et al. Sleep abnormalities in type 2 diabetes may be associated with glycemic control. *Acta Diabetol.* 2008;45:225–229.

99. Knutson KL, Cauter EV, Zee P, et al. Cross-sectional associations between measures of sleep and markers of glucose metabolism among subjects with and without diabetes. *Diabetes Care.* 2011;34:1171–1176.

100. Donga E, Van Dijk M, Van Dijk JG, Partial sleep restriction decreases insulin sensitivity in type 1 diabetes. *Diabetes Care.* 2010;33:1573–1577.

101. O'Donnell AB, Araujo AB, McKinlay JB. The health of normally aging men: the Massachusetts Male Aging Study (1987–2004). *Exp Gerontol.* 2004;39:975–984.

102. Cappuccio FP, D'elia L, Strazzullo P, et al. Quantity and quality of sleep and incidence of type 2 diabetes: a systematic review and meta-analysis. *Diabetes Care.* 2010;33:414–420.

103. Chin-Chance C, Polonsky KS, Schoeller DA. Twenty-four-hour leptin levels respond to cumulative short-term energy imbalance and predict subsequent intake. *J Clin Endocrinol Metab.* 2000;85:2685–2691.

104. van der Lely AJ, Tschop M, Heiman ML, et al. Biological, physiological, pathophysiological, and pharmacological aspects of ghrelin. *Endocr Rev.* 2004;25:426–457.

105. Spiegel K, Tasali E, Penev P, et al. Brief communication: sleep curtailment in healthy young men is associated with decreased leptin levels, elevated ghrelin levels, and increased hunger and appetite. *Ann Intern Med.* 2004;141:846–850.

106. Jauch-Chara K, Schmid SM, Hallschmid M, et al. Altered neuroendocrine sleep architecture in patients with type 1 diabetes. *Diabetes Care.* 2008;31:1183–1188.

107. Young T, Blustein J, Finn L, et al. Sleep-disordered breathing and motor vehicle accidents in a population-based sample of employed adults. *Sleep.* 1997;20:608–613.

108. Pillar G, Shehadeh N. Abdominal fat and sleep apnea: the chicken or the egg? *Diabetes Care.* 2008;31(suppl 2):S303–S309.

109. Young T, Evans L, Finn L, et al. Estimation of the clinically diagnosed proportion of sleep apnea syndrome in middle-aged men and women. *Sleep.* 1997;20:705–706.

110. Erman MK, Stewart D, Einhorn D, et al. Validation of the ApneaLink for the screening of sleep apnea: a novel and simple single-channel recording device. *J Clin Sleep Med.* 2007;3(4):387–392.

111. Babu AR, Herdegen J, Fogelfeld L, et al. Type 2 diabetes, glycemic control, and continuous positive airway pressure in obstructive sleep apnea. *Arch Intern Med.* 2005;165:447–452.

112. Phillips BG, Kato M, Narkiewicz K, et al. Increases in leptin levels, sympathetic drive, and weight gain in obstructive sleep apnea. *Am J Physiol Heart Circ Physiol.* 2000;279:H234–H237.

113. Harsch IA, Konturek PC, Koebnick C, et al. Leptin and ghrelin levels in patients with obstructive sleep apnoea: effect of CPAP treatment. *Eur Respir J.* 2003;22:251–257.

114. Jauch-Chara K, Hallschmid M, Gais S, et al. Hypoglycemia during sleep impairs consolidation of declarative memory in type 1 diabetic and healthy humans. *Diabetes Care.* 2007;30:2040–2045.

115. Wagner U, Hallschmid M, Rasch B, et al. Brief sleep after learning keeps emotional memories alive for years. *Biol Psychiatry.* 2006;60:788–790.

116. Tattersall RB, Gill GV. Unexplained deaths of type 1 diabetic patients. *Diabetic Med.* 1991;8:49–58.

117. Tanenberg RJ, Newton CA, Drake AJ. Confirmation of hypoglycemia in the "Dead-in-Bed" syndrome as captured by a retrospective continuous glucose monitoring system. *Endocr Pract.* 2010;16:244–248.

118. Jones TW, Porter P, Sherwin RS, et al. Decreased epinephrine response to hypoglycemia during sleep. *N Engl J Med.* 1998;338. 1657–1662.

119. Bainbridge KE, Hoffman HJ, Cowie CC. Diabetes and hearing impairment in the United States: audiometric evidence from the National Health and Nutrition Examination Survey, 1999 to 2004. *Ann Intern Med*. 2008;149:1–10.

120. Bainbridge KE, Hoffman HJ, Cowie CC, Risk Factors for Hearing Impairment Among U.S. Adults With Diabetes. National Health and Nutrition Examination Survey 1999–2004. *Diabetes Care*. 2011;34:1540–1545.

121. Frisina ST, Mapes F, Kim S, et al. Characterization of hearing loss in aged type II diabetics. *Hear Res*. 2006;211(1–2)103–113.

122. Mohr PE, Feldman JJ, Dunbar JL, et al. The societal costs of severe to profound hearing loss in the United States. *Int J Technol Assess Health Care*. 2000;16(4):1120–1135.

123. Wackym PA, Linthicum FH Jr. Diabetes mellitus and hearing loss: clinical and histopathologic relationships. *Am J Otol*. 1986;7:176–182.

124. Makishima K, Tanaka K. Pathological changes of the inner ear and central auditory pathway in diabetics. *Ann Otol Rhinol Laryngol*. 1971;80:218–228.

125. Bogardus ST, Yeuh B, Shekelle PG. Screening and management of adult hearing loss in primary care. *JAMA*. 2003;289(25):1986–1990.

126. Agrawal Y, Carey JP, Della SCC, et al. Diabetes, vestibular dysfunction, and falls: analyses from the National Health and Nutrition Survey. *Otol Neurotol*. 2010;31(9):1445–1450.

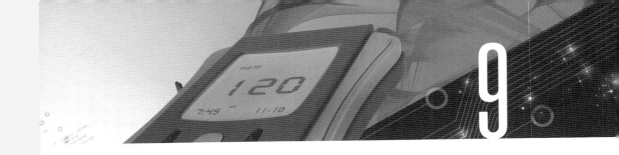

Comanaging Mental Illness in Patients with Diabetes

Our life is what our thoughts make it.
—*Marcus Aurelius, Roman emperor and*
 Stoic philosopher (121–180 AD)

Introduction: The Link between Mind and Body

Unless one's health is acutely compromised, patients with mental illness coexisting with diabetes should always have the affective disorder stabilized before attempting to improve the metabolic status. Patients who have bipolar depression, schizophrenia, and other forms of affective disorders have a significantly higher rate of suicide. If one is unable to think clearly or make reasonable decisions about one's personal care, how could one take on the added responsibility of managing a complicated disease such as diabetes? Most patients with diabetes will need to take not only medications for glycemic control but also aspirin, a statin, and multiple antihypertensive agents. Lifestyle interventions such as exercise, dietary modification, home blood glucose monitoring, compliance with appointments, and even picking up prescription refills at the pharmacy in a timely fashion are crucial to successful diabetes management.

Patients with psychiatric disorders have difficulty functioning at work and within their family unit. Productivity and employment are adversely affected by bipolar disorder (BPD) and schizophrenia. Many of these patients are unemployable. More than 60% of patients in the Stanley Center Bipolar Disorder Registry were unemployed, despite the fact that 30% of these individuals had actually successfully completed college.[1] The devastating impact of the effects of mental illness in patients with bipolar depression is reflected by the suicide rate, which is 20 times higher than that in the general population and is more likely to occur after repeated episodes of depression.[2]

Patients with any degree of disabling mental illness will be unable to perform even the basic self-management skills. Therefore, until their emotional status improves and their decompensated mental capacity is stabilized, metabolic control of coexisting diabetes will be virtually impossible. Major depression, schizophrenia, and bipolar depression all increase the risks for diabetes and coronary artery disease (CAD). Because of the undeniable link between emotional unrest and diabetes, patients with mental illness should be screened for coexisting diabetes and vice versa. Treatment for patients with both mental illness and diabetes should focus first and foremost on improving the psychiatric illness with the use of appropriate pharmacologic and behavioral interventions. As one's cognitive functioning improves, focus may be directed toward treating the metabolic parameters (weight, lipids, blood pressure, glycemic control) to their individualized targets. By comanaging both the mental and physical aspects of the disease state, long-term survivability will be enhanced.

Depression and Diabetes

Although many newly diagnosed patients with T2DM relate the onset of their depression with the time they were initially diagnosed with diabetes, in reality, 80% of patients with diabetes have had a major depressive episode predating their metabolic diagnosis by 6 to 8 years.[3] A longitudinal study evaluating more than 11,000 nondiabetic adult depressed patients aged 48 to 67 years determined that those individuals who were most symptomatic had a 63% chance of developing T2DM within 6 years compared with the least symptomatic patients.[4]

Depression is the most studied psychosocial factor in adolescents with both T1DM and T2DM. The prevalence of depressive symptomatology in this challenging patient population is reported to be between 14% and 33%.[5,6] As adolescents with T1DM transition into adulthood, nearly 50% will develop major depression or general anxiety disorder.[7] Primary care providers must be trained to screen, and if necessary, initiate appropriate management of younger patients who have coexisting mental illness and diabetes.

Diabetes negatively impacts the health-related quality of life (HRQOL) of patients with T2DM. Interestingly, men with T2DM who experience depression and anxiety have a statistically increased likelihood of mortality versus women who report similar symptoms.[8] Instruments that measure HRQOL such as the RAND-36 questionnaire that assesses nine aspects of health status, including physical functioning, role limitations due to physical health problems, bodily pain, general health, vitality, social functioning, role limitations due to emotional problems, mental health, and health change may be useful screening tool in clinical practice. (http://www.rand.org/health/surveys_tools/mos/mos_core_36item_survey.html). The nine categories in RAND-36 may be subdivided into physical (PCS) and mental (MCS) component summaries. Low PCS scores are suggestive of substantial limitations in self-care, physical and social activities, severe body pain, or frequent fatigue. Low MCS scores suggest psychological distress as well as substantial social and role limitations due to emotional dysfunction.[9]

Patients with diabetes frequently have coexisting affective disorders that may directly affect self-management skills, cardiovascular risk factors, metabolic abnormalities, morbidity, and mortality. Fifteen percent of patients with T2DM meet the diagnostic criteria for an affective illness (depression and anxiety).[10] Twice as many women as men have affective disorders.[6,11] Major depression disorder (MDD) has been found to be a chronic or recurrent illness in most patients with T2DM. Over a 5-year period, 80% of patients with MDD and T2DM have at least one episode of relapsing depression.[12] Compared with patients with diabetes alone, those with depression and diabetes demonstrate poorer self-management skills (following diet and exercise regimens, performing home blood glucose monitoring) and more often fail to refill their prescribed medications.[13] Smoking, obesity, sedentary lifestyle, and higher A1C levels are also more common in depressed patients with diabetes.[14]

Depressed patients frequently adopt a lifestyle that promotes cardiovascular disease. For example, patients with depression tend to be overweight, are physically inactive, and abuse nicotine more than do age-matched controls.[3,15] Depressed patients who are overweight [body mass index (BMI) greater than 30 kg per m²] may have poorer long-term outcomes related to diabetes, as these individuals tend to be more resistant to entering weight-loss programs or beginning an exercise regimen.[16]

Cigarette smoking increases insulin resistance and is a risk factor for progression of many of the microvascular and macrovascular complications of diabetes. Smokers with a history of depression are likely to become even more symptomatic when they attempt smoking cessation, unless they are initially screened and treated for depression.[17]

Inflammatory mediators also influence the association between depression and diabetes. Patients with major depressive disorders have elevated levels of interleukin (IL)-6 and C-reactive protein (CRP), inflammatory cytokines that are known to cause endothelial cell dysfunction.[18] Experimental infusion of another inflammatory cytokine, tumor necrosis factor-α, induced depressive symptoms in human subjects.[19,20]

Obesity, a precursor to diabetes, is marked by reduced levels of adiponectin. As adiponectin levels decrease, insulin resistance increases, predisposing genetically susceptible individuals to β-cell failure. Inflammatory cytokines released by the liver can reduce the expression of adiponectin.[21,22] The elevation in inflammatory cytokines may have a direct influence on future cardiac risk in depressed patients. A study that measured levels of CRP 2 months after depressed patients were discharged from an acute coronary care unit noted that those individuals receiving statins had lower levels of CRP than did patients who were not taking a statin.[23]

Patients who have major depression have difficulty achieving an A1C level of less than 8%, resulting in a higher incidence of morbidity and mortality, with more frequent and costly hospitalizations. Elevated A1C levels are associated with depression in younger patients. With the exception of elderly patients, improving depression across all age groups has been associated with a significant reduction in glycemic control.[24]

Although men may experience major depression less often than women, major complications related to diabetes are more often seen in men with coexisting depression and diabetes. As glycemic control deteriorates and complications begin to develop, women appear to be able to bring a more flexible range of coping strategies to the surface, whereas men are more likely to become more passive and accepting of their ultimate fate.[25] As patients age and develop more diabetes-related complications, their likelihood of developing depressive symptoms tends to increase as they become more disabled by their disease and face the realization that reversal of their symptoms is unlikely. Older patients become depressed as diabetes begins to have an impact on their quality of life. Difficulty with balance, neuropathic pain, vision problems, sexual dysfunction, and syncope, along with an increasing dependence on additional therapeutic modalities, ultimately cause many patients to realize that their symptoms are irreversible and unmanageable while becoming increasingly more expensive. MDD (major depressive disorder) has been shown to be associated with a 2.3-fold increased risk in mortality for patients with T2DM.[26] Patients with coexisting depression and diabetes have more ambulatory care visits, higher pharmacy costs, and incur lifetime medical expenses that are 4.5 times higher than those of individuals with diabetes who are not clinically depressed.[27]

The biologic mediators that appear to link depression with long-term diabetes-related complications are shown in Table 9-1.

To be successfully treated, the disorders of the mind and the body must both be addressed. Failure to recognize the link between mental illness and diabetes can lead to a higher incidence of diabetes-related complications, especially CAD. Patients with severe mental illness may also be at risk for successful completion of a suicide attempt. Because coexisting diabetes and mental illness is so common, one should consider screening patients with mental illness for diabetes and vice versa. Comanagement with a mental health provider is certainly appropriate for high-risk patients. The use of pharmacotherapeutic agents is warranted in patients with clinical depression. Initially, medications are used to induce remission, whereas the long-term treatment goal should be to reduce the likelihood of symptom recurrence.

• Depression, Diabetes, Microvascular, and Macrovascular Complications: The Metabolic Link

One may question why patients with coexisting depression and diabetes have a higher risk of morbidity and mortality when compared with patients with no clinical evidence of affective disorder. Speculation suggests that depression directly affects the hypothalamic-pituitary-adrenal (HPA) axis.[28,29] Some, but not all, depressed patients have elevated levels of corticotrophin-releasing factor (CRF) in their cerebrospinal fluid. This increase in CRF stimulates the HPA to produce high levels of plasma cortisol and induce adrenal hypertrophy. Cortisol, as a counterregulatory hormone, promotes insulin resistance. Patients who have normal pancreatic β-cell function simply produce and secrete more insulin to maintain euglycemia during this enhanced state of insulin resistance. In contrast, patients with prolonged and significant depression, who are obese, physically inactive, and genetically

TABLE 9-1. Mediators of Diabetes Risk, Depression, and Their Possible Link to Long-term Complications

Diabetes Risk Measure	Depression Effect	Effect on Complications
Obesity	Increased weight	Reduced adiponectin Hypertension Hyperlipidemia Proteinuria Elevated CRP and other inflammatory cytokines Insulin resistance Prothrombotic state Proinflammatory state Increase in counterregulatory hormones (glucagon, catecholamines, cortisol)
Physical inactivity	Increased fatigue Obesity Increase in neuropathic pain symptoms Reduced quality of life Sleep disturbance	Insulin resistance Hypertension Hyperlipidemia Elevated CRP Prothrombotic state Proinflammatory state
Nicotine addiction	Increased use	Insulin resistance Hypertension Proinflammatory state Prothrombotic state Increased thromboxane and platelet adhesion Vasospasm Reduced NO synthetase
HPA axis hyperactivity	Increased CRF Increased serum cortisol	Insulin resistance Obesity Hyperlipidemia Hypertension
Increased sympathetic autonomic tone	Increased norepinephrine	Hypertension Insulin resistance Proteinuria Enhanced prothrombotic state Increased vascular tone/vasospasm
Decreased parasympathetic autonomic tone	Reduced heart rate variability	Exercise intolerance Increased risk of sudden death Symptomatic fatigue Insulin resistance Obesity Osteopenia Dyslipidemia
Inflammation	Increased cytokines: IL-6 Tumor necrosis factor-α CRP	Insulin resistance Endothelial cell destruction Prothrombotic state Proinflammatory state
Genetic	Susceptibility genes	Genes can influence the expression of diabetes-related complications

Adapted from Unger J. Managing mental illness in patients with diabetes. *Pract Diabetol.* 2006;25:44–53.

predisposed, will eventually be unable to produce sufficient levels of endogenous insulin to maintain a euglycemic state. As hyperglycemia becomes more severe, pancreatic β-cell function further deteriorates. Patients begin to experience symptoms of chronic hyperglycemia, including polyuria, nocturia, fatigue, visual loss, sexual dysfunction, and neuropathic pain. The physical and emotional stressors associated with major mood disorder and persistent hyperglycemia may lead patients into feeling discouraged about their general state of well-being. They become even more depressed, believing that they are simply prone to developing symptoms associated with the normal aging process for which nothing can be done. Left undiagnosed and untreated, patients' physical and emotional states of well-being deteriorate rapidly. Fortunately, successful recognition and management of depression can reduce plasma cortisol levels, reverse insulin resistance, and restore the HPA to normal function.[29]

Depression also is associated with stimulation of the sympathetic nervous system and higher levels of circulating plasma norepinephrine levels. Resting heart rates are increased, heart-rate variability is enhanced, QT intervals are altered, and baroreflex dysfunction is noted more often in patients with depression when compared with nondepressed controls.[30] This suggests that the autonomic derangement in depressed individuals predisposes them to dyslipidemia, insulin resistance, obesity, fatigue, CAD and a higher risk of sudden death.[31]

Depressed patients have platelet abnormalities that promote a prothrombotic state.[32] Drugs that are useful in treating depression, such as serotonin reuptake inhibitors, appear to play a role in limiting this prothrombotic effect.[31]

Heart disease flourishes within the metabolic milieu of insulin resistance, endothelial cell dysfunction, altered autonomic function, and a proinflammatory state fueled by poor lifestyle and behavioral choices. Excuses abound as to why patients are unable or unwilling to increase their level of physical activity. Nonadherence to treatment protocols is common. As depression worsens and concentration becomes impaired, job performance and family issues deteriorate. Coping mechanisms are lost as life simply becomes too stressful for many patients to manage. Some patients enter into a downward spiral, losing their jobs, health insurance, and depleting their savings accounts. Because diabetes is an expensive disease, patients are quick to discontinue medications that may not directly affect the way that they "feel." As antihypertensive medications, statins, and even oral hypoglycemic agents are stopped, the metabolic status of the patient rapidly worsens, resulting in irreversible microvascular and macrovascular disease.

• Defining and Screening for Major Depressive Disorder

The *Diagnostic and Statistical Manual of Mental Disorders* (DSM) specifies a set of conditions that must be met to make the diagnosis of MDD.[11] Depression is a syndrome consisting of a group of symptoms that occur together, are severe, interfere with normal functioning, and persist daily over a period of at least 2 weeks. One of the symptoms must be depressed mood or anhedonia (absence of pleasure from the performance of acts that would otherwise be pleasurable). The diagnostic criteria for MDD are listed in Figure 9-1. Note that symptoms must be present during the majority of the day, for at least half of the previous 14 days. Bereavement, organic disease, and medication adverse effects must be ruled out as causes of symptoms that may simulate MDD.

MDD is a serious medical disorder that quickly becomes an all-encompassing and incapacitating condition for the patient. Alterations in sleeping and eating patterns result in deterioration in cognitive functioning. Patients are unable to think rationally, much less follow directions on complex treatment protocols. Deterioration of the patient's mental status often coincides with deterioration of glycemic control and loss of overall metabolic stability. Severely depressed patients are unable to revert to euthymia (a normal functional mood state) without medical intervention. The longer one has unrecognized depression, especially in conjunction with a deterioration in metabolic status, the more likely the patient is to lose the will to live. The potential benefits for recognizing and treating depression in patients with diabetes are listed in Table 9-2.

The early diagnosis and management of depression in our diabetic population can reduce morbidity, mortality, and medical expenses. Unfortunately, nearly everyone would agree that time

1. **One of the following:**
   - Depressed mood (Children and adolescents may be noted to be irritable)
   - Marked diminished interest or pleasure in almost all activities

2. **Four of the following:**
   - Significant weight loss when not dieting or weight gain (e.g., a change of more than 5% of body weight in a month), or decrease or increase in appetite nearly every day. (Children may not achieve expected weight benchmarks)
   - Insomnia or hypersomnia nearly every day
   - Being fidgety, restless, or a significant reduction in any movement
   - Fatigue
   - Reduced concentration (cannot read, write, understand work assignments, TV shows, perform simple tasks that required minimal efforts in the past)
   - Suicidal ideation

Note: Symptoms must be present most of the day. Symptoms must be present on more than 50% of the days over the past 2 weeks. Symptoms must not be attributable to an organic disorder, bereavement, or side effect from a medication. The symptoms cause clinically significant distress or impairment in social, occupational, or other important areas of functioning.

Figure 9-1 • **Diagnostic Criteria for Major Depressive Disorder.**
(APA. *Diagnostic and Statistical Manual of Mental Disorders*, 4th ed. Washington, DC: American Psychiatric Association; 1994.)

TABLE 9-2. Potential Benefits of Screening for, Diagnosing, and Treating Depression in Patients with Diabetes in the Primary Care Setting

Improved adherence with prescribed treatment regimen
Improved glycemic control with lowered A1C toward targeted levels
More acceptance by the patient of medically managing coexisting hypertension and hyperlipidemia with behavioral and pharmacologic intervention
Improved compliance related to scheduled office visits with PCP, specialists, and educators
Reduction in anxiety
Restoration of normal sleep patterns
Reduction in severity of chronic pain related to diabetic peripheral neuropathy
Willingness by patient to participate in healthy lifestyle choices such as exercise, smoking cessation, and dietary intervention
Enhanced sexual functioning
Increased likelihood that patient may be willing to participate in community events sponsored by the American Diabetes Association
Increased likelihood that patient will become a more active participant in his or her own diabetes self-management
Increased likelihood that patient will be willing to perform self–blood glucose monitoring
Increased likelihood that patient would be willing to increase the level of intensity of his or her diabetes management, even switching from oral agents to injectable drugs
Promote healthy lifestyle choices and prolong life

PCP, primary care physician.
Adapted from Unger J. Managing mental illness in patients with diabetes. *Pract Diabetol.* 2006;25:44–53. Copyright by R.A. Rapaport Publishing, Inc.

restraints and reimbursement issues limit one's ability to practice behavioral intervention in the office setting. PCPs should use effective yet proven means to diagnosis MDD, before embarking on a successful intervention program.

Although not all patients with diabetes are depressed, many initially demonstrate clues that are strongly associated with coexisting MDD. Patients with a history of depression, anxiety, or substance abuse or a family history of mental illness should undergo periodic screening for MDD. Patients experiencing frequent unexplained hypoglycemia or those who choose to focus on somatic complaints rather than on concerns related to glycemic control should also undergo screening. Patients with diabetic peripheral neuropathic pain often develop sleep disturbances, sexual dysfunction, anxiety disoders, and difficulty maintaining their balance. In time, their neuropathic dysfunction becomes all encompassing, driving their depressive and somatic complaints.

A screening test for depression that has been used effectively for years in the primary care setting is the PRIME-MD (Fig. 9-2). This questionnaire can be completed by the patient with or without assistance from the medical assistant before being seen by the physician. If five of the eight questions are noted to be positive for more than 50% of the days over the previous 2-week period, the patient can be diagnosed as having depression. Further direct questions can then inquire about (a) a history of depression; (b) the age at onset of the first episode of significant depression; (c) a history of suicide ideation or attempt; (d) a family history of mental illness such as depression, bipolar depression, or schizophrenia; (e) what, if any, medications have been used in the past to treat the patient's depression and for how long the patient was treated; and (f) a history of alcohol

1. Over the last 2 weeks, how often have you been bothered by any of the following problems?

	Not at all	Several days	More than half the days	Nearly every day
a. Little interest or pleasure in doing things	☐	☐	☐	☐
b. Feeling down, depressed, or hopeless	☐	☐	☐	☐
c. Trouble falling or staying asleep, or sleeping too much.	☐	☐	☐	☐
d. Feeling tired or having little energy	☐	☐	☐	☐
e. Poor appetite or overeating	☐	☐	☐	☐
f. Feeling bad about yourself—or that you are a failure or have let yourself or your family down	☐	☐	☐	☐
g. Trouble concentrating on things, such as reading the newspaper or watching television	☐	☐	☐	☐
h. Moving or speaking so slowly that other people could have noticed? Or the opposite—being so fidgety or restless that you have been moving around a lot more than usual	☐	☐	☐	☐
i. Thoughts that you would be better off dead or of hurting yourself in some way	☐	☐	☐	☐

Figure 9-2 • Screening for Depression in Primary Care by Using the PRIME-MD. The PRIME-MD can be used to screen patients for depression. The screening tool has a high sensitivity (73%) and specificity (98%) for the diagnosis of major depression. The criteria for major depression require the patient to have at least 2 weeks of five or more depressive symptoms present for more than half of the days. Note: Developed by Drs. Robert Spitzer and colleagues with an educational grant from Pfizer, Inc. (ris8@columbia.edu). PRIME-MD is a trademark of Pfizer, Inc. (Used from Spitzer R, Kroenke K, Williams J. Validation and utility of a self-report version of PRIME-MD: the PHQ primary care study: Primary Care Evaluation of Mental Disorders: Patient Health Questionnaire. *JAMA*. 1999;282:1737–1744, with permission.)

or substance abuse. Patients with a positive PRIME-MD should be considered strong candidates for behavioral and/or pharmacologic intervention for depression. Treatment should last for at least 1 year, and possibly longer if (a) the patient had a history of depression, (b) the first episode of depression occurred during the teenage years, (c) the patient had a previous suicide attempt, and (d) the patient has a family history of suicide or depression.

In patients aged 13 and older who are clinically depressed, the Beck Depression Inventory (BDI)[33] may be used to assess the severity of the symptoms. The BDI is a self-administered, 21-item, 4-point rating scale that evaluates mood, pessimism, sense of failure, self-dissatisfaction, guilt, punishment, self-dislike, self-accusation, suicidal ideas, crying, irritability, social withdrawal, indecisiveness, body-image change, work difficulty, insomnia, fatigability, loss of appetite, weight loss, somatic preoccupation, and loss of libido. The BDI is interpreted as follows:

- 0 to 9, Minimal depression
- 10 to 16, Mild depression
- 17 to 29, Moderate depression
- 30 to 63, Severe depression

The BDI can be downloaded at http://www.psych.upenn.edu/courses/psych001_601_Fall2002/bdi.doc.

Management of Depression in Patients with Diabetes

Once depression has been diagnosed in a patient with diabetes, the importance of medical intervention should be emphasized (Table 9-2). Most patients will be reassured knowing that a physiologic relationship between diabetes and depression is well known, and that depression most often precedes the onset of diabetes by a number of years. Depression is not a permanently curable disease; therefore, goals of therapy must be directed initially at inducing remission and, over the long term, reducing the likelihood of recurrence. Partial remissions tend to increase the chance of recurrence, implying that patients should be treated until they are free of depression symptoms and maintained at this level for a minimum of 1 year.[3]

Depression should *not* be viewed as a consequence of diabetes. Simply attempting to improve glycemic control in an attempt to resolve the depressive state is most often unsuccessful.[3] The behavioral approaches that may be helpful and self-motivating for depressed patients with diabetes include the following:

- Begin a regularly scheduled exercise program. Try an "exercise date night" with their significant other, complete with a personal trainer for motivation. Patients should exercise for at least 30 to 45 minutes each day.
- Join the American Diabetes Association (ADA) and attend community events targeting patients with diabetes. Become a community activist for diabetes.
- Keep family and friends involved with their daily diabetes care. Allow them to assist in any way possible. Perhaps they can help bring the patient to appointments, remind them to take medications, help prepare meals, rub their feet, assist with self blood glucose monitoring, help administer injections, and join in exercise routines.
- The physician should encourage patients to develop a positive attitude toward diabetes self-management. Discouraged patients should be reminded that they are attempting to "think like a pancreas," a process that is rarely forthcoming, often discouraging, yet absolutely necessary to master to the best of one's ability. Treating oneself to failure is not an option.
- Medical personnel should always find at least one positive attribute that warrants praise during each patient visit. One should never scold a patient, especially those who are making an effort in diabetes self-management programs. Praising patients will offer them hope and encouragement. Labeling patients as "noncompliant" implies that we have failed in

our role of medical educators and health-care providers. A patient who consistently fails to show improvement in treatment parameters will often become depressed and discouraged. Such a patient should be helped to think "outside the box" to find other treatment modalities that could be more effective. Ask a colleague or a thought leader in your community for help with the difficult-to-manage patients.

- Partnering with a certified diabetic educator (CDE) is certainly warranted for many patients with diabetes. Some patients may have cognitive deficiencies that require "special education skills," which CDEs are trained to develop. The more patients learn about their diabetes or depression, the more likely they may be to follow the treatment recommendations.

- Push patients to break out of their depressive patterns of life. Find something to do that is positive. They can join a club at their church or synagogue, volunteer for a charity or at a local school, or even take a class at a local senior center. Remind patients that they are ultimately responsible for their own happiness in life and that the doctor does not always have a "pill" for everything that ails them. Ultimately, successful management of major depression will depend upon the partnership between the physician and the patient in finding a common ground toward successful interventional strategies.

- Don't do diabetes alone. Many educational opportunities are available for anyone with diabetes. The ADA has an excellent Web site that can assist patients in getting started on their successful self-management program (http://www.diabetes.org).

- The physician should place patients on the medical regimen that will most likely result in treatment success rather than promote failure. For example, a patient with T1DM who is having difficulty with glycemic control while taking four daily injections of insulin may do much better on an insulin pump. Once patients perceive that their day-to-day diabetes management is improving, they will be more willing to continue as active participants in diabetes self-care.

- Always intensify therapy for patients who are symptomatic. Patients will not feel energetic with an A1C of 11%, especially if they are urinating six times a night, are unable to see clearly, and have lost the ability to obtain or maintain an erection. Continuing patients on oral therapy is bound to worsen their symptoms and their depression. These individuals should be placed on insulin therapy, either by inhalation or by injection.

- Depression can occur in anyone whether or not they have coexisting diabetes. However, patients with diabetes may also experience sleep disorders, chronic pain, disordered eating, sexual dysfunction, and even mood disorders as an adverse effect of medications used to treat hypertension, pain, or glaucoma. Low testosterone levels may also contribute to major depression as can illicit drugs and alcohol. Therefore, patients and physicians must have open communication as to the way they are feeling both physically and emotionally so that any depressive symptoms may be aggressively identified and managed.

- Always educate patients and their families regarding the link between the mind and the body, depression, and chronic illness. For example, chronic kidney disease results in elevated plasma levels of nitric oxide (NO). High levels of NO can cause sexual dysfunction, weight loss, psychomotor retardation, indecisiveness, and irritability.[34] Patients, family members, and coworkers should understand that some behaviors and actions have physiologic etiologies. This explains why most patients with a chronic illness cannot simply "snap out of it" of their own volition without professional guidance. Always remember that major depression is a neurochemically mediated disease state. Once normal neurotransmission is reestablished, major depression and other forms of mental illness should improve.

- Good sleep and daily exercise are the least expensive yet most cost-effective forms of antidepressant therapy. Patients should get at least 7 hours of uninterrupted sleep each night. Fragmented sleep, insomnia, sleep apnea, shift work, and circadian rhythm (advanced phase and delayed sleep phase disorders) can adversely affect the neuroendocrine sleep axis, which will increase insulin resistance and cause weight gain. (See chapter on associated sleep disorders.)

- Remind patients that although diabetes is a chronic progressive disease, the good news is that most individuals will live their entire life without experiencing any major disrupting event secondary to the disorder. The incidence of eye and kidney disease in the United States is rapidly declining. The likelihood of anyone requiring a limb amputation is very low. The treatment of diabetes today is much more advanced compared to 10 years ago.

Some patients may benefit from cognitive behavioral therapy (CBT), in which they are instructed by psychologists to recognize and remove patterns of negative thought processes that perpetuate depression (e.g., "I am terrible, my life is miserable, and I have no future."). CBT has been shown to be effective in achieving remission in 85% of patients with T2DM over a 10-week course, and 70% of these patients remained free of depression at the 6-month follow-up visit.[35,36]

Another example of where CBT may be effective is when patients realize they have a doctor's appointment in a week, but "all of the blood glucose values are terrible." They believe that there is "nothing that the doctor can do for me and I will most certainly go blind or lose an eye." In reality, CBT teaches patients that this is unlikely to happen with today's array of medical therapies. Most diabetes-related complications may be prevented, delayed, or even reversed if treated intensively. Formation of an optimistic partnership between the PCP, behavioralist, CDE, and family members is an integral aspect of cognitive behavioral therapy. "Doing diabetes alone" is not wise for anyone, whether or not they have any type of mental illness.

CBT shifts the focus away from what patients are doing "wrong each day" to how they are actually being successful with their diabetes self-management. An example of successful CBT was a 71-year-old retired family physician with a 51-year history of T1DM. The patient feared having ANY blood glucose values greater than 160 mg per dL. While using an insulin pump, the patient would monitor his blood glucose levels 8 to 10 times each day. Any blood glucose level greater than 160 mg per dL would be managed with a correction bolus to "get the blood sugar below 100 mg per dL." The physician experienced episodes of severe hypoglycemia at least three times weekly over the past 6 months necessitating the administration of glucagon by his wife. Despite proudly boasting an A1C of 6.1%, the patient had developed cognitive impairment, which interfered with the safe operation of his insulin pump. Figure 9-3 shows this patient's continuous glucose sensor tracing prior to entering into CBT. After reviewing the result of the continuous glucose sensor tracing, the patient and his wife understood the implications of his aggressive attempts to avoid "hyperglycemia." His physician noted that despite having significant glycemic variability and T1DM for over 50 years, the patient's only complication

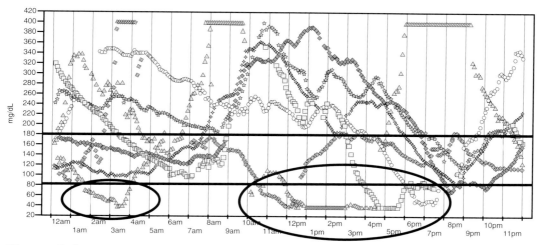

Figure 9-3 • **Continuous Glucose Sensor Tracing of a Patient with Severe Nocturnal and Diurnal Hypoglycemia Due to Insulin Stacking.** These hypoglycemic events would last up to 5 hours and occurred multiple times each week, resulting in hypoglycemia awareness autonomic failure and dementia. (Case supplied courtesy of Jeff Unger, MD.)

was hypoglycemia awareness autonomic failure. Perhaps focusing his attention on everything he has done right over the past 5 decades rather than dwelling on the ill effects of hyperglycemia may be in the patient's best interest. The patient agreed to purchase a continuous glucose sensor monitor that alarmed when his glucose level dropped below 80 mg per dL. He was also warned to stop giving inappropriate correction boluses of insulin as this could affect his own safety as well as others around him. The doctor even threatened to discontinue his insulin pump prescription if he did not follow his prescribed treatment plan.

Figure 9-4 shows the improvement in the patient's glycemic control at his 2-month follow-up visit. One year after initiating the use of his sensor and avoiding insulin stacking, the patient's dementia has resolved and his quality of life has dramatically improved.

Although these self-help techniques may relieve depression (especially minor depression) in some cases, most patients with MDD will require antidepressant medication and/or talk therapy for optimal control of their mental illness. Successful depression treatment was associated with significant improvement in glycemic control in studies using fluoxetine and sertraline.[37,38] Interestingly, obese patients treated with fluoxetine have been shown to have improved insulin resistance while requiring lower doses of exogenous insulin for maintenance of good glycemic control.[38,39] Side effects may limit the utility of some antidepressant medications in the diabetic population. Tricyclic antidepressants can cause dry mouth, urinary hesitancy, orthostatic hypotension, blurred vision, and weight gain. Mood stabilizers (valproic acid) cause weight gain and gastric reflux. Monoamine oxidase inhibitors, which are highly effective agents in patients with treatment-resistant depression, have dangerous drug and food interactions (duloxetine, meperidine, over-the-counter cold remedies, tyramine), making this class of drugs very risky in the diabetic population. Because of their more favorable side effect profiles, the selective serotonin reuptake inhibitors (SSRIs) and serotonin norepinephrine reuptake inhibitors (duloxetine, venlafaxine) are the most appropriate antidepressant drugs for managing depression in diabetes patients. Bupropion and mirtazapine are also acceptable choices.

Before initiating pharmacologic treatment for depression, the clinician should consider possible side effects associated with the most commonly prescribed medications. Sexual dysfunction and weight gain may become apparent within 1 month of starting a patient on an SSRI. More than 50% of patients with MDD will have sexual dysfunction as a symptom of their depression.[40] Determining whether sexual dysfunction exists before initiating antidepressant therapy is an important step in managing depression. Patients who report a change in sexual functioning within 8 to 12 weeks of starting treatment with an antidepressant are most likely experiencing a side effect of the medication rather than a core symptom of the depression. Although sexual dysfunction is generally not

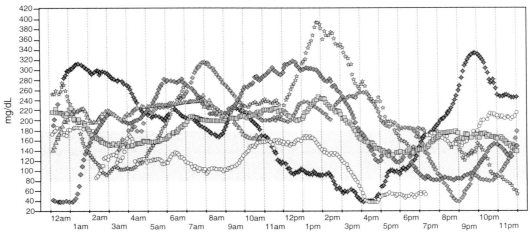

Figure 9-4 • Patient's A1C has Increased from 6.1 to 7.4. His hypoglycemic events are still present but are less frequent and prolonged. Only a single nocturnal event over the past 7 days has been recorded.

a major problem in urgent treatment of depression, a persistence in symptoms frequently leads to early discontinuation of treatment.

Although a low incidence of sexual side effects (less than 15%) is stated on the product labeling for the most commonly prescribed antidepressants, a review of published studies between 1986 and 2000 suggests that 30% to 60% of SSRI-treated patients may experience some form of treatment-induced sexual dysfunction.[41] The SSRIs and venlafaxine extended release are related to higher rates of sexual dysfunction than are bupropion, nefazodone, and duloxetine.[42]

Several treatment options are available for patients whose major depression has improved while taking an antidepressant, but in whom sexual dysfunction developed during their course of therapy:

1 / **Wait for tolerance to develop.** Sexual dysfunction that becomes apparent soon after therapy is initiated with an antidepressant agent may improve spontaneously. A patient who no longer presents with symptoms of depression may also show improvement in his glycemic control, which is also likely to improve sexual function.

2 / **Reduce the dose of the antidepressant.** Although reducing the dose may improve sexual performance, it may reduce the therapeutic efficacy of the drug. Patient education is critical. Providing the male patient with a phosphodiesterase type 5 inhibitor might be an option for these patients.

3 / **Take a drug holiday.** Patients may be advised to hold their antidepressant medications after their Thursday dose and restart on Sunday over the course of four successive weekends. In a small open-label clinical trial, 30 patients who were instructed on using such a drug holiday reported improved sexual performance and no changes in their depression scores with this protocol.[43]

4 / **Switch medications.** Patients who experience sexual dysfunction on an SSRI or another antidepressive agent might show symptom improvement when changed to either duloxetine or bupropion SR (slow release). These medications have a lower incidence of sexual side effects than do other antidepressant medications.[44]

Weight gain may complicate therapy with antidepressants in patients with diabetes. Weight gain during antidepressant treatment may be associated with improvement in patients who have weight loss as a symptom of depression. However, some patients with persistent depression may overeat when they become more desperate. Weight gain that continues after depressive symptoms have resolved is likely to be a side effect of the medication and frequently leads to premature discontinuation of therapy that provided an otherwise favorable response. Some of the newer antidepressants (duloxetine and bupropion) are considered weight neutral.

Several steps can be initiated to manage treatment-emergent weight gain associated with antidepressant therapy:

1 / **Improve diet and initiate exercise program.** Solutions for Wellness is a 6-month program designed to assist patients in incorporating healthy dietary and exercise habits into their daily routines. This program is free of charge and is available at http://www.solutionsforwellness.info/Custom/home/home.asp

2 / **Use weight-neutral medications in high-risk patients.** Table 9-3 lists the antidepressants that are most likely to cause weight gain. Patients who are obese may do best with a drug considered to be weight neutral.

3 / **Consider adding adjunctive therapy to the primary antidepressant.** Adding bupropion, 100 to 150 mg per day, or topiramate, 25 to 50 mg at bedtime, may mitigate weight gain in some patients.[45]

Once pharmacologic treatment for depression is initiated, follow-up should be scheduled within 4 weeks to evaluate the following treatment parameters:

1. Is the patient showing clinical improvement related to the mood disorder?
2. Are any significant adverse side effects from the medications present (delayed ejaculation, loss of sexual desire, fatigue, headache, weight gain)?
3. Are signs of developing suicidality noted, warranting immediate psychiatric referral?

TABLE 9-3. Effect of Antidepressant Therapy on Weight Gain

Drug (Generic Name)	Effect
Monoamine oxidase inhibitors	Weight gain
Tricyclic compounds	Weight gain
SSRIs	• Fluoxetine may cause weight loss when used for <6 mo, but weight gain when used for >6 mo • Paroxetine weight gain is greater in patients being treated for major depression than in those being treated for generalized anxiety disorders • Weight gain is more likely to occur with paroxetine than with other SSRIs
Nefazodone	Weight neutral
Bupropion	May cause weight loss
Mirtazapine	Weight gain, but fewer TCAs
Venlafaxine	Weight neutral
Duloxetine	Weight neutral
Escitalopram	Weight neutral
Desvenlafaxine	Weight neutral
Milnacipran	Weight neutral

TCAs, tricyclic antidepressants.
Adapted from Deshmukh R, Franco K. Managing weight gain as a side effect of antidepressant therapy. *Cleve Clin J Med.* 2003;70:614–623.

4. What is the pattern of the glycemic response to pharmacologic management of the major depression?
5. What, if any, lifestyle interventions have been adopted by the patient since the previous visit?
6. Is a need for "talk therapy" apparent in addition to pharmacologic intervention?
7. Reinforce the fact that antidepressant medications must be continued for a prolonged period and should not be abruptly discontinued under any circumstances. Medications should be tapered slowly over a 1- to 2-week period to avoid emotional decompensation.

The PRIME-MD (Fig. 9-2), which was used to screen patients for depression initially, may also be used to evaluate the patient's response to treatment. Those individuals who demonstrate no response to therapy may require an increase in dose, combination therapy with a mood stabilizer (valproate or topiramate), and possibly a psychiatric consultation to assist in pharmacologic management. Communication between the PCP and the psychiatric team is critical because the mental health personnel may be unfamiliar with the principles involved in managing metabolic anomalies such as hyperglycemia, hypertension, and hyperlipidemia. The best outcomes for both mental illness and metabolic disorders can be achieved if the mental illness is stabilized first. After patients' cognitive functioning improves, they can begin to play a more active role in their own diabetes self-management program.

Unfortunately, recurrent depression rates in patients with diabetes are high. Only 40% of patients remain free of MDD in the year after successful treatment, with symptom recurrence often seen in association with deterioration in glycemic control.[38] Therefore, long-term management with both pharmacologic and behavioral interventions (such as exercise) is usually necessary to prolong the depression-free interval and stabilize glycemic control. Lustman et al.,[39] by using meta-analysis data, determined that treatment of depression in diabetes could increase the proportion of patients in good glycemic control from 41% to 58%. The projected improvement in optimal glycemic control would have significant individual and societal benefits in terms of outcomes related to complications, quality of life, and health-care expenditures.

Schizophrenia and Diabetes

Schizophrenia is a cross-cultural illness occurring in 1% of the worldwide population. Approximately 30% to 40% of homeless individuals have schizophrenia.[46] Age at onset occurs between late adolescence and the third decade, often after an insidious premorbid course of subtle psychosocial difficulties. The prodromal phase, which may begin years before the syndrome becomes manifest, is characterized by losses of functioning in home, society, and occupation. Patients exhibit poor school or work performance, have deterioration in their appearance and hygiene, and display decreasing emotional connections with friends, family members, or coworkers. An abrupt onset of hallucinations and delusional, bizarre, or disorganized thinking in patients who previously functioned normally may result in a better intermediate and long-term outcome. Initially, treatment may be complicated further by the presence of alcohol or drug intoxication. Substance abuse among patients with schizophrenia is common, with nicotine, alcohol, and stimulants being the most commonly used. Excessive use of these stimulants, alcohol, and nicotine by patients who commonly have comorbid metabolic abnormalities contributes to their shortened lifespan. Ten percent of patients with schizophrenia commit suicide.[47] Schizophrenia cannot be cured; the prognosis is dependent on the patient's response to antipsychotic medication rather than the severity of the symptoms.

The diagnosis of schizophrenia is based on the presence over the prior month of two or more of the following psychiatric conditions[48]:

- **Delusions:** Bizarre or illogical false beliefs, which often have a paranoid, grandiose, persecutory, or religious flavor
- **Hallucinations:** Typically auditory (visual or tactile strongly suggest organic etiology), often involving evil or taunting voices commenting on the patient's actions or character, often with a sexual flavor, giving commands (i.e., command hallucinations); two or more voices discussing or arguing with each other; audible thoughts; thought withdrawal (feeling that thoughts are being removed from the head), thought broadcasting, or thought interference by outside agent
- **Disorganized speech:** Tangential, incoherent, rambling speech; neologisms (new word creation); loosening of associations
- **Behavior:** Grossly disorganized or catatonic
- **Negative symptoms:** Depression; lack of speech (alogia); complete lack of energy, spontaneity, or initiative (avolition); or loss of interest and pleasure in activities once enjoyed (anhedonia)

Other psychiatric conditions such as bipolar depression and major mood disorder as well as organic disease (endocrine disorders, electrolyte imbalance, neoplasm, seizure disorder, drug intoxication) must be excluded before the diagnosis of schizophrenia is made.

• Schizophrenia May be Considered an Independent Risk Factor for the Development of T2DM

The link between schizophrenia and diabetes was first postulated[49] in 1920, long before the introduction of pharmacologic therapies, which have been linked to treatment-emergent hyperglycemia. A recent study of patients with schizophrenia in the United States Veterans Administration health-care system found that the rate of diabetes was 6.2% to 8.7%, compared with 1.1% in U.S. men aged 20 to 39 years without schizophrenia.[50] The Canadian Diabetes Association lists schizophrenia as an independent risk factor in the development of diabetes.[51] Patients hospitalized with schizophrenia are twice as likely to have hyperglycemia than are individuals from the general population.[52] Just as depression tends to precede the onset of T2DM by a number of years, patients with schizophrenia often have metabolic abnormalities that precede their first episode of emotional decompensation. Ryan et al.[53] evaluated the metabolic parameters of 26 treatment-naive schizophrenic patients who presented to the emergency department during their initial episode of psychotic decompensation. When compared with age- and sex-matched control subjects, these individuals had higher levels of serum cortisol, increased insulin resistance, and higher fasting glucose levels, suggesting an inherent abnormality in their hypothalamic-pituitary axis.[53]

Schizophrenia is an inherently stressful disease state. To understand how truly stressful this disorder can be, put yourself for just a few seconds into the mind of someone with schizophrenia. You could be walking down a street, becoming increasingly aware of people staring at you. This begins to make you very angry. At that very moment you begin hearing voices telling you to "run off the sidewalk into oncoming traffic." You know that is likely to cause injury, and you are doing everything in your power to avoid shutting the voices down and acting on their commands. You begin to tremble, talk back to the voices, and run to avoid being chased by people who have been watching you on your way home.

Perhaps this is why the treatment-naive patients in Ryan's study had elevated serum cortisol levels. Serum cortisol raises plasma glucose. Patients with schizophrenia are chronically exposed to stress. This results in chronic stimulation of the hypothalamic-pituitary axis, leading to insulin resistance that progresses to clinical diabetes in genetically prone individuals.

Patients with schizophrenia have a severe, disabling, and chronic illness often complicated by coexisting metabolic abnormalities that increase their risks for diabetes and heart disease. Whereas suicidality may be a well-known cause of premature death in severe mental illness, the fact that their underlying metabolic disorders may contribute to morbidity and mortality is often overlooked. Because patients with schizophrenia are at high risk of CAD (two to three times higher than age-matched controls), PCPs should become familiar with the psychiatric, metabolic, and pharmacologic treatment issues of these challenging patients.[54]

Unfortunately, management of their coexisting metabolic abnormalities in an outpatient setting is extremely challenging unless the mental illness is first stabilized. Because some mental health-care providers fear that antipsychotic medication may worsen metabolic parameters and "cause diabetes," the drugs that are the most efficacious in the treatment of schizophrenia and bipolar depression may not be used for the most mentally ill patients.

One of the major problems we face in managing patients with mental illness is premature discontinuation of prescribed medications, which can lead to frequent hospital admissions, dysfunctional or antisocial behavior, and increased risk of suicide. The Clinical Antipsychotic Trial of Intervention Effectiveness (CATIE Trial) demonstrated that 74% of patients with schizophrenia prematurely discontinued their antipsychotic medications because of either lack of efficacy or intolerable side effects.[55] A study by Liu-Siefert[56] demonstrated that patients with schizophrenia were three times more likely to discontinue their antipsychotic medications because of lack of efficacy rather than issues related to intolerability.

The benefits of a particular medication for a specific person may outweigh the potential risks, even when those risks include diabetes, weight gain, and dyslipidemia. Once the psychiatric condition is stabilized, patients may become active and successful participants in their own lifestyle interventions and diabetes self-management programs. Controlling psychotic illnesses with appropriate pharmacotherapy can often lead to improved insight into medical diagnosis, enhanced adherence to medical recommendations, and improved medical outcomes.[57]

Pharmacologic Interventions

Since being introduced more than 50 years ago, antipsychotic medications have been the cornerstone of treatment for psychotic illnesses. These drugs are also used in a variety of other off-label conditions[58] such as migraine, chronic pain, attention deficit disorder, stuttering, fibromyalgia, autism, post-traumatic stress syndrome, aggressive behavior, acute agitation, sleep disorders, and dementia. Although these drugs are certainly useful in patients with bipolar depression or schizophrenia, their off-label use in some patients has resulted in an increased risk of mortality. The U.S. Food and Drug Administration (FDA) has determined that treating behavioral disorders in elderly patients with dementia with second-generation antipsychotic medications (olanzapine, aripiprazole, risperidone, or quetiapine) was associated with a 1.6 times increased risk of mortality compared with patients using placebo drugs for the same disorder. Nevertheless, for patients who respond well, antipsychotic medications can mean the difference between remaining disabled and living a full and engaging social life.

The first-generation (also called "conventional" or "typical") antipsychotics are effective in treating the positive symptoms of schizophrenia, most notably hallucinations, delusions, aggression, and hostility (Table 9-4). Their primary disadvantage has been the lack of response toward improvement in negative symptoms (apathy, social isolation and withdrawal, and lack of motivation). First-generation antipsychotic agents also exhibit a high rate of extrapyramidal side effects such as dystonia, akathisia (an inability to sit still), and tardive dyskinesia. Tardive dyskinesia is characterized by repetitive, involuntary, purposeless movements. Features of the disorder may include grimacing, tongue protrusion, lip smacking, puckering and pursing of the lips, and rapid eye blinking.

Both the efficacy and adverse effects of these drugs are associated with antagonism at the D2 receptors. Efficacy is associated with at least 60% occupancy of these receptors, yet

TABLE 9-4. Antipsychotic Drugs

Generic Name	Brand Name	Urgent Treatment Daily Dose (mg/d)	Maintenance Daily Dose (mg/d)	Geriatric Daily Dose (mg/d)	IM Dose for Acute Agitation
"Conventional" Antipsychotic Agents					
Chlorpromazine	Thorazine	300–1,000	300–600	25–75	25–50 mg 3–4/d
Perphenazine	Trilafon	30–100	30–60	2–8	
Thiothixene	Navane	15–20	15–30	2–6	
Haloperidol	Haldol	6–20	6–12	2–4	2.5–5 mg q 4–6 h
Fluphenazine	Prolixin	6–20	6–12	2–4	
"Atypical" Second–Generation Antipsychotic Agents					
Clozapine	Clozaril	200–800	200–800[a]	25–50	
Risperidone	Risperdal	4–10	4–10	1–2	
Olanzapine	Zyprexa	10–20	10–20	5–10	10 mg IM × 1, repeat in 2 h and 6 h prn; max, 30 mg/24 h; info: use 5 mg IM × 1 in elderly or 2.5 mg × 1 if debilitated
Quetiapine	Seroquel	200–800	200–800	50–200	
Ziprasidone	Geodon	80–160	80–160	80–160	10 mg q 2 h up to 40 mg/d
Aripiprazole	Abilify	10–30	10–30	5–10	
Paliperidone[b]	Invega	3–9	6–12	6–12[b]	
Olanzepine/Fluoxetine Symbyax		3/25–12/50	6/25	3/25	

[a]Therapeutic plasma level is 350 μg/L.
[b]Adjust dose for renal insufficiency (consult prescribing information).
h, hour; IM, intramuscular; prn, as needed; q, every.

when the receptor occupancy exceeds 80%, extrapyramidal symptoms and hyperprolactinemia occur.[59]

Although the first-generation antipsychotic agents are effective at treating the positive symptoms of psychosis (hallucinations and delusions), the negative symptoms (withdrawal, apathy, speech impairment), as well as depressive symptoms and cognitive impairment, are better managed with the second-generation drugs. All antipsychotic drugs have the potential of causing extrapyramidal side effects in clinically effective doses, although these uncomfortable adverse effects are experienced in up to 60% of patients using first-generation drugs. These side effects—which include dystonic reactions, drug-induced parkinsonism, tardive dyskinesia, and akathisia (restlessness, inability to sit still)—can make treatment intolerable for many patients, reducing compliance, worsening psychotic symptoms, and increasing the likelihood that an urgent hospital readmission will be necessary.

The second-generation drugs are better tolerated and overall more effective in managing schizophrenia and BPD. Clozapine is the most effective antipsychotic agent, but because of the drug's potential to induce agranulocytosis, is used only when other drugs have failed or in patients at high risk of suicide.[60]

One of the primary concerns expressed by patients and physicians when using second-generation antipsychotic drugs is treatment-emergent weight gain. The amount of weight one gains varies from 0.5 to 5.0 kg over the course of 10 weeks. The patients who gain the most weight appear to do so while augmenting their daily caloric intake, which in some cases may already be excessive, in conjunction with minimal energy expenditure in the form of exercise.

Among the atypical antipsychotic medications, varying degrees of weight gain have been reported. The relative tendency to cause weight gain is as follows: clozapine > olanzapine > risperidone = quetiapine > ziprasidone = ariprazole.[60]

The reason that patients gain weight while using these drugs is uncertain. One theory suggests that blocking histamine receptors will induce weight gain. Drugs that have the highest affinity toward histamine-receptor blockade, such as olanzapine, are associated with the most weight gain, whereas ziprasidone and ariprazole demonstrate the least weight gain and have limited histamine-receptor activity.[61] Blockade of the serotonin receptor subtypes 5-HT2C has been associated with increased appetite and obesity in animal models. Most atypicals do block this receptor, which may explain the increase in appetite patients experience while using atypical antipsychotics.[59]

Treatment-emergent diabetes is another concern for patients using second-generation antipsychotic medications. Most cases of treatment-emergent T2DM occur within the first 6 months of treatment and are always associated with significant weight gain or obesity. Patients with a family history of T2DM are also at high risk for developing treatment-emergent diabetes and must be screened for hyperglycemia when starting antipsychotic medication.

As with weight gain, variability exists among the specific atypical antipsychotic as to which agents are most likely to be associated with treatment-emergent diabetes. Olanzapine and clozapine are associated with a higher rate of diabetes than are risperidone and quetiapine.[62] However, the risk of developing diabetes is inherently higher in patients with mental illness than in the general population.[63]

Patients treated with olanzapine and clozapine have higher fasting and postprandial insulin levels than do those treated with first-generation antipsychotic agents, even after adjusting for body weight, indicative of insulin resistance.[60] Clozapine and olanzapine, which produce the greatest weight gain, are associated with the greatest increases in total cholesterol, low-density lipoprotein cholesterol, and triglycerides and with decreased high-density lipoprotein cholesterol. However, these two drugs are the most powerful with regard to symptom stabilization in patients with bipolar depression and schizophrenia.[64]

Several mechanisms of glucose dysregulation have been proposed to explain the association between the use of atypical antipsychotics and treatment-emergent hyperglycemia. First, the medications that cause the most weight gain also are associated with the highest risk of diabetes. However, some patients develop diabetes while using atypicals in the absence of weight gain. Other etiologies, such as a disruption in hypothalamic regulation of glucose regulation through dopamine antagonism, might be one possible mechanism. Second, patients treated with clozapine and olanzapine have elevated insulin levels, suggesting a link between atypical antipsychotics and insulin resistance. Finally, atypical drugs that have the highest anticholinergic activity may alter the ability of pancreatic β-cells to secrete insulin in response to a normal glycemic stimulus, as demonstrated in animal models.[65]

When choosing to use an antipsychotic medication, the following individual factors should be considered:

- What are the nature and severity of the patient's psychiatric condition? The more severe the mental illness, the more important appropriate drug utilization becomes.
- What are the treatment target signs and symptoms? Patients with negative symptoms, especially those with anxiety and sleep disorders, would probably gain most benefit from a second-generation agent.
- What is the patient's history of drug response, both therapeutic and adverse? Patients should be treated with the drug that will allow them not only to have the best chance of restoring function but also encourage them to remain with the medication for the long haul without premature discontinuation. Potential adverse events should be discussed in detail with both the patient and family members. Concerns regarding these medications should be addressed at each visit. Important potential adverse events that should be discussed include treatment-emergent diabetic ketoacidosis (DKA), weight gain, extrapyramidal symptoms, drowsiness, and changes in metabolic status. The signs and symptoms of DKA that should be discussed include

  ■ Rapid onset of

Polyuria, polydipsia
Weight loss
Nausea, vomiting
Dehydration
Altered consciousness/coma
Rapid respiration

- What is the most appropriate formulation to use in any given patient? Second-generation drugs may be given orally, via oral disintegrating tablets (olanzapine zydis), or as an intramuscular agent for acute symptom stabilization (Table 9-4). Patient preference should be considered.
- When choosing a second-generation drug, consider the metabolic influences each drug may have on an individual (Table 9-5). Patients with preexisting metabolic conditions may use the second-generation drugs. However, these individuals should be carefully monitored, as is discussed later.
- All patients who are initiated on antipsychotic therapy should be screened and followed up periodically, as suggested by the American Diabetes Consensus Development Conference on Antipsychotic Drugs and Obesity (Table 9-6).[56,60]
- The basic premise should be to focus initial management on stabilization of the mental illness. Any treatment-emergent metabolic abnormalities that become apparent over time should be aggressively managed with appropriate lifestyle and pharmacologic interventions.

Bipolar Depression and Diabetes

Although BPD is one of the most distinct syndromes in psychiatry, in more than 70% of patients, the disorder is initially misdiagnosed. On average, each patient will experience 3.5 misdiagnoses

TABLE 9-5. Second-generation Antipsychotic Drugs and Metabolic Abnormalities

Drug	Weight Gain	Risk for Diabetes	Worsening Lipid Profile
Clozapine	+ + +	+	+
Olanzapine	+ + +	+	+
Risperidone	+ +	D	D
Quetiapine	+ +	D	D
Aripiprazole[a]	±	–	–
Ziprasidone[a]	±	–	–
Olanzapine/Fluoxitine	+++	+	+
Paliperidone	+	+	–

+ = increase effect; – = no effect; D = discrepant results.
[a]Newer drugs with limited long-term data.
From American Diabetes Association. Consensus development conference on antipsychotic drugs and obesity and diabetes. *Diabetes Care.* 2004;27:596–601 and prescribing information websites for each drug. Accessed November 11, 2011.

and 4 consults before receiving an accurate diagnosis.[66] The unique hallmark of BPD is mania, characterized by an elevated, euphoric mood, and reduced need for sleep so extreme that one's judgment may be impaired. Manic patients are sometimes disinhibited in their sexual actions, which may endanger their marriage. The manic behavior, which may develop gradually over a period of weeks or months, is distinct from the patient's true personality and is often recognized as atypical by family members and coworkers. A single manic episode is sufficient for the diagnosis of bipolar illness, assuming that the symptoms of mania are not due to an underlying medical disorder such as Graves disease, amphetamine abuse, or pheochromocytoma. A manic episode, which occurs at a young age, may be followed by intermittent periods of depression. Patients who have four or more episodes of mania or depression per year are considered to be "rapid cyclers," a condition that may be treatment refractive.[67]

TABLE 9-6. Monitoring Protocol for Patients on Second-generation Antipsychotic Agents

	Baseline	4 wk	8 wk	12 wk	Quarterly	Annually	Every 5 y
Personal/family history[a]	X					X	
Weight (BMI)[b]	X	X	X	X	X	X	
Waist circumference[c]	X					X	
Blood pressure	X			X		X	
Fasting plasma glucose[d]	X			X		X	
Fasting lipid profile	X			X			X

[a]Ask a patient at baseline as well as annually about a personal or family history of diabetes or impaired glucose tolerance.
[b]A BMI ≥ 30 kg/m² is considered obesity.
[c]A waist circumference of >35 inches (female) or >40 inches (male) is suggestive of android (upper body) obesity. This type of obesity is prominently seen in diabetes, coronary artery disease, as well as in schizophrenia phenotypes.
[d]A patient with a fasting plasma glucose level >100 mg/dL should undergo a 2-h glucose challenge to determine whether he or she has diabetes. After an overnight fast, the patient consumes a 75-g glucose test drink; 2 h later, a blood glucose level is determined. Blood glucose levels: (a) <140 mg/dL is considered normal; (b) 140–199 mg/dL, impaired glucose tolerance; and (c) ≥200 mg/dL is diagnostic of diabetes. If a patient is not initially seen fasting, obtain a random blood glucose level. Any glucose ≥ 140 mg/dL is abnormal and warrants further investigation.
[e]Lipid profiles should be obtained more frequently if clinically warranted.
From American Diabetes Association. Consensus development conference on antipsychotic drugs and obesity and diabetes. *Diabetes Care.* 2004;27:596–601.

The lifetime prevalence of BPD is 1%, in comparison to 10% to 25% of individuals who develop major depression over the course of their lifetime.[68] BPD affects one's ability to work, socialize, and appropriately function within the family unit. Ten to fifteen percent of patients with BPD will successfully commit suicide.[2] Sixty percent have coexisting substance abuse.[69] Women with BPD suffer a greater amount of difficulty in social and family life, whereas men have more problems with the justice system, including increased time spent in jail and more criminal convictions.[70] Women with BPD have a higher risk of suicide, irrational behavior, mania, and substance abuse during the postpartum period.[67]

Adding to the difficulties associated with diagnosing and managing patients with BPD is the unfortunate reality that the rate of baseline obesity is disproportionate in patients with chronic psychiatric illness[71]; 68% of patients with BPD and schizophrenia are estimated to be overweight or obese at the time of their initial diagnosis.[72,73] Obesity in the psychiatric population may be due to poor nutritional choices, sedentary lifestyle, lower socioeconomic status, and a genetic predisposition toward this metabolically active phenotype. Increased weight is related to low self-esteem and a negative self-image, even in individuals not suffering from a mental disorder. These emotions profoundly impact the quality of lives of those suffering from mental illness and obesity. This is important for the clinician to understand, because medications used for the treatment of BPD tend to further increase one's weight. Once the patient's emotional status becomes stabilized, the PCP should begin a "full court press" emphasizing healthy lifestyle choices and increased levels of physical activity in order to minimize any additional weight gain.

When parents accompany their 22-year-old daughter to the doctor's office for the treatment of BPD, they will ask the question, "Doctor, when can we get our daughter back to the way she used to be?" If a patient gains 5 to 7 lbs on an atypical antipsychotic agent, yet is able to become fully employed while resuming a normal family or social life, there is an excellent chance that adherence to the drug therapy will continue. However, if the patient gains no weight but shows no improvement emotionally, patients will more than likely discontinue use of their antipsychotic drugs. Efficacy surpasses tolerability as the primary goal of pharmacologic intervention for patients with any psychiatric illness.[56]

• Diagnosing Bipolar Disorder

When evaluating a patient for BPD, physicians should review the following historical factors:

1. Early age at onset of patient's initial symptoms (typically younger than 25 years) with an episodic presentation
2. Family history of mental illness (in particular, bipolar illness)
3. Prior history of suicide attempts
4. History of substance or alcohol abuse
5. Multiple treatment failures with "antidepressants"
6. A rapid response to an SSRI (a patient who begins to feel "better" within a few days after starting an SSRI may have had an induction of acute mania. Most patients with major depression require a 2- to 4-week response time before they perceive improvement in depressive symptoms while on an SSRI.)
7. Is the patient experiencing racing thoughts, periods of insomnia, difficulty with concentration, or anxiety?
8. Does the patient have a history of going several days without requiring much sleep? During these times, did the patient feel energetic enough to begin several new projects, yet complete none of them?
9. Has the patient ever been treated for "attention deficit disorder," yet not responded positively to stimulant therapy?
10. Has the patient ever been evaluated by a mental health worker? If so, what was the diagnosis? What medications were prescribed? How did the patient respond to those medications?
11. Has the patient ever been incarcerated?
12. Does the patient experience frequent mood swings that may be affecting family members and coworkers?

INSTRUCTIONS: Please answer each question as best you can.   YES   NO

1. Has there ever been a period of time when you were not your usual self and...

    ...you felt so good or so hyper that other people thought you were
        not your normal self or you were so hyper that you got into trouble?   ○   ○

    ...you were so irritable that you shouted at people or started fights
        or arguments?   ○   ○

    ...you felt much more self-confident than usual?   ○   ○

    ...you got much less sleep than usual and found that you really didn't
        miss it?   ○   ○

    ...you were more talkative or spoke much faster than usual?   ○   ○

    ...thoughts raced through your head or you couldn't slow your mind
        down?   ○   ○

    ...you were so easily distracted by things around you that you had
        trouble concentrating or staying on track?   ○   ○

    ...you had much more energy than usual?   ○   ○

    ...you were much more active or did many more things than usual?   ○   ○

    ...you were much more social or outgoing than usual, for example,
        you telephoned friends in the middle of the night?   ○   ○

    ...you were much more interested in sex than usual?   ○   ○

    ...you did things that were unusual for you or that other people might
        have thought were excessive, foolish or risky?   ○   ○

    ...spending money got you or your family in trouble?   ○   ○

2. If you checked YES to more than one of the above, have several of these   ○   ○
   ever happened during the same period of time?

3. How much of a problem did any of these cause you—like being able to work;
   having family, money, legal troubles; getting into arguments or fights?

    ○ No problem   ○ Minor problem   ○ Moderate problem   ○ Serious problem

4. Have any of your blood relatives (i.e., children, siblings, parents, grandparents, ○   ○
   aunts, uncles) had manic-depressive illness or bipolar disorder?

5. Has a health professional ever told you that you have manic-depressive   ○   ○
   illness or bipolar disorder?

Figure 9-5 • Mood Disorder Questionnaire for Bipolar Depression. Note: This tool is for *screening* purposes only and does not establish a diagnosis of bipolar depression. Positive screen requires all of the following: (a) seven of thirteen positive (yes) responses; (b) Question 2: must be answered yes; and (c) Question 3: must be answered "moderate" or "serious." (Used from Hirschfeld RM, Williams JB, Spitzer RL. Development and validation of a screening instrument for bipolar spectrum disorder: the Mood Disorder Questionnaire. *Am J Psychiatry.* 2000;157:1873–1875, with permission.)

13. Inquire about specific psychiatric risk factors, such as a history of physical, verbal, or sexual abuse directed toward the patient during childhood; a family history of substance or alcohol abuse; and a history of parental divorce, separation, or abandonment during childhood.

Those patients in whom a diagnosis of BPD is suspected should be asked to complete the Mood Disorder Questionnaire (MDQ). This brief validated, self-reporting questionnaire may help to determine if a patient has had a manic episode during his or her lifetime (Fig. 9-5). Table 9-7 lists symptoms differentiating mania and depression in patients with BPD.

TABLE 9-7. Symptoms of Bipolar Mania and Bipolar Depression

Symptoms of Mania

Increased physical and mental activity and energy
Heightened mood, exaggerated optimism, and self-confidence
Excessive irritability, aggressive behavior
Decreased need for sleep without experiencing fatigue
Grandiose delusions, inflated sense of self-importance
Racing speech, racing thoughts, flight of ideas
Impulsiveness, poor judgment, distractibility
Reckless behavior
In the most severe cases, delusions and hallucinations

Symptoms of Depression

Prolonged sadness or unexplained crying spells
Significant changes in appetite and sleep patterns
Irritability, anger, worry, agitation, anxiety
Pessimism, indifference
Loss of energy, persistent lethargy
Feelings of guilt, worthlessness
Inability to concentrate, indecisiveness
Inability to take pleasure in former interests, social withdrawal
Unexplained aches and pains
Recurring thoughts of death or suicide

(Adapted from APA. *Diagnostic and Statistical Manual of Mental Disorders*, 4th ed. Washington, DC: American Psychiatric Association; 1994.)

Screening Protocols for Patients Using Antipsychotic Medications

The strong association between diabetes and mental illness, coupled with the fact that in some patients, treatment-emergent diabetes may develop while they are using atypical antipsychotic medications, has prompted the ADA to issue guidelines for screening and surveillance of these high-risk individuals (see Table 9-6).

Close follow-up of patients with mental illness is imperative from both a psychiatric and a metabolic perspective. The patient's weight should be reassessed monthly after initiating or changing antipsychotic therapy. Healthy eating practices, exercise prescriptions, and encouragement for patients to join support groups that may help meet their social goal should be enforced at each visit. Patients who gain 5% or more of their initial weight at any time during therapy, or those gaining more than 5 kg during the first month, may need to be switched to a different therapeutic agent after tapering off the original drug. Rapid discontinuation of antipsychotic agents may lead to serious psychosis and suicidal feelings. All patients with symptomatic or asymptomatic hyperglycemia (greater than 300 mg per dL) should be referred for immediate metabolic management to the PCP or specialist.

Patients who are being treated for mental illness may rapidly gain weight from sources other than the use of second-generation antipsychotic medications. Drugs that may result in weight gain include SSRIs, hormones, tricyclic antidepressants, mood stabilizers, and corticosteroids (Table 9-8). Rapid weight gain may also be due to pregnancy. Therefore, a pregnancy test should be performed on women of childbearing age who rapidly gain weight while taking antipsychotic medications.

TABLE 9-8. Medications That Can Result in Weight Gain

Drug Class	Gain		
	1%–3%	4%–10%	>10%
Tricyclic antidepressants			X
SSRIs		X	
Sulfonylureas		X	
Thiazolidinediones	X		
Insulin			X
Anticonvulsants			
• Divalproex, gabapentin		X	
• Oxcarbazepine	X		
Prednisone, Cortef			X
SERMS- Raloxifene		X	

SERMS, selective estrogen-receptor modulators; SSRIs, selective serotonin reuptake inhibitors
From www.keepitoff.com/physician/medications_that_cause_weight_gain.pdf. Accessed and verified February 25, 2007.

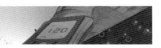

SUMMARY

Mental illness and diabetes are coexisting disorders. Depression often precedes clinical manifestations of diabetes by 6 to 8 years. The link between depression and diabetes is most likely due to adverse lifestyle conditions, such as obesity, poor dietary habits, inactivity, and cigarette smoking. Inflammatory cytokines are elevated in depression and obesity. For this reason, patients with obesity are prone to developing not only diabetes, depression, schizophrenia, and bipolar depression, but also CAD.

Patients with bipolar depression and schizophrenia are at high risk for diabetes, and bipolar depression and schizophrenia are linked to diabetes. Patients with these forms of mental illness are two to four times more likely to have coexisting diabetes. Again, lifestyle plays a large role in the anticipated comorbidities of these individuals. The 20% premature death in patients with bipolar depression and schizophrenia, which have been linked to an increase in suicide, may actually be due to a higher rate of sudden death from CAD. The second-generation antipsychotic agents are powerful medications that have the potential of stabilizing the emotional states of these disabled individuals. However, the use of these drugs may significantly alter the baseline metabolic status of many of these individuals. Therefore, when second-generation antipsychotic drugs are used in any patients, PCPs and psychiatrists should consider the following ADA Consensus Panel recommendations:

1. Consider metabolic risks when starting second-generation antipsychotic drugs
2. Provide patient, family, and caregiver education regarding potential adverse effects of these agents
3. Perform baseline screening on all patients
4. Regularly monitor and record all suggested metabolic parameters
5. Refer to specialized services when appropriate

When prescribing a second-generation antipsychotic agent, a commitment to baseline screening and follow-up monitoring is essential to limit the likelihood of developing CAD, treatment-emergent diabetes, metabolic syndrome, or other diabetes-related complications.

Finally, for patients with severe, disabling mental illness or family members who remain skeptical about using an antipsychotic medication for fear of experiencing weight gain, the physician should consider using the following paradigm:

If a patient comes in with a cough, and his chest radiograph shows a 7-cm tumor in the right lung, we most likely will need to come up with some therapeutic options. These might include radiation, surgery, or chemotherapy. If I then tell that patient that I could use a pill that would very likely shrink the size of his tumor by 80% within 4 months, yet may cause him to lose his hair, do you think for a moment that patient would ask me to find another treatment alternative? In other words, we are using medications that are highly likely to improve short- and long-term disabilities. Treatment may be associated with some weight gain. However, we will work with you on methods that may be helpful in reducing the amount of weight you gain. Most of the weight gain will occur within the first 6 months that these drugs are used.

Controlling psychotic illnesses with appropriate antipsychotic medications can lead to improved insight into medical diagnoses, enhanced adherence to medical and behavioral recommendations, and improved medical outcomes.

For patients with coexisting mental illness and diabetes, the first priority is to *always* fix the mental illness first. There is no way that patients can intensify their metabolic management when they are hallucinating or emotionally incapacitated. Consultation with a certified behavioral therapist should be considered when appropriate.

REFERENCES

1. Unger J. Managing mental illness in patients with diabetes. *Pract Diabetol*. 2006;25:44–53.
2. Goodwin FK, Fireman MA, Simon GE, et al. Suicide risk in bipolar disorder during treatment with lithium and divalproex. *JAMA*. 2003;290:1467–1473.
3. Lustman PJ, Clouse RE. Practical considerations in the management of depression in diabetes. *Diabetes Spectrum*. 2004;17:160–166.
4. Golden SH, Williams JE, Ford DE, et al. Depressive symptoms and the risk of type 2 diabetes. *Diabetes Care*. 2004;27:429–435.
5. Hood KK, Huestis S, Maher A, et al. Depressive symptoms in children and adolescents with type 1 diabetes: association with diabetes specific characteristics. *Diabetes Care*. 2006;29:1389–1391.
6. Anderson BJ, Edelstein S, Abramson NW, et al. Depressive symptoms and quality of life in adolescentswith type 2 diabetes. Baseline data from the TODAY study. *Diabetes Care*. 2011;34:2205–2207.
7. Kovacs M, Obrosky DS, Goldston D, et al. Major depressive disorder in youths with IDDM: a controlled prospective study of course and outcome. *Diabetes Care*. 1997;20:45–51.
8. Landman GWD, van Hateren KJJ, Kleefstra N, et al. Health-related quality of life and mortality in general and elderly population of poatients with type 2 diabetes (Zodiac-18). *Diabetes Care*. 2010;33(11): 2378–2382.
9. Ware JE, Jr, Kosinski M. SF-36 *Physical and Mental Health Summary Scales: A Manual for Users of Version 1*, 2nd ed. Lincoln, RI: QualityMetric Inc; 2005.
10. Anderson RJ, Freedland KE, Clouse RE, et al. The prevalence of comorbid depression in adults with diabetes: a meta-analysis. *Diabetes Care*. 2001;24:1069–1078.
11. American Psychiatric Association. *Diagnostic and Statistical Manual of Mental Disorders*. 4th ed. Washington, DC: American Psychiatric Association, 1994.
12. Katon W, von Korff M, Ciechanowski P, et al. Behavioral and clinical factors associated with depression among individuals with diabetes. *Diabetes Care*. 2004;27:914–920.
13. Lustman PJ, Griffith LS, Clouse RE. Depression in adults with diabetes: results of 5-yr follow-up study. *Diabetes Care*. 1988;11:605–612.

14. Lin EH, Katon W, von Korff M, et al. Relationship of depression and diabetes self-care, medication adherence, and preventive care. *Diabetes Care.* 2004;27:2154–2160.

15. Katon WJ, Lin EH, Russo J, et al. Cardiac risk factors in patients with diabetes mellitus and major depression. *J Gen Intern Med.* 2004;19:1192–1199.

16. Marcus M, Wing R, Guare J, et al. Lifetime prevalence of depression and its effect on treatment outcome in obese type 2 diabetic patients. *Diabetes Care.* 1992;15:253–255.

17. Dierker L, Avenevoli S, Stolar M, et al. Smoking and depression: an examination of mechanisms of comorbidity. *Am J Psychiatry.* 2002;159:947–953.

18. Danner M, Kasl SV, Abramson JL, et al. Association between depression and elevated C-reactive protein. *Psychosom Med.* 2003;65:347–356.

19. Kop WJ, Gottdiener JS. The role of immune system parameters in the relationship between depression and coronary artery disease. *Psychosom Med.* 2005;67(suppl 1):S37–S41.

20. Kop WJ, Gottdiener JS, Tangen CM, et al. Inflammation and coagulation factors in persons > 65 years of age with symptoms of depression but without evidence of myocardial ischemia. *Am J Cardiol.* 2002;89:419–424.

21. Lesperance F, Frasure-Smith N, Theroux P, et al. The association between major depression and levels of soluble intercellular adhesion molecule 1, interleukin-6, and C-reactive protein in patients with recent acute coronary syndromes. *Am J Psychiatry.* 2004;161:271–277.

22. Matsuzawa Y, Funahashi T, Kihara S, et al. Adiponection and metabolic syndrome. *Arterioscler Thromb Vasc Biol.* 2004;24:29–33.

23. Lanquillon S, Krieg J, Bening-Abu-Shach U, et al. Cytokine production and treatment response in major depressive disorder. *Neuropsychopharmacology.* 2000;22:370–379.

24. Lustman PJ, Freedland KE, Griffith LS, et al. Fluoxetine for depression in diabetes: a randomized double-blind placebo-controlled trial. *Diabetes Care.* 2000;23:618–623.

25. Unruh J, Ritchie J, Merskey H. Does gender affect appraisal of pain and coping strategies? *Clin J Pain.* 1999;15:31–40.

26. Katon WJ, Rutter C, Simon G, et al. The association of comorbid depression with mortality in patients with type 2 diabetes. *Diabetes Care.* 2005;28:2668–2672.

27. Egede LE, Zheng D, Simpson K. Comorbid depression is associated with increased health care use and expenditures in individuals with diabetes. *Diabetes Care.* 2002;25:464–470.

28. Gillespie CF, Nemeroff CB. Hypercortisolemia and depression. *Psychosom Med.* 2005;67(suppl 1):S26–S28.

29. Gold PW, Chrousos GP. The endocrinology of melancholic and atypical depression: relation to neurocircuitry and somatic consequences. *Proc Assoc Am Physicians.* 1998;111:22–34.

30. Carney RM, Freedland KE, Veith RC. Depression, the autonomic nervous system, and coronary heart disease. *Psychosom Med.* 2005;67(suppl 1):S29–S33.

31. Schins A, Honig A, Crijns H, et al. Increased coronary events in depressed cardiovascular patients:5-HT2A receptor as missing link? *Psychosom Med.* 2003;65:729–737.

32. Bruce EC, Musselman DL. Depression, alterations in platelet function, and ischemic heart disease. *Psychosom Med.* 2005;67(suppl 1):S34–S36.

33. Beck AT, Steer RA, Garbin GM. Psychometric properties of the Beck Depression Inventory: twenty-five years of evaluation. *Clin Psychol Rev.* 1988;8:77–100.

34. Papageorgiou G, Grapsa E, Christodoulou NG, et al. Association of serum nitric oxide levels with depressive symptoms: a study with end-stage renal failure patients. *Psychother Psychosom.* 2001;70:216–220.

35. Williams MM, Clouse RE, Lustman PJ. Treating depression to prevent diabetes and its complications: understanding depression as a medical risk factor. *Clin Diabetes.* 2006;24:79–86.

36. Lustman PJ, Griffith LS, Freedland KE, et al. Cognitive behavior therapy for depression in type 2 diabetes: a randomized controlled trial. *Ann Intern Med.* 1998;129:613–621.

37. Williams MM, Clouse RE, Rubin EH, et al. Evaluating late-life depression in patients with diabetes. *Psychol Ann.* 2004;34:305–312.

38. Daubresse J-C, Kolanowski J, Krzentowski G, et al. Usefulness of fluoxetine in obese non insulin-dependent diabetics: a multicenter study. *Obes Res.* 1996;4:391–396.

39. Lustman PJ, Anderson RJ, Freedland KE, et al. Depression and poor glycemic control: a meta-analytic review of the literature. *Diabetes Care.* 2000;23:434–442.

40. Hirschfield RMA. Management of sexual side effects of antidepressant therapy. *J Clin Psychiatry.* 1999;60(suppl 14):27–30.

41. Gregorian RS, Golden KA, Bahoe A, et al. Antidepressant-induced sexual dysfunction. *Ann Pharmacother.* 2002;36:1577–1589.

42. Clayton AH, Pradko JF, Croft HA, et al. Prevalence of sexual dysfunction among newer antidepressants. *J Clin Psychiatry.* 2002;63:357–366.

43. Rothschild AJ. Selective serotonin reuptake inhibitor-induced sexual dysfunction: efficacy of a drug holiday. *Am J Psychiatry.* 1995;152:1514–1516.

44. Clayton AH. Duloxetine has less effect on male sexual function than escitalopram: presentation to the American Psychiatric Association Annual Meeting, Toronto, Canada. Presented May 24, 2006.

45. Deshmukh R, Franco K. Managing weight gain as a side effect of antidepressant therapy. *Cleve Clin J Med.* 70;614–623.

46. Carpenter WT Jr, Buchanan RW. Schizophrenia. *N Engl J Med.* 1994;330:681–689.

47. Axelsson R, Lagerkvist-Briggs M. Factors predicting suicide in psychotic patients. *Eur Arch Psychiatry Clin Neurosci.* 1992;241:259–266.

48. National Institute of Mental Health Web Site: http://www.nimh.nih.gov/healthinformation/ schizophrenia-menu.cfm. Accessed January 30, 2006.

49. Lorenz WF. Sugar tolerance in dementia praecox and other mental disorders. *Arch Neurol Psychiatry.* 1922;8:184–196.

50. Sernyak MJ, Douglas DL, Alarcon RD, et al. Association of diabetes mellitus with use of atypical neuroleptics in the treatment of schizophrenia. *Am J Psychiatry.* 2002;159:561–566.

51. The Canadian Diabetes Association website: http://www.diabetes.ca/Section_About/atrisk.asp. Assessed January 28, 2006.

52. Cassidy F, Ahearn E, Carroll BJ. Elevated frequency of diabetes mellitus in hospitalized manic-depressive patients. *Am J Psychiatry.* 1999;156:1417–1420.

53. Ryan MC, Collins P, Thakore JH. Impaired fasting glucose tolerance in first-episode, drug-naïve and drug-free patients with schizophrenia. *J Obes Relat Metab Disord.* 2002;26:137–141.

54. Cohen LJ, Test MA, Brown RL. Suicide and schizophrenia: data from a prospective community treatment study. *Am J Psychiatry.* 1990;147:602–607.

55. Lieberman JA, Stroup TS, McEvoy JP, et al. Effectiveness of antipsychotic drugs in patients with chronic schizophrenia. *N Engl J Med.* 2005;353:1209–1223.

56. Liu-Seifert H, Adams DH, Kinon BJ. Discontinuation of treatment of schizophrenic patients is driven by poor symptom response: a pooled post-hoc analysis of four atypical antipsychotic drugs. *BMC Med.* 2005;3:1–10.

57. Yu BP, Ortiz T, Chong YS, et al. Use of novel antipsychotic medications in diabetes: a retrospective review. *Drug Benefit Trends.* 2002;14:42–45.

58. Weiss E, Hummer M, Koller D, et al. Off-label use of antipsychotic drugs. *J Clin Psychopharmacol.* 2000;20:695–698.

59. Llorente MD, Urrutia V. Diabetes, psychiatric disorders, and the metabolic effects of antipsychotic medications. *Clin Diabetes.* 2006;24:18–24.

60. American Diabetes Association. Consensus development conference on antipsychotic drugs and obesity and diabetes. *Diabetes Care.* 2004;27:596–601.

61. Wirshing DA, Wirshing WC, Kysar L, et al. Novel antipsychotics: comparison of weight gain liabilities. *J Clin Psychiatry.* 1999;100:3–16.

62. Koro CE, Fedder DO, L'Italien GJ, et al. Assessment of independent effect of olanzapine and risperidone on risk of diabetes among patients with schizophrenia: population based nested case-control study. *Br Med J.* 2002;325:243–247.

63. Fuller MA, Shermock KM, Secic M, et al. Comparative study of the development of diabetes mellitus in patients taking risiperidone and olanzapine. *Pharmacotherapy.* 2003;23:1037–1043.

64. Melkersson KI, Hultin A-L, Brismar KE. Different influences of classical antipsychotics and clozapine on glucose-insulin homeostasis in patients with schizophrenia or related psychoses. *J Clin Psychiatry.* 1999;60:783–791.

65. Johnson DE, Yamazaki H, Ward KM, et al. Inhibitory effects of antipsychotics on carbachol-enhanced insulin secretion from perfused rat islets: role of muscarinic antagonism in antipsychotic-induced diabetes and hyperglycemia. *Diabetes.* 2005;54:1552–1558.

66. Manning JS. Management of bipolar disorder in primary care versus psychiatric settings: Primary care companion. *J Clin Psychiatry.* 2004;6:222–223.

67. Belmaker RH. Bipolar disorder. *N Engl J Med.* 2004;351:476–486.

68. Merikangas K, Yu K. Genetic epidemiology of bipolar disorder. *Clin Neurosci Res.* 2002;2:127–141.

69. Manning JS. Primary care companion. *J Clin Psychiatry.* 2002;4:142–150.

70. Calabrese JR, Hirschfeld RM, Reed M, et al. Impact of bipolar disorder on a U.S. community sample. *J Clin Psychiatry.* 2003;64:425–432.

71. Elmslie JL, Silverstone JT, Mann JI, et al. Prevalence of overweight and obesity in bipolar patients. *J Clin Psychiatry.* 2000;61:179–184.

72. Homel P, Casey D, Allison DB. Changes in body mass index for individuals with and without schizophrenia, 1987–1996. *Schizophr Res.* 2002;55:277–284.

73. Fagiolini A, Frank E, Houck PR, et al. Prevalence of obesity and weight change during treatment in patients with bipolar I disorder. *J Clin Psychiatry.* 2002;63:528–533.

Diagnosis and Management of T2DM

You can tell a lot about a fellow's character by his
way of eating jelly beans.

—Ronald Reagan, 40th U.S. president

Introduction Type 2 diabetes (T2DM) is a metabolic disorder characterized by abnormalities at multiple organ target sites, including the pancreatic β-cell, skeletal muscles, adipose tissue, kidneys, brain, gut, and liver. The hyperglycemia characteristic of T2DM develops slowly over time as the pancreatic β-cells fail to produce insulin in response to a glucose stimulus. The resulting elevated plasma glucose levels become cytotoxic, leading to the loss of β-cell function and mass.

An estimated 25.8 million Americans or 8.3% of the population have diabetes, with estimates between 90% and 95% having T2DM.[1] Approximately 90% of patients with diabetes are managed by primary care physicians (PCPs), many of whom have had little education in screening for, diagnosing, and managing this complex metabolic disorder.[2] Successful management of T2DM requires an understanding of the disease pathogenesis, a strategy to promote and encourage lifestyle modifications, surveillance for identifying and preventing long-term diabetes-related complications, knowledge of intensive pharmacologic intervention options, and professional skills for providing customized patient education. Pursuing an ambitious approach to diabetes care can lead to positive treatment outcomes as well as to improvement in the quality of life for these patients and their families.

Screening for and Diagnosing T2DM

Screening for diabetes should be performed by a health-care provider at 3-year intervals beginning at the age of 45 years in asymptomatic individuals. An asymptomatic adult of *any age* having a BMI ≥ 25 kg per m² or greater and at least one additional risk factor as noted in Table 10-1 should also be screened for diabetes.[3] A patient who screens negative for prediabetes or diabetes should be rescreened after 3 years (Fig. 10-1).

The ADA discourages screening for diabetes in a nonmedical environment because patients with positive findings may not be provided with appropriate follow-up instructions, repeated testing, or care.

Mathematical modeling studies suggest that screening independent of risk factors beginning at age 30 or 45 is highly cost-effective (less than $11,000 per quality adjusted life-year gained).

TABLE 10-1. Risk Factors That Place Patients at High Risk for Developing T2DM

- Physical inactivity
- First degree relative with T2DM
- High-risk ethnicity: African American, Hispanic, Native American, Asian American, Pacific Islander
- Women who delivered a baby weighing ≥ 9 lb
- Women with a history of gestational diabetes
- History of hypertension (blood pressure ≥ 140/90 mm Hg or on medication for hypertension)
- Atherogenic hyperlipidemia (HDL-C < 35 mg/dL and/or a triglyceride level > 250 mg/dL
- Women with a history of polycystic ovary syndrome
- Prior history of glycemic values consistent with the diagnosis of prediabetes: A1C > 5.7%, fasting plasma glucose 100–125 mg/dL or 2-h postprandial glucose 140–200 mg/dL
- Clinical evidence of acanthosis nigricans, which is associated with IR (see Fig. 10-1)
- History of cardiovascular disease

From American Diabetes Association. Standards of medical care in diabetes—2012. *Diabetes Care.* 2012;35(suppl 1):S14.

Prediabetes and diabetes meet established criteria for conditions in which early detection is appropriate. Both conditions are endemic and impose significant global public health burdens. A long presymptomatic phase precedes the clinical diagnosis of T2DM during which cost-effective and nonpharmacologic measures can be utilized to delay or reverse diabetes progression. Simple testing is available to detect preclinical disesase. Finally, the duration of one's exposure to chronic hyperglycemia correlates with one's microvascular and macrovascular outcomes. Thus, simple, inexpensive glycemic testing employed during the preclinical phase of diabetes can prevent disease progression and minimize economic burden.[4]

A pharmacoeconomic analysis by Torgdon and Hylands suggested that the cost of managing diabetes increases one's annual medical expenditures by $158.[5] These costs are in addition to baseline increases associated with medical expenditures with aging. Thus, not only does diabetes increase medical expenditures at any age, the effect grows by $158 each year.

As clinicians attempt to prevent long-term complications by encouraging earlier pharmacologic interventions, patients feel the crunch of higher annual prescription drug costs. A growing diabetes epidemic and introduction of new treatment options could increase drug costs by 70% by 2013.[6] With a surge in pharmacy spending, health plans are likely to increase cost sharing with enrollees by raising copays and coinsurance rates. Higher costs passed on to patients may increase the likelihood of medication nonadherence. In a national survey of 875 older adults with diabetes, 19% reported cutting back on the use of their medications because of cost, 11% reported cutting back on their diabetes medications, and 7% reported cutting back on their diabetes medications at least once a month. In order to pay for their medications, 20% reported foregoing food and other essentials, 14% increased credit card debt, and 10% borrowed money from family or friends.[7]

The rate of medication adherence is typically low in patients with chronic conditions, especially in patients with T2DM. A review of the literature by Cramer showed that patient adherence to treatment with oral hypoglycemic agents ranged from 36% to 93% and adherence to insulin therapy was 62% to 64%.[8]

Medication nonadherence accounts for more than 10% of all hospitalizations and 23% of all nursing home admissions each year.[9] The estimated cost of medication nonadherence to the healthcare system is approximately $100 billion a year.[10]

The incidence of T2DM within the pediatric population is increasing in ethnic minority groups although the disorder remains rare within the general pediatric and adolescent population. The

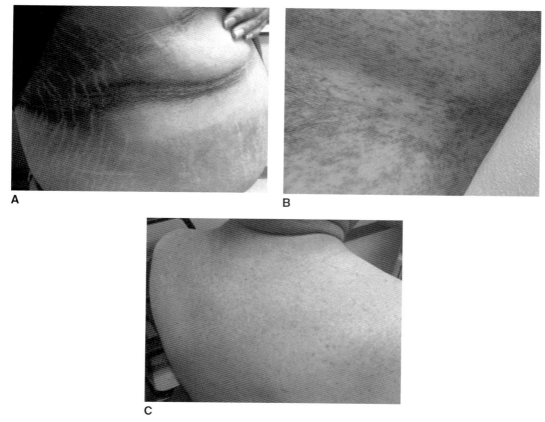

Figure 10-1 • Acanthosis Nigricans. A. A 24-year old Latino male patient with newly diagnosed T2DM and acanthosis nigricans on his chest and abdomen. **B**. A 58-year-old man with poorly controlled T2DM (A1C = 9.9%). He developed acanthosis nigricans while taking daily prednisone as adjunctive treatment for cancer chemotherapy. As diabetes therapy was intensified (with insulin) the acanthosis improved significantly over a period of 5 months (Fig. 10-1C). **C**. Acanthosis nigricans (AN) is a dermatologic condition commonly seen in patients with diabetes and IR. Histologically, AN is characterized by the proliferation of epidermal keratinocytes and fibroblasts. Patients with AN experience hyperpigmented lesions and dark-brown thickened plaques on the neck, axillae, and abdomen. As patients lose weight, experience improvement in their IR or diabetes, the pigmentation of the AN tends to lighten as shown in Figures 10-1B and C.

ADA has published guidelines for screening asymptomatic children for T2DM as summarized in Table 10-2. Screening should be performed every 3 years in high-risk children and adolescents.

For decades, clinicians have relied upon fasting and 75-g glucose challenge testing to screen and diagnose diabetes. In 2010, the ADA adopted the recommendations of an International Expert Committee, which set the A1C of 6.5% as the diagnostic threshold for diabetes.[11] The A1C may also be used to screen patients for prediabetes as reviewed in Tables 10-1 and 10-2.

Any test result that is diagnostic of diabetes should be repeated to rule out laboratory error, unless the patient has classic signs and symptoms of hyperglycemia (thirst, frequent urination, weight loss, blurred vision, fatigue, paresthesias, dry skin, or a random plasma glucose level greater than 200 mg per dL). If the abnormal lab test is repeated and found to be consistent with the previous value, the diagnosis of diabetes is confirmed. The diagnosis of diabetes can also be presumed based upon the presence of two different test results both of which are above the diagnostic threshold. For example, an A1C of 7.8% coupled with a random plasma blood glucose of 201 mg per dL does establish the diagnosis of T2DM. If two screening tests are discordant, the ADA suggests repeating the result that is above the diagnostic cut point prior to diagnosing the patient as having

TABLE 10-2. American Diabetes Association Recommendations for Glycemic Screening in High-risk Asymptomatic Children

Children at high risk for developing prediabetes and diabetes have the following criteria:
• Overweight (BMI) >85th percentile for age and sex, weight for height >85th percentile, or weight > 120% of ideal for height)

Plus any two of the following risk factors:
- Family history of T2DM in first- or second-degree relative
- Race/ethnicity (Native American, African American, Latino, Asian American, Pacific Islander)
- Signs of IR or conditions associated with IR (acanthosis nigricans, hypertension, dyslipidemia, polycystic ovary syndrome, or small-for-gestational-age birth weight)
- Maternal history of diabetes or gestational diabetes during the child's gestation
  - Initiate screening in children at age 10 or at onset of puberty
  - Screening should be conducted every 3 years.

From American Diabetes Association. Standards of medical care in diabetes—2012. *Diabetes Care.* 2012;35(suppl 1):S14.

prediabetes or diabetes. For example, a patient is suspected of having prediabetes. The patient's A1C is 6.2% but his 2-hour 75-g postglucose challenge is 135 mg per dL. The repeated A1C performed 3 months later is now 6.4%. Based on the fact that the patient has had two consistently abnormally elevated A1C values that surpass the diagnostic cut point for prediabetes, the diagnosis is made and lifestyle interventions are immediately initiated.

Prevention of T2DM by Using Intensive Lifestyle Intervention

Both genetic and environmental factors contribute to the development and progression of T2DM. Specific at-risk population groups have a high prevalence of T2DM, as do individuals with an afflicted first-degree relative. The most dominant determinant in the development of diabetes appears to be one's BMI.[12] An estimated 65% of Americans have a BMI of 25 kg per m² or more and are thus labeled "overweight" by U.S. standards.[13] The direct relation between obesity and the increasing prevalence to T2DM suggests that lifestyle interventions for weight reduction and improvement in physical activity participation could slow or prevent the progression from normoglycemia to prediabetes and beyond. Weight reduction and physical activity can improve insulin-mediated glucose disposal, reduce postprandial hyperglycemia, delay β-cell death (apoptosis), and slow the progression of glucose intolerance to T2DM.[14,15] Table 10-3 summarizes the landmark clinical trials that have demonstrated the important role of lifestyle modification in delaying and preventing T2DM.

The most comprehensive clinical trial that evaluated the importance of lifestyle modification as a deterrent to diabetes was the Diabetes Prevention Program (DPP).[16] This $174 million National Institutes of Health (NIH) study enrolled 3,234 individuals with impaired glucose tolerance (IGT). Patients were randomly assigned to receive intensive lifestyle intervention or metformin at 27 U.S. centers. The lifestyle-intervention group participated in walking or other moderate-intensity exercise averaging 150 minutes per week. These subjects lost on average

TABLE 10-3. Published Studies Demonstrating the Importance of Lifestyle Modification in the Prevention of T2DM

Trial	RCT	Intervention	Population	Results
Malmo Feasibility Trial[a]	No	Diet + exercise	232 Swedish men aged 47–49 with early T2DM or IGT. Studied over a 5-y period	Diet + exercise normalized glycemia in >50% of subjects with IGT.
Da Qing IGT Study[11]	Yes	Diet, exercise, or both	577 Chinese men and women (average age, 45) with IGT. Studied for 6 y	Diet, exercise, or both decreased progression to T2DM 31%–46%. Efficacy equal in both diet and exercise groups. No added benefit with combining exercise + dietary intervention. High-risk **nonobese** subjects reduced risk as well with diet and exercise.
Finnish Diabetes Prevention Study[10]	Yes	Dietary instruction + personalized exercise program	522 obese Finnish men and women, mean age, 55 ± 7 y, with IGT	Diet + exercise reduced progression to T2DM by 58%.
The Nurses' Health Study	Yes	Weight loss + exercise or metformin	3,234 ethnically diverse U.S. men and women, mean age, 50.6 y ± 10.7 y, with IGT	Diet + exercise decreased progression to T2DM by 58%.
Diabetes Prevention Program 10-Y Follow-up	No	All active DPP patients were offered group-implemented lifestyle intervention. Metformin 850 mg b.i.d was continued in the original group	Diabetes incidence in the 10 years since DPP randomization was reduced by 34% in the lifestyle group and 18% in the metformin group.

[a]Eriksson KF, Lingarde F. Prevention of type 2 (non-insulin dependent) diabetes mellitus by diet and physical exercise: the 6-year Malmo feasibility study. *Diabetologia.* 1991;34:891–898.
IGT, impaired glucose tolerance; RTC, randomized clinical trial; T2DM, T2DM mellitus.
From Diabetes Prevention Program Research Group. 10-year follow-up of diabetes incidence and weight loss in the Diabetes Prevention Program Outcomes Study. *Lancet.* 2009;374(9702):1677-1686.

5% to 7% of their initial body weight while reducing their risk of diabetes progression by 58% (Fig. 10-2). Forty-five percent of the subjects came from high-risk minority groups who have disproportionate numbers of T2DM (African Americans, Hispanics, Asian Americans, Pacific Islanders, and Native Americans). Other high-risk subjects in the DPP included patients older

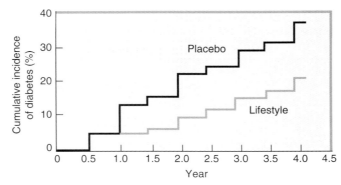

Figure 10-2 • Modest Weight Loss Prevents Diabetes in Overweight and Obese Persons with IGT. Modest weight loss can prevent the development of T2DM. This figure shows data from the Diabetes Prevention Program Research Study, which examined the effect of lifestyle intervention (reducing energy intake and increasing physical activity) on the incidence of diabetes. At the initiation of the study, the participants were 51 years old, had a BMI of 34 kg per m^2, and comprised 68% women and 45% ethnic minorities. The average follow-up was 2.8 years. Participants treated with the lifestyle-modification program experienced a 6% weight loss and 58% decrease in the incidence of diabetes compared with placebo ($p < 0.001$). (Adapted from Knowler WC, Barrett-Connor E, Fowler SE, et al., and the Diabetes Prevention Program Research Group. Reduction in the incidence of T2DM with lifestyle intervention or metformin. *N Engl J Med.* 2002;346:393–403.)

than 60, women with a history of gestational diabetes, and individuals with a first-degree relative with T2DM.

DPP subjects were randomized into one of three treatment arms: (a) intensive individualized lifestyle intervention with the aim of reducing weight by 7% through low-fat diet and exercising 150 minutes per week, (b) treatment with metformin (850 mg twice daily), or (c) a standard group taking placebo pills in place of metformin. The metformin and placebo groups also received information about the importance of diet and exercise. A fourth arm of the study, using troglitazone combined with standard diet and exercise recommendations, was discontinued in June 1998 because of the potential for liver toxicity. DPP participants ranged in age from 25 to 85 years, with an average of 51 years. On entry into the trial, all had IGT, as measured by an oral glucose tolerance test (OGTT), and all were overweight, with an average BMI of 34 kg per m^2.

Lifestyle intervention worked well in men and women as well as in all ethnic groups regardless of their baseline BMIs.[15] In subjects older than 60 years, lifestyle intervention reduced the progression to diabetes by 71%. Metformin was not as effective as lifestyle intervention in reducing diabetes risk in the population older than 60 years or in those who were less obese.

Ten years following the initial randomization within the DPP, the modest weight loss within the metformin cohort was maintained. Diabetes incidence in the 10 years since DPP randomization was reduced by 34% in the lifestyle group and 18% in the metformin group compared with placebo. The DPP extension proves that the prevention or delay of diabetes with lifestyle intervention or metformin can persist for at least 10 years.[17] The use of metformin in both the DPP and the ADOPT trial was found to be associated with β-cell preservation.[18]

Diets that include mono- or polyunsaturated fatty acids may alter the composition of membrane phospholipids and improve insulin sensitivity. Specific dietary patterns that are high in fruits, vegetables, and whole grains and low in red or processed meat, sugars, and high-fat dairy products also appear to reduce the risk of T2DM.[15]

Physical activity improves insulin sensitivity independent of its effect on weight loss or improvement of fat distribution.[19] A study of Pima Indians showed that the incidence of T2DM, as determined by OGTT, was lower in more active individuals regardless of their BMI.[20]

Effects of Pharmacotherapies on Reversing T2DM in Newly Diagnosed Patients

Pharmacotherapies that have proven to be effective or deleterious to high-risk patients are discussed in detail in Chapter 2.

Can intensive insulin therapy initiated shortly after one is diagnosed with T2DM reverse the disease course by establishing "β-cell rest" whereby insulin secretory function is preserved and islet mass is maintained? Several studies have demonstrated that intensive reversal of hyperglycemia, glucotoxicity, and lipotoxicity favors recovery of β-cell function.

Intensive insulin treatment can decrease the secretory demand on β-cells to near zero levels, providing the β-cells with a resting phase and lowering the likelihood of further loss of β-cell mass. Weng et al.[21] demonstrated that normalization of hyperglycemia improved β-cell function after 2 weeks of active therapy regardless of treatment with multiple daily injections of insulin, insulin pumps or orally administered hypoglycemic agents. The study was performed on patients with newly diagnosed T2DM rather than in patients with prediabetes. The remission rates 1 year off medications were 51%, 45%, and 27% in the insulin pump, MDI, and oral agent groups, respectively. Prolonged β-cell improvement was noted in both insulin groups but not in those patients using oral agents. The duration of intensive insulin therapy needed to achieve β-cell rest is unknown. The ultimate efficacy of insulin therapy at preserving β-cell function may be dependent on the actual duration of prediabetes and the number of recoverable β-cells present at the time the insulin is initiated.

Intensive insulin pump therapy also appears to restore β-cell secretory function. Li et al.[22] recruited 138 newly diagnosed patients with T2DM having fasting glucose levels greater than 200 mg per dL. All patients were hospitalized for 2 weeks and placed on intensive insulin pump therapy. Optimal glycemic control was attained within 6.3 ± 3.9 days in 126 patients. The remission rates (percentage of participants maintaining near-normal glucose levels) at the 3rd, 6th, 12th, and 24th months were 72.6, 67.0, 47.1, and 42.3%, respectively. Those patients in remission for greater than 1 year had greater recovery of β-cell function compared with the nonremission group as demonstrated by favorable proinsulin:insulin ratios in the long-term remission group. Under normal circumstances, small amounts of proinsulin are secreted concurrently with insulin; the result is a plasma proinsulin:insulin ratio of approximately 0.1. Conditions characterized by inflammation or dysfunction of β-cells are associated with increased levels of proinsulin, resulting in an increased ratio of proinsulin to insulin.[23]

In summary, early intensive insulin treatment in patients with newly diagnosed T2DM may be effective in retarding the progressive dysfunction of β-cells in patients by reducing glucotoxicity and lipotoxicity. Incretin mimetics and TZDs result in maintenance and improvement of β-cell function during their active use; yet continued efficacy appears to diminish once the drugs are stopped. Use of pioglitazone in high doses for diabetes prevention can result in unwanted side effects such as weight gain and edema.

Prevention and Reversal of T2DM with Metabolic Surgery

• The Definition, Epidemiology, and Pathogensis of Obesity-related Insulin Resistance

Obesity, typically measured as body mass index (BMI) ≥ 30 kg per m², has three subclasses: obesity 1 (30 to 34.9 kg per m²); obesity 2 (35 to 39.9 kg per m²); and clinically severe (extreme) obesity (greater than 40 kg per m²).[24] A BMI of more than 40 kg per m² corresponds to being 100 lb above ideal body weight or more than 200% of ideal body weight.[25] From 1986 to 2000, the prevalence of individuals with extreme obesity having of BMI ≥ 50 kg per m² has increased fivefold.[26]

Obesity is a major independent risk factor for the development of T2DM and is associated with the rapid increase in the prevalence of T2DM. In the United States, the majority diagnosed with T2DM are overweight, with 50% obese (i.e., BMI greater than 30 kg per m²) and 9% severely obese (BMI greater than 40 kg per m²).[27] The primary risk factor for T2DM is obesity, and 90% of all patients with T2DM are overweight or obese. The relative risk of diabetes increases about 42-fold in men as the BMI increases from 23 to 35 kg per m² and approximately 93-fold in women as BMI increases from 22 to 35 kg per m².[18,28]

Intensive lifestyle intervention programs with diet therapy, behavior modification, exercise prescription, and pharmacotherapy are known to preserve β-cell function and restore normal glucose tolerance in high-risk patients.[29] With rare exceptions, clinically significant weight loss is generally modest and transient, especially in patients with extreme obesity. In one study, 80 adults with moderate obesity (BMI 30 to 35 kg per m²) were randomized to nonsurgical intervention (very-low-calorie diet, orlistat, and lifestyle intervention) or to gastric banding.[30] At 2 years, the surgical group demonstrated a weight loss of 87.2% versus 21.8% for the nonsurgical group. However, long-term maintenance of weight loss is difficult for all patients, especially those practicing lifestyle intervention.[31]

The development of T2DM is strongly associated with obesity and the accumulation of visceral fat that is linked to insulin resistance (IR), inflammation, and lipotoxicity of pancreatic β-cells. Adipose tissue in obese patients with diabetes is characterized by increased production and secretion of inflammatory cytokines such as tumor necrosis factor-α, interleukin-6, transforming growth factor-b, monocyte chemotactic protein-1, and plasminogen activator inhibitor-1, and C-reactive protein. Weight loss improves inflammatory status in obesity and subsequent comorbidities by decreasing numbers of circulating inflammatory cytokines.[32]

The mechanisms underlying the dramatic effects of malabsorptive surgery on insulin sensitivity and β-cell function are poorly understood. Caloric restriction and changes in glucagon-like peptide-1 (GLP-1) release have been implicated as important mediators toward restoration of NGT in the early postoperative state. However, skeletal muscle insulin sensitivity mediated by changes in gene expression is thought to play a major role in reversing diabetes after metabolic surgery.[33]

Of considerable interest for extremely obese patients with diabetes is the observation that euglycemia and normal insulin levels occur within days after surgery, long before there is any significant weight loss.[34] Although extreme obesity is associated with profound IR and marked insulin hypersecretion, the dynamics of β-cell function (i.e., β-cell glucose sensitivity, rate sensitivity, and potentiation) are preserved. Metabolic surgery improves peripheral insulin sensitivity two- to threefold before any substantial weight loss is observed.[35]

Metabolic Surgical Procedures

Bariatric (also known as "metabolic surgery") consists of several well-defined procedures. Restrictive surgeries, such as laparoscopic adjustable gastric banding (LAGB) and vertical banded gastroplasty (VBG), reduce the volume of the stomach by 85% to decrease food intake and induce early satiety. VBG is also known as sleeve gastrectomy. LAGB is considered a minimally invasive intervention in which a restrictive band is placed around the upper stomach to partition a small proximal pouch. Initially, these bands were designed for open surgical placement and were not adjustable. However, further refinement of these devices now enables surgeons to place the adjustable appliance laparoscopically. Malabsorptive procedures, such as biliopancreatic diversion (BPD), shorten the small intestine to decrease nutrient absorption. Combined procedures, such as the Roux-en-Y gastric bypass (RYGB) incorporate both restrictive and malabsorptive elements. RYGB surgery is the current gold standard treatment for severe obesity. Both BPD and RYGB alter the secretion of gut hormones that affect satiety.[32]

Historically, RYGB had been the most common bariatric surgical procedure performed in the United States. However, since 2009 gastric banding procedures have exceeded RYGB for the reasons listed in Table 10-4. The Roux-en-Y procedure is named after the surgeon who first described the

TABLE 10-4. Advantages and Disadvantages of Different Metabolic Surgical Procedures

Metabolic Surgical Procedure	Advantages	Disadvantages	Complications	Approximate Cost per Procedure
Gastric Bypass	• Rapid initial weight loss • No device insertion	• Stomach is cut, stapled and intestines rerouted • Difficult procedure to reverse • Nonadjustable	• Dumping syndrome can occur • Vitamin deficiencies can occur	$25,000 plus 2 nights in hospital
Sleeve Gastrectomy Gastric sleeve Pylorus Resected stomach	• Rapid initial weight loss • No device insertion	• Cutting and stapling of stomach are required • Prolonged hospital stay • Nonadjustable procedure • Portion of stomach is removed, which maintains vitamin B_{12} production and absorption	• Deep vein thrombosis (5%) • nonfatal pulmonary embolism (0.5%) • Pneumonia (0.2%) • Acute respiratory distress syndrome (0.25%) • Splenectomy (0.5%) • Gastric leak and fistula (1.0%) • Death (0.25%) • Total mortality rate (0.8%)	$20–$25,000 Plus 5 d in hospital
Lap Banding	• No stomach cutting, stapling or redirecting of intestinal anatomy • Easily reversible • Few complications • Outpatient procedure	• Device is placed on stomach during procedure • Band may slip or leak • Risk of internal infection • Abdominal pain if patient overeats • Requires periodic "adjustment" of banding volume postoperatively through a subcutaneous port • Nutritional deficiencies during liquid diet • Patients who do not adhere to postoperative lifestyle instructions may not lose anticipated weight	• Gastric perforation (1%) • Anastomotic strictures (0.7%)	$10–$15,000 as outpatient plus $150 per adjustment of lap band as an office procedure

operation in 1993 and the "Y" shape produced by the redirected intestines as food is redirected around the stomach. The surgeon creates a walnut-sized pouch (1 to 2 tablespoons) on the proximal area of the stomach and "bypasses" the remaining stomach by attaching a section of the small bowel to the pouch. Although the stomach does not receive any nutrients, gastric enzymes continue to be produced. The gastric pouch is anastomosed to a Roux-en-Y proximal jejunal segment, bypassing the remaining stomach, duodenum, and a small portion of jejunum. The standard Roux (alimentary) limb length is about 50 to 100 cm, and the biliopancreatic limb is 15 to 50 cm. The Roux limb allows the gastric content to mix with nutrients entering from the gastric pouch and bypassing the stomach. Patients experience very rapid fullness with this procedure and significant weight loss. The gallbladder is typically removed during this procedure, as patients who experience rapid weight loss have a higher incidence of cholelithiasis.[36] The major benefits of RYGB include rapid weight loss and early improvement or remission of T2DM, independent of weight loss. RYGB is associated with increased operation times, longer hospital stays, and increased risk of complications.

During the Lap-Banding procedure, a silicone band filled with saline is wrapped around the proximal portion of the stomach. This restricts the amount of food one could consume and induces satiety. An injection port allows subcutaneous access to the lap band through which saline may be added or removed postoperatively depending upon the patient's level of satiety.

The sleeve gastrectomy creates a thin vertical staple line across the stomach. The lower portion of the stomach is amputated, leaving the patient with a gastric capacity of 10% of its normal volume. With minimal gastric capacity, patients quickly develop satiety and weight loss ensues. No rerouting of intestinal anatomy is required.

The anticipated weight loss associated with each procedure can vary based upon several factors. Patients can increase their weight reduction by following the nutritional consumption guidelines provided by their surgical team. Periodic adjustment in gastric band tightening might be necessary to increase satiety and limit the amount of food that enters the gastric pouch in lap-banded patients.

Metabolic surgical studies report results as "mean percent excess body weight loss" calculated as the percent of body weight above the stated upper limit of normal BMI of 25 kg per m^2.

The mean percent excess body weight loss after lap banding in published series is 46%, and the mean resolution in diabetes is 56%,[37] both substantially lower than after RYGB.[37] Studies that directly compare the RYGB and LAGB also suggest substantially greater weight loss and resolution of comorbidities after RYGB.[38] There are no studies to date suggesting that the LAGB has a specific effect on T2DM beyond that of inducing caloric restriction and subsequent weight loss.

The long-term expected body weight loss observed with three different metabolic surgical procedures is shown in Table 10-5.

Data from larger LAGB studies show that morbidity rates remain uniformly low, whereas RYGB and VBG retain a higher risk of morbidity than LAGB, even with considerable numbers of patients

 TABLE 10-5. Reported Weight Loss as a Percentage of Excess Body Weight^a Following Metabolic Surgery

Metabolic Surgical Procedure	Weight Loss at 1–2 Y (% of Excess Body Weight)	Weight Loss at 3–6 Y (% of Excess Body Weight)	Weight Loss at 7–10 Y (% of Excess Body Weight)
RYGB	48–85	53–77	25–68
Sleeve gastrectomy	33–58	66	—
Lap banding	29–87	49–72	14-60

^{a}Dividing the excess body weight by 2 provides the clinician with an "estimation" of the approximate percentage of total body weight from baseline that each patient has lost. For example, a patient who has lost 50% of their excess body weight with metabolic surgery has reduced their total body weight approximately 25% from their presurgical baseline. Weight loss after metabolic surgery reaches a peak within 12 to 18 months postoperatively. Within 10 years patients experience an average of 10% regain of weight.
From Mechanick JI, Kushner RF, Sugerman HJ, et al. American Association of Clinical Endocrinologists, The Obesity Society, and American Society for Metabolic and Bariatric Surgery medical guidelines for clinical practice for the perioperative nutritional, metabolic, and nonsurgical support of the bariatric surgery patient. *Endocr Pract.* 2008;14(suppl 1):3–83.

being treated.[39] The main complications of LAGB are related to misplaced or inadequately secured devices.[39]

One must always consider the risk:benefit for each patient who is considering metabolic surgery. A study by Keidar has suggested that weight loss surgery reduces diabetes-related mortality by 90%.[40] As many as 14,300 lives can be saved in the United States over 5 years through metabolic surgical intervention.[40]

Improvements in hyperglycemia are observed almost immediately after surgery. Fasting plasma glucose levels often normalize before hospital dismissal and before weight loss is observed. Insulin-treated patients note a decrease in insulin requirements while some who have been severely insulin resistant may be able to discontinue insulin within 6 weeks after surgery. However, the longer one has had T2DM, the less likely he or she is to be able to discontinue insulin use.[41] Patients undergoing gastric bypass surgery tend to achieve remission of diabetes faster than those undergoing lap banding, although both procedures are highly successful at normalizing glycemia (Fig. 10-3).[36]

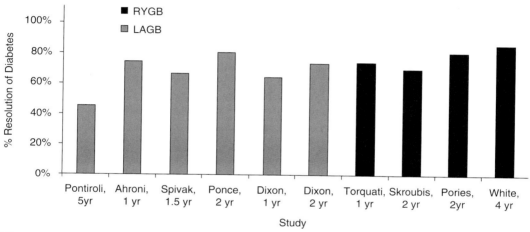

Figure 10-3 • Resolution of Diabetes Following Laparoscopic Banding and Gastric Bypass Procedures. The remission rate attributable to metabolic surgery is dependent upon the type of procedure performed. A higher percentage of patients achieve diabetes resolution 1 to 2 years postoperatively following the RYGB versus the LAGB.

References

1. Pontiroli AE, et al. Laparoscopic gastric banding prevents type 2 diabetes and arterial hypertension and induces their remission in morbid obesity: a 4-year case-controlled study. *Diabetes Care*. 2005;28(11):2703–2709.
2. Ahroni JH, et al. Laparoscopic adjustable gastric banding: weight loss, co-morbidities, medication usage and quality of life at one year. *Obes Surg*. 2005;15(5):641–647.
3. Spivak H, et al. Weight loss and improvement of obesity-related illness in 500 U.S. patients following laparoscopic adjustable gastric banding procedure. *Am J Surg*. 2005;189(1):27–32.
4. Ponce J, et al. Effect of Lap-Band-induced weight loss on type 2 diabetes mellitus and hypertension. *Obes Surg*. 2004;14(10):1335–1342.
5. Dixon JB, et al. Health outcomes of severely obese type 2 diabetic subjects 1 year after laparoscopic adjustable gastric banding. *Diabetes Care*. 2002;25(2):358–356
6. Torquati A, et al. Is Roux-en-Y gastric bypass surgery the most effective treatment for type 2 diabetes mellitus in morbidly obese patients? *J Gastrointest Surg*. 2005;9(8):1112–1116; discussion 1117–1118.
7. Skroubis G, et al. Roux-en-Y gastric bypass versus a variant of biliopancreatic diversion in a non-superobese population: prospective comparison of the efficacy and the incidence of metabolic deficiencies. *Obes Surg*. 2006;16(4):488–489.
8. Pories WJ. *Presented at NAASO. The Obesity Society Annual Scientific Meeting*. October 24–28, 2006; Boston, MA.
9. White MA, et al. Gender, race, and obesity-related quality of life at extreme levels of obesity. *Obes Res*. 2004;12(6):949–955.
10. Dixon JB, et al. Adjustable gastric banding and conventional therapy for type 2 diabetes: a randomized controlled trial. *JAMA*. 2008;299(3):316–323.

TABLE 10-6. Preoperative Factors Positively Predicting Diabetes Resolution Following Metabolic Surgery in Severely Obese Patients with T2DM

- Baseline A1C 6.5%–7.9% (77% remission rate vs. 50% remission for baseline A1C > 10%)
- Duration of diabetes of ≤ 5.5 y
- Baseline C-peptide > 3 ng/mL (suggestive of severe IR)
- Baseline BMI > 45 kg/m^2
- Significantly elevated basal and 2-h postprandial insulin levels

From Schernthaner G, Brix JM, Kopp HP, et al. Cure of type 2 diabetes by metabolic surgery? A critical analysis of the evidence in 2010. *Diabetes Care.* 2011;34(suppl 2):S355–S360.

Factors that predict resolution of diabetes following metabolic surgery are listed in Table 10-6. Patients with better preoperative control of their diabetes and those with shorter duration of diabetes and higher degrees of IR are more likely to be euglycemic for 1 to 2 years postprocedure.

Obesity and diabetes may also be associated with an increased risk of cancer and cancer-related mortality (see Chapter 8).[42] In the SOS study, metabolic surgery resulted in a sustained mean weight reduction of 19.9 kg over 10 years, in contrast to a weight gain of 1.3 kg in the control group.[43] The number of first-time cancers after inclusion was significantly lower in the surgery group than in the controls, with the modest reduction in cancer risk favoring women over men. Whether metabolic surgery clearly reduces cancer risk in severely obese patients with T2DM is unknown.

Although, the evidence suggests that metabolic surgery is a successful long-term treatment of obesity for people with diabetes, the procedure is expensive, with costs exceeding $13,000 per patient.[44] A study by Hoerger et al.[44] evaluated the cost-effectiveness of metabolic surgery in severely obese adults with diabetes relative to usual diabetes care. Cost analysis was performed on patients with T2DM of less than 5 years duration as well as greater than 10 years. Table 10-7 lists the conclusions from this study.

Table 10-8 lists the inclusion and exclusion criteria for metabolic surgery candidates based upon the 2008 American Association of Clinical Endocrinologists/The Obesity Society/American Society for Metabolic and Metabolic Surgery Medical Guidelines for Clinical Practice.[36]

Additional inclusionary characteristics for patients who may be considered strong candidates for metabolic surgery are shown in Table 10-9.[45]

TABLE 10-7. Benefits of Metabolic Surgery in Severely Obese Patients with T2DM

- 1.72 life-years gained in patients with history of diabetes for < 5 y prior to surgery
- Patients with BMIs 30–34 kg/m^2 had the most cost-effective outcomes over time
- Cost-effectiveness ratio of $7,000–$12,000 per quality-adjusted life year gained
- Cost savings were greatest in patients ages 65–74 y having diabetes for < 5 y
- Metabolic surgery resulted in a remission rate of ˜40–80 (see Fig. 10-3)
- Following metabolic surgery the likelihood of diabetes relapse is 8% annually
- Systolic blood pressure is reduced 11.25% during the first 2 y followed by an additional 1.4% reduction until year 10 after which no further improvement in blood pressure is observed.
- Total cholesterol is reduced 16.1% during the first 2 y followed by a 1.2% reduction each year thereafter until year 10.
- HDL-cholesterol improves 10% during the first 2 y, then decreases by 0.05% through year 10

From Hoerger TJ, Zhang P, Segel JE, et al. Cost-effectiveness of metabolic surgery for severely obese adults with diabetes care. *Diabetes Care.* 2010;33:1933–1939.

TABLE 10-8. The AACE Metabolic Surgical Selection Criteria for Patients with Severe Obesity

Selection Factor	Criteria
Weight	BMI ≥ 40 kg/m² with no comorbidities BMI ≥ 35 kg/m² with obesity-associated comorbidity
Children/Adolescent selection criteria	>95th percentile of weight for age + severe comorbidity
Weight Loss History	Failure of previous nonsurgical attempts at weight reduction, including nonprofessional programs (Weight Watchers, Jenny Craig, personal trainer, etc.).
Commitment	Realistic expectation that patient will adhere to postoperative care and instructions
Exclusion	• Any potentially reversible endocrine disorder that could result in obesity • Severe psychiatric dysfunction • Current drug or alcohol abuse • Lack of comprehension of risks or understanding of personal commitment to postoperative care

From Mechanick JI, Kushner RF, Sugerman HJ, et al. American Association of Clinical Endocrinologists, the Obesity Society and American Society for Metabolic and Metabolic surgery Medical Guidelines for Clinical Practice for the Perioperative, Nutritional, Metabolic and Nonsurgical Support of the Metabolic Surgery Patient. *Endocr Pract.* 2008;14 (suppl 1):1–83.

A patient who is considering metabolic surgery should be counseled on the risks and benefits of the different types of available procedures. Specific contraindications to metabolic surgery are few. They include mental or cognitive impairment that limits the patient's ability to understand the procedure and thus precludes informed consent. Very severe coexisting medical conditions, such as unstable coronary artery disease (CAD) or advanced liver disease with portal hypertension, may in some instances render the risks of surgery unacceptably high.

When scrutinizing reports of complications related to metabolic surgeries, the reader should consider the following. First, most surgical outcome studies include very small cohorts, usually less than 100 subjects. Second, surgeons do not always perform the exact type of procedure on each bypass or lap-band patient. For example, some bypass procedures are performed laparoscopically, whereas others are performed as open procedures. Thus, including all complications as being directly related to a single bypass procedure would be inappropriate. Next, not all lap bands are

TABLE 10-9. Selection Characteristics That Should be Considered Prior to Bariatric Surgery

• BMI > 40 or >35 kg/m² with significant obesity-related comorbidities

• Age 16 to 65 y

• Acceptable operative risk

• Documented failure at nonsurgical approaches for weight loss

• Psychologically stable patient with realistic expectations

• Well-informed and committed patient

• Supportive family/social environment

• Resolution of alcohol/substance abuse

From Bult MJ, van Dalen T, Muller AF. Surgical treatment of obesity. *Eur J Endocrinol.* 2008;158(2):135–145.

equal. Several companies produce the devices, including Johnson and Johnson and Allergan. The surgical techniques are different for each device. Finally, some "centers of excellence" for metabolic surgery, may actually only perform a handful of procedures each month. Unlike cardiovascular centers of excellence, a surgeon who performs only 15 to 20 procedures each year may not be considered as expert in a given surgical procedure as a cardiac surgeon who has performed hundreds of coronary artery bypass grafts.

Postoperative complications include gastrointestinal leak, deep vein thrombosis, bleeding, anastomotic stricture, incisional or internal hernia, marginal ulceration, vitamin and protein malnutrition, gallstone formation, and wound infections. The more adept a surgeon is at performing gastric bypass procedures, the fewer complications the patient experiences.[46] Postoperative patients must be evaluated frequently for deficiencies in calcium, iron, thiamine, folate, and vitamin B_{12}.

On average, metabolic surgery is associated with a mortality risk in the range of 0.3%. Significant or major complications occur in just over 4% of patients.[47] Studies have demonstrated that the likelihood of postoperative complications is significantly associated with annual surgical experience. The risks are greatest when surgeons perform fewer than 25 operations and hospitals host fewer than 50 operations per year, and the risks are lowest when surgeons perform more than 100 operations and hospitals host more than 150 operations per year.[48,49] Studies suggest that lap banding is perhaps the safest of all the metabolic surgical procedures available in the United States.[50,50a]

The reason for the effectiveness of metabolic surgery in reversing T2DM is uncertain. Food intake, transit, and absorption are regulated by a complex network including the gastrointestinal system, the liver, and the brain. Thus, many factors may influence the physiologic and metabolic outcomes that are commonly observed following metabolic surgery. GLP-1 potentiates insulin release following the consumption of a meal in a glucose-dependent manner. In patients with T2DM as well as individuals who are obese, GLP-1 responses to glucose or mixed meals are impaired or patients exhibit evidence of resistance at the sites of targeted receptors. Serum levels of GLP-1 increase early after both RYGB and BPD procedures, which is believed to contribute to both improvement and hypertrophy of pancreatic β-cells postoperatively.[51] Excessive stimulation of the β-cells following RYGB can induce a condition known as nesidioblastosis that can present clinically as postabsorptive hypoglycemia.[52] Gastric bypass procedures may result in distention of the stomach, which, in turn, stimulates the release of central GLP-1 via vagal stimulation inducing satiety.[53]

Metabolic surgery heightens the dynamic responsivity of β-cells and appears to improve β-cell function. Whether β-cell function is fully restored is dependent principally upon the severity of diabetes relative to duration of the disease, the degree of metabolic control, and the intensity of ongoing antidiabetes treatment.[54,55]

Table 10-10 summarizes facts related to metabolic surgery procedures in the United States.

Two recently published randomized, controlled trials suggest that metabolic surgery can be a more efficient means than either standard or intensive medical treatment alone in managing obese patients with diabetes. Mingrone et al. assigned patients to undergo gastric bypass, gastric sleeve, or standard medical therapy.[55a] After 2 years, diabetes remission had occurred in 75% of the gastric bypass group, 95% of the gastric sleeve group, and none of the medical therapy group. The average baseline A1C of 8.65% decreased in all groups at 2 years, but was most improved in the surgical groups (average A1C at study end: 7.69 for the medical therapy group, 6.35 in the gastric bypass group, and 4.95 for the gastric sleeve group).

In another study, Schauer et al. compared intensive medical therapy with gastric bypass or sleeve gastrectomy.[55b] After 1 year, the primary end point, an A1C of 6% or less, was achieved in 12% of patients in the medical therapy group versus 42% in the gastric bypass group and 37% in the sleeve gastrectomy cohort.

The studies by Mingrone et al. and Schauer et al. suggest that metabolic surgery should probably be considered sooner in obese patients with diabetes and severe IR. Within 1 to 2 years following surgical intervention, more patients are able to attain remission of their diabetes and normalize their A1Cs than if prescribed intensive medical therapies. Patients with T2DM in whom recommended

TABLE 10-10. Metabolic Surgery Fact Sheet

1. Metabolic surgery treats clinically severe obesity and obesity-related conditions by (a) limiting the amounts of nutrients the stomach can hold and/or (b) reducing the gastric volume to a few ounces, thereby limiting caloric absorption.

2. Indications for metabolic surgery include a BMI of ≥40 kg/m² or a BMI of 35–40 kg/m² with an obesity-related disease such as diabetes, heart disease, or sleep apnea. Patients with obesity-induced physical limitations such as joint disease and limitation of ambulation may also benefit from surgical intervention.

3. 220,000 patients underwent metabolic surgery in 2009. 15 million Americans have clinically severe obesity, yet <1% are being referred for and treated with metabolic surgery. Costs of the procedure, low financial credit scores, insurance restrictions, and lack of understanding related to metabolic surgical procedures among primary care referral health-care professionals are believed to be responsible for sluggish growth of the surgical market.

4. Metabolic surgery costs are $10,000–$25,000 per procedure.

5. The most commonly performed procedures are lap banding, gastric bypass, and sleeve gastrectomy.

6. Metabolic surgical procedures can improve or reverse T2DM, heart disease, sleep apnea, hypertension, and hyperlipidemia in most patients.

7. Preoperative factors that positively predict diabetes resolution following metabolic surgery include; short duration of T2DM, high BMI, lower A1C and high degree of IR.

8. Gastric bypass resolves T2DM rapidly in nearly 90% of patients

9. Gastric banding resolves T2DM more slowly in 73% of patients

10. Metabolic surgery reduces the risk of CAD by 50%

11. Metabolic surgery resolves obstructive sleep apnea in more than 85% of patients

12. The risks of death from metabolic surgery is 0.17%. The overall likelihood of a major complication is 4%

13. Metabolic surgery improves life expectancy by 89% vs. nonsurgical interventions

14. Metabolic surgery reduces the risk of premature death by 30%–40%

15. Metabolic surgery reduces the risk of all cause mortality from T2DM by 92%, from cancer by 60% and CAD by 56%

16. Maximum weight loss occurs within 1–2 y postoperatively with improvement in obesity-related comorbidities for years afterward

17. Patients lose 30%–50% of their excess weight 6 months postoperatively and 77% of their excess weight within the first year.

18. Long-term studies performed 10–14 y following surgery demonstrate that clinically severe obese patients who underwent metabolic surgery maintained much greater weight loss and more favorable levels of blood glucose control, lipid and hypertension as compared to nonsurgical aged matched controls.

From American Society of Metabolic and Metabolic Surgery Fact Sheet: http://www.asmbs.org/Newsite07/media/ASMBS_Metabolic_Bariatric_Surgery_Overview_FINAL_09.pdf. Accessed June 3, 2011.

glycemic targets are not reached with available medical therapies, especially when the individual has major coexisting illnesses such as sleep apnea, hypertension, and dyslipidemia, should be provided with the option of bariatric surgery.

In summary, metabolic surgery appears to be the only long-term effective therapy in reducing morbidity and mortality related to the comorbidities observed with obese T2DM. Operative selection algorithms have attempted to match specific patients with a specific operation in order to, among other factors, minimize surgical complications. The different types of surgeries appear to be cost-effective as they tend to reverse all-cause mortality, prolong life, improve lipids and hypertension, and reverse diabetes. Ideal patients for metabolic surgery are those having preoperative A1Cs less than 7.9%, duration of diabetes less than 5.5 years, BMI greater than 45 kg per m,[2] and evidence of severe IR. Patients who cannot comprehend the nature of the surgical intervention and the lifelong measures required to maintain an acceptable level of health should not be offered these procedures. Partnering with local metabolic surgeons would be an appropriate initial step to allow obese patients with T2DM to receive a timely surgical consult.

▌Pathogenesis of T2DM

Although the "core defects" of T2DM are pancreatic β-cell failure and IR, other systems appear to play unique and contributory roles in the progressive nature of the disease. Genetic and environmental susceptibility certainly increase the likelihood of developing T2DM. In addition, abnormalities in adipocytes (accelerated lipolysis), neuroprotective mechanisms (resulting in excessive appetite), changes in kidney absorption of glucose (involving the SGTL2 transport system), incretin resistance in the GI tract, and excessive hepatic glucose production in spite of a threefold increase in β-cell secretion of insulin all contribute to chronic hyperglycemia, oxidative stress, and long-term complications. When patients state that "they are doing the best they can" to control their glucose values, one should remain cognizant of the complex highway on which these paths will likely intersect clinical diabetes. Whether an individual remains euglycemic or advances toward the hyperglycemic pathway is ultimately determined by the ability of one's pancreatic β-cells to produce and secrete enough insulin to maintain normoglycemia.

The hallmark of the metabolic dysfunction associated with T2DM includes a reduction in insulin secretion as well as altered insulin action, resulting in hyperglycemia. Unlike autoimmune T1DM, the progression to T2DM occurs over a period of 7 to 10 years (Fig. 10-4). In the prediabetes states of impaired fasting glucose (IFG) and IGT, pancreatic β-cells excrete increasing amounts of insulin in an attempt to maintain normal glycemia. The higher insulin output is accompanied by reduced

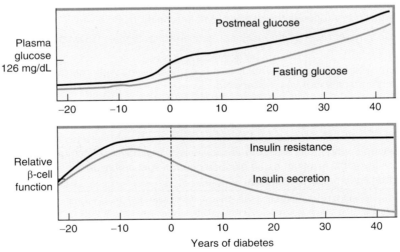

Figure 10-4 • Progressing from Normoglycemia to Diabetes is a Process Taking Many Years.
Approximately 7 years before the diagnosis of clinical diabetes, patients may have postprandial glucose levels greater than 140 mg per dL. Just before the diagnosis of diabetes, the fasting glucose levels increase greater than 126 mg per dL. β-cells produce a high level of insulin to overcome insulin resistance that occurs at the liver, adipose tissue, and skeletal muscle cells. At the time of diagnosis of diabetes, IR is prominent, yet endogenous insulin production by β-cells is reduced by 50%. When only 20% of the β-cell mass remains functioning, patients require exogenous insulin therapy.

insulin activity in the liver, adipose tissue, and skeletal muscles, resulting in diminished intracellular glucose disposal. A further decline in β-cell insulin secretion and an increase in hepatic glucose production lead to overt diabetes with fasting and postprandial hyperglycemia. Patients proceed through a spectrum of abnormal glucose states, including IFG and IGT, until ultimately progressing to diabetes. Based upon a mathematical model of patients in the United Kingdom Prosepective Diabetes Study (UKPDS), the traditional belief has been that a newly diagnosed patient with T2DM has approximately 50% of their β-cell functioning remaining.[56]

Pancreatic β-cell failure appears to occur much earlier in the natural history of T2DM and is more severe than previously thought. The San Antonio Metabolism (SAM) study evaluated patients with normal glucose tolerance and T2DM.[57] Patients received an OGTT with plasma glucose and insulin concentrations measured every 15 minutes to evaluate overall glucose tolerance and β-cell function. An insulin clamp technique was used to measure insulin sensitivity. Patients with "impaired glucose tolerance" who had a 2-hour postprandial glucose level of 180 to 199 mg per dL were found to have lost 80% to 85% of their β-cell function. Thus, by the time the diagnosis of clinical diabetes is made and therapeutic interventions are initiated, patients have already lost at least 80% of their β-cell function and are maximally insulin resistant. The SAM study suggests that intensive pharmacologic intervention may be reasonable for patients with both prediabetes and newly diagnosed T2DM.

In postmortem analysis, Butler et al.[58] determined that β-cell mass is significantly decreased in patients with T2DM and that the underlying mechanism for this is β-cell apoptosis (genetically mediated cell death). Obese individuals in Butler's study had a 63% deficit in relative β-cell volume compared with nondiabetic obese individuals. Thus, patients with prediabetes tend to lose β-cell function and mass prior to being clinically diagnosed with T2DM.

Multiple mechanistic anomalies have been implicated in the progression from euglycemia to clinical diabetes (Fig. 10-5). The pancreas, liver, muscle, kidneys, brain, gut, and adipose cell appear to be "team players" in driving susceptible individuals into chronic hyperglycemia. The individual

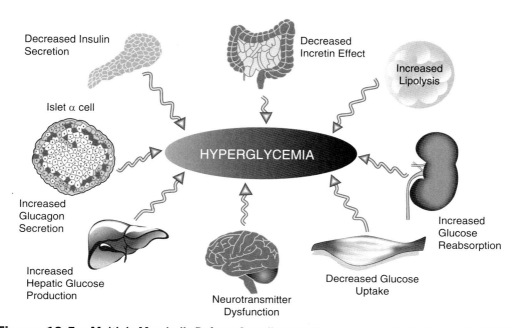

Figure 10-5 • Multiple Metabolic Defects Contribute to Hyperglycemia in Patients with T2DM.
T2DM develops over time as a result of metabolic defects originating from multiple organ systems. This process is referred to as "The Ominous Octet." (Adapted from DeFronzo RA. From the triumvirate to the ominous octet: a new paradigm for the treatment of type 2 diabetes mellitus. *Diabetes*. 2009;773–795.)

pathways that appear to favor IR, β-cell destruction, and progression from prediabetes to clinical diabetes are discussed below.

• β-cell Failure and Apoptosis

Patients with IGT have lost over 80% of their β-cell function and 50% of their β-cell mass.[57] These patients are maximally insulin resistant and have a 10% incidence of diabetic retinopathy.[59] Some would argue that patients with prediabetes should be treated intensively in order to preserve any remaining β-cell function.[60]

Multiple mechanisms have been proposed that appear to target progressive β-cell failure. Advancing age plays an important role in β-cell failure. Well-established observational studies confirm the incidence of diabetes increases with advancing age.[61]

Vitamin D (25-hydroxyvitamin D [25(OH)D]) may have a direct influence on diabetes pathogenesis and β-cell function. Several mechanistic pathways have provided researchers with circumstantial evidence linking vitamin D to β-cell preservation. Vitamin D3 may be obtained directly from the diet or by means of the sunlight-induced photochemical conversion of 7-dehydrocholesterol to previtamin D3. D3 must be hydroxylated twice to produce the biologically active form of the hormone. The first hydroxylation process occurs in the liver. This conversion produces 25-hydroxyvitamin D [25(OH)D], which is the major circulating form of vitamin D used by clinicians to determine vitamin D status. This form of vitamin D is biologically inactive and must be converted once again in the kidneys by 1 α-hydroxylase to the biologically active form of vitamin D 1,25-dihydroxyvitamin D [1,25(OH)2D].[62] β-cells contain both vitamin D receptors and express activity of 1 α-hydroxylase.[63] This suggests that the 1 α-hydroxylase enzyme plays a role in vitamin D signaling within the islet as well as in other organs such as the kidneys.[64] (b) Vitamin D improves β-cell function by stimulating insulin release and restoring impaired insulin secretion in vitamin D-deficient mice.[63] (c) Vitamin D is known to improve insulin action by stimulating expression of the insulin receptor and enhancing responsiveness for glucose transport.[65] The Nurses' Health Study of 83,779 women with 20-year follow-up revealed 4,843 new cases of T2DM. However, patients who consumed greater than 1,000 mg per day of calcium and greater than 800 mg per day of vitamin D had a 33% lower risk of developing T2DM."[66] (d) Mutations in genes coding for 1 α-hydroxylase may explain an association between obesity, T2DM, and low level of serum vitamin D.[67] Unfortunately, no well-conducted randomized, controlled trials with adequate vitamin D doses have been conducted to determine if vitamin D supplementation could reduce the incidence of T2DM in adults.[68] In light of the widespread prevalence of both vitamin D insufficiency and T2DM, the potential relationship between both disorders could hold tremendous public health implications.

IGT in association with elevated free fatty acids (FFAs) can induce oxidative stress. Intracellular oxidative stress occurs when the production of reactive oxygen species (ROS) (by-products of normal metabolism) exceeds the capacity of the cell's antioxidants to neutralize them. Oxidative stress can be minimized by optimization of metabolic control. Stress-induced pathways such as NF-κB, stress kinases, and hexosamines tend to promote not only β-cell apoptosis but also pathways leading to long-term diabetes-related complications[69]

Glucotoxicity (chronically elevated plasma glucose levels) also influences the functionality and survivability of pancreatic β-cells. Short-term exposure of β-cells to increasing glucose concentrations initially induces proliferation of β-cell mass in a concentration-dependent manner.[70] Over time, the proliferative capacity of β-cells is suppressed as demonstrated by Leahy et al. His team noted that cultured human islets undergo linear acceleration of β-cell apoptosis when exposed to glucose concentrations ranging 99 to 594 mg per dL.[70]

Insulin secretion from the pancreas occurs in two phases. The first-phase insulin response represents an acute release of insulin from the β-cells (Fig. 10-6). Normally, this insulin release occurs as β-cells excrete preformed insulin for 10 to 20 minutes after a glucose stimulus. The second-phase

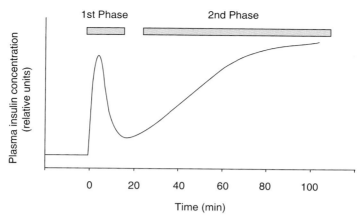

Figure 10-6 • Normal First and Second Phase Insulin Responses to Oral Glucose Challenge by Pancreatic β-Cells. In response to an initial glucose stimulation, the pancreatic β-cell produces an "acute" insulin response followed by a slower secondary release of insulin, which will be maintained as long as necessary in order to maintain euglycemia. The first phase insulin response is reduced or absent in patients with T2DM, leaving a delayed and/or exaggerated second phase insulin release.

insulin release will continue until the blood glucose level returns to normal, approximately 90 to 180 minutes after eating. First-phase insulin response is genetically predetermined and frequently abnormal in subjects with a first-degree relative with diabetes.[71] (First-phase insulin response is also impaired because of the effects of chronic hyperglycemia on β-cell function and postreceptor signaling, which promote intracellular glucose transport.[72,73](Direct β-cell death resulting from an elevation in FFA levels will also impair first-phase insulin response.

To summarize, hyperglycemia plays a central role among the factors that contribute to loss of β-cell function. Vitamin D deficiency may predispose susceptible patients to glucose intolerance, altered insulin secretion, and progression to clinical diabetes. Initially, transient postprandial hyperglycemia may induce β-cell proliferation in insulin-resistant individuals. Over time this adaptive mechanism will fail as β-cell dysfunction and death ensue in those who are genetically or environmentally at risk. Aging β-cells may also be more prone to apoptosis. Chronic glucotoxicity induces intracellular oxidative stress when inflammatory cytokine production further impairs the β-cell's production and insulin secretory capacity. T2DM does not occur in the absence of progressive β-cell failure, although IR is well established early during the natural course of the disease.

Considering the taxing global projections of patients who will eventually develop T2DM, novel strategies and agents will need to be developed that can halt the progression and perhaps either induce a β-cell rest or restore normoglycemia to high-risk patients. Clinical and mathematical assessments of β-cell function will allow investigators to determine the success or failure of pharmacologic interventions designed for β-cell rescue and preservation. Table 10-11 lists several of the commonly used assessment tools for determining β-cell function in clinical trials.

• Increased Lipogenesis and Free Fatty Acid Production

Fat cells play a pivotal role in the pathogenesis of T2DM. In fact, one may assume that the path toward T2DM will not become activated "until the fat cells begin to sing!" The fat cells travel with an entourage that includes the liver, muscle, and the β-cells. The damaged done metabolically by these four players are rarely detected until patients have been subject to microvascular or macrovascular complications for several years before treatment is initiated.

FFAs are responsible for antagonizing insulin action, promoting IR, reducing β-cell responsiveness to ambient hyperglycemia, and inducing β-cell apoptosis. At the cellular level, FFAs inhibit

TABLE 10-11. Clinical Tests That Assess β-cell Function

β-cell Function Clinical Assessment Tool	Clinical Application	Comment
C-peptide	• Can be used to diagnose insulinomas and detect factitious hypoglycemia. When hypoglycemia is due to surreptitious insulin injection, insulin concentrations are high, but C-peptide levels are low because C-peptide is not found in commercial insulin preparations and exogenous insulin suppresses β-cell function. • Elevated C-peptide levels result from increased β-cell activity as seen in insulinomas, thyrotoxicosis, Cushing syndrome, hypokalemia, pregnancy, acromegaly and chronic kidney disease • Fasting reference range = 1–3 ng/mL	• Human insulin and C-peptide originate as a single polypeptide chain known as proinsulin in the pancreatic β-cell. Proinsulin is cleaved proteolytically to form equimolar amounts of insulin and C-peptide that are released into the portal vein. • C-peptide binds the A and B chains of human insulin • C-peptide has no biologic role other than to act as a "connector" for the 2 insulin chains • C-peptide levels ≥3 ng/mL is predictive of cardiovascular risk in patients with multiple components of the metabolic syndrome • Low C-peptide levels are expected when endogenous insulin secretion is decreased (T1DM), or suppressed as a normal response to exogenous insulin injections. Thiazide diuretics and alcohol ingestion also suppress C-peptide levels • Half-life of C-peptide is 30 vs. 5 min for insulin. Thus, C-peptide provides a semi-quantitative assessment of endogenous insulin secretion
Acute Insulin Response to Glucose (AIRg)	• Evaluates loss of first phase insulin response in patients with T2DM	• Loss of first phase insulin response is one of the early defects observed in β-cell response to glucose stimulation • AIRg is the mean increment in insulin concentration during the first 5 to 10 min after a standardized amount of glucose (0.3 g/kg of body weight) has been delivered intravenously as a bolus

(Continued)

TABLE 10-11. Clinical Tests That Assess β-cell Function *(Continued)*

β-cell Function Clinical Assessment Tool	Clinical Application	Comment
Proinsulin-to-Insulin Ratio	The proinsulin:insulin ratio has been used as an indirect marker of β-cell function. For example, elevation of the proinsulin:insulin ratio correlates with a decreased acute insulin response to glucose in T2DM • Fasting proinsulin levels > 5 pmol/L in conjunction with hypoglycemia (plasma blood glucose <45–60 mg/dL) suggests the presence of insulinoma due to endogenous hyperinsulinemia	• In euglycemic individuals, small amounts of proinsulin are secreted concurrently with insulin, resulting in a plasma proinsulin:insulin ratio of ~0.1. • Inflammation of β-cells, β-cell dysfunction, and β-cell stress will increase proinsulin:insulin ratios • IR and T2DM may result in an increase in proinsulin relative production. Thus, a rise in proinsulin levels suggests β-cell stress
Homeostasis Model Assessment-β-Cell (HOMA-B)	• HOMA can be used to assess longitudinal changes in β-cell function and IR in patients with diabetes in order to examine the natural history of diabetes and to assess the effects of treatment. • HOMA can also be used to track changes in insulin sensitivity and β-cell function longitudinally in individuals. • (HOMA) estimates steady state β-cell function (%B) and insulin sensitivity (%S), as percentages of a normal reference population.	• HOMA is a method for assessing β-cell function and IR from basal (fasting) glucose and insulin or C-peptide concentrations. • HOMA is a measure of basal insulin sensitivity and β-cell function and, is not intended to give information about the stimulated state of β-cells unlike clamp studies. • HOMA cannot be used to test β-cell sensitivity in patients treated with exogenous insulin therapy • HOMA calculator can be found online at: http://www.dtu.ox.ac.uk/homacalculator/index.php

From Kim ST, Kim BJ, Lim DM, et al. Basal C-peptide level as a surrogate marker of subclinical atherosclerosis in type 2 diabetic patients. *Diabetes Metab J.* 2011;35(1):41–49; Henry JB. *Clinical Diagnosis and Management by Laboratory Methods.* 18th ed. Philadelphia, PA: WB Saunders Co.; 1991; Mykkanen L, Haffner SM, Hales CN, et al. The relation of proinsulin, insulin, and proinsulin-to-insulin ratio to insulin sensitivity and acute insulin response in normoglycemic subjects. *Diabetes.* 1990;46(12):1990–1995; Vezzosi D, Bennet A, Fauvel J, et al. Insulin, C-peptide and proinsulin for the biochemical diagnosis of hypoglycaemia related to endogenous hyperinsulinism. *Eur J Endocrinol.* 2007;157:75–83; Wallace TM, Levy JC, Matthews DR. Use and abuse of HOMA modeling. *Diabetes Care.* 2004;27(6):1487–1495.

insulin-mediated glucose uptake by interfering with the translocation of the glucose transport protein, GLUT-4, to the plasma membrane, effectively blocking glucose uptake by muscle cells and increasing peripheral IR (Fig. 10-7). Elevated FFAs prevent the peripheral uptake of glucose by skeletal muscles and inhibit insulin-mediated suppression of glycogenolysis and gluconeogenesis effectively increasing hepatic glucose production.[74,75] Animal studies suggest that β-cell failure and death are preceded by an increase in plasma FFAs, accompanied by an accumulation of triglyceride within the β-cell.[76–78] Figure 10-8 summarizes the relationship between lipotoxicity and T2DM pathogenesis.

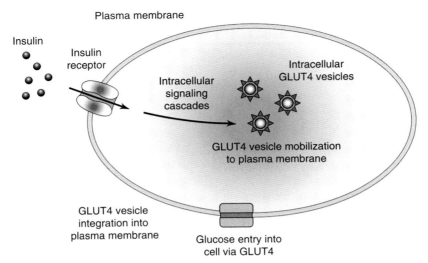

Figure 10-7 • Insulin Action in Muscle and Fat Cells. Insulin binds to the insulin receptor on the cell membrane. The binding induces a long series of intracellular molecular actions, which mobilize GLUT4 transporter protein to the cell surface. Glucose gains entry into the cell via the GLUT4 transport mechanism. IR may involve mutations of the insulin receptor or alterations in normal intracellular insulin signaling.

Several prospective epidemiologic studies have evaluated the link between elevated plasma concentrations of FFAs and the development of diabetes. In the Pima study, subjects with the highest plasma FFA levels had a 2.3-fold higher risk of developing diabetes than subjects in the lowest decile.[79] In the Paris Prospective Study, higher FFA levels were also associated with progression from normal glucose tolerance at baseline to clinical diabetes.[80]

Approximately 80% of body fat is located within the subcutaneous adipose tissue, while 20% is stored within visceral (abdominal) adipose tissue (VAT).[81] Individuals with a high accumulation of VAT, as measured by CT imaging, are at increased risk for developing T2DM, dyslipidemia, and coronary heart disease.[82] Visceral fat produces higher levels of FFA, which explains the link between obesity and the progression to T2DM. Adipocytes in obese individuals are resistant to the antilipolytic effects of insulin. Both T2DM and obesity are characterized by an elevation in the mean day-long plasma FFA concentration as well as increased triglyceride levels within muscle, liver, and β-cells further promoting IR. Figure 10-9 summarizes the mechanisms by which lipotoxicity depicts the cellular mechanisms by which FFA heightens IR.

Decreased levels of cardiovascular fitness (as reflected by low VO_{2max} during graded exercise testing) is associated with increased VAT in offspring of patients with T2DM who have evidence of impaired insulin sensitivity.[83,84] Whether or not obese patients with a strong family history of T2DM may have a form of genetically impaired exercise intolerance is pure speculation. Other studies have proven that intentional weight loss of 25 lb via diet and exercise modulation can result in a 30% to 35% reduction in total body VAT mass.[85] Moreover, consumption of a diet high in saturated fat can acutely increase plasma FFA levels in obese, insulin-resistant patients. Dietary elevation of FFA levels for as little as 48 hours markedly impairs both first- and second-phase insulin secretion in genetically predisposed individuals, further impairing insulin secretion and peripheral disposal.[86]

In summary, lipotoxicity increases IR in patients with visceral adiposity. Increased FFA production impairs insulin secretion by promoting β-cell death and blocks insulin action within myocytes and hepatocytes heightening IR. Ninety percent of patients with T2DM are considered obese. Dietary consumption that is high in saturated fat increases visceral adiposity that impairs first- and second-phase insulin secretion, peripheral glucose disposal within the skeletal

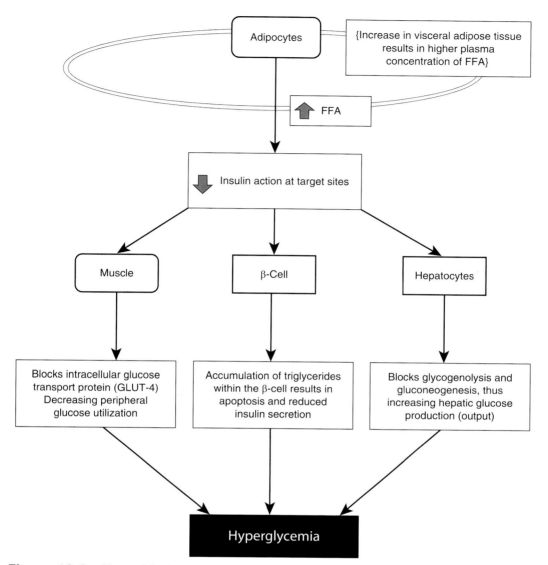

Figure 10-8 • Lipotoxicity Impacts Severely Impacts IR at Multiple Target Sites.
An increase in activity within VAT results in elevated plasma levels of FFAs. The FFAs effectively block intracellular glucose transport within skeletal muscle cells, increase hepatic glucose production, and cause pancreatic β-cell failure. The ultimate result is progressive hyperglycemia in genetically predisposed patients.

muscles, and increases hepatic glucose production. The resultant IR is the hallmark of T2DM pathogenesis.

• Insulin Resistance

Both the liver and skeletal muscles are severely resistant to insulin action in patients with T2DM. Excessive hepatic glucose production in patients with T2DM adds an additional 30 g of glucose to the systemic circulation of an 80-kg person each night. The initial response of the β-cell is to accelerate insulin production and secretion to compensate the rise in hepatic glucose output. Even at endogenous insulin secretion rates that exceed threefold normal levels, hepatic glucose production

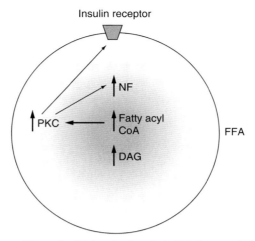

Figure 10-9 • Mechanism of IR at the Molecular Level via FFA Accumulation in Skeletal Muscle Cells.
Once FFAs accumulate in skeletal muscle cells, fatty acyl coenzyme A (CoA) and diacylglycerol (DAG) accumulate and activate the protein kinase C (PKC) pathway. High levels of PKC alter the structure of the insulin receptor on the cell membrane, resulting in IR. An increase in DAG is accompanied by activation of the nuclear factor (NF) pathway. NF has been linked to the pathogenesis of CAD, which may explain the increased prevalence of heart disease in obese patients with T2DM. (Adapted from Petersen KF, Shulman GI. Etiology of insulin resistance. *Am J Med.* 2006;119(5 suppl 1):S10–S16.)

continues to increase unabated. This leads credence to the belief that 90% of IR is due to defects in the peripheral uptake of glucose in skeletal muscle tissue.[87]

The skeletal muscles are responsible for absorbing and processing glucose in the postabsorptive state. Patients with T2DM exhibit defective insulin receptor binding and postreceptor signaling.[88,89] (As glucose clearance in the peripheral skeletal muscle is reduced, IGT and chronic postabsorptive hyperglycemia replace the normal euglycemic state (Fig. 10-7).

IR may be the best predictor of future T2DM risk. The likelihood that a patient has IR can be assessed by calculating the ratio of one's plasma triglycerides to HDL-C. A level greater than 3.5 is strongly associated with IR.[90] For example, if a patient's lipid profile demonstrates a triglyceride level of 500 mg per dL and a HDL-c of 30 mg per dL, the TG:HDL ratio is 17:1. This patient is at increased risk of developing T2DM and should be encouraged to minimize his or her saturated fat intake, initiate a weight reduction diet, eliminate any alcohol consumption, and start a comprehensive exercise program.

To summarize, IR results from defective glucose utilization within peripheral target organs, specifically skeletal muscle cells. Hepatic glucose production rises despite an initial threefold increase in endogenous insulin production. Eventually, the ability of the β-cells to continue their quest toward producing optimal insulin levels will end as their exposure to increasing plasma levels of hyperglycemia result in apoptosis.

• Hyperglucagonemia

Basal plasma glucagon concentration is elevated in patients with T2DM and their hepatocytes appear to be hypersensitive to the stimulatory effect of glucagon in inducing gluconeogenesis.[91]

Glucagon is normally secreted from pancreatic α cells located around the periphery of the islet in response to a hypoglycemic trigger. The protective mechanism of glucagon activates hepatic gluconeogenesis and glycogenolysis, thereby raising ambient glucose levels (Fig. 10-10). Under normal conditions, a postprandial increase in glucose concentration is associated with a corresponding reduction in glucagon. As plasma glucose levels decrease, glucagon levels increase, resulting in a 60% increase in hepatic glucose production and output through gluconeogenesis.[92] Glucagon secretion is regulated, in part, by endogenous insulin secretion. Insulin action results in the storage of

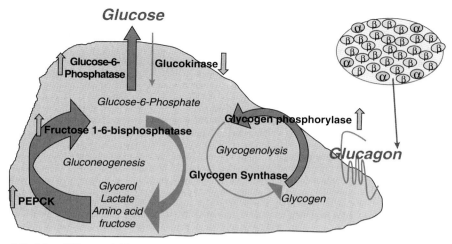

Figure 10-10 • Effects of Glucagon on Hepatocytes. Glucagon opposes the action of insulin in peripheral tissues, predominantly in the liver. Although meals generally suppress glucagon secretion from normal α cells, patients with diabetes exhibit disordered control of glucagon secretion leading to excess hepatic glucose production. Glucagon release is stimulated by hypoglycemia and inhibited by hyperglycemia, insulin, and somatostatin. GLP-1 also inhibits glucagon secretion. Once released, glucagon increases hepatic glucose production by activating glycogenolysis and gluconeogenesis pathways.

glycogen within hepatocytes. IR, insulinopenia, or an increase in glucagon output signals the liver to depolymerize glycogen, resulting in a rise in plasma glucose concentration. Paradoxically, glucagon secretion is substantially elevated in the fasting state and is not suppressed during the postabsorptive phase in patients with both prediabetes and clinically apparent diabetes. The hypersensitivity of glucagon toward promoting gluconeogenesis in T2DM promotes chronic hyperglycemia and intensifies IR.

Drugs that inhibit glucagon secretion or antagonize the glucagon receptor, such as exenatide and liraglutide, are effective in treating patients with type 2 and possibly T1DM.[93–95]

Fasting hyperglucagonemia is an early defect in the pathogenesis of T2DM. Analysis of islet hormones in young obese adolescent subjects demonstrated significantly increased levels of fasting glucagon, particularly in obese individuals with IR or IGT. Glucagon secretion was appropriately suppressed by glucose or insulin in these subjects.[96]

• Impaired Incretin Effect

The incretin effect refers to a phenomenon in which oral glucose administration elicits a much higher insulin secretory response than an equimolar intravenous infusion of glucose.[97] In humans, the incretin effect is mediated by two peptide hormones, GLP-1 and glucose-dependent insulinotropic polypeptide (GIP).

Contradicting information has been published regarding the secretion of GLP-1 in response to oral glucose in T2DM patients. Both elevated and reduced postchallenge responses have been described.[94] The plasma levels of dipeptidyl peptidase 4 (DPP-4), which rapidly degrades GLP-1 following its meal-stimulated release from the small and large intestinal L-cells, are similar in euglycemic individuals and patients with diabetes.[94] As a consequence of the action of DPP-4, as well as rapid renal clearance, the half-life of GLP-1 is 1 to 2 minutes and that of GIP is approximately 7 minutes.[94] Basal (fasting) concentrations of GLP-1 are approximately 5 pmol per L, while peak concentrations of approximately 15 to 40 pmol per L are observed 1 hour after eating.[94] Although small reductions in postprandial GLP-1 secretion may occur in patients with T2DM, these observations do not appear to have a meaningful physiologic effect on glucose metabolism and insulin secretion.[98]

The effects of both GLP-1 and GIP are expressed by specific receptors present on β-cells and other target tissues. GLP-1 and GIP increase insulin secretion from β-cells in a glucose-dependent manner. In rodents, GLP-1 and GIP also enhance β-cell mass by increasing rates of proliferation and decreasing rates of apoptosis.[99] This effect, however, has not been observed in humans. GLP-1 suppresses glucagon secretion, slows gastric emptying, and enhances satiety. GIP has a direct effect on adipocytes to promote triglyceride storage.[99] Taken together, the incretin hormones provide a physiologic response to meals of variable sizes allowing for optimal metabolic control of nutrients.

In patients with T2DM, the incretin effect is reduced by approximately 50% compared with euglycemic subjects.[99] The defect appears to be secondary to impairments in incretin hormone action (resistance) rather than secretion because most studies have found comparable circulating concentrations of GLP-1 and GIP in response to nutrient challenges in subjects with T2DM and normal controls.[99] The glucodynamic effects observed in GLP-1–deficient patients may be overcome by infusing native GLP-1 subcutaneously to achieve "pharmacologic" plasma levels.[100] However, pharmacologic replacement of GIP does not appear to restore glycemic control to patients with IGT.

Interestingly, GLP-1 resistance in some individuals may be secondary to a genetic defect affecting the receptor binding site. Defective GLP-1 receptor binding may result in loss of intracellular signaling and reduced expression of hormonal action. A single nucleotide polymorphism (SNP) in which methionine is substituted for threonine at position 149 of GLPIR on the receptor binding site has been identified.[101] When present, this defect results in an altered insulin secretory response to GLP-1 infusion.

Glucose toxicity may down-regulate GLP-1 receptor expression.[99] However, improvement in glucose control and reversal of glucose toxicity with both DPP-4 inhibitors and GLP-1 analogues can restore β-cell function and perhaps receptor responsiveness to endogenous GLP-1.[94]

In summary, resistance to the stimulatory effects of the gut hormone actions on insulin secretion and glucagon suppression (Fig. 10-11) suggest that GLP-1 and GIP contribute to the pathogenesis of T2DM.

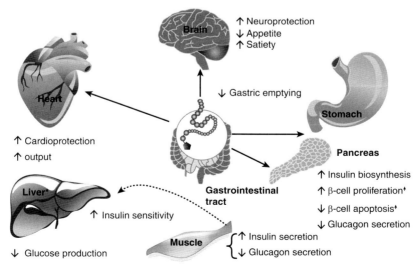

Figure 10-11 • Role of GLP-1 on Glycemic Regulation. Once secreted from the intestines in response to an oral stimulus, GLP-1 slows gastric emptying, decreases glucagon secretion (which lowers hepatic glucose production), and stimulates the secretion of endogenous insulin from the pancreatic β-cell in a glucose dependent manner. GLP-1 also increases satiety, promotes glucose uptake in skeletal muscles, and appears to be cardioprotective.

• Renal Influence on Insulin Resistance

The role of the kidneys in maintaining normoglycemia, through the filtration and reabsorption of glucose as well as gluconeogenesis, is well established. Euglycemic individuals filter approximately 180 L of plasma and 180 g of glucose through the kidneys daily.[102]

Under normal conditions, the ability of the kidneys to reabsorb glucose from the glomerular filtrate is extremely effective with less than 0.5 g per day of the filtered glucose ultimately appearing in the urine. However, in patients with hyperglycemia, the amount of filtered glucose reabsorbed increased in proportion to the plasma glucose concentration until the resorptive capacity of the proximal convoluted tubules of the glomerulus is exceeded. At this point, the excess glucose is excreted into the urine and is detected as glycosuria

Glucose reabsorption is accomplished via the active high-capacity transport protein sodium–glucose transporter-2 (SGLT 2). SGLT2 is expressed predominantly in the kidneys and is located in the brush border membrane of the S1 segment of the proximal tubule. The remainder of the glucose is reabsorbed from the distal S3 segment of the proximal tubule by the low-capacity sodium glucose cotransporter-1 (SGLT1).[103] (see Fig. 10-12).

In patients with diabetes, the SGLT 2 transport mechanism is as potent as in euglycemic individuals. This appears to be an adaptive response by the kidneys to conserve glucose, which is required to meet the energy demands of the brain and cardiovascular system in the presence of severe IR. Thus, an individual with IR is incorrectly "marked" as developing intracellular starvation of nutrients. In an attempt to correct this pathologic defect, the kidneys reabsorb excessive amounts of glucose hoping that this energy source will ease the burden of the brain,

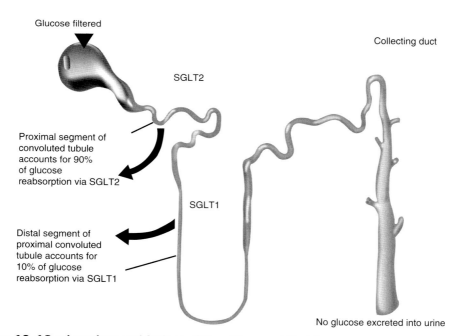

Figure 10-12 • Locations and Actions of Renal Transport Proteins.
Within the glomerulus glucose molecules are reabsorbed via active transport mechanisms within the proximal convoluted tubule rather than being lost in the urine. Two glucose transporters, SGLT2 and SGLT1 are responsible for the reabsorption of glucose in the proximal convoluted tubule. The majority of the glucose (90%) is reabsorbed via SGLT2. Patients with diabetes continue to reabsorb glucose from the plasma despite experiencing ambient hyperglycemia. This further raises plasma glucose and increases IR. Drugs that block the ability of SGLT2 to reabsorb glucose while causing the excessive glucose to be excreted in the urine can be effective in lowering blood glucose.

skeletal muscle, and cardiovascular system all of which appear to be unable to transport glucose intracellularly.

Drugs that are able to normalize plasma glucose levels by antagonizing the action of proximal tubule protein transporters appear to be an attractive pharmacologic target for both T1DM and T2DM. Simply increasing urinary glucose excretion without causing weight gain, negatively affecting β-cell function while minimizing the risk of hypoglycemia should offer positive therapeutic options to many patients.

• Impaired Neuroprotection

Few would argue that the current epidemic of diabetes is driven by the epidemic of obesity. Could the IR seen in peripheral tissues also extend into the central nervous system?

The direct administration of GLP-1 into the third cerebral ventricle of rats augments glucose-stimulated insulin secretion as the brain attempts to overcome a state of acute hyperglycemia.[104] In addition, when GLP-1 is directly administered into the arcuate nucleus of the hypothalamus hepatic glucose production is reduced.[105] Food intake is reduced when GLP-1 was injected directly into the paraventricular nucleus.[106] Thus, GLP-1 receptor expression is based upon their unique location within the brain. Stimulation of those receptors within the arcuate nucleus lowers basal and postprandial glucose levels, whereas expression of GLP-1 receptors in the paraventricular nucleus will induce satiety.

Functional magnetic resonance imaging (MRI) has been used to evaluate the cerebral response to an ingested glucose load in obese subjects.[107] Following glucose ingestion, the ventromedial nuclei and the paraventricular nuclei demonstrated consistent inhibition. These are the key centers in the brain that regulated appetite. Whether the impaired functional MRI response in obese subjects contributes to or is a consequence of IR and weight gain is unclear. However, these results suggest that in patients with impaired glucose metabolism, the brain may not only be insulin resistant, but may also have additional defects in GLP-1 expression and secretion.[108]

In summary, the pathogenesis of T2DM is multifactorial. Genetically or environmentally "challenged" individuals begin the transformation from euglycemia toward clinically apparent T2DM as their skeletal muscles and hepatocytes exhibit evidence of IR. Initially, pancreatic β-cells attempt to compensate for the IGT by overproducing insulin. Perhaps patient's appetites are increased at this early phase of prediabetes. As their meal portions increase, so does the secretion of GLP-1, resulting in β-cell hypertrophy. Over time, other metabolic defects appear that tend to aggravate the existing state of hyperglycemia. Accelerated adipocyte-centered lipolysis heightens plasma levels of circulating FFA, thereby promoting IR and β-cell apoptosis. As glycemic control deteriorates, the renal threshold for glucose excretion is exceeded. SGLT2 levels are elevated and the renal absorption of glucose is paradoxically increased as if the kidneys believed that the body required additional glucose to meet energy demands. Meanwhile, neuroprotective mechanisms within the central nervous system are also flawed as the brain is unable to minimize hepatic glucose production or induce satiety. At the cellular level, defective receptor signaling and glucose transport have occurred. Glucose is unable to enter or provide fuel for skeletal muscle cells. Hyperglycemia tends to favor GLP-1 receptor resistance. As a result, meal-stimulated GLP-1 production by the intestinal L-cells cannot effectively stimulate insulin secretion by the pancreatic β-cells. Due to the theoretical communication between β-cells and α-cells, a defect in β-cell function may result in inappropriate glucagon production that would stimulate hepatic gluconeogenesis.

▌ Genetic Susceptibility for T2DM and MODY

The development of T2DM diabetes is strongly influenced by genetics. Thirty-nine percent of patients with T2DM have at least one parent with the disease.[109] **The lifetime risk for a first-degree relative of a patient with T2DM diabetes is 5 to 10 times higher than that of age- and**

weight-matched subjects without a family history of diabetes.[110] Among monozygotic twin pairs with one affected twin, T2DM eventually develops in 60% to 90% of unaffected twins.[109] First-degree relatives of patients with T2DM often have IGT, delayed first-phase insulin response, and β-cell dysfunction years before diabetes develops.[111,112]

Approximately 2% to 5% of patients with T2DM who are first seen at a young age have mild disease and show autosomal dominant transmission. This condition was formerly called maturity-onset diabetes of the young (MODY). In 2006, the International Society of Pediatrics and Adolescent Diabetes renamed MODY "monogenetic diabetes."[113] In the new classification, the MODY subtypes have been eliminated and replaced by specific descriptions of the known genetic defects. Six different genetic abnormalities have been identified. The currently recognized genetic defects of β-cell function are described in Table 10-12.

MODY is an autosomal dominant *single* gene phenotype of youth-onset diabetes occurring typically prior to age 25, whereas T2DM is of polygenic origin. MODY can occur at any age resulting in the *limited* release of insulin in response to a glucose stimulus. Unlike MODY patients, individuals with T2DM have evidence of IR including central obesity, low HDL-c, elevated triglycerides, acanthosis nigricans, and hypertension. Patients with MODY are nonketotic and noninsulin dependent.

TABLE 10-12. MODY Classification, Characteristic Metabolic Defects, and Suggested Treatments

MODY Type	Pattern of Inheritance	Genetic Defect	Clinical Presentation
MODY1	Autosomal dominant	• HNF-4 α Expressed in the liver, kidney, intestines, and islets	• Hyperinsulinemia in fetal and neonatal life, progressing to insulin-deficient diabetes in later years • Sulfonylureas may be effective for years • Decreased apolipoproteins and triglycerides suggesting the role of the transcription factor HNF on regulating genes within hepatocytes • Deficient insulin secretion in response to an arginine stimulus • Uncommon cause of MODY (~5%)
MODY2	Autosomal dominant	• Glucokinase molecule (GK) • Decreased β-cell sensitivity to glucose. Insulin is released at increased glucose concentrations	• Nonprogressive (mild) insulinopenia • Intervention may not be needed except in the homozygous state that causes more significant hyperglycemia. Treat only if A1C > 6.5% or fasting glucose > 126 mg/dL. • In the future, glucokinase activator drugs might be a useful option • Few, if any complications • Slight increase in fasting and postprandial glucose values • A1C is near the upper limits of normal • "Neonatal diabetes." Birth weight may be decreased by 500 g • Accounts for 22% of all MODY cases

(Continued)

TABLE 10-12. MODY Classification, Characteristic Metabolic Defects, and Suggested Treatments *(Continued)*

MODY Type	Pattern of Inheritance	Genetic Defect	Clinical Presentation
MODY3	Autosomal dominant	• HNF-1 α (TCF1) Expressed in hepatocytes and β-cells	• Progressive insulinopenia with increasing age. • May regulate β-cell growth • Common cause of 58% of all MODY. • Can be treated with sulfonylureas and low-carbohydrate diet
MODY4	Autosomal dominant/ autosomal recessive (pancreatic agenesis)	• IPF-1 (Insulin Promotor Factor-1) • This is also a pancreatic transcription factor	• Later onset of diabetes • Strong history of diabetes on both sides of family
MODY5	Autosomal dominant	HNF-1 B (TCF2)	• Neonatal diabetes is possible • Renal cysts, vaginal/uterine malformations, abnormal liver functions, nondiabetic kidney disease is present Accounts for only 2% of MODY cases
MODY6	Autosomal dominant and spontaneous	• KATP channel (NEUROD1) • Most have a mutation in the tRNA gene. Many other genes may also be abnormal. • Affects the function of the mitochondria, resulting in a mitochondrial diabetes phenotype • Mitochondria normally link glucose detection to insulin secretion. Decreased energy production results in hypoinsulinism	• MELAS syndrome: mitochondrial myopathy, encephalopathy, lactic acidosis and stroke. May also present with seizures, diabetes, hearing loss, cardiac disease, short stature, endocrinopathies and neuropsychiatric dysfunction • Treat with CoQ10, riboflavin, dichloroacetate, and vitamin K. • Very rare form of MODY

From Mehrazin M, Shanske S, Kaufmann P, et al. Longitudinal changes of mtDNA A3243G mutation load and level of functioning in MELAS. Am J Med Genet A. 2009;149A(4):584–587. Fajans SS, Bell GI. MODY: history, genetics, pathophysiology and clinical decision making. *Diabetes Care.* 2011;34:1878–1884.

Patients are typically lean and white.[114] The presence of autoantibodies, such as GAD, IA-2 autoantibodies and insulin autoantibodies are pathognomonic for T1DM.

MODY patients display a variable course in severity and rate of progression of hyperglycemia and loss of endogenous insulin production. In many MODY families, microvascular and macrovascular complications occur in a frequency similar to the pattern observed in patients with T2DM.[115]

Patients with MODY3 have a genetic mutation in their glucokinase gene (HNF1A).[116] Glucokinase (expressed in both hepatocytes and pancreatic islet cells) performs as an intracellular glucose sensor and plays a crucial role in regulating insulin secretion in response to plasma glucose concentrations. Normal functioning glucokinase levels will allow maintenance of one's blood glucose levels in the fasting state between 85 and 99 mg per dL. A mutation in the glucokinase (GK) gene will cause the ambient glucose level to rise to greater than 100 mg per dL. Most often, fasting blood glucose levels are mildly elevated (110 to 140 mg per dL) and recognizable in the perinatal period. Postprandial hyperglycemia is minimal. Patients lack progression of diabetes, demonstrate an absence of insulin requirement, and do not develop vascular complications.[115]

Five other types of MODY have been identified involving mutations in transcription factor genes that control the way that insulin is produced by the pancreatic β-cells (HNF-1 α, HNF-1 β, HNF-4α, IPF-1, and NEURO-D1). Each form of MODY produces a slightly different clinical form of diabetes.[115]

A typical MODY patient may present between 12 and 30 years of age with slowly advancing abnormal glucose tolerance. In some patients with MODY, T2DM may NOT become apparent unless endogenous insulin requirements substantially increase such as during superimposed obesity, pregnancy, or periods of prolonged physical inactivity. Patients are nonobese. Both a parent and a grandparent will have diabetes. MODY patients are typically asymptomatic and may have been misdiagnosed with T1DM years prior due to their young age. Any young patient who appears to have T1DM, a strong family history of diabetes, has measurable C-peptide levels, yet tests GAD-65 (autoantibody) negative should undergo genetic testing to determine the presence of MODY.[117] Genetic testing will disclose whether MODY is present and will distinguish between a subtype of MODY, providing clues to both prognosis and treatment. Once a diagnosis for MODY is established, other family members, whether or not they are symptomatic, should be screened for the family-specific mutation and possible abnormalities of carbohydrate metabolism associated with that anomaly. Patients should also be screened with the following tests: A1C, fasting plasma glucose, 2-hour postglucose levels, 1-hour postglucose levels, and OGTT.[115] Further information regarding MODY testing may be obtained through Athena Diagnostics (http://www.athenadiagnostics.com/content/diagnostic-ed/endocrinology/mody).

Other genetic influences for the development of T2DM may be entirely "nonspecific." For example, genes that regulate appetite, energy expenditure, and intra-abdominal fat accumulation may increase the likelihood of a patient becoming obese. These "diabetes-related genes" would enhance the progression of euglycemia toward IGT and β-cell dysfunction under the influence of certain environmental factors (smoking, alcohol, reduction in serum vitamin D levels, increased BMI, loss of incretin response, etc).[118] An individual with a specific mutation in the insulin receptor gene may develop IR sooner than a patient who does not have this genetic defect. Thus, the heterogeneous nature of T2DM often makes genetic determination of pathogenesis very complex.

Patients with MODY1 and 3 may be treated with sulfonylureas.[119] Early intensive intervention with sulfonylureas appears to slow the decline of β-cell mass that occurs in these patients.[115] Diets low in carbohydrates, and intensive exercise will improve peripheral glucose uptake. Glinides may reduce the risk of hypoglycemia in patients with MODY.[120]

Glucokinase (GK) would be an excellent therapeutic target. GK is an intracellular glucose sensor in pancreatic β-cells and a rate-controlling enzyme for hepatic glucose clearance and glycogen synthesis. These metabolic processes are defective in T2DM. Patients with T2DM appear to have a reduction in GK function. Within hepatocytes, GK expression is severely reduced because the actions of GK are entirely insulin dependent.[121] In euglycemia, hyperglycemia induces GK expression in the β-cells 5- to 10-fold, resulting in insulin synthesis and secretion. Glucokinase activators (GKAs) have been shown to potentiate the glucose-stimulated release of insulin by β-cells. They also augment the receptor action of GLP-1 on target organs, thereby increasing glucose stimulation and insulin biosynthesis.[122] GKAs lower hepatic glucose production in normal and diabetic rats.[123] Some concerns related to the GKA drug class include hypoglycemia induction, fatty liver infiltration, and hyperlipidemia. The GKAs that are currently in development are shown in Table 10-13.

GLP-1 analogues such as exenatide and DPP-4 inhibitors may be a useful therapeutic option for patients diagnosed with MODY1. Clinically, such individuals develop progressive insulinopenia with advancing age, although initially sulfonylureas are effective at maintaining euglycemia.

TABLE 10-13. GKAs in Clinical Development

Drug	Pharmaceutical Sponsor	Phase/Clinicaltrials.gov Identifier:
LY2599506[a]	Eli Lilly and Company	II/ NCT01029795
LY2608204	Eli Lilly and Company	I/ NCT01313286
LY2608204	Eli Lilly and Company	I/ NCT01247363
Oral ZYGK1	Cadila Healthcare Limited	I/ NCT01472809

[a]Study was terminated due to "nonclinical safety findings."
From www.clinicaltrials.gov. Accessed March 8, 2012.

First-phase insulin response is absent and lipid panels are abnormal (low apo C2, apo C3, Lp (a), and triglycerides). GLP-1 analogues appear to enhance first-phase insulin release and may prove beneficial in patients identified with this form of monogenetic diabetes.[124,125]

Pharmacologic Intervention for T2DM

• Defining Therapeutic Goals

When lifestyle interventions including weight reduction and exercise fail to reduce glycemia to the desirable range, oral antihyperglycemic agents should be initiated. Nine years after randomization, only 9% of obese patients with T2DM in the United Kingdom Prospective Diabetes Study (UKPDS)[126] were able to maintain an A1C of less than 7%.

Because of the progressive nature of the disease, nearly all patients with T2DM will eventually require insulin to treat their hyperglycemia (see Chapter 12). Additionally, T2DM is associated with metabolic abnormalities such as hypertension, hyperlipidemia, endothelial inflammation, and procoagulation, all of which increase one's risk of early cardiovascular morbidity and mortality. The assessment and management of these comorbid conditions are imperative. One can understand how T2DM is in no way "a simple form of diabetes," as many patients are led to believe.

The goals of pharmacologic intervention in T2DM are to normalize hyperglycemia, improve insulin sensitivity, preserve β-cell function, reduce hepatic glucose output, improve peripheral glucose utilization, and delay or prevent microvascular and macrovascular complications. To that end, health-care providers should strive to treat patients as quickly as possible, as safely as possible, to the lowest glycemic targets as possible, for as long as possible, and to use pharmacologic interventions as rationally as possible. The many factors that must be considered when designing treatment programs for patients with T2DM may be reviewed in Table 10-14.

Just as the prevalence and economic burden of diabetes have increased, so too has the complexity of management. Such a process is a dynamic one that occurs partly in response to the availability of new drugs and therapeutic classes. Several studies have documented changes in the use of diabetes therapies over time.[127] Although sulfonylureas and human insulins were the mainstay of diabetes therapy before 1995, many new pharmacotherapy options have been introduced in the past decade, including glitinides, AGIs, biguanides, incretins, DPP-4 inhibitors, amylin analogues, glitazones (thiazolidinediones), insulin analogues, and GLP-1 agonists. These new compounds, although more costly than their older counterparts, are marketed on the basis of their potential promise of greater convenience and enhanced ability to achieve glycemic control.

Randomized controlled clinical trials such as the Diabetes Control and Complications Trial for patients with T1DM as well as the UK Prospective Diabetes Study and Kumamoto Study for those with T2DM have established the glycemic therapeutic goals that appear to minimize the risk of long-term complications.[56,128,129]

TABLE 10-14. Patient-Centered Care for T2DM Should Address the Following Historical, Physical, and Metabolic Characteristics

- The age and gender of the patient
- Duration of disease
- Coexisting metabolic abnomalities (i.e., hyperlipidemia, hypertension, obesity, infertility, thyroid disorder, sleep apnea, proteinuria, renal insufficiency)
- Personal or family history of microvascular or macrovascular complications
- History of hypoglycemia or hypoglycemia unawareness
- Socioeconomic status and ability to cover the costs of the medications as well as self-diabetes care
- Formulary status
- Type of employment as well as work hours (sleep dysfunction or erratic sleep schedules may complicate the ability of the patient to achieve targeted A1C levels)
- Lifestyle variables: smoking, alcohol, or substance-abuse history, activity level, meal schedule
- Preconception planning
- Concerns about weight
- Prior history of adverse events associated with a given treatment regimen
- Prior treatment successes and failures
- Prior history of exposure to a given therapeutic regimen within a clinical trial whether or not the study was performed prior to FDA approval of the drug
- Presence or absence of mental illness (If present, target treatment of mental illness first before attempting to intensify diabetes management as discussed in Chapter 9
- Cultural influences on therapeutic options (see Chapter 14)

Neither the DCCT nor the UKPDS was successful in maintaining A1C levels within their intensively treated cohort at less than 7%, which is four standard deviations above the nondiabetic norm. Recently published randomized clinical trials have attempted to intensify patients' A1C to a target of less than 6.5% using a variety of interventions. The Action to Control Cardiovascular Risk in Diabetes (ACCORD) had the primary objective of decreasing cardiovascular disease in "high-risk patients" with glycemic interventions targeting an A1C level at less than 6.0% versus treatments aimed at a more conservative A1C of less than 7.9%.[130] The intensively treated cohort showed excess cardiovascular mortality suggesting that patients with preexisting cardiovascular disease, those with hypoglycemic unawareness, elderly patients, and those who lived alone may be managed less aggressively. Otherwise, the American Diabetes Association continues to suggest that the majority of patients with diabetes can safely be treated to a target of 6.5% to 7%.[131] Thus, PCPs should consistently stress the importance of individualization of glycemic goals for all patients with diabetes.

In addition, health-care providers should consider the importance of "clinical inertia" when managing all patients with diabetes. Diabetes intensification refers to "any improvement in glycemic control" while minimizing the risk of adverse complications, especially hypoglycemia. Thus, a patient who presents to the office who is treatment naïve with a baseline A1C of 11% is considered as having been intensively managed even if their A1C does not drop below 9% after 4 months. The fact that the patient has experienced a 2% reduction in A1C implies that they also have likelihood of developing heart disease, stroke, chronic kidney disease, and neuropathy. These patients, and their physicians, should be congratulated, rather than chastised, for a job well done.

Metrics other than A1C are important to evaluate and manage in order to minimize one's risk for long-term diabetes-related complications. Hirsch and Brownlee suggested that one's A1C and duration of diabetes (glycemic exposure) accounts for only 11% of the total risk in the retinopathy cohort in TIDM patients studied in the DCCT.[132] The remaining 89% of one's likelihood of developing microvascular complications may be derived from genetics, environmental factors, poorly controlled lipids, and hypertension. Thus, although targeting ideal glycemic control in our patients is a noble goal, one must never forget the complex metabolic nature of T2DM. Normalization of lipids, blood pressure, and renal function cannot be overshadowed by one's attempts at becoming a "glycemic perfectionist." Chronic diabetes self-management requires that emphasis be placed on weight control, avoidance of nicotine, adherence to medication use, and participation in physical activity.

Several expert consensus panel guidelines have been published and subsequently revised that provide a framework for initiating and titrating pharmacologic therapies for patients with T2DM. The American Academy of Family Physicians has yet to publish any consensus guidelines on diabetes management. This is unfortunate considering that family physicians see patients of all ages and cultures. Our cradle to the grave patient cohort encompasses every possible type of published diabetes subclass. We see patients who are pregnant as well as those who are planning conception. We follow patients within the hospital setting, nursing homes, homeless shelters, and as part of hospice care. No specialist is better at identifying patients at risk for having prediabetes and even progression to clinical diabetes. Families having multiple generations of T2DM may actually have MODY. We are trained to manage the complex transition from adolescent diabetes toward adult care. Unlike endocrinologists, family physicians may actually perform a preoperative evaluation on a patient and actively participate in the perioperative care of that individual. Our services toward diabetes patients are certainly unique and customized guidelines should be written to address the needs of our diverse and growing population. Each of our patients is a unique entity with individual concerns, fears, and abilities to address their given disease state. As such, PCPs must never lose sight of directing care toward what is safe and efficacious for each patient and family.

The American Diabetes Association has now endorsed "patient-centered care" defined as an approach that ensures that patient values guide all clinical decisions.[132a] At the time of the encounter, clinicians should determine the patient's level of involvement. Therapeutic choices should be explored, shared, and prescribed with full cooperation and understanding of the engaged patient. Pharmacologic intensification that involves patient cooperation and interaction may enhance adherence to therapy.

Not all individuals with diabetes benefit from aggressive glucose management. Yet, *most* patients with A1Cs of 7% or greater should intensify their treatment regimens to achieve an A1C as close to the nondiabetic range (≤6%) as possible or, at a minimum, strive to lower their A1C to less than 7% (Table10-15). In most patients, this targeted goal will reduce the incidence of microvascular disease.[132a] Ideally, fasting and premeal glucose should be maintained at less than 130 mg per dL and

TABLE 10-15. Glycemic Targets for Adults with Diabetes Based on Guidelines Published by the American Diabetes Association (ADA) and the American Association of Clinical Endocrinologists (AACE)

Parameter	Target: ADA Guidelines	Target: AACE Guidelines
A1C	<6% (individual goal)[a] <7% (general goal)[a]	≤6.5%[a]
Fasting plasma glucose	90–130 mg/dL	<110 mg/dL
Postprandial plasma glucose	<180 mg/dL	<140 mg/dL

Notes: The AACE recommends a more rigorous A1C goal for all patients than the ADA's general recommendation of less than 7.0%. Instead, AACE advocates a goal of ≤6.5%, based on the epidemiologic analysis of the United Kingdom Prospective Diabetes Study (UKPDS) data, which showed that the risk for both microvascular and macrovascular complications of diabetes increased at A1C values ≥6.5%. These guidelines may be modified for individual patients whose functional state or risk for other adverse treatment effects (e.g., hypoglycemia) is thought to outweigh the benefits of optimal glucose control. In addition, AACE recommends treatment targets for FPG and 2-hour PPG of less than 110 and less than 140 mg per dL, respectively. These targets are based on the increased cardiovascular risk associated with plasma glucose values above these levels.
[a]Upper limit of "normal" is 6% using a Diabetes Control and Complications Trial-based assay.
Data from American Diabetes Association. *Diabetes Care.* 2006;29(suppl):S4–S42; and American Association of Clinical Endocrinologists. *Endocr Pract.* 2002;8(suppl):5–11.

the postprandial glucose should be less than 180 mg per dL. More stringent A1C targets (e.g., 6% to 6.5%) might be warranted in patients with short disease duration, long life expectancy, and no significant coronary heart disease if hypoglycemic events and treatment-emergent weight gain can be minimized. Conversely, less stringent A1C goals (e.g., A1C 7.5% to 8% or higher) are appropriate for patients with a history of hypoglycemia-associated autonomic failure (HAAF), limited life expectancy, elderly patients, those with advanced complications, and those in whom the glycemic target is difficult to attain despite intensive self-management education and effective doses of glucose-lowering agents.

Clinicians should continue to emphasize lifestyle intervention at each office visit as physical activity and food intake do impact glycemic control. Modest weight loss (5% to 10% from baseline) contributes meaningful improvement in A1C. Thus, establishing a goal of weight reduction or even weight maintenance is recommended by the ADA.[132a] At diagnosis, highly motivated patients with A1C levels near target (less than 7.5%) could be given the opportunity to engage in lifestyle intervention for 3 to 6 months prior to beginning pharmacologic therapy. However, treatment-naïve patients might also be offered the option of beginning both metformin and intensive lifestyle intervention concurrently.

The best outcomes for T2DM management have been noted when intensive treatment is initiated early in the course of the disease.[56,133] Although the method by which one targets normoglycemia is less important than actually safely achieving the desired goals, clinicians should be mindful of their many treatment options as shown in Figure 10-13

- Metformin should be initiated concurrent with lifestyle intervention at the time of the diagnosis. Because T2DM is a metabolic disorder in which the level of hyperglycemia

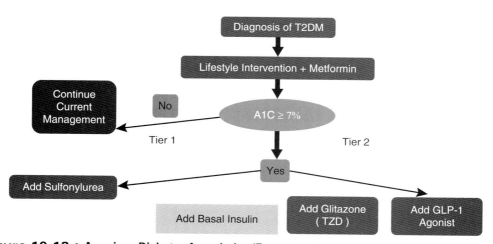

Figure 10-13 • American Diabetes Association/European Association for the Study of Diabetes Consensus Panel Guidelines for Management of Patients with T2DM.
Inzucchi SE, Bergenstal RM, Buse JB, et al. Management of hyperglycemia in type 2 diabetes: a patient-centered approach. Position statement of the American Diabetes Association (ADA) and the European Association for the Study of Diabetes (EASD). *Diabetologia* 2012. DOI 10.1007/s00125-012-2534-0)
Moving from top to bottom, the figure lists potential sequences of diabetes therapy beginning with lifestyle intervention and adding metformin monotherapy when appropriate (unless contraindicated). If A1C target is not achieved after approximately 3 months, consider adding additional agents to metformin. This could include a sulfonylurea, TZD, DPP-4 inhibitor, GLP-1 receptor agonist or basal insulin. (The order of the drugs presented on the chart is determined by the drug's historical introduction into the diabetes marketplace as well as route of administration. No specific preference is implied by the ordering of the drug sequence). Pharmacologic intervention should be based upon likelihood of achieving one's individualized glycemic targets as well as minimizing treatment emergent adverse effects such as weight gain and hypoglycemia. Basal insulin should be used before moving to more complex insulin strategies as discussed in Chapter 12. One could opt to rapidly progress from a two-drug combination to multiple daily insulin injections for those patients with severe hypoglycemia (A1C ≥ 10% to 12%). One could also begin MDI in patients with A1Cs ≥ 9%.

mirrors the progressive failure of β-cell function, lifestyle interventions fail to achieve and maintain targeted glycemic goals in most patients.

- Metformin is an excellent choice as the initial pharmacologic therapy because of its effect on glycemia, absence of weight gain or induction of hypoglycemia, generally well accepted side effect profile, low cost, and broad-based formulary acceptance.
- When metformin is initiated as monotherapy, titrate to the maximum effective dose over 1 to 2 months as tolerated. Supplement with additional glucose-lowering drugs in the setting of persistent hyperglycemia.
- When adding a second agent to metformin, consider which agent will most likely allow the patient to achieve his or her targeted A1C level.
- Consider initiating insulin therapy for patients having an A1C greater than 8.5%, especially if they have symptomatic hyperglycemia.

Although the means to intensify T2DM therapy may be unique for each patient, the ultimate goals for all patients are similar:

- Achieve and maintain normal glycemia.
- Once T2DM is diagnosed, begin lifestyle intervention and metformin.
- Rapidly add other medications to a patient's treatment regimen when glycemic targets are not achieved or sustained.
- Insulin should be added sooner (as opposed to later) to the patient's treatment regimen if the A1C cannot be maintained below 7% on oral agents or if the patient has symptomatic hyperglycemia.[134] The basal insulin analogues (glargine, detemir, and degludec) are more expensive than NPH but are associated with less nocturnal hypoglycemia than human insulin.[134a]

If basal insulin is initiated, continuing a secreatagogue (sulfonylurea) may minimize the initial deterioration of glycemic control. However, secreatagogues should be stopped once prandial insulin regimens are begun. TZDs should be reduced in dosage or discontinued to avoid edema or weight gain. Incretin therapy, where appropriate considering cost, should be continued.

Patient-centered therapy should focus on other specific targets and characteristics of each individual:

- *Age*: The younger the age at the onset of diabetes, the greater the cumulative exposure to hyperglycemia and risk for complications; the older the age at onset, the higher the probability of existing comorbid conditions and the shorter the expected life span. The ACCORD trial reported a trend toward lower all-cause mortality among participants younger than 65 years at baseline who were randomly assigned to receive standard treatment, whereas the ADVANCE trial reported lower rates of combined major macro- and microvascular events in younger participants in the intensive therapy group. However, neither finding was statistically significant. In a VADT substudy, patients aged 57 to 64 years with lower coronary calcium scores at baseline (suggestive of less atherosclerosis) had fewer coronary events with intensive control. No trial data on patients younger than 45 years with newly diagnosed T2DM are available. Yet, a near-normal A1C target range appears appropriate for younger patients who are unlikely to have established atherosclerosis.[134b]
- *Duration of disease*: Participants in the UKPDS had newly diagnosed T2DM, whereas those in ACCORD, ADVANCE, and VADT had T2DM for 8 to 11.5 years. The long-term followup of the UKPDS showed fewer micro- and macrovascular events in patients intensively treated. Participants in the VADT with established CHD had T2DM for 2 years longer than those without established CHD implying that intensive treatment is more likely to be beneficial when initiated sooner rather than later.[134b]
- *Presence of macrovascular disease*: Patients with T2DM and a history of MI are at a high risk for recurrent events. Among patients enrolled in ACCORD, ADVANCE, and VADT,

32% to 40% had a history of a CHD event and demonstrated greater mortality. Intensive intervention did NOT reduce the incidence of new CVD events or mortality. Therefore, a higher A1C target in these patients may certainly be appropriate.[134b]

- *Presence of microvascular disease*: ACCORD demonstrated that intensive control decreased the progression of retinopathy and neuropathy. A microvascular complication in an organ often suggests that other complications may be present or evolving. More intensive glycemic control may therefore be considered in the presence of microalbuminuria and normal serum creatinine or in patients with early retinopathy. Strict glycemic control does NOT appear to alter progression of renal disease once the serum creatinine exceeds 2.5 mg per dL.[134b]

- *History of HAAF*: Intensive therapy increases the risk of severe hypoglycemia two- to three-fold and is more common in elderly patients with dementia. Hypoglycemia events may increase one's risk of myocardial ischemia or arrhythmia. Both ACCORD and ADVANCE reported higher mortality rates in patients with one or more episodes of severe hypoglycemia although no direct cause and effect relationship was established because CGMS was not performed in these studies. Less-intensive A1C targets are therefore appropriate for patients with a history of recent severe hypoglycemia or HAAF.[134b]

- *Psychosocial concerns*: Clinicians should consider factors such as treatment-emergent weight gain, drug interactions, costs, cognitive status, frequency of self-blood glucose monitoring, and patient motivation or lack thereof when prescribing patient-centered therapies.

In summary, younger patients with relatively recent onset of T2DM should be managed more intensively in an attempt to target near-normal glycemic levels. Rational pharmaceutic intervention should always be prescribed based upon one's psychosocial characteristics. Older patients with established disease of long duration and evidence of micro- or macrovascular risk factors should have their glycemic targets adjusted with emphasis and considerations based on safety, comfort, and psychosocial values. Glycemic targets should be viewed as flexible and may be adjusted based upon changes in the patient's health status and living conditions.

In 2009, the American Association of Clinical Endocrinologists (AACE) published an algorithm designed to assist PCPs, endocrinologists, and other health-care providers to manage adult, non-pregnant patients with T2DM (Fig. 10-14).[135]

The AACE algorithm is conceptually simple. A patient with an A1C of ≤ 6.5% may be managed effectively with monotherapy. Patients with A1C levels between 7.5% and 9% should be placed on dual combination therapy using the options listed in Figure 10-14B. Triple therapeutic options should be utilized in **asymptomatic** patients with A1C levels greater than 9%. However, insulin should be initiated in symptomatic patients whose A1C levels are ≥ 9%. Insulin should also be used in patients in whom triple combination therapy fails to reduce A1C levels to less than 9%. AACE favors insulin analogues over human insulins (NPH and regular) in order to minimize the risk of hypoglycemia.

AACE recognizes the commonly observed adverse complications associated with intensification of diabetes therapy weight gain and hypoglycemia. As such, the rational use of pharmacologic therapies that minimize weight gain and hypoglycemic events is emphasized. Unlike the ADA consensus panel guidelines, AACE endorses the safety and efficacy of DPP-4 inhibitors in improving glycemic control, and minimizing weight gain while reducing one's risk of developing treatment-emergent hypoglycemia.

"Boutique drugs," such as colesevelam and AGIs, although rarely used by diabetologists, may be appropriate in a limited number of cases. Their use is limited by adverse side effects, frequency of dosing requirements, and minimal effect on A1C reduction.

When reviewing the AACE algorithm, one should focus on the statement, "safety and efficacy trump cost," as medication accounts for only a small part of the overall cost of diabetes care."

The AACE algorithm suggests that although cost of care is important to consider, the safety and efficacy of drugs always take precedence. Prescribing an inexpensive sulfonylurea to an elderly

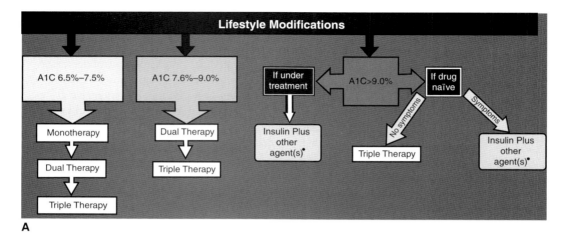

A

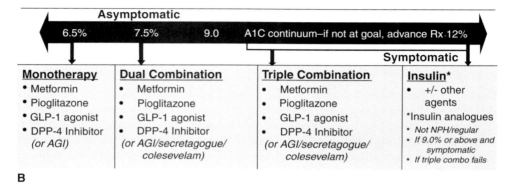

B

Figure 10-14 • A. AACE Algorithm for Achieving Glycemic Control in Patients with T2DM.
AACE Guideline Bullet Points for Rational Treatment of Hyperglycemia:

- Consider use of medications that minimize the risk and severity of hypoglycemia.
- Consider use of medications that minimize the likelihood or severity of weight gain.
- Quick therapeutic interventions (every 2 to 3 months) should be considered until the targeted A1C is attained.
- Lifestyle modification should be emphasized at each visit. Smoking is unacceptable. Encourage patient to call: 1800-Quit-NOW.
- Combination therapy with complimentary mechanisms of action is often required to achieve glycemic goals.
- When using insulin, maintain use of metformin if tolerated.
- Cost is important, but SAFETY TRUMPS COST.

B. GLP-1, Glucagon like peptide-1 agonist; DPP-4, dipeptidyl peptidase-4 inhibitor; AGIs, α-glucosidase inhibitors. (Adapted from Rodbard HW, Jellinger PS, Davidson JA, et al. Statement by an American Association of Clinical Endocrinologist/American College of Endocrinology Consensus Panel on T2DM Mellitus: An Algorithm for Glycemic Control. *Endocrine Pract.* 2009;15(6):541–559.)

woman who lives alone places her at high risk for severe hypoglycemia. A patient with stage 4 chronic kidney disease should avoid using metformin due to a higher risk of developing lactic acidosis. Hypoglycemia and weight gain are observed more often in patients taking regular human insulins than in those using analogues.

Physicians often persist in their desire to provide the "least expensive" therapies to their patients knowing that oral agents and GLP-1 agonists will likely all lower the baseline A1C by 0.6% to 2.0%. Criticism may be directed at pharmaceutical companies for continuing to develop novel therapies that are likely to be more expensive than those that are on the Walmart $4.00 formulary list. However, physicians who manage patients with diabetes would prefer to have every tool available on their plates regardless of price. We can look at this extensive, and growing menu, and help our patients choose the best options available to reduce glucotoxicity and protect β-cell mass and function, while minimizing adverse events that may occur as we work together to achieve their individual metabolic targets. Patients are counting on their health-care providers to become advocates for their future health and welfare. The best physicians among us can always find a way to incorporate the safest and most effective drugs into one's treatment regimen.

Whereas 50% of the nation's health-care costs related to diabetes are derived from hospital admissions ($97 billion), only 8% ($12.7 billion) are derived from prescription drug costs.[136] Yet, diabetes is a progressive disease state often necessitating the use of polypharmacy and dose titrations to allow patients to successfully achieve their glycemic targets. As one gets closer to the ADA-recommended glycemic target, the rate of hypoglycemic events as well as severity of weight gain increases.[18,126] Patients with cardiovascular risk factors may experience an increase in cardiovascular mortality when exposed to polypharmacy, increased weight, and increased risk of hypoglycemic events.[130] Safe, effective, and durable drugs must be prescribed based on one's customized and clearly defined metabolic targets.

Prior to initiating or intensifying pharmacologic therapies, health-care providers should discuss a verbal "informed consent" options package for each patient (Table 10-16). This is considered by many physicians as time well spent, as patients are allowed to participate in choosing their own therapeutic interventions.

TABLE 10-16. Discussion Points to Address When Initiating or Intensifying Therapy for Patients with T2DM

1. Why intensification or initiation of therapy is necessary at this time. Remind patient that diabetes is a progressive disorder and that the need to intensify or initiate therapy in no way implies guilt on behalf of the individual for killing his or her remaining β-cells.

2. Maintaining A1C levels of 6.0%–6.5% for 4–6 y soon after one is diagnosed with diabetes may induce either "metabolic memory" or the "legacy effect" implying that one's future risk of developing long-term complications will be significantly reduced even if A1C rises.

3. Treatment options are based on one's duration of diabetes. Long duration diabetes patients are likely to have less β-cell function and mass and may require combination therapy or insulin. Newly diagnosed patients may do well with monotherapy.

4. The frequency, timing, and route of administration of medication should be clearly defined.

5. Discuss the benefits and most commonly observed side effects of suggested medications.

6. The frequency of blood glucose monitoring following initiation of a given glucose lowering agent should be defined.

7. An excellent composite metabolic endpoint would be to achieve the ADA recommended A1C of 6.5%, without gaining weight or inducing hypoglycemia.

8. If insulin is the best therapeutic option, will the duration of treatment be temporary or permanent?

9. How can lifestyle interventions be used most effectively as adjunctive therapies with pharmacologic agents?

10. What would happen if the patient decides to maintain his/her current course of therapy *without* initiating or intensifying therapy?

Patient:
Date:

Medication	Dose	When to Take the Dose	Reason

Timing of self-blood glucose monitoring (circle desired timing and frequency)

Timing		Frequency
Fasting		Daily
Fasting and Bedtime		First 7 days of each month
Fasting and before each meal		For the next 7 days
3 AM		
Other (Exercise, driving)		
Before a designated meal and 2 hours after eating		Designated meal: • Breakfast • Lunch • Dinner

Blood glucose targets:
• Fasting:
• 2-hours after eating:
• Bed:

Figure 10-15 • **Customized Diabetes Management Plan.**

Finally, once a therapeutic option is agreed upon, patients should be provided with customized written instructions (Fig. 10-15). Remember, many of our patients are obtaining drugs from several providers. Some of these drugs may even be duplicates (two statins or two sulfonylureas). Providing a patient with a written protocol for their medications and self-monitoring will avoid confusion and instill confidence in the patient to successfully achieve their metabolic targets.

Current Pharmacologic Therapies for Patients with T2DM

Today, 11 distinct classes of medications are available for the management of T2DM (see Table 10-17). Each drug promotes improved glycemia when used alone or in combination therapy. Initiation of an oral agent should be guided by the targeted metabolic defect that must be managed at any given time.

For the anxiety-prone clinician who feels overwhelmed by the number of pharmaceutical agents currently on the market, don't expect to catch a break any time soon. Over 21 agents targeting different metabolic deficits of T1DM and T2DM are currently in development. This list does not include several new formulations of DPP-4 inhibitors, GLP-1 agonists, insulin analogues, ultrafast-acting prandial insulins, concentrated (low volume) basal insulins, or combinations of GLP-1 analogues with basal insulins. The world of diabetes pharmacology is just about to become very crowded!

TABLE 10-17. Classes of Medications That Can Be Used in the Management of Patients with T2DM

Oral agents	Sulfonylureas Biguanides Meglitinides AGIs Thiazolidinediones (glitazones) DPP-4 inhibitors BAS Dopamine agonists
Systemic agents	Amylin analogues GLP-1 analogues Insulin
Therapeutic agents in development	• G-protein–coupled receptor 40 agonists • SGLT2 inhibitors • Dual PPAR agonists • Bile receptor agonist • 11-β-hydroxysteroid dehydrogenase type 1 • GLP-1 receptor agonists • Glucokinase activators • Recombinant human hyaluronidase (rHuPH20) • Fatty acid transport protein inhibitors • Phosphatase inhibitors • Calcium channel agonists • Aldose reductase inhibitors • Protein tyrosine phosphatase inhibitors • Insulinotropin agonists • Gene therapy • Growth factor agonists • Gluconeogenesis inhibitors • Islet amyloid polypeptide aggregation • Inhibitors • Adenylate cyclase stimulants • Mitochondrial function enhancers • GAD65 vaccine • Insulin B chain vaccine • r-metHuLeptin

From Drugs in Development for Diabetes: http://www.diabetes-mellitus.org/dmrx.htm#5. Accessed March 9, 2012.

Once oral hypoglycemic therapy is initiated, patients must become active participants in diabetes self-management. Contrary to the belief held by many patients, T2DM is certainly not a "mild form of diabetes." Blood glucose self-monitoring, medical nutrition therapy, enhancing one's active lifestyle, and professional surveillance to determine if the targeted metabolic goals are being achieved are all necessary to lessen the impact associated with diabetes-related complications. Patients should be aware of the potential risks and clinical benefits of the different types of oral hypoglycemic agents. Some medications may increase weight or induce hypoglycemia, whereas others must be held before undergoing certain diagnostic procedures. The continued use of oral hypoglycemic agents in the acute hospital setting may be detrimental.[137] Insulin is the preferred drug for patients with diabetes admitted to the hospital for acute illness. Insulin may also be necessary in certain situations that complicate the management of T2DM, such as during the concomitant use of corticosteroids, for patients requiring surgery, for patients with restricted oral intake, or in those patients who become pregnant while taking oral agents.

Sulfonylureas

The first oral agents for treating T2DM were initially marketed in 1957 as sulfonylureas. Although the first-generation sulfonylureas (orinase, tolinase, and diabinese) can improve hyperglycemia, potential drug interactions resulting in hypoglycemia make these drugs less attractive than the second-generation drugs. The second-generation sulfonylureas (glipizide and glyburide) were first introduced in 1984, and glimepiride followed in 1996. During the 11-year period from 1990 to 2001, a 3.9-fold increase (from 23.4 million to nearly 92 million) occurred in the dispensing of outpatient prescriptions for oral antidiabetic drugs.[138] Only 21.5 million prescriptions were dispensed in 1986.[139] This rapid increase in prescriptions coincides with the increase in the incidence of T2DM diabetes in the United States.

Sulfonylureas are known as "secretagogues" because their binding to pancreatic β-cell receptors results in an increase in insulin production and secretion through a complex series of intracellular events. Once bound to the sulfonylurea receptor (SUR) on the pancreatic β-cell plasma membrane, the potassium channel closes. This reduces the exit of potassium from the β-cell, resulting in depolarization, allowing calcium influx through the plasma membrane and a prompt release of insulin into the plasma.[140]

Sulfonylureas may not be equal in regard to their efficacy and safety profile. Glimepiride has been shown to improve first- and second-phase insulin output,[141] whereas other sulfonylureas are thought to improve only second-phase insulin response. Glimepiride has been shown in a European study to have many fewer incidents of hypoglycemia than glibenclamide, a European sulfonylurea.[142] Although long-term therapy with any sulfonylurea can result in weight gain, a meta-analysis study of more than 14,000 patients demonstrated far less weight gain with glimepiride in comparison with other sulfonylureas.[143]

Treatment with sulfonylureas generally results in a 1% to 2% reduction in A1C levels.[144,145] Sulfonylureas are effective as monotherapy or in combination with other oral agents having complementary mechanisms of action as well as with insulin.[146] Side effects of sulfonylureas include weight gain, which could be significant when used in patients who are already struggling with obesity.[147]

Hypoglycemia is a major concern for users of sulfonylureas. Magnitude and severity of sulfonylurea-induced hypoglycemia range widely across studies. In an observational study, the annual risk for a first hypoglycemia diagnosis associated with sulfonylurea use was 1.8% (1,800 per 100,000 person-years); long-acting formulations, renal impairment, older age, and incidental use of sulfonylureas were associated with a higher hypoglycemia risk.[148] A nested cased-control analysis using a UK General Practice Research Database to identify patients with T2DM who used oral agents determined a 1.5-fold increased risk of hypoglycemia in those using sulfonylureas vs. metformin.[149] Risk of hypoglycemia was greater in patients with renal insufficiency as well as in those in the early phase of diabetes therapy, whereas obesity and smoking appeared to protect patients against sulfonylurea treatment–emergent hypoglycemia.

In a 2007 meta-analysis, glyburide was compared with other antidiabetic medications, including insulin, to determine whether the drug was associated with a higher risk of hypoglycemia.[150] The meta-analysis, which included 21 studies, revealed a 52% higher risk of hypoglycemia in patients receiving glyburide compared with those taking other insulin secretagogues. In addition, glyburide posed an 83% higher risk of hypoglycemia compared with other sulfonylureas. Interestingly, the A1C levels of patients using glyburide in the meta-analysis were similar to those of patients using other sulfonylureas, suggesting that the high risk of hypoglycemia was not associated with lower A1Cs.[150]

Although glyburide is the least safe of all sulfonylureas, the drug is recommended for women with gestational diabetes who may not necessarily require insulin but who are unable to achieve their targeted glycemic goals with lifestyle intervention.[151] These recommendations are based largely on a randomized unblinded trial that compared the use of glyburide with that of insulin in women with gestational diabetes mellitus. This study found no difference in rates of glycemic control between the two treatment groups.[152]

When sulfonylureas are used in combination with insulin or TZDs, risks of weight gain, fluid retention, and congestive heart failure are increased.[135] The package insert for sulfonylureas also includes a boldprint warning mandated by the FDA regarding possible cardiovascular risk associated with this class of oral agents. A retrospective analysis of patients with diabetes who had balloon angioplasty after myocardial infarction reported increased early mortality (odds ratio 2.7 after adjustment for a number of covariates) in 67 persons taking sulfonylureas vs. 118 using insulin or lifestyle therapy alone.[153] Although the types of sulfonylureas in this study were not specified, glyburide was most commonly used by patients undergoing the balloon angioplasties.

The proposed underlying mechanism for this increased risk of cardiovascular mortality in patients with T2DM treated with sulfonylureas may be due to "myocardial ischemic preconditioning" (Fig. 10-16). Thus, sulfonylureas potentially have an increased likelihood of cardiovascular mortality in high-risk patients with preexisting cardiovascular disease as well as in those individuals who are prone to developing hypoglycemia.[154]

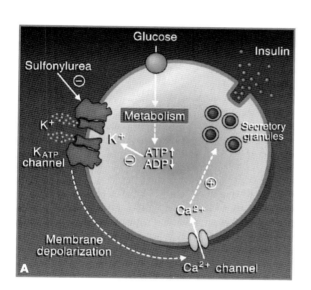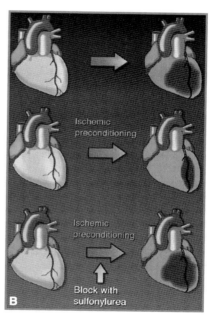

ADP = adenosine diphosphate; ATP = adenosine triphosphate; Ca^{2+} = calcium ion; K^+ = potassium ion; K_{ATP} channel = ATP-sensitive potassium channel.

Figure 10-16 • During myocardial ischemia, the opening of cardiac KATP channels causes potassium efflux, reductions in action potential duration and alterations in repolarization, which favor the induction of malignant arrhythmias. However, transient ischemia (angina) prompts the myocardium into a protective mode, which affords myocytes greater protection against a subsequent acute coronary event. Within myocytes, KATP channel **activation** promotes the production of reactive oxygen species (ROS). The free radicals provide oxygen to the myocardial cells thereby protecting the muscle against infarction **(B)**. Some sulfonylureas (tolbutamide and glyburide) block this protective effect by binding to KATP channels located both within myocardial cells and in β-cells **(A)**. Sulfonylurea inhibition of the KATP channels within β-cells blocks calcium uptake thereby inducing insulin synthesis and secretion. The selectivity of KATP channel inhibition among different sulfonylureas may have an affect on ischemic preconditioning. (Seino S, Takahashi H, Takahashi T, et al. Treating diabetes today: a matter of selectivity of sulphonylureas. *Diabetes Obesity Metab.* 2012;14(Suppl 1):9–13.)

Zeller et al.[155] reported an analysis of data collected from a French registry evaluating mortality rates of patients with T2DM hospitalized for acute myocardial infarction. Early mortality rates were almost three times higher (7.5 vs. 2.7%) for patients taking glyburide than those taking glimepiride or gliclazide (2 sulfonylureas that appear to lack direct cardiac effects).

Zoungas et al.[156] examined the associations between severe hypoglycemia and the risks of death among 11,140 patients with T2DM treated within the Action in Diabetes and Vascular Disease: Preterax and Diamicron Modified Release Controlled Evaluation (ADVANCE) study. Interestingly, the median time from the first episode of severe hypoglycemia (an event requiring assistance of another person to normalize glucose) was 1.6 years. Inclusion criteria for participating in ADVANCE included individuals with T2DM ≥ 55 years of age with a history of major macrovascular or microvascular plus one additional risk factor for vascular disease.[157] Thus, these subjects were at high risk for having a secondary cardiac event prior to entry into the study. Sixty percent of the patients in ADVANCE were using sulfonylureas, including 57% of patients in the conventional group. Severe episodes of hypoglycemia occurred more often in the intensive versus control group (2.7 vs. 1.8) including one fatal episode in the control group.

The frequency of severe hypoglycemia tends to increase in relation to one's duration of the disease.[158] As diabetes is a progressive disorder, pancreatic β-cell mass and function deteriorate. A signaling defect between the β-cells and α-cells may account for failure to mount an acceptable counterregulatory response in a hypoglycemic state. With the loss of glucose-dependent β-cell insulin secretion, signaling pathways between the α- and β-cells appear to be disrupted. Loss of glucagon secretory response to hypoglycemia is a key feature of HAAF.[159] Thus, any drug that is likely to increase one's risk of developing severe hypoglycemia or possibly impair ischemic reconditioning should not be used in patients with T2DM. The AACE consensus panel guidelines suggest that sulfonylureas are low-priority agents due to their risk of inducing hypoglycemia, weight gain, and short-term effective pharmacologic durability of only 1 to 2 years.[135]

A Diabetes Outcome Progression Trial (ADOPT) was a randomized, double-blind, controlled study designed to evaluate the effectiveness and durability of glycemic control as initial treatment for newly diagnosed patients with T2DM.[18] Patients were randomized to receive monotherapy with TZD (rosiglitazone), metformin, or glyburide. Monotherapy failure occurred earliest with glyburide and latest with rosiglitazone, although glyburide produced more improvement in A1C than the comparators. Similarly, patients using glyburide in the UKPDS demonstrated more rapid loss of glycemic control relative to metformin.[160] However, patients taking the long-acting sulfonylurea, chlorpropamide, had the greatest persistence of glycemic control relative to metformin. Although ADOPT was not intended to identify medical outcomes, safety findings were reported. Glyburide caused the most hypoglycemia and 1.6-kg weight gain (vs. a 4.8-kg gain with rosiglitazone and weight loss with metformin), but serious cardiovascular events were, if different at all, less frequent with glyburide (26 events) than with metformin (46 events) or rosiglitazone (49 events). We must wonder what ADOPT might have shown had glimepiride or extended-release formulations of gliclazide or glipizide been studied instead of glyburide!

Until randomized placebo-controlled studies are performed comparing the safety and efficacy of newer sulfonylureas (gliclazide, glimepiride, or glipizide) with metformin and older agents (glyburide), concerned physicians should lean toward eliminating glyburide from their treatment regimen for T2DM. Again, safety and efficacy should always trump cost in high-risk populations. Patients who are at risk for hypoglycemia and cardiovascular events should not receive glyburide as other drugs are safer and equally effective for such high-risk individuals.

Substantial evidence indicates that patients with T2DM have an increased risk of cancer and cancer mortality[161] (see Chapter 8). T2DM appears to be linked to IR, hyperinsulinemia, obesity, environmental factors, and elevated levels of IGF-1 that promote tumor cell growth. Oral agents that lower glucose levels in patients with T2DM may also influence cancer occurence and mortality. One study demonstrated that patients using sulfonylureas as monotherapy had a 20% increase in cancer mortality when compared with patients using metformin monotherapy.[162]

Agents that increase circulating insulin levels may influence cancer-related mortality in patients with T2DM. A cohort of 10,309 treatment-naïve patients with T2DM followed for 5 years were found to have increased cancer-related death when initiated on sulfonylureas (4.9% or 162 of 3,340 subjects) versus metformin (3.5% or 245 of 6,969 subjects) as well as insulin (5.8% or 85 of 1,443) versus metformin.[163] Still unclear is the duration of exposure of medications from any class that may impact risk. Some drugs within a single class may reduce oxidative stress and protect cells from undergoing mitogenic transformation.[164] Therefore, the true story regarding sulfonylureas and cancer risk remains to be elucidated.

Sulfonylureas should be initiated at low doses and increased weekly until target fasting blood glucose levels are less than 110 mg per dL. For best efficacy, sulfonylureas should be given 1 hour before breakfast (to improve first-phase insulin release) and/or at bedtime (to reduce overnight hepatic glucose production).[2]

Patients first seen with "newly diagnosed T2DM" and blood glucose levels more than 300 mg per dL could be started on glipizide XL, 20 mg at bedtime, and monitored for glycemic improvement. Usually, blood glucose levels and diabetes-related symptoms improve dramatically within 3 to 4 days. After 2 weeks, assuming glucose control is improved, the dose of the glipizide can be reduced and metformin initiated. Another option would be to continue the same high-dose glipizide while adding metformin to the treatment regimen.[2] Long-duration hyperglycemia can induce β-cell toxicity, which may not respond to low-dose secretagogue therapy. Higher-dose sulfonylureas might therefore be more appropriate in these patients.

Meglitinides

Although patients with T2DM may have high fasting insulin levels and a reduction in insulin action, a blunted or absent first-phase insulin response to a glycemic challenge is also present. Most sulfonylureas (except glimepiride) increase pancreatic β-cell insulin secretion as well as plasma insulin concentrations, yet fail to improve first-phase insulin release. The meglitinides do increase early insulin response, allowing improved postprandial glycemic control.[165] Drugs in this class include nateglinide (Starlix) and repaglinide (Prandin). Both agents are rapid-acting insulin secretagogues. When the drugs are taken 15 minutes before a meal, postprandial glucose excursions can be minimized. This is important because significant postprandial hyperglycemia has been associated with cardiovascular morbidity.[166–168] In randomized placebo-controlled clinical trials, repaglinide appears to reduce the A1C more significantly than nateglinide (−1.9% at 6 months vs. 1% at 24 weeks).[169,170] Side effects are similar to those of sulfonylureas and include weight gain. Hypoglycemia is less common with meglitinides than with sulfonylureas,[171] because the stimulation of insulin release is rapid, easily reversible, and glucose dependent from β-cells.[172] In low doses, these drugs may prove beneficial in slowing the progression from IGT to diabetes by reducing postprandial hyperglycemia.[173] However, their use in patients with IGT may result in more frequent hypoglycemia, suggesting that the lowest doses of meglitinides should be used in prediabetes.

Meglitinides are more expensive than sulfonylureas. Both repaglinide and nateglinide are approved for use as monotherapy and in combination with TZDs and metformin. Although long-term outcome data are unavailable for this drug class, their effects on improving diabetes-related complications are likely to be at least similar to those observed with sulfonylureas.

α-Glucosidase Inhibitors

AGIs block the action of a-glucosidase enzymes at the brush border of the intestine. The inhibition slows the breakdown of dietary oligosaccharides and disaccharides. The delayed digestion of carbohydrates decreases postprandial glucose concentrations.[174] The two members of this drug class include acarbose (Precose) and miglitol (Glyset). In placebo-controlled trials, AGIs have been shown to reduce

AIC levels by only 0.5% to 1.0%[175–178] and are therefore considered less effective than other oral agents. AGIs are approved for use as monotherapy and in combination with sulfonylureas and metformin.

The use of AGIs in managing diabetes has been limited in the United States because of the side effects, which include abdominal bloating, cramping, and flatulence. Patients will frequently discontinue use of these drugs because of these uncomfortable side effects. The use of acarbose has been shown to reduce the incidence of T2DM by 25% over a 3.3-year period compared with placebo, regardless of age, sex, or BMI.[179] In post hoc analysis of data from the Study to Prevent Non–Insulin-Dependent Diabetes Mellitus trial (Stop NIDDM), acarbose was observed to have an impressive effect on risk of myocardial infarction, supporting the view that postprandial hyperglycemia has a greater influence on cardiovascular events than does fasting glucose.[180]

Metformin

Metformin, a biguanide, is commonly referred to as an "insulin sensitizer" because glucose levels improve without stimulation of insulin secretion. Metformin acts by decreasing hepatic glucose production, decreasing glucose absorption, and increasing glucose uptake into skeletal muscle.[181,182] As circulating glucose levels are reduced, peripheral IR at the skeletal muscle site and adipose tissue may also improve. At the molecular level, metformin appears to improve glucose transport into skeletal muscle cells. This action appears to be additive in the presence of insulin, suggesting an insulin-dependent enhancement to the drug's effect.[183]

Metformin as monotherapy has numerous beneficial effects on metabolic parameters and diabetes prevention. In the DPP, patients with IGT or IFG receiving metformin, 850 mg twice daily, had a 31% reduction in progression toward diabetes. Those individuals randomized to lifestyle intervention (exercising 150 minutes per week and weight loss of 7% of baseline body weight) had a reduction of 58%. Metformin was found to be most effective in reducing progression toward diabetes[16] in subjects younger than 45 as well as in individuals with a BMI greater than 35 kg per m². The diagnosis of the primary outcome, diabetes, was based either on a 75-g OGTT with FPG or 2-hour glucose exceeding 125 or 199 mg per dL, respectively, or on 6-month FPG, exceeding 125 mg per dL. Metformin was particularly effective in decreasing diabetes among individuals with FPG exceeding 110 mg per dL, whereas the lifestyle intervention was similarly effective in persons above and below this level. Half of those treated with metformin experienced GI side effects, and some reduced the dose to 850 mg once daily. No evidence indicates whether combined lifestyle-metformin treatment would have an additive benefit. Patients with prediabetes who are unable to or unwilling to participate in lifestyle-intervention programs might benefit from pharmacologic therapy using metformin.

Metformin has been shown to improve inflammatory markers linked to cardiovascular risk. The drug reduces triglyceride levels by 10% to 30%,[184] LDL-C and total cholesterol by 5% to 10%,[185] while having no significant influence on HDL-C levels.[186] Metformin has no effect on blood pressure.[184] Levels of fibrinogen[187] and CRP[188] are also lower in metformin-treated patients.

The UKPDS showed that obese patients using metformin as monotherapy had a lower risk of myocardial infarction and stroke when compared with subjects taking metformin with a sulfonylurea.[189] Although the risk of vascular disease was slightly higher when metformin was used in combination with a sulfonylurea, most authorities believe these numbers to be statistically insignificant.[190]

In placebo-controlled trials,[191–193] metformin consistently lowers A1C by 1% to 2%, similar to secretagogues. Metformin is approved for use alone or in combination with all other antidiabetic agents, as well as exenatide and pramlintide. Patients with polycystic ovary syndrome who take metformin have improved ovulatory function and show a reduction in parameters suggestive of IR.[194]

Extended-release metformin (Glucophage XR, Fortamet, Glumetza) offers the option of giving the drug as a single daily dose with the largest meal of the day. Improvements in glycemic control have been shown to be similar in patients taking once-daily extended-release metformin or the traditional twice-daily dosing schedule, whereas the gastrointestinal side effects were equal in both groups over a 24-week period.[195]

Gastrointestinal side effects of metformin are common and can be minimized by slow-dose titration and by taking the medication while in the process of eating. Because of the rare risk of lactic acidosis (characterized by elevated blood lactate levels more than 5 mmol per L, an increased lactate-to-pyruvate ratio, and an increased anion gap), several contraindications limit this drug's use, including renal and liver dysfunction, heart failure, dehydration, and alcohol abuse.

Metformin therapy has been considered inappropriate if the baseline serum creatinine level is 1.5 mg per dL or more for men or 1.4 mg per dL or more for women. Adverse-event reports suggest that the incidence of metformin-associated lactic acidosis is between 1 in 10,000 and 1 in 100,000 patient-years.[196] However, few reports have assessed the impact of renal insufficiency on metformin clearance during long-term use. One study concluded that metformin can be efficiently cleared in mild–moderate CKD.[197] Older patients (aged 70 to 80 years) were administered metformin 850 or 1,700 mg per day based on a CrCl of 30 to 60 or 60 mL per minute. After 2 months, metformin remained in the therapeutic range and lactate within the reference limits in all participants. In addition, the measured levels of metformin and lactate were not statistically different between those with and without renal impairment.

Many of the early pharmacokinetic studies with metformin actually relied on 24-hour creatinine clearance rather than glomerular filtration rate (GFR). The GFR is more predictive of chronic kidney disease and is based upon muscle mass, age, race, and gender (see Chapter 6). How well serum creatinine or creatinine clearance predicts one's ability to actually clear metformin is unknown.[198] Therefore, the recommendations that metformin be discontinued if a serum creatinine or creatinine clearance is elevated should be brought into question. In fact, although metformin is renally cleared and plasma accumulation of the drug may conceivably lead to lactic acidosis, there currently is limited systematic evidence to substantiate continued reliance on the creatinine-based contraindications in use in the U.S. Estimated GFR (eGFR) appears to be a more reliable estimate of true renal dysfunction in patients with diabetes. Metformin-associated lactic acidosis is exceedingly rare and the use of metformin has not been comprehensively assessed in patients with chronic kidney disease. Discontinuation of metformin in patients with mild to moderate chronic kidney disease may predispose individuals to loss of glycemic control and increased risk of cancer-related mortality.[198,199] Based on current recommendations from the FDA, off-label use of metformin is extremely common, suggesting that many "high-risk patients" are exposed to dangerous plasma levels of metformin, yet never develop lactic acidosis. Despite the warnings regarding treatment-emergent lactic acidosis associated with the use of metformin, 22% to 54% of patients taking the drug have an absolute or relative contraindication to its use.[196,200] Hospitalized patients taking metformin often do not have the drug discontinued despite having at least one risk factor for lactic acidosis developing.[201] A review of patients discharged from the hospital with a diagnosis of congestive heart failure and diabetes found that 11% were given a prescription for metformin.[202]

Based upon review of current literature related to lactic acidosis and the pharmacokinetics of metformin use in patients with chronic kidney disease, the American Diabetes Association in 2011 published suggested parameters for initiating and titrating doses of metformin in patients with CKD as noted in Table 10-18. Additional caution is required in patients with anticipated significant fluctuations in renal status or those at risk for abrupt deterioration in kidney function, based on previous history, other comorbidities, albuminuria, and medication regimen (e.g., potent diuretics or nephrotoxic agents, IV contrast material). Because metformin is a generic drug, the U.S. Food and Drug Administration is unlikely to reconsider the current metformin-prescribing guidelines, although emerging evidence suggests the drug is actually safer within the clinical setting than originally reported.

The use of iodinated contrast material for studies including intravenous pyelography, intravenous cholangiography, angiography, and computed tomography (CT) scanning may induce acute renal failure, resulting in lactic acidosis in metformin-treated patients. Metformin should be temporarily stopped immediately before the planned procedure and withheld for 48 hours once the procedure is completed. The patient's renal status should always be reassessed before resuming metformin.

Approximately 10% of patients using metformin will develop a vitamin B_{12} deficiency. Although megaloblastic anemia is rarely seen in metformin users, the risk of developing vitamin B_{12} deficiency correlates with the duration of use as well as the dose of the drug. Patients should be monitored on

TABLE 10-18. American Diabetes Association Recommendations for Metformin Dose Initiation and Titration in Patients with Chronic Kidney Disease

eGFR (mL/min per 1.73 m²)	Metformin Dose for Initiation and Titration	Recommended Monitoring Frequency of Renal Function
>60	No adjustments required	Routine follow-up
<60	Metformin may be initiated or continued	Monitor eGFR every 3–6 mo
<45	Do not initiate metformin. Reduce metformin dosage by 50% or to 1/2 maximal dose	Monitor eGFR every 3 mo
<30	Discontinue metformin	Routine renal surveillance

From Lipska KJ, Bailey CJ. Use of metformin in the setting of mild-to-moderate renal insufficiency. *Diabetes Care.* 2011;34:1431–1437.

an annual basis and provided with vitamin B_{12} supplementation (either via subcutaneous injection or intranasal spray) if necessary.[203,204]

Metformin has been found to be associated with a reduced risk of cancer-related mortality. (Fig. 10-17). A prospective study following patients using metformin for 9.6 years found that cancer mortality was reduced by approximately 50% versus patients not taking metformin at baseline.[199] Higher doses of metformin also appeared to impart greater protection against mortality as the hazard ratio for cancer mortality decreased by 42% for every 1 g increase in metformin dose. Patients with

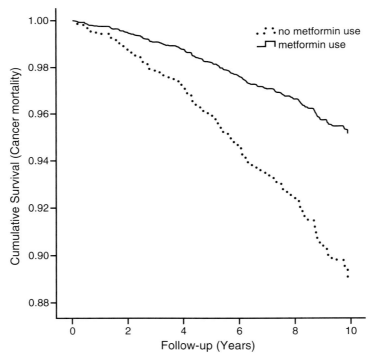

Figure 10-17 • **Cumulative Survival Curves for Cancer Mortality in T2DM Patients Using Metformin versus Nonmetformin Users.**
Cumulative cancer survival rates were approximately 50% greater over 10 years with the use of metformin vs. nonmetformin use in patients with T2DM. Sulfonylureas and insulin usage was not significantly associated with increased mortality rates in this study. (Used from Landman GWE, Kleefstra N, Van Hateren KJJ, et al. Metformin associated with lower cancer mortality in T2DM. ZODIAC-16. *Diabetes Care.* 2010;33:322–326, with permission.)

T2DM who were not taking metformin demonstrated an increased cancer mortality ratio compared with that of the general population, whereas the use of metformin inferred a mortality risk equal to that of the general population. Therefore, assuming there are no issues with tolerability, initiating and continuing metformin as baseline therapy in all patients with T2DM appears to be a safe and cost-effective therapeutic option. Metformin may be used in combination with all other pharmacologic options including insulin.

Thiazolidinediones

Thiazolidinediones (TZDs) act (a) by stimulating the PPAR-γ receptor, which promotes insulin-sensitizing effects on skeletal muscle and adipose tissue, and (b) by inhibiting hepatic gluconeogenesis. Stimulation of the PPAR receptors modulates the activity of the cell's genes and helps to regulate both carbohydrate and lipid metabolism. In adipose tissue, PPAR-γ activation causes preadipocytes to differentiate into mature fat cells while promoting lipid synthesis.[205]

TZDs enhance the effects of insulin on the liver, thereby reducing hepatic glucose production (gluconeogenesis and glycogenolysis).[206] FFA suppression by TZDs can improve insulin sensitivity while preserving pancreatic β-cell function. TZDs suppress both fasting and postprandial levels of FFA, which can significantly improve IR affecting the liver and skeletal muscles.[206,207]

Adiponectin also plays an important role in the modulation of glucose and lipid metabolism. Low levels of circulating adiponectin have been linked with human obesity[208] as well as IR and dyslipidemia.[209] Plasma adiponectin levels are significantly lower in patients with T2DM but can be increased rapidly when TZDs are initiated.[210] In addition, plasma adiponectin levels in diabetes patients with evidence of CAD are lower than those in diabetes patients without CAD, suggesting that adiponectin may be cardioprotective as well as endothelial cell protective.[211]

PPAR-γ activation by TZDs promotes the differentiation of small adipocytes into larger adipocytes, resulting in weight gain and an absolute increase in adipose cell mass. As a result, patients who use TZDs may experience modest weight gain in association with improvement in their blood glucose and lipid levels. TZDs have been postulated to improve insulin sensitivity by redistributing fat from visceral to subcutaneous adipose tissue.[212] PPAR-γ is expressed at highest concentrations in adipose tissue and at much lower concentrations in liver and muscle,[213] suggesting that the primary action of TZDs is on adipose tissue.

IR occurs in association with a number of metabolic abnormalities that improve when TZDs are added to the therapeutic regimen. For example, patients with IR tend to have a predominance of small, dense, atherogenic LDL particles that are susceptible to oxidation, an important step in the atherosclerotic process. TZDs increase the ratio of large, buoyant LDL to small, dense LDL particles, reducing the degree of atherogenesis.[214,215] Small, dense LDL particles easily lodge themselves into vessel walls that have been damaged by inflammation, where they become oxidized. Large, buoyant LDL particles are too hefty to become wedged within the vessel walls and instead simply "bounce" through the blood vessels, causing minimal harm. Although lipid profiles tend to improve with the use of TZDs, patients older than 40 with diabetes should still be provided with statins.[216]

Pioglitazone may decrease the concentration of conjugated oral contraceptives (COCs). Therefore, patients taking pioglitazone and COCs should be informed of this potential interaction.[217] Additionally, TZDs may cause resumption of ovulation in premenopausal anovulatory women.[218]

In summary, activation of PPAR-γ results in higher expression of adiponectin from adipose tissue, reducing plasma levels of FFA, thereby improving IR and redistributing fat from metabolically active VAT to metabolically inactive subcutaneous fat. In diabetes, as FFA levels increase, IR worsens, within both the liver and the skeletal muscle sites, causing the pancreatic β-cells to produce more endogenous insulin. Individuals with a genetic predisposition for diabetes cannot produce and secrete enough endogenous insulin to maintain euglycemia. TZDs appear to improve IR by directly affecting PPAR-γ activation in adipose tissue, hepatocytes, and skeletal muscle cells. The metabolic effects of the TZDs are displayed in Table 10-19.

TABLE 10-19. Summary of Effects of Thiazolidinediones on Cardiovascular Risk Factors

Parameter	Outcome	Effect
Insulin sensitivity/ β-cell function	Insulin sensitivity/peripheral glucose utilization	++
	Glucose uptake in skeletal muscles	++
	Glucose uptake in cardiac muscle	++
	Glucose uptake in subcutaneous fat	++
	Improve fasting insulin and C-peptide levels	+
Glucose metabolism	Sustained reduction in fasting plasma glucose levels	++
	Lowers A1C levels	+
	Improves postprandial hyperglycemia	+
Lipid metabolism	Improves free fatty acid levels	+
	Improves triglyceride levels	+
	Improves HDL-C levels	+
	Changes small, dense atherogenic LDL-C particles to large, buoyant LDL particles	+
	Redistributes adipocytes from visceral fat to less metabolically active subcutaneous fat	+
Weight gain	Increases weight when used as monotherapy	+
	Increases weight when used in combination with insulin	++
	Increases weight when used in combination with metformin	++
	Increases weight when used with a secretagogue	
Cardiovascular system	Reduces blood pressure	+
	Promotes vasodilatation	+
	Improves urinary albumin:creatinine	+
	Limits fibrinogen and clot activation	+
	Improves levels of emerging inflammatory markers (CRP, PAI-1, TNF)	++
	Increases levels of adiponectin	++

+, positive effect; ++, strong positive effect; CRP, C-reactive protein; HDL-C, high-density lipoprotein cholesterol; LDL, low-density lipoprotein; LDL-C, low-density lipoprotein cholesterol; PAI-1, plasminogen-activator inhibitor-1; TNF, tumor necrosis factor.
Adapted from Seufert J, Lubben G, Dietrich K, et al. A comparison of the effects of thiazolidinediones and metformin on metabolic control in patients with type 2 diabetes mellitus. *Clin Ther.* 2004;26:805–818.

The currently marketed TZD (pioglitazone) is equipotent in reducing A1C levels as metformin and sulfonylureas. Pioglitazone may be used as monotherapy and in combination with other agents, including metformin, sulfonylureas, and insulin. Side effects include weight gain (range, 0.9 to 2.6 kg) and edema. The weight gain tends to occur early and is not associated with a prolonged upward trend. TZDs should not be used in patients with advanced heart-failure symptoms (New York Heart Association class III or IV).[219]

Patients with diabetes are twice as likely to have hypertension as are those individuals with normoglycemia.[220] The UKPDS blood pressure substudy revealed a significant reduction in microvascular and macrovascular complications when blood pressure is controlled in patients with diabetes. Pioglitazone appears to reduce systolic and diastolic blood pressures by 5 to 6 mm Hg in patients with T2DM.[221]

A direct correlation exists between IR, T2DM, and increased levels of plasminogen activator inhibitor type-1 (PAI-1). Elevation of PAI-1 inhibits fibrinolysis, thereby increasing one's risk of arterial thrombosis. Higher A1C levels correlate with higher PAI-1 levels.[222] Patients with suboptimal diabetes control therefore are at higher risk of vascular thrombosis. Whereas sulfonylureas increase PAI-1 levels, TZDs in combination with sulfonylureas appear to decrease PAI-1 activity by more than 33%.[223] TZDs may play a critical role in reducing endothelial damage by improving fibrinolytic activity, leading to lowered cardiovascular risk in patients with T2DM.

CRP is an independent marker of vascular inflammation. Elevated CRP levels are associated with an increased cardiovascular risk as well as IR. TZDs reduce CRP levels by 30% and improve endothelial cell function.[224,225] Table 10-19 summarizes the effects of TZDs on cardiovascular risk factors.

The current available clinical data show that no hepatotoxicity occurs with pioglitazone. However, patients using a TZD should have liver function tests performed on initiation of the drug. TZDs should not be started if a patient has evidence of active liver disease or if the ALT levels are greater than 2.5 times the upper limits of normal. Patients with normal liver function tests should have an ALT performed every 2 months for the first year, followed by "periodic testing." If at any time during treatment with a TZD the ALT levels exceed three times the upper limits of normal, complete liver function testing should be repeated immediately. If on repeated testing, the ALT remains three or more times the upper limits of normal, the drug should be discontinued. Liver enzymes should also be checked if a patient experiences symptoms suggesting hepatic dysfunction while taking the TZDs.[226]

Use of TZDs should begin early in the course of diabetes treatment and, in most patients, be considered cornerstone therapy. TZDs improve insulin sensitivity, hyperglycemia, and pancreatic β-cell function. Lipid profiles, vascular dynamics, inflammatory markers, fibrinolysis, blood pressure, and endothelial cell function are all positively affected with TZD therapy. TZDs have also been useful in delaying the onset of diabetes in high-risk patients (TRIPOD Study)[227] while improving the likelihood of ovulation in patients with PCOS.

The ADOPT evaluated the efficacy of a thiazolidinedione (rosiglitazone), metformin, and glyburide as initial treatments for patients newly diagnosed with T2DM.[18] The 4,360 patients treated in this randomized placebo controlled trial were treated for a median period of 4 years. The primary outcome was the time to monotherapy failure (defined as a confirmed FPG greater than 180 mg per dL). Secondary outcomes included levels of FPG and A1C, insulin sensitivity, and β-cell function. Patients randomized to the rosiglitazone arm demonstrated a 32% risk of treatment failure compared with metformin and a 63% reduction in risk of failure compared with glyburide over 4 years. Rosiglitazone was associated with weight gain. On average, patients gained 6.9 kg compared with metformin and 2.5 kg compared with glyburide. Cardiovascular events were similar in the rosiglitazone and metformin arms but lower in the glyburide arm. Rosiglitazone was most effective, probably because of its effects on insulin sensitivity and β-cell function. Rosiglitazone is no longer marketed in the United States.

Since 2006, evidence of bone loss possibly induced by TZDs began appearing in the medical literature. The bone loss is most likely secondary to activation of PPARγ receptors, which drives the bone marrow allocation of stem cells toward adipocytes at the expense of osteoblasts. This may, in turn, result in loss of bone matrix and a reduction in bone density.[228] Although the original reports were based on preclinical studies, concerns were expressed as to whether the TZD class as a whole could have similar effects on human subjects. Since 2006 more reports have linked both rosiglitazone and pioglitazone to increased fracture risk among diabetic women. Short-term clinical trials with TZDs also demonstrated substantial bone loss with TZD usage.[229] The time to first fracture in women subjects who participated in the ADOPT study was 1.81 (95% CI: 1.17, 2.80) when using rosiglitazone versus metformin and 2.13 increased in subjects taking rosiglitazone vs. glyburide (95% CI: 1.30, 3.51).[18] However, the risk of fracture for men was not increased for patients using rosiglitazone versus either metformin or glyburide.

With the published report of increased fracture risk in the rosiglitazone arm of ADOPT, Takeda Pharmaceuticals, IL, USA, the manufacturer of pioglitazone, reviewed their clinical trial databases and, in a letter to health-care providers in 2007, reported an increased fracture risk with pioglitazone treatment in women, but not men.[230] The databases included 24,000 years of follow-up for over 8,100 patients treated with pioglitazone and over 7,400 patients in the comparison group. In these trials, the maximum duration of pioglitazone use was only 3.5 years. The magnitude of the increased risk reported for all clinical fractures was similar to the ADOPT results with a fracture rate of 1.9

per 100 person years in those using pioglitazone compared with a rate of 1.1 per 100 person years in those using placebo or an active comparator drug. The relative risk for men was not reported but was stated to be not statistically significant.

Still unclear is how to define a high risk group among female TZD users. Menopausal status does not appear to correlate with fracture risk. The ADOPT results indicate that not appear that increased fracture risk extends to those who are premenopausal as well as postmenopausal. Both premenopausal and postmenopausal women have been shown to lose bone density with TZD treatment.[231,232] A possible explanation for the lack of effect on the skeleton in men is the higher estrogen levels found in older men compared with older women. There are no studies to date on treatments that might prevent TZD-induced bone loss.

A link between pioglitazone and bladder cancer first appeared in preclinical studies and was initially reported on the U.S. pioglitazone label in 1999. Although experimental studies suggested that the association may be a rat-specific phenomenon, a large PROactive (PROspective pioglitAzone Clinical Trial In macroVascular Events) study demonstrated 14 cases of bladder cancers in the pioglitazone arm (0.5%) versus 6 in the placebo arm (0.2%).[233] In September 2010 the FDA mandated that possible risk of tumor Takeda conduct a 10-year observational study to address the possible risk of bladder cancer in humans exposed to pioglitazaone.[234]

On June 9, 2011, The French drug regulatory authority, AFSSAPS, suspended the marketing of pioglitazone following the recommendation of its Commission d'Autorisation de Mise sur le Marche (AMM) and National Commission on Pharmacovigilance. The decision was made after a study requested by AFSSAPS confirmed a small increase in bladder cancer among patients treated with the diabetes drug. AFSSAPS had sent a letter on April 19 to physicians alerting them of the potential cancer risk. A subsequent review of pharmacovigilance data presented to the commission in recent months had led the AMM to conclude that the risks associated with pioglitazone use exceed its benefits.[235]

An Adverse Event Reporting System (AERS) analysis of antidiabetic drugs used between 2004 and 2009 retrieved 93 reports of bladder cancer linked to 138 drugs and combinations of agents.[236] The reporting odds ration demonstrated a significant relationship between bladder cancer and pioglitazone (4.30 [95%CI 2.82 to 6.52]) and weaker risk for patients taking glyburide and acarbose. The authors concluded that the AERS analysis "is consistent with an association between pioglitazone and bladder cancer" and suggested additional studies be performed urgently to further define this association.

On June 13, 2011, the FDA announced that patients who have used the highest dose of pioglitazone for more than 1 year should be aware of the association between bladder cancer and high dose pioglitazone therapy.[237] The directive noted that patients using pioglitazone for more than 1 year showed a 40% higher risk of bladder cancer, although the FDA review of five-year interim results of an ongoing, 10-year epidemiologic study described in FDA's September 2010 ongoing safety review, showed that there was no overall increased risk of bladder cancer with pioglitazone. Consequently, the FDA recommends that no patient with urinary bladder cancer or a prior history of such a malignancy be started on pioglitazone or maintained on it without thorough evaluation and consideration by the treating physician. Continuation of pioglitazone therapy in patients without bladder cancer is a matter for individual consideration by patients and physicians, according to the FDA.

D2-Dopamine Agonist (Bromocriptine)

Recently, timed-release bromocriptine (Cycloset), a sympatholytic dopamine D2 receptor agonist, has been approved by the FDA for the treatment of T2DM. Bromocriptine is a centrally acting agent that reduces plasma glucose, triglycerides and FFA levels. A 1-year prospective study also demonstrated that the drug reduced cardiovascular events.[238]

Bromocriptine is unique among oral agents in that the drug binds to no target receptor.Instead, the drug works by resetting dopaminergic and sympathetic tone within the central nervous system.[239] The mechanism of action of bromocriptine has been deduced primarily from animal studies. During the state of IR basal lipolytic activity increases, further promoting IR and sparing glucose uptake by skeletal muscles. Fat oxidation becomes the predominant energy source for the periphery, while hepatic glucose production and gluconeogenesis increase to provide the central nervous system with energy during prolonged fasts. Two areas within the hypothalamus, suprachiasmatic nucleus (SCN) and the ventromedial hypothalamus (VMH) have been implicated in the transition from insulin-sensitive to insulin-resistant state.[239] The VMH has multiple neuronal connections with other hypothalamic nuclei and plays a pivotal role in modulating autonomic nervous system function, hormonal secretion, peripheral glucose/lipid metabolism, and feeding behaviors.[240] Serotonin and noradrenergic levels and activity are increased during the state of IR and decreased with return to insulin sensitivity in hibernating animals.[241] Conversely, dopamine levels are low during the insulin-resistant state and increase to normal following return of the insulin-sensitive state.[242] Finally, selective destruction of dopaminergic neurons within the CNS results in severe IR.[243]

Both systemic and intracerebral administration of bromocriptine into insulin resistant animals normalizes VMH noradrenergic and serotonergic levels, resulting in a decline in hepatic glucose production, gluconeogenesis, reduced lipolysis, and improved IR.[239] The proposed mechanism of action of bromocriptine is summarized in Figure 10-18.

Cycloset has a rapid release mechanism allowing for peak concentrations to be achieved within 60 minutes of ingestion. The starting dose is 0.8 to 1.6 mg per day with dose titrations to a maximum of 4.6 mg per day. Cycloset should be administered once daily within 2 hours of awakening because patients with T2DM are believed to have a reduction in early AM dopaminergic tone that increases IR.[244] Plasma prolactin concentrations of lean euglycemic individuals peak at night during sleep.

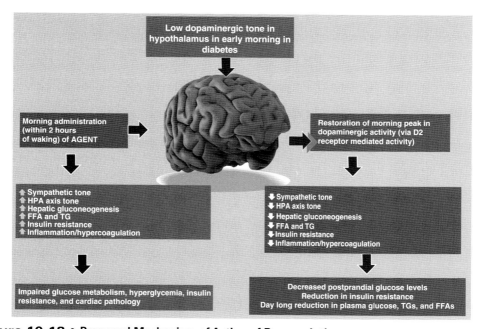

Figure 10-18 • Proposed Mechanism of Action of Bromocriptine.
Bromocriptine has a central mechanism of action. By "resetting" the endogenous production rhythm of dopamine that is produced in the hypothalamus in patients with T2DM, IR, and glucose toxicity appears to improve. Bromocriptine improves dopaminergic tone within the hypothalamus. As a result, postprandial glucose levels improve as do FFA and triglycerides. Bromocriptine does NOT increase endogenous insulin secretion. Dopaminergic neurotransmission is thought to affect both glucose and lipid metabolism. Patients with T2DM experience an early morning decline in hypothalamic dopaminergic tone leading to an increase in sympathetic tone, activation of the hypothalamic–pituitary–adrenal axis, and a potentiation of systemic low-grade inflammation. These actions precipitate abnormal glucose metabolism, IR and cardiovascular pathology. When administered within two hours of awakening, bromocriptine is believed to restore physiologic dopaminergic activity via its D2 mediated action. Clinically, patients note improvement in postprandial glucose levels without increasing insulin secretion. Triglycerides and FFAs are also reduced. (FFA, free fatty acids; HPA, hypothalamic–pituitary–adrenal axis; TG, triglycerides; D2, Dopamine 2 receptor; HGP, Hepatic glucose production.)

Obese insulin-resistant patients demonstrate a twofold day time increase in plasma prolactin levels consisted with reduced dopaminergic tone.[239] Dosing bromocriptine within 2 hours of awakening reduces the elevated prolactin levels by restoring dopaminergic activity to normal. Normalization of dopamine activity results in improvement in postprandial plasma glucose, triglyceride and FFA concentrations *without* increasing endogenous insulin secretion.

Four phase 3 trials have evaluated the efficacy of bromocriptine versus placebo in the treatment of T2DM.[239] Given as monotherapy, bromocriptine can be expected to reduce A1C from baseline by 0.5% to 0.6%. When bromocriptine is added to metformin or a sulfonylurea, A1C can be reduced up to 0.9% from baseline over 9 weeks. Fasting and postprandial FFA and triglyceride concentrations also improve, yet there is no change in body weight or serum insulin levels.[239] In clinical trials, the most common adverse events observed in greater than 5% of bromocriptine versus placebo patients are nausea, asthenia, constipation, and dizziness. Thirteen percent of bromocriptine versus only 3% to 5% of placebo treated patients across the clinical trials. Bromocriptine causes no increase in hypoglycemia when compared to placebo treated patients.

In 52-week cardiovascular safety trial, bromocriptine reduced A1C by 0.6% (p, 0.0001), blood pressure by 2/1 mm Hg (p, 0.02 heart rate by only 1 bpm ($p = 0.02$), and plasma triglyceride by only 1.44 mg per dL ($p = 0.02$). However, the study demonstrated a 40% reduction in composite cardiovascular outcomes. The mechanism as to the cardiovascular risk improvement is uncertain.

In summary, the quick release formulation of bromocriptine used as either monotherapy or in combination with other oral agents can reduce A1C from baseline by 0.5% to 0.9%. The drug appears to work through normalization of dopamine release within the hypothalamus. Dopamine release is disordered in patients with IR. When taken 2 hours of rising each day, postprandial glucose levels improve secondary to reversal of abnormal "dopaminergic tone." The drug does not cause the release of endogenous insulin, induction of hypoglycemia, or weight gain. Adverse events are minimal and for unclear reasons, a cardiovascular safety trial demonstrated a 40% reduction in composite outcomes.

Bile Acid Sequestrants

Although bile acid sequestrants (BASs) were originally formulated as lipid-lowering agents, recently published studies suggest that colesevelam is also beneficial in improving glycemic control in patients with T2DM.[245] Colestimide is approved in Japan, yet colesevelam is the only BAS approved in the United States for improving glycemic control in adults with T2DM.

The glycemic lowering mechanism of BAS therapy remains uncertain. BASs may affect secretion of incretin hormones, particularly GLP-1 and GIP. In patients with T2DM and hypercholesterolemia, treatment with 1,500 mg per day colestimide increased fasting GLP-1 levels.[246] Similarly, treatment with 3.75 g per day colesevelam was shown to increase fasting GLP-1 levels as well as postprandial GLP-1 and GIP levels.[247]

Colesevelam can lower both A1C and LDL-C levels in patients with T2DM who were uncontrolled on a metformin-based regimen. The addition of colesevelam ($n = 79$) to preexisting metformin monotherapy achieved a significant mean reduction in A1C levels of 0.47% relative to placebo ($p < 0.0024$).[248] Further, the total colesevelam treatment group, when treated with either metformin monotherapy or metformin-combination therapy, achieved significantly greater reductions in A1C levels compared to placebo (mean reduction of 0.54%, $p < 0.001$). The study also demonstrated that the total colesevelam treatment group achieved significantly lower LDL-C levels compared to the placebo group (mean reduction of 15.9%, $p < 0.001$).[248]

Two other studies demonstrated similar results in A1C reductions when colesevelam was added to either sulfonylurea-based therapy or insulin-based therapy.[249,250]

The most common drug-related adverse effects (AEs) with colesevelam were gastrointestinal in nature (mainly constipation) and often mild or moderate in severity. Gastrointestinal AEs are common with BAS treatment, since these agents bind to bile acids within the intestine. The drug is considered weight neutral and is unlikely to induce hypoglycemia.

Colesevelam is indicated to improve glycemic control in patients with T2DM. Currently, the drug is only indicated for use in combination therapy with metformin or metformin and a sulfonylurea.[251] The drug is NOT approved for monotherapy, nor in combination with a DPP-4 drug or a TZD. The recommended dose of colesevelam is either 6 tablets (625 mg each= 3.75 g per day) once daily with food or three tablets twice daily. Oral suspension packets (dosing strengths 3.75 and 1.875 g) are also available.

The drug may be useful in patients with prediabetes in whom the goal of therapy is directed both toward salvaging β-cell function and reducing LDL-cholesterol levels to a predefined target of less than 100 mg per dL.[252] Post hoc analysis of data from a 24-week study showed that 3.75 g per day colesevelam reduced LDL cholesterol (placebo-corrected change from baseline: −13.2%; $p < 0.001$) and FPG (placebo-corrected change from baseline: −4.0 mg per dL) in patients with hypercholesterolemia and prediabetes.[253]

One might also consider the use of colesevelam as adjunct therapy for patients with T2DM who are not achieving both glycemic and LDL-cholesterol targets while using metformin, a sulfonylurea or insulin as background therapy. Patients with multiple cardiovascular risk factors might benefit from the fact that colesevelam does not induce hypoglycemia or weight gain and can reduce LDL levels in patients with T2DM. However, cholesevelam has not directly been shown to reduce cardiovascular risk in patients with diabetes.[251]

■ DPP-4 Inhibitors and GLP-1 Agonists

The hypothetical existence of gut hormones capable of stimulating a hormonal release from pancreas in response to nutrient ingestion was postulated in the early 1900s.[254,255] In 1965, the administration of oral glucose was noted to induce a significantly greater increase in plasma insulin levels than equimolar infusion of intravenous glucose.[256] This physiologic activity was subsequently referred to as the intestinal secretion of insulin, or incretin effect and accounts for approximately 50% to 70% of the total insulin secreted following oral glucose administration. Two hormones, glucose-dependent insulinotropic polypeptide (GIP) and GLP-1 are responsible for the incretin effect and are expressed in the pancreas, central and peripheral nervous system, heart, endothelium, kidneys, lungs, and gastrointestinal tract.[257] GLP-1 receptor activation within the pancreatic β-cells results in release of insulin in a "glucose-dependent manner" (Fig. 10-19). Glucose dependent insulin release implies the effects of the drug are prominent only in the presence of hyperglycemia. In contrast to incretin hormones, sulfonylureas and insulin are "glucose independent agents" meaning that glucose levels will continue to fall even if the patient becomes hypoglycemic as long as the absorption glucodynamic action of the drug continues.

Although secretion of GIP remains relatively normal in T2DM subjects, its effect on insulin secretion is severely impaired.[258] Conversely, despite the reduced secretion of GLP-1 or presence of GLP-1 resistance, its insulinotropic and glucagon-suppressive actions remain intact.[259] Thus, pharmacologic efforts to develop medications that mimic the actions of GLP-1 have become a target for improving chronic hyperglycemia.

The GIP receptor is predominantly expressed in pancreatic islet β-cells, whereas GLP-1 receptors are expressed in islet α- and β-cells, as well as in the central and peripheral nervous systems, heart, lungs, kidneys, and gastrointestinal tract.[260]

Activation of the GIP and GLP-1 receptors on the β-cells results in insulin production and exocytosis in a glucose-dependent manner that minimizes risk of hypoglycemia. Sustained activation of these receptors results in enhanced levels of insulin biosynthesis, β-cell proliferation, resistance to β-cell apoptosis, and enhanced β-cell survival in both humans and rodents.[260] Table 10-20 presents the glucose homeostatic actions of both GIP and GLP-1 in a euglycemic individual.

Once released from the gut in response to a meal stimulus, GLP-1 and GIP are rapidly degraded by DPP-4, an enzyme that is expressed in many tissues including the liver, lungs, kidneys, intestines, lymphocytes, and endothelial cells (Fig. 10-20).[257] If DPP-4 were NOT present and active, GLP-1 release would cause hyperstimulation of pancreatic β-cells likely resulting in islet hyperplasia and chronic hyperglycemia. Therefore, DPP-4 serves as a means by which the body may maintain optimal glucose stimulated insulin release with each meal. The physiologic actions directed against both

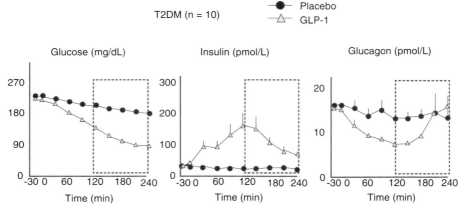

Figure 10-19 • Glucose-dependent Effects of GLP-1.
In this study, the effect of a GLP-1intervenous infusion on measures of β-cell function was investigated in 10 patients with T2DM. Within 4 hours of GLP-1 treatment, plasma glucose (left) had fallen to normal fasting levels, while insulin levels increased significantly early as reflected by rising C-peptide levels, and then dropped as plasma glucose reached normal. Similarly, glucagon levels were significantly reduced during the GLP-1 infusion and fell to baseline once plasma glucose approached fasting levels. The glucose-dependent activity of GLP-1 is evident in the return of insulin and glucagon to basal levels when glucose reached normal fasting levels, despite continued infusion of GLP-1 (*dotted boxes*). GLP-1, Glucagon-like peptide-1. (Adapted from Nauck MA, Kleine N, Ørskov C, et al. Normalization of fasting hyperglycaemia by exogenous GLP-1 (7-36 amide) in type 2 (non–insulin-dependent) diabetic patients. *Diabetologia.* 1993;36:741–744.)

GLP-1 and GIP are swift and efficient. Only 60% of the GLP-1 remains available for pancreatic β-cell receptor activation within 2 minutes of release from the L cells of the intestines due to immediate DPP-4 degradation.[261] Pharmacologic inhibition of DPP-4 would prolong the physiologic effect of GLP-1 at the targeted receptor site while increasing the level of endogenous GLP-1.

 TABLE 10-20 Effects of GIP and GLP-1 on Physiologic Glucose Homeostasis

Action	Gastric Inhibitory Polypeptide	GLP-1
Site of origination upon ingestion of food	K cells of duodenum	L cells of distal ileum and colon
Stimulates production and secretion of insulin from pancreatic β-cells in a glucose-dependent manner	Yes	Yes
Slows gastric emptying	No significant effect	Yes
Induces satiety, thereby reducing caloric intake	No significant effect	Yes
Inhibits glucagon secretion	No significant effect	Yes
Plasma glucose levels reduced in patients with T2DM2	No	Yes
Insulinotropic effect preserved in patients with T2DM	No	Yes
Expression may be enhanced by activation of PPAR-γ receptors	Possibly	Unknown

Adapted from: Unger J, Parkin CG. Type 2 diabetes: An expanded view of pathophysiology and therapy. *Postgr Med.* 2010;122(3):145–157; Gupta D, Peshavaria M, Monga N, et al. Physiologic and pharmacologic modulation of GIP receptor expression in ss-cells by PPARγ signaling: possible mechanism for the GIP resistance in type 2 diabetes. *Diabetes.* 2010;59:1445–1450.

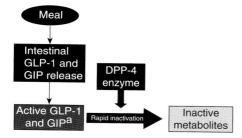

Figure 10-20 • Mechanism Of GLP-1 and GIP Degradation.
Once released by the intestines in response to an oral nutrient stimulus, the incretin hormones are rapidly degraded by DPP-4.

aThe half-life of GLP-1 is approximately 2 minutes; GIP- approximately 5 minutes.

Patients with prediabetes and T2DM demonstrate a significant reduction in insulinotropic effect of GLP-1. Patients with T2DM also show a small but significant decrease in their GLP-1 response to a meal, indicative of GLP-1 receptor site resistance. Endogenous glucagon secretion in T2DM paradoxically increases and plasma levels are refractory to glucose administration. However, glucagon is suppressed by GLP-1 replacement therapy. GLP-1 deficiency and resistance may contribute to the persistent and predictable decline in β-cell function and mass observed in progressive T2DM. Exogenous GLP-1, but not GIP, exerts potent glucose-lowering activity in patients with the disease The potential benefits of restoring GLP-1 physiologic function has made the peptide a focus of efforts to correct the multiple metabolic abnormalities in patients with T2DM.[262]

Among the newest approved classes of antidiabetes medications are incretin-based therapies. GLP-1 agonists (exenatide, exenatide extended-release, liraglutide) and DPP-4 inhibitors (sitagliptin, saxagliptin and linagliptin) are currently FDA approved for use as adjunctive therapy to diet and exercise in patients with T2DM.

The GLP-1 agonists and DPP-4 inhibitors have differing mechanisms of actions, side effect profiles, and glucose lowering effects. However, they are unique within the diabetes pharmacology class of agents by having low risk of hypoglycemia and weight gain. The incretin class of drugs has demonstrated favorable cardiovascular biomarker profiles in clinical trials.[263] Evidence supports that the GLP-1 receptor agonists exert positive beneficial effects on the β-cells and suggests that they are capable of preserving β-cell function, thereby limiting disease progression and the development of its micro- and macrovascular complications.[264]

GLP-1 agonists work by binding to receptors on β-cells, resulting in production and secretion of endogenous insulin (Fig. 10-21). GLP-1 agonists are NOT denatured by DPP-4 and are therefore capable of prolonged receptor activation. Bound receptors are activated by either pharmacologic binding of the agonist or physiologic binding of the native GLP-1 gut hormone. An injection of a GLP-1 agonist effectively "floods" the receptor binding sites to a much greater degree than will DPP-4 inhibition that will only slightly raise endogenous GLP-1 levels above baseline. Thus, DPP-4 inhibitors tend to have less effect on weight reduction, gastric emptying, and A1C reduction than the GLP-1 agonists.[265]

Exenatide is a synthetic form of exendin 4, a naturally occurring GLP-1 receptor agonist found in the salivary secretions of the Gila monster. Exendin-4 is 53% homologous with human GLP-1 and binds to the mammalian GLP-1 receptor with affinity equal to that of native GLP-1, producing many of the same glycoregulatory effects. Exenatide is resistant to degradation by DPP-4 and detectable in the circulation for up to 10 hours after administration, allowing for twice-daily administration in the treatment of patients with T2DM.[94]

Short-acting exenatide has been available since 2005 and is approved for monotherapy or as part of combination therapy as an adjunct to diet and exercise. The drug is approved for use in combination with basal insulin. Clinical trials showed that exenatide 5 to 10 µg injected subcutaneously twice a day lowers HbA1c by almost a percentage point (0.8%) and at the same time is associated with weight loss of 3 to 6 lb over 30 weeks. The greatest weight loss was obtained when exenatide was used with metformin.[266]

The most potent glucose-lowering effects occurred when exenatide was used in combination with metformin and a thiazolidinedione.[267] Subsequent studies have shown HbA1C reductions

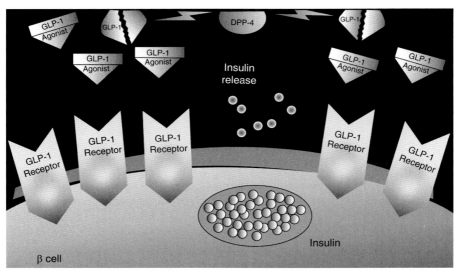

Figure 10-21 • GLP-1 Mechanism of Action.
GLP-1 agonists bind to GLP-1 receptors on the surface of pancreatic β-cells, resulting in the production and secretion of endogenous insulin. Patients with T2DM have deficient levels of native GLP-1 and resistance of GLP-1 action at the receptor site. In addition, unlike GLP-1 agonists, native GLP-1 is rapidly denigrated once released by the intestinal L cells. The efficiency of GLP-1 agonist receptor binding adds to the "physiologic" benefits of this drug class.

of –1.3% and –1.6% at 9 and 12 months, respectively. In a "real world study," a progressive reduction of weight (about 10 lb) was also observed.[268] The primary effect of short-acting GLP-1 agonists such as exenatide is the lowering of postprandial glucose levels.[269] Nausea occurs in 44% of exenatide users but is likely to diminish over time.[270] To minimize nausea and maximize efficacy, exenatide should be administered via a designated 5 to 10 μg or 10 μg pen injector within 1 hour of eating. If nausea is significant, the clinician might suggest slowing dose titration by using the drug once daily at 5 μg until the nausea subsides or by continuing with the twice daily dosing for more than 4 weeks before titrating to the 10 μg dose. Nausea, which resumes once the patient has successfully been titrated to the highest therapeutic dose, should be managed by either reducing the dose to 5 μg twice daily or switching to a different GLP-1 agent.

Twice daily exenatide or placebo injections were added to insulin glargine (± metformin in combination with pioglitazone) in T2DM patients with A1C levels of 7.1% to 10.5%.[270a] During this 30-week parallel, randomized, placebo controlled trial, patients on glargine having a prerandomization A1C of less than 8% were advised to reduce their dose of insulin by 20%. Those with an A1C greater than 8% maintained their prestudy dose of glargine to which exenatide or placebo was subsequently added. The dose of glargine was subsequently titrated in both cohorts based on a predefined treat-to-target protocol. The A1C level decreased by 1.74% with exenatide and 1.04% with placebo, a placebo corrected difference of –0.7%. The weight decreased by 1.8 kg with exenatide and increased by 1.0 kg with placebo, a between group difference of –2.7 kg favoring exenatide + glargine over placebo + glargine. Thirteen exenatide recipients and 1 placebo recipient discontinued the study because of adverse events ($P < 0.010$); rates of nausea (41% vs. 8%), diarrhea (18% vs. 8%), vomiting (18% vs. 4%), headache (14% vs. 4%), and constipation (10% vs. 2%) were higher with exenatide than with placebo. No increase in hypoglycemia occurrence was noted in the exenatide + glargine group. Exenatide is FDA approved for use with insulin.[270]

Exenatide extended-release (bydureon) uses a proprietary technology for long-acting medications that encapsulates active medication into polymer-based microspheres made of polylactide co-glycolide. The microspheres are injected into the subcutis where the are slowly degraded releasing exenatide in a controlled manner and providing a continuous therapeutic drug level in the plasma.[271]

Exenatide b.i.d reaches median peak plasma concentrations in 2.1 hours, has a mean terminal half-life of 2.4 hours, and is primarily eliminated by the kidneys. With exenatide once weekly injections, mean plasma concentrations rise gradually over 6 weeks with greater time to peak plasma and steady-state concentrations compared to exenatide b.i.d.[272]

DURATION, which stands for "Diabetes therapy Utilization: Researching changes in A1C, weight and other factors Through Intervention with exenatide ONce weekly," is an acronym for the overall exenatide extended-release once weekly clinical program. The DURATION program was designed to test the safety and efficacy of exenatide once weekly to other medications in the treatment of T2DM.

To directly compare the two dosing methods, a 30-week, randomized, noninferiority study (DURATION-1), was completed using exenatide extended-release 2 mg once weekly versus traditional dosing of exenatide 10 mcg twice daily in 295 patients with uncontrolled T2DM on one or more oral agents.[273] There were no differences in baseline A1C, fasting blood glucose, BMI or duration of diabetes between the groups. The weekly exenatide group demonstrated a significantly greater reduction from baseline in A1C (–1.9% vs. –1.5%) and fasting blood glucose (–42 vs. –25 mg per dL) compared to the group dosed twice daily. In addition, a greater percentage of patients on the weekly regimen (77% vs. 61%) achieved an A1C level ≤ 7%. Weight loss did not differ between the groups and nausea was significantly lower (26.4% vs. 34.5%) in the group dosed weekly.

The DURATION-2 trial directly compared exenatide once weekly and maximum approved doses of sitagliptin (DPP-4 inhibitor) and pioglitazone (thiazolidinedione) in patients with T2DM not achieving adequate glycemic control on metformin alone.[274] This 26-week randomized, double-blind, double-dummy (meaning that each patient received a pill and an injection, but were blinded to the content of their medication), superiority trial consisted of 491 patients with T2DM and baseline A1C 8.5%. Exenatide once weekly produced significantly greater A1C reduction (–1.5%) compared to sitagliptin (–0.9%) or pioglitazone (–1.2%). Significantly more patients achieved A1C targets of 7.0% or less with exenatide than with sitagliptin or pioglitazone. All treatments improved fasting plasma glucose (–32, –16.2, and –27 mg per dL with exenatide, sitagliptin and pioglitazone respectively), although the treatment differences were only significant versus sitagliptin.

DURATION-3 was a 26-week, open-label randomized parallel study comparing exenatide extended-release to insulin glargine. At 26 weeks, mean reduction in A1C was significantly greater in the exenatide extended-release group than with insulin glargine (–1.5% vs. –1.3%, treatment difference).[275] More patients treated with exenatide extended-release than with insulin glargine achieved a target A1C of less than 7.0% (60% vs. 48%). Exenatide extended-release was also associated with a decrease in body weight, whereas insulin glargine was associated with weight gain (–2.6 vs. +1.4 kg). The most frequently reported adverse events were nausea and diarrhea with exenatide and nasopharyngitis and headache with insulin glargine. Three patients (one taking exenatide extended-release and two taking insulin glargine) had an episode of hypoglycemia that required assistance of another person, but did not involve loss of consciousness or lead to study discontinuation. Minor hypoglycemia was reported in 19 (8%) of exenatide extended-release patients (46 events) compared with 58 (26%) of insulin glargine patients (135 events). Hypoglycemia was reported most often in patients receiving concomitant sulphonylurea; however, incidence was consistently lower with exenatide extended-release than with insulin glargine.

The DURATION-4 26-week double-blind, randomized, four-arm parallel study examined exenatide extended-release as a monotherapy treatment compared to either metformin, sitagliptin, or pioglitazone (thiazolidinedione).[276] 820 patients with T2DM uncontrolled on diet and exercise were randomized to either exenatide extended-release (2 mg, once-a-week injection, n = 248), metformin (dose escalated up to 2,500 mg per day, n = 246), pioglitazone (dose escalated up to 45 mg per day, n = 163) or sitagliptin (100 mg per day, n = 163). Exenatide extended-release produced significantly greater reduction in A1C compared to sitagliptin (–1.5% vs. 1.2%). Exenatide extended-release was noninferior to metformin (both drugs lowered A1C –1.5%) but inferior to pioglitazone (–1.5 for exenatide extended-release vs. –1.6 for pioglitazone). Exenatide once weekly resulted in significantly greater reduction in body weight than sitagliptin or pioglitazone (–4.5, –1.7, and +3.3 lb, respectively) and was similar to metformin (–4.4 lb). There were no major hypoglycemic events in any treatment group and the frequency of minor hypoglycemia was low.

The DURATION-5 trial, a randomized, open-label, parallel-group, comparator-controlled, multicenter study, evaluated the glycemic effects, safety and tolerability of exenatide once weekly (2 mg once weekly) compared to exenatide b.i.d (5 µg b.i.d for 4 weeks followed by 10 µg b.i.d) in 252 subjects with T2DM managed with diet and exercise alone or with oral antidiabetic medications.[277] At 24 weeks, exenatide extended-release produced significantly greater changes from baseline compared to exenatide b.i.d in A1C (–1.6 vs. –0.9) and mean fasting plasma glucose (–35 ± 5 mg per dL vs. –12). Reductions in mean body weight from baseline to week 24 were similar between the two groups (–2.3 ± 0.4 kg and –1.4 ± 0.4 kg). Both treatments were generally well tolerated with no episodes of major hypoglycemia in either group. The most common adverse event was transient and predominantly mild to moderate nausea that occurred less with exenatide extended-release (14%) compared with exenatide b.i.d (35%). Injection site reactions were more common with exenatide extended-release.

DURATION-6 was a 26-week head-to-head open-label superiority trial comparing exenatide extended-release 2 mg weekly or liraglutide force titrated to 1.8 mg daily in patients using metformin, a sulfonylurea, metformin plus pioglitazone, or metformin plus sulfonylurea. More than 85% of the 900 patients in the treatment arms completed the study. The mean reduction in A1C was –1.3% for exenatide extended-release versus –1.5% for liraglutide. Injection site nodules occurred more frequently among BYDUREON users (10%) compared with Victoza users (1%). There were no major hypoglycemia events in either treatment group. Exenatide extended-release did not meet the prespecified endpoint of noninferiority vs. liraglutide, although GI side effects were more common within the liraglutide cohort.[278]

Exenatide once weekly reduces systolic blood pressure by about 5 mm Hg, which is significantly more than sitagliptin and similar to exenatide b.i.d. Compared to sitagliptin and pioglitazone, exenatide extended-release is the only medication that lowers total cholesterol, LDL, triglycerides and raises HDL.[273,275,279] While pioglitazone significantly reduces triglycerides and raises HDL more than exenatide extended-release TC and LDL are increased with pioglitazone whereas all parameters have shown improvement with exenatide extended-release.

Long-acting GLP-1 receptor agonists have been shown to activate thyroid C cells in some rodent models, resulting in increased secretion of calcitonin, a marker of thyroid C cell hyperplasia and medullary carcinoma. Calcitonin was measured in both the DURATION-3 and DURATION-5 trials with no mean changes in calcitonin concentrations noted and no events of thyroid neoplasms reported. These results are consistent with observations in primate models and in patients with T2DM treated for 2 years with liraglutide.[280]

In summary, exenatide extended-release is well tolerated by patients and produces a statistically greater reduction in A1C than sitagliptin and exenatide b.i.d. Treatment emergent reductions in A1C are similar to those of insulin glargine and metformin. Weight loss with exenatide extended-release is equal to exenatide and metformin while superior to glargine and pioglitazone. Patients who are unable to use either metformin or pioglitazone may have a favorable therapeutic response to exenatide extended-release. No clinical trials evaluating the efficacy and safety of exenatide extended-release and insulin are on going.

Another GLP-1 agonist, liraglutide, is approved for use as adjunctive therapy in patients with T2DM who are unable to achieve their targeted glycemic goals with lifestyle intervention. The drug may be used as monotherapy in patients who are metformin intolerant. Combination with other oral agents is acceptable. The combination of sulfonylurea and liraglutide may result in a higher risk of hypoglycemia. Therefore, the dose of the sulfonylurea should be reduced by 50% when both drugs are used concomitantly.

Dose titration begins with a nontherapeutic dose of 0.6 mg injected once daily. After 1 week, the patient increases the dose to 1.2 mg daily. Fasting glucose levels should be monitored daily. Although not indicated in the label, most experts prefer to increase the dose of liraglutide to 1.8 mg if the patient is unable to achieve consistent fasting glucose levels within the ADA recommended range of 90 to 130 mg per dL.

Liraglutide has been studied in a head-to-head, 26-week randomized trial evaluating 464 subjects with T2DM.[281] Patients were randomized to treatment with either liraglutide 1.8 mg once daily or exenatide 10 μg twice daily, both as an add-on to their existing treatment consisting of metformin and/or a sulfonylurea. Patients taking liraglutide experienced significantly less minor hypoglycemia compared with exenatide (2 vs. 2.5 per patient-year), with no episodes of major hypoglycemia for liraglutide. Although nausea was the most common side effect for both treatment arms, the percentage of patients reporting nausea with liraglutide decreased to 8% after 5 weeks and 4% after 10 weeks. The exenatide group reported nausea of greater than 10% for greater than 20 weeks. Weight loss was equal between the 2 incretins (~2 to 3 kg). However, β-cell function as a measure by homeostatic model assessment (HOMA) percentage from baseline (32.1% vs. 2.7%) was significantly greater with liraglutide versus exenatide. Finally, the percentage of patients achieving A1C levels less than 7% on liraglutide was 54% versus 43% using exenatide.

The study also had a 14-week extension phase during which subjects who were taking exenatide twice daily were switched to doses of either 1.2 or 1.8 mg of liraglutide.[282] These studies suggested that liraglutide provided statistically significant improvements in glycemic control compared with exenatide when used in combination with oral antidiabetic therapy. Liraglutide demonstrated superiority over exenatide regarding pancreatic β-cell function. However, weight reduction was equal with both drugs in the primary study. When patients were switched from exenatide twice daily to once daily liraglutide, A1C was further reduced by 0.3%. The improvement in A1C after one is switched to the long acting GLP-1 is thought to be secondary to sustained levels of receptor binding achieved with liraglutide over the biphasic receptor activation observed with exenatide.

In April 2012, the FDA approved the use of liraglutide and basal insulin in combination.[282a] The safety and efficacy of liraglutide in combination with insulin detemir were evaluated in a 26-week open label trial enrolling 988 subjects.[282b] At baseline, patients had an A1C of 7-10% on metformin alone or inadequate control with a A1C of 7% to 8.5% on metformin + a sulfonylurea. During a 12-week run-in phase, the sulfonylurea was discontinued while patients began receiving liraglutide and titrating their dose to 1.8 mg once daily. At the conclusion of the run-in period, 50% of these patients had already achieved an A1C of less than 7% with liraglutide plus metformin and continued in the nonrandomized observational arm of the study. 167 (17%) of the patients withdrew during the run in phase, with nearly half doing so secondary to nausea. The remaining 323 patients with A1C levels greater than 7% (33%) were randomized to receive once daily insulin detemir + liraglutide + metformin or simply continue liraglutide + metformin. The initial dose of detemir was 10 U once daily. At trial's end, the mean dose of insulin detemir 39 U. Treatment with detemir added on to liraglutide resulted in a further reduction A1C reduction of 0.5% from baseline. No change in A1C was noted in the liraglutide + metformin cohort. The FPG was reduced 39 versus 9 mg per dL favoring detemir + liraglutide. Most importantly, 43% of patients in the more intensive cohort were able to achieve an A1C of less than 7% versus 17% of those who continued to take liraglutide + metformin. Weight reduction occurred in both groups: −0.3 kg in detemir + liraglutide + metformin versus −1.1 kg for the liraglutide + metformin group. No major hypoglycemia events were recorded and the rates of minor hypoglycemia were also low.

Although acute pancreatitis has occurred in a small number of patients treated with GLP-1 agonists, a causal relationship has not been established. A retrospective analysis of a large health plan using data from 2005 to 2008 assessed the risk of pancreatitis in patients treated with exenatide or sitagliptin compared with patients treated with metformin or glyburide.[283] The estimated risk of developing pancreatitis over 1 year of follow-up was 0.13% with exenatide, 0.12% with sitagliptin, and was comparable to that of patients treated with metformin or glyburide (exenatide relative risk, 1; 95% confidence interval, 0.6 to 1.7).[283]

The safety of GLP-1 receptor agonists has been evaluated using meta-analysis data from published and unpublished data of global, randomized, placebo-controlled clinical trials.[284] When used as monotherapy, GLP-1 receptor agonists do not increase one's risk of developing hypoglycemia. However, when used in combination with a sulfonylurea, the risk of hypoglycemia increases threefold. The most common adverse events associated with GLP-1 receptor agonists are nausea, vomiting, and diarrhea No case of acute pancreatitis has been reported in trials studying GLP-1 receptor agonists.[284]

Dipeptidyl Peptidase 4 Inhibitors

DPP-4 inhibitors mimic many of the actions ascribed to GLP-1 agonists including stimulation of insulin, inhibition of glucagon secretion, and preservation of β-cell mass through stimulation of β-cell proliferation and inhibition of apoptosis. By contrast, DPP-4 inhibitors are not associated with slowing of gastric emptying or weight loss, as these drugs only double endogenous GLP-1 levels in the postprandial state to 15 to 25 pmol per L.[265] The degree of activation of the GLP-1 receptor by a GLP-1 agonist is at least equivalent to if not greater than the degree of activation with endogenous GLP-1.[285] GLP-1 receptor activation is approximately fourfold greater 2 hours postprandial when compared with receptor activation generated by DPP-4 inhibitors.[265]

Two-hour postprandial levels of GLP-1 in patients with T2DM are in the range of 5 to 7 PM. Use of sitagliptin will double the levels of endogenous 2-hour postprandial levels to 15 PM.[265] The "pharmacologic" receptor activation achieved with GLP-1 agonists far exceeds the "physiologic" activation observed with DPP-4 inhibitors. DPP-4 inhibitors elevate the levels of endogenous GLP-1 closer to what they should be in euglycemic individuals. The actions of GLP-1 agonists and DPP-4 inhibitors are compared in Table 10-21.

 TABLE 10-21. Comparison of Pharmacologic Actions of GLP-1 Agonists and DPP-4 Inhibitiors

| | Incretin Mimetic | | |
Pharmacologic Action	Exenatide	Liraglutide	DPP-4 Inhibitors[a]
Glucose-dependent stimulation of insulin secretion from pancreatic β-cells	Yes	Yes	Yes
Improve first phase insulin secretion from pancreatic β-cells	Yes	Yes	Yes
Postprandial glucose-dependent suppression of glucagon secretion from pancreatic α-cells	Yes	Yes	Yes
Decelerates gastric emptying, reducing postprandial hyperglycemia	Yes	Yes	No
Suppresses appetite and induces satiety	Yes	Yes	No
Effects on body weight from baseline	Favors weight loss	Favors weight loss	Favors weight neutrality
Inhibition of programmed β-cell death (apoptosis) in animal and in vitro models	Yes	Yes	Animals only
Increases β-cell mass (animals) and markers of β-cell function (humans)	Yes	Yes	Animals only
Lowers blood pressure	Yes	Yes	No
Reduces hepatic biomarkers	Yes	Not reported	Not significant
Reduces cardiovascular biomarkers	Yes	Yes	Not significant
Reduces visceral fat	Unknown	Yes	No

[a]Information provided based on sitagliptin data only.
Adapted from Unger J, Parkin CG. T2DM: An expanded view of pathophysiology and therapy. *Postgr Med.* 2010;122(3):145–157.

Table 10-22 Dose Adjustment of DPP-4 Inhibitors Based upon Renal Function

Drug	Mild Renal Insufficiency	Severe Renal Insufficiency or Disease Requiring Dialysis
Linagliptin	No dose adjustment required	No dose adjustment required
Saxagliptin	No dose adjustment required	Reduce dose to 2.5 mg/d
Sitagliptin	50 mg/d	25 mg/d

Mild RI, Creatinine clearance ≥ 50 mL per minute, serum creatinine ≤1.7 (men) and ≤ 1.5 mg per dL (women).
Severe RI, Creatinine clearance < 30 mL per minute, serum creatinine > 3.0 (men) and > 2.5 (women).
From Januvia prescribing information: http://www.merck.com/product/usa/pi_circulars/j/janumet/janumet_pi.pdf. Accessed July 1, 2011.
Onglyza prescribing information: http://packageinserts.bms.com/pi/pi_onglyza.pdf. Accessed July 1, 2011.
Tradjenta prescribing information: http://bidocs.boehringer-ingelheim.com/BIWebAccess/ViewServlet.
ser?docBase=renetnt&folderPath=/Prescribing±Information/PIs/Tradjenta/Tradjenta.pdf. Accessed July 1, 2011.

Sitagliptin became the first DPP-4 inhibitor to gain FDA approval for treatment of T2DM in 2006. Commercial dose availability includes 25, 50, and 100 mg tablets. Sitagliptin is also available in a combination product with metformin and metformin XR. A polypill combining sitagliptin with simvastatin (Juvisync) is also commercially available). The usual recommended dose of sitagliptin is 100 mg per day. Renal function studies should be performed prior to initiating sitagliptin and periodically during the course of therapy. Dose adjustments should be made for patients with renal insufficiency (Table 10-22).

Sitagliptin appears to be most efficacious when initiated in combination with metformin and pioglitazone in treatment naïve patients with T2DM. The A1C difference from placebo adjusted mean in these individuals is −2.4%, allowing 60% of treated patients to achieve the American Diabetes Association target of ≤ 7%. As pancreatic β-cell function deteriorates over time, adding a DPP-4 inhibitor to one's treatment regimen provides a 0.6% to 0.8% reduction from baseline in most patients. Sitagliptin is the only DPP-4 inhibitor that is currently FDA approved for use in combination with insulin.

On average, saxagliptin will lower one's A1C from on average 0.43 to 1.17 from baseline.[286] As with sitiglipin, glycemic efficacy is improved when metformin is combined in a single pill rather than used separately. Speculation as to the reasons for improved efficacy with combination therapy include the following: (a) metformin upregluates GLP-1 secretion thereby enhancing the incretin effect of the DPP-4 inhibitor, (b) metformin is an insulin sensitizing agent which potentiates the insulin secretagogue effect of DPP-4 inhibitors, and (c) taking a single drug rather than two may enhance adherence to a treatment regimen as patients are responsible for a single copay.

Saxagliptin is excreted by both renal and hepatic pathways with 75% being eliminated in the urine and 22% in the feces.[287] Saxagliptin is approved as monotherapy or in combination with extended release metformin (500 to 1,000 mg) as an adjunct to diet and exercise to improve glycemic control in adults with T2DM. The drug is also approved for use as add-on therapy with insulin (with or without metformin).[288]

The recommended dosage of saxagliptin is 2.5 or 5 mg once daily administered regardless of meals. The 2.5 mg dose is preferred in patients with severe renal impairment (CrCl less than 50 mL per min) as well as in patients receiving strong CYP3A4/5 inhibitors (ketoconazole, clarithromycin, atazanavir, indinavir, itraconazole, nefazodone, nelfinavir, ritonavir, saquinavir, and telithromycin. Assessment of renal function is required prior to initiation of saxagliptin and periodically once the drug has been utilized. No dose adjustment is required for hepatic impairment. Due to a heightened risk of hypoglycemia, the sulfonylurea dose should be reduced when used in combination with saxagliptin. Results of six double blind-controlled clinical studies have not shown any differences in safety and effectiveness between adult patients and those age ≥ 65 years of age.[289] Still, one should be mindful about the possibility of renal insufficiency in the aged population and adjust the dose of saxagliptin accordingly.

As with other drugs in the DPP-4 class, saxagliptin is very well tolerated. The most commonly observed adverse events include upper respiratory infections, urinary tract infections, headache and nasopharyngitis. Although the drug is considered "weight neutral" significant increases in body weight have been observed with saxagliptin is combined with glyburide.[290]

In clinical trials up to 24-weeks duration, saxagliptin as monotherapy reduces A1C by 0.4% to 0.9%. In treatment naïve patients and in patients inadequately controlled with metformin monotherapy, saxagliptin–metformin combination was found to be more effective in reducing glycemic parameters as compared with metformin alone.[291] Adding saxagliptin to TZDs in patients not achieving glycemic control with TZDs alone is well tolerated and results in improvement in glycemic parameters (–0.66% for 2.5 mg + TZD and –0.94% for 5 mg + TZD vs. –0.30% for placebo + TZD).[292] Saxagliptin + metformin might be most appropriate for treatment naïve patients with no evidence of renal insufficiency. The study by Jadzinsky et al. has demonstrated a mean adjusted reduction of A1C of –2.5% over 24 weeks in this population while 60.3% of patients achieved an A1C less than 7% when using this combination.[291]

Linagliptin is the third DPP-4 to be marketed in the United States. Although glycemic endpoints appear to be similar to both sitigliptin and saxagliptin, linagliptin appears to have a safety advantage in patients with moderate and severe renal insufficiency. A pooled analysis of three global studies evaluated the effect of renal function on the efficacy and safety of linagliptin in 2,141 T2DM patients with and without declining renal function.[293] After 24 weeks of treatment no difference in safety or glycemic endpoints were noted in any of patients grouped according to renal function ("normal renal function" defined as a GFR ≥ 80 mL per minute, "mild renal insufficiency" defined as a GFR 50 to 80 mL per minute, and moderate renal insufficiency" defined as a GFR 30 to 50 mL per minute).

DPP-4 inhibitors have an excellent safety profile as a class. The three most commonly reported adverse reactions reported in clinical trials are nasopharyngitis, upper respiratory tract infections, and headache. During postmarketing surveillance, acute pancreatitis was reported in 88 patients taking sitagliptin or metformin + sitagliptin between October 2006 and February 2009. Twenty-one percent of the reported cases occurred within 30 days of drug initiation and upon discontinuation of the drug, 53% resolved.[286] Interestingly, other risk factors for acute pancreatitis, including hypercholesterolemia, hypertriglyceridemia, and obesity were present in 51% of the reported cases.[294] A direct causative effect between sitagliptin and acute pancreatitis has never been established.

Rashes may also occur with DPP-4 inhibitors. Drug hypersensitivity reactions from DPP-4 inhibitors may present a challenging diagnostic dilemma for the clinician. A patient who is taking eight concomitant medications should discontinue the drug that is thought to be the one most likely to be the cause of the hypersensitivity reaction. Most patients will note improvement in their rash within 5 to 7 days of drug cessation. After 2 weeks, the patient may be re-challenged with the alleged offending agent. If the rash recurs, that medication, as well as other drugs within that class should be avoided in the future.

None of the DPP-4 inhibitors have demonstrated a positive effect on cardiovascular outcomes, although randomized, placebo controlled trials to assess cardiovascular endpoints are currently underway. (Sitagliptin Cardiovascular Outcome Study (0431-082 AM1) (TECOS), CAROLINA: Cardiovascular Outcome Study of Linagliptin Versus Glimepiride in Patients with T2DM, Does Saxagliptin Reduce the Risk of Cardiovascular Events When Used Alone or Added to Other Diabetes Medications (SAVOR- TIMI 53). The reporting dates for the primary endpoints of these studies will be between 2014 and 2018.

The manufacturer of linagliptin has now added metformin to the product to enhance efficacy. The newly marketed drug known as jentadueto, is available in doses of metformin 500, 850, and 1,000 mg with linagliptin 2.5 mg and is taken twice daily. The placebo corrected A1C of jentadueto 2.5 per 1,000 b.i.d after 24 weeks was –1.5%. When using jentadueto, the patient's renal function should be assessed at baseline and verified as being normal. Patients with evidence of renal insufficiency should use only linagliptin rather than the drug in combination with metformin to minimize the risk of lactic acidosis.[295] Dosing of jentadueto should be customized based on tolerability to metformin, efficacy of the drug to achieve the desired glycemic targets and the patient's prior exposure to metformin therapy. Patients who are metformin naïve should initiate therapy with jentadueto 2.5 per 500 b.i.d. Patients may be also converted to jentadueto based on their current daily dose of metformin. Those who are using metformin 850 or 1,000 mg b.i.d should be switched to jantadueto 2.5 per 850 or 1,000 b.i.d with meals.

Table 10-22 lists the dose adjustments of DPP-4 inhibitors that should be considered in patients with renal insufficiency. Table 10-23 displays the clinical efficacy of DPP-4 inhibitors based upon registration trials submitted to the FDA for product approval.

TABLE 10-23 Efficacy of DPP-4 Inhibitors in Clinical Practice

Drug	A1C Difference from Placebo Adjusted Mean (%)[a]	FPG Difference from Placebo Adjusted Mean (mg/dL)	% of Patients Achieving A1C < 7%	2-h PPG Change from Baseline (mg/dL)[b]
Sitagliptin monotherapy	−0.6	−20	36	−49
Sitagliptin 50 mg b.i.d + metformin 500 mg b.i.d	−1.6	−47	43	−93
Sitagliptin 50 mg b.i.d + metformin 1,000 mg b.i.d	−2.1	−64	43	−117
Sitagliptin 100 mg + pioglitazone	−0.7	−17	45	
Sitagliptin 100 mg + pioglitazone (treatment naïve)	−2.4	−63	60	−114
Sitagliptin 100 mg + glimepiride (≥ 4 mg/d)	−0.6	−19	11	—
Sitagliptin 100 mg + glimepiride (≥ 4 mg/d) + metformin (≥ 1,500 mg/d)	−0.9	−8	26	—
Sitagliptin 100 mg + insulin (± metformin)[c]	−0.7	−18	14	−39
Saxagliptin monotherapy 5 mg	−0.6	−21	38	−37
Saxagliptin 5 mg + metformin ≥ 1,500 mg	−0.8	−23	44	−40
Saxagliptin 5 mg + metformin > 1,500 mg (treatment naïve patients)	−2.5	−13	60	−41
Saxagliptin 5 mg ± metformin + insulin	−0.4	−4	11	−27
Saxagliptin 5 mg + TZD[d]	−0.6	−15	42	−50
Saxagliptin 5 mg + glyburide 7.5 mg	−0.7	−10	23	−42
Linagliptin 5 mg monotherapy	−0.7	−8.5	25	−33.5

(Continued)

TABLE 10-23 Efficacy of DPP-4 Inhibitors in Clinical Practice *(Continued)*

Drug	A1C Difference from Placebo Adjusted Mean (%)[a]	FPG Difference from Placebo Adjusted Mean (mg/dL)	% of Patients Achieving A1C < 7%	2-h PPG Change from Baseline (mg/dL)[b]
Linagliptin 5 mg + metformin (≥1,500 mg/d)	−0.6	−10.7	28.3	−48.9
Linagliptin 2.5 mg b.i.d + metformin 500 mg b.i.d	−1.3	−43	31	
Linagliptin 2.5 + metformin 1,000 mg b.i.d	−1.7	−60	54	
Linagliptin 5 mg + pioglitazone 30 mg	−0.5	−32.6	42.9	—
Linagliptin 5 mg +sulfonylurea	−0.5	−8.2	15.2	—
Linagliptin 5 mg + metformin ≥ 1,500 mg/d + sulfonylurea	−0.7	−4.6	31.2	

[a]The Food and Drug Administration considers an A1C placebo adjusted mean reduction of ≥0.5% as being clinically significant.
[b]2-hour PPG change from baseline does not include the difference with the active comparator.
[c]Study evaluated sitagliptin added on to patients using premixed, intermediate or basal insulin. The median dose of insulin was 40 U. 75% of patients were also using metformin at doses ≥1,500 mg per day.
[d]To qualify for enrollment, patients were required to be on a stable dose of pioglitazone (30 or 45 mg per day) or rosiglitazone (4 or 8 mg per day) for 12 weeks.
PPG, postprandial glucose.
From Januvia prescribing information: http://www.merck.com/product/usa/pi_circulars/j/janumet/janumet_pi.pdf. Accessed July 1, 2011.
Onglyza prescribing information: http://packageinserts.bms.com/pi/pi_onglyza.pdf. Accessed April 2, 2012.
Tradjenta prescribing information: http://bidocs.boehringer-ingelheim.com/BIWebAccess/ViewServlet. ser?docBase=renetnt&folderPath=/Prescribing±Information/PIs/Tradjenta/Tradjenta.pdf. Accessed July 1, 2011.
Jantadueto prescribing information: http://bidocs.boehringer-ingelheim.com/BIWebAccess/ViewServlet. ser?docBase=renetnt&folderPath=/Prescribing+Information/PIs/Jentadueto/Jentadueto.pdf. Accessed April 2, 2012.

The pharmacologic actions of all drugs used to treat patients with T2DM are compared in Table 10-24, and selected dosing comparisons are presented in Table 10-25.

Some clinicians believe that use of clinically relevant composite outcome data provides important guidance toward determining which therapeutic interventions may prove to be the safest and most effective for a given patient. One such composite endpoint suggests determining the percentage of patients in a clinical trial who achieve a predefined A1C, while avoiding weight gain and hypoglycemia. A prespecified meta-analysis was performed on 26-week patient-level data from seven trials (N = 4,625) evaluating liraglutide with commonly used therapies for T2DM: glimepiride, rosiglitazone, glargine, exenatide, sitagliptin or placebo, adjusting for baseline A1C and weight, for a composite outcome of HbA1c of less than 7.0%, no weight gain, and no hypoglycemic events. At 26 weeks, 40% of the liraglutide 1.8 mg group, 32% of the liraglutide 1.2 mg group, and 6% to 25% of comparators (6% rosiglitazone, 8% glimepiride, 15% glargine, 25% exenatide, 11% sitagliptin, 8% placebo) achieved this composite outcome. In this meta-analysis, the odds ratios favored liraglutide 1.8 mg by 2- to 10.5-fold over the comparators, suggesting that liraglutide was superior to other commonly used therapies. However, the long-term clinical impact of these observations has not been addressed.

TABLE 10-24. Pharmacologic Comparisons of Available Agents for Treating T2DM[a]

Drug	Class	Mode of Action	Alerts
Glyburide (Micronase, Diabeta) Glipizide (Glucotrol) Glipizide-GITS (Glucotrol XL) Glyburide micronized (Glynase) Glimepiride (Amaryl)	Sulfonylurea	Insulin secretagogue	Hypoglycemia especially in the elderly and those with renal insufficiency, weight gain, increase cancer risk, interference with ischemic preconditioning
Metformin (Glucophage) Metformin XL (Fortamet) Metformin XR (Glucophage XR, Glumetza) Metformin oral suspension	Biguanide	Decreases hepatic glucose production, decreases glucose absorption from the GI tract, and increases peripheral utilization of glucose	Must take with food to avoid gastritis and GI side effects. Caution in elderly patients and in those with eGFR <45 mL/min. Withhold prior to contrast studies and for
Acarbose (Precose) Miglitol (Glyset)	AGIs	By inhibiting α-glucosidase enzymes, slows gut absorption of carbohydrates	Contraindicated in inflammatory bowel disease, malabsorption syndromes and partial bowel obstructions May induce hypoglycemia when used in combination therapy. Oral glucose (dextrose) whose absorption is not inhibited by AGIs, should be used instead of sucrose (cane sugar). Hypoglycemia will also respond to glucagon injection.
Pioglitazone (Actos)	Thiazolidinedione	Enhance tissue sensitivity to insulin in skeletal muscles by activating intracellular PPAR receptors	May cause resumption of ovulation in anovulatory premenopausal women. Weight gain average of 0.9–2.6 kg. Do not use in any patient with advanced heart failure (NYHA Class III–IV). Liver function testing at baseline, every 2 mo for the first year, then periodically thereafter. Increased fracture risk in women. Do not use in any patient with a history of bladder cancer.

(Continued)

TABLE 10-24. Pharmacologic Comparisons of Available Agents for Treating T2DM[a] *(Continued)*

Drug	Class	Mode of Action	Alerts
Repaglinide (Prandin) Nateglinide (Starlix)	Meglitinides	Rapid-acting insulin secretagogues with short duration of action (1–2 h) Same mechanism of action as sulfonylureas but with a different binding site to pancreatic β-cells Less risk of hypoglycemia than sulfonylureas due to rapid kinetics	More effective at lowering postprandial blood glucose than metformin, sulfonylureas, and thiazolidinediones Must take 15 min before meals Approximately one month of therapy is required before a decrease in fasting blood glucose is seen May be either weight neutral or result in a slight weight increase
Bromocriptine (Cycloset)	D2-Dopamine Agonist	Resets dopaminergic and sympathetic tone within the central nervous system.	Reduces glucose, triglycerides, and IR in patients with T2DM. Can be used with all oral agents and insulin Take within 2 h of rising each morning Only oral agent with a label indication for cardiovascular risk reduction for patients with T2DM.
Colesevelam (Welchol)	BASs	Uncertain mode of action. May affect secretion GLP-1	Not indicated as monotherapy in T2DM. Can be used with metformin or metformin + sulfonylurea. May consider off label use in patients with prediabetes in order to reduce LDL to < 100 mg/dL and preserve β-cell function Can consider use in T2DM with elevated LDL cholesterol
Sitagliptin (Januvia) Saxagliptin (Onglyza) Linagliptin (Tradjenta)	DPP-4 inhibitors	Block action of DPP-4 enzyme, resulting in a 2- to 3-fold increase in plasma levels of endogenous GLP-1	Only sitagliptin is approved for use in combination with insulin Most common side effects are rash and rhinitis Dose of sitagliptin and saxagliptin must be reduced for patients with renal insufficiency (see Table 10-26)

(Continued)

TABLE 10-24. Pharmacologic Comparisons of Available Agents for Treating T2DM[a] *(Continued)*

Drug	Class	Mode of Action	Alerts
Exenatide (Byetta) Liraglutide (Victoza) Exenatide Extended-release (Bydureon)	GLP-1 agonists	Enhance nutrient-stimulated insulin secretion via activation of GLP-1 R on pancreatic β-cells Inhibits glucagon secretion Delays gastric emptying Reduces appetite	Favors weight loss Favorable effect on cardiovascular biomarkers Low rates of hypoglycemia Favors preservation of β-cell function GLP-1 infusion studies demonstrate favorable effects on endothelial cell function in humans Direct link to acute pancreatitis has not been demonstrated Do not use in patients with a personal or family history of medullary thyroid carcinoma or multiple endocrine neoplasia II (medullary thyroid cancer + pheochromocytoma) Most common adverse effect is nausea. This can be avoided by making certain the **patient does not eat beyond the point of satiety** When used with a secretagogue (sulfonylurea or insulin, reduce dose of secretagogue to minimize the likelihood of inducing hypoglycemia) Exenatide is injected twice daily within 1 h of eating. Liraglutide is injected once daily without regard to meals. Exenatide extended-release can be injected once weekly. Do not use in patients with a history of pancreatitis. Discontinue use in patients suspected of having pancreatitis. Exenatide extended-release may cause injection nodules

[a]Insulin and pramlintide are discussed in Chapters 10 and 12.
GLP-1, glucagon-like peptide-1; GIP, glucose-dependent insulinotropic polypeptide.

TABLE 10-25. Dosing Comparisons

Drug	Available Dose	Daily Dose	Dose/d	Dose Timing
GLP-1 Analogues				
Exenatide (Byetta)	5 and 10 mg	10 mg maximum	b.i.d	Inject within 1 h of scheduled meal time
Liraglutide (Victoza)	0.6, 1.2, and 1.8 mg	1.8 mg	Qd	Inject once daily without regard to meals
Exenatide extended-release (Bydureon)	2 mg	2 mg	One injection weekly	Inject once weekly without regard to meals
DPP-4 Inhibitors				
Sitagliptin (Januvia)	25, 50, and 100 mg	CrCl 30–50 mL/min: 50 mg PO qday CrCl <30 mL/min: 25 mg PO qday ESRD: 25 mg PO qday regardless of hemodialysis	Once daily	Once daily with or without food
Sitagliptin/metformin (Janumet)	50/500 mg and 50/100 mg	Patients who are metformin naïve: initial dose is 50/500 b.i.d Patient who are currently on metformin: 50/1,000 b.i.d	Twice daily	Twice daily with meals to minimize nausea (Contraindicated in males with serum creatinine ≥ 1.5 mg/dL and women with serum creatinine ≥ 1.4 mg/dL)
Saxagliption (Onglyza)	2.5 and 5 mg	5 mg is suggested dose Use 2.5 mg for patients with moderate, severe, or end-stage renal function (CrCl ≤50 mL/min) or for patients also taking strong cytochrome P450 3A4/5 (CYP3A4/5) inhibitors (e.g., ketoconazole)	Once daily	Once daily with or without meals

Drug	Available strengths	Dose	Frequency	Administration
Saxagliptin/metformin XR (Kombiglyze XR)	5/500 mg 5/1,000 mg 2.5/1,000 mg	Patients who are metformin naïve: titrate from initial dose of 5/500 mg to maximum of 5/1,000 mg. Maximum daily dose should not exceed saxagliptin 5 mg and metformin XR (as individual components) Patients who are on metformin can be initiated on 5/1,000 mg/d Patients who need 2.5 mg saxagliptin in combination with metformin extended release may be treated with 2.5/1,000 mg/d	Once daily	Once daily with evening meal
Linagliptin (Tradjenta)	5 mg	5 mg	Once daily	With or without food
Jentadueto (Linagliptin + metformin)	−2.5 mg linagliptin/500 mg metformin		b.i.d	With meals
	−2.5 mg linagliptin/850 mg metformin		b.i.d	With meals
	−2.5 mg linagliptin/1,000 mg metformin		b.i.d	With meals
D2-Dopamine Agonist −Bromocriptine (Cycloset)	0.8 mg	0.8–1.6 mg/d increasing to maximum of 4.6 mg/d	Once daily	Take within 2 h of rising in AM
Bile Acid Sequestrant **Colesevelam (Welchol)**	Tablets: 625 mg	3.75 mg	=	Should be taken with food and a liquid.
	Oral suspension: 3.75 g packet, 1.875 g packet		Choices: 6 tabs daily 3 tabs b.i.d Or 1 3.75 oral suspension packet daily Or 1 1.875 mg oral suspension packet b.i.d	Oral suspension must be added to 4–8 oz of water and stirred completely prior to drinking

Cardiovascular Safety of T2DM Therapeutic Agents

The traditional pathway for new drug development in diabetes involved 6 to 12 month studies focusing on a product's ability to reduce A1C. The FDA now takes a particularly hard look at drugs for conditions for which we already have safe and effective treatments, particularly if the incremental benefits appear to be small. The FDA comes under intense pressure to raise preapproval safety standards. The pressure is a direct result of controversies over such widely used drugs as rosiglitazone and rofecoxib, which have led the press, government agencies, and Congress to question the transparency and completeness of safety reporting, as well as the effectiveness of the FDA's oversight.

Although clinicians and patients need to know more about the safety and effectiveness of pharmaceutical products, simply demanding larger quantities of traditional preapproval safety information will raise the cost of bringing a drug to market. Some may argue that postmarketing surveillance of large numbers of patients using approved medications in real clinical settings would be more cost-effective and allow newer agents to be introduced in a timely manner.

In 2008, the FDA mandated that sponsors of new antidiabetic therapies for managing patients with T2DM demonstrate that their agents will "not result in an unacceptable increase in cardiovascular risk."[296] The recommendations published by the FDA are described in Figure 10-22.

In summary, preapproval of new diabetes therapeutic agents must rule out a greater than 1.8-fold increase in hazard ratio of cardiovascular events in order to submit for a new drug application. Postmarketing trials must show a hazard ratio of less than 1.3 to satisfy the FDA safety requirements on cardiovascular risk.

---

1. An independent cardiovascular endpoints committee should prospectively adjudicate in a blinded fashion cardiovascular endpoints during all phases 2 and 3 trials. The endpoints include cardiovascular mortality, MI, stroke, hospitalizations for acute coronary syndrome, and urgent revascularization procedures.
2. Phases 2 and 3 studies should be designed to include higher risk patients with relatively advanced disease including elderly patients and some degree of renal impairment.
3. Meta-analysis should be performed for all placebo-controlled trials, add-on trials, and active-controlled trials. Active comparator trials may need to last for a minimum of 2 years to provide cardiovascular outcome data.
4. Meta-analysis of all trials should be performed on cardiovascular outcomes across all phase 2 and phase 3 trials to evaluate similarities or differences between subgroups (sex, age, race)
5. The incidence of important cardiovascular events occurring with the investigational drug versus the control group should have a risk ratio of less than 1.8 bound by the two-sided 95% confidence interval before submission of the new drug application.
6. If the premarketing application contains data showing that the upper bound of the two-sided 95% confidence interval for the risk ratio is 1.3 to 1.8 a postmarketing trial will be needed to show that the risk ratio is less than 1.3. Premarketing data showing a risk ratio of less than 1.3 does not require additional postmarketing studies.

Reference: http://www.fda.gov/downloads/Drugs/GuidanceComplianceRegulatoryInformation/Guidances/ucm071627.pdf. Accessed March 10, 2012.

Figure 10-22 • FDA Guidance Regarding Cardiovascular Safety Evaluation of New Antidiabetic Therapies for Patients with T2DM.

TABLE 10-26 Ongoing Postmarketing Cardiovascular Outcome Studies

Drug	Study Name	ClinicalTrials.gov Identifier
Tradjenta	CAROLINA	NCT01243424
Saxagliptin	SAVOR-TIMI	NCT01107886
Liraglutide	LEADER	NCT00393718
Exenatide extended-release	EXSCEL	NCT01144338
Alogliptin	EXAMINE	NCT00968708
Itca 650 (Exenatide)	Intarcia Therapeutics	NCT01455896
Canagliflozin	CANVAS	NCT01032629
BI 10773	Boehringer Ingelheim	NCT01131676

Table 10-26 lists the ongoing postmarketing cardiovascular studies that are adequately powered for safety and designed to show superiority rather than noninferiority. All toll, these studies need to recruit 56,986 high risk patients and obtain data for primary endpoints for up to 8 years in order to satisfy the regulatory mandate of the FDA.

The costs of performing these studies is substantial. As a comparator, the 5-year ACCORD Study, funded by the NIH, cost $300 million and included 10,108 patients.[297] However, many companies donated drugs, equipment and supplies to the research sites. Postmarketing cardiovascular outcomes trials are privately funded and tightly regulated by the FDA. One can clearly see that before a new drug is approved, the costs related to research, development, and regulatory affairs are astronomical.

Cardiovascular outcome data are available for many of the antihyperglycemic drugs currently marketed to treat T2DM as noted in Table 10-27. Metformin, both as monotherapy and in combination with other medications, has the highest benefit–risk profile. The safety of some of the newer agents such as DPP-4 inhibitors and GLP-1 agonists cannot be determined. Long-term outcome studies on these agents are pending. Most drug combinations have similar effects on glycemic control, with some having advantages by inducing less treatment emergent weight gain and hypoglycemia.

TABLE 10-27 Comparitive Cardiovascular Outcome Data for T2DM Antihyperglycemic Drugs

Drug	A1C Reduction	Hypoglycemia Risk	Weight Change	Outcome Study Reference	Outcome Data
Metformin	1.5	No	Neutral	UKPDS	In UKPDS metformin intensive patients showed a 39% risk reduction in MI vs. 21% risk reduction in the sulfonylurea/insulin intensive group
				Lamauna Meta-analysis	Metformin monotherapy is likely associated with improved survival
					Metformin + sulfonylurea is associated with reduced survival

(Continued)

TABLE 10-27 Comparitive Cardiovascular Outcome Data for T2DM Antihyperglycemic Drugs *(Continued)*

Drug	A1C Reduction	Hypoglycemia Risk	Weight Change	Outcome Study Reference	Outcome Data
Sulfonylureas	1.5	Yes	Gain	Shramm, et al.	*Patients without previous MI*: Glimepiride, glipizide, glyburide, tolbutamide showed higher hazard ratio for mortality than metformin Patients *with* previous MI: Glimepiride, glipizide, glyburide and tolbutamide had higher hazard ratio for mortality than metformin
Thiazolodin-ediones	0.5–1.4	No	Gain	Bennett Meta-analysis	Higher risk of heart failure when compared with sulfonylureas
GLP-1 agonists	0.5–1.0	No	Loss	None	
Nateglinide	0.5–0.8	Rare	Gain	NAVIGATOR	Addition of nateglinide to patients with T2DM increased risk of hypoglycemia but did not improve cardiovascular outcomes
Repaglinide	1–1.5	Yes	Gain	Shramm, et al.	In patients with previous MI, patients on repaglinide had similar hazard ratio for mortality as metformin
α-Glucosidase inhibitor	0.5–0.8	No	Neutral	None	
DPP-4 inhibitors	0.6–0.8	No	Neutral	None	
Bile acid sequestrant	0.5	No	Neutral	None	
Bromocriptine	0.7	No	Neutral	Gaziano et al.	HR was reduced vs. placebo (HR) 0.55 two-sided 95% CI 0.39–0.98, $p < 0.05$).

References
UKPDS Group. *Lancet*. 1998;352:854–865.
Lamauna et al. *Diabetes Obes Metab*. 2011;221–228.
Schramm et al. *Eur Heart J*. 2011;1900–1908.
NAVIGATOR Study Group. *N Engl J Med*. 2010;362(16):1477–1490.
Bennett, et al. *Ann Int Med*. 2011;154(9):602–613.
Gaziano et al. *Diabetes Care*. 2010;33:1503–1508.

The FDA mandate requiring sponsors to include high-risk patients in their phase 2 and phase 3 clinical trials will allow us to evaluate clinical outcomes in different ethnic groups, older individuals, and in those with multiple comorbid conditions.

Combination Therapies

Combination therapy involving agents with complementary mechanisms of action is not only logical but also frequently necessary to achieve the targeted A1C level of 7% or less.[298,299]

The AACE algorithm for achieving glycemic control recommends dual or triple drug therapy for patients unable to achieve an A1C less than 7.5% further justifying the simplistic nature of initiating or titrating medications that are provided as fixed dosed combinations.[135]

A meta-analysis study published by Jonas et al.[300] the addition of metformin to any other drug produced statistically greater reductions in A1C compared to monotherapy with any of their respective components.

Practical Management of T2DM—A Patient's Perspective

Patients who are initially diagnosed with T2DM are often overwhelmed by the changes that are required to comply with the "rules and regulations" of living with diabetes. Dr. Bill Polonsky of the Behavioral Diabetes Institute in San Diego, CA explains that patients with diabetes should not "freak out" at the prospect of having to be scrutinized by the "diabetes police" throughout the rest of their living days. Dr. Polonsky explains that the well meaning "police officers" may be family member, coworkers, supervisors, even children who are constantly looking over the shoulder of the sugared soul trying to catch a glimpse of his or her blood glucose meter reading. "Oh, my gosh," says Sargeant Perfect when she spots the "156 mg/dL" on the *diabetes criminal's* meter. "You know, you really shouldn't be eating that entire sandwich? Oh, and you really should eat more fruits and vegetables rather than those tomatoes and cottage cheese! And while we're at it, what are you going to do about that yellow toenail of yours? You don't really want to lose your foot do you?"

As physicians, we base our therapeutic interventions on "evidence-based medicine," outcome trials, and consensus panel guidelines. What we really should be doing is working toward individualizing the management goals of each patient we see. What should the priorities be in our patients' diabetes care? Should we enforce "lifestyle intervention," make certain that our patients are checking their blood glucose readings multiple times each day, and, make certain that we are carefully documenting all of our meaningful use outcome measurements?

In 2004, The Diabetes Monitor published a monograph entitled "The Importance of Diabetes Treatment and Management."[301] This document lists 74 different steps that a patient with diabetes should take in order to self-manage his or her diabetes. If one were to read this publication, there is a high probability that both the patient and his spouse would "freak out!" The Monitor suggests that patients "check feet for sores and calluses every day, wear shoes that fit properly, and get a comprehensive foot exam at least once per year with a health-care professional *since people with diabetes are at a higher risk for foot problems that can be caused by neuropathy (nerve damage) or poor blood flow to the feet.*" Really? Less than 1% of all patients in the UKPDS experienced an amputation despite having suboptimal glycemic control.[302] The number of lower extremity amputations in the United States is actually on the decline. In 1997, 65,000 patients lost a limb secondary to diabetes. In 2006 only 65,700 nontraumatic amputations were performed in the United States, but under 30,000 were actually related to diabetes.[303,304]

Although diabetes has the potential of causing devastating consequences, medical science has made tremendous advances over the past 50 years. Diabetes is no longer a death sentence for our patients. Therefore, when one is first informed of diagnosis, the patient should be reassured, "Don't freak out!" In reality, patients and providers should focus on five primary goals in order to assure success in diabetes management (Table10-28).

TABLE 10-28 The Top 5 Goals for Managing Diabetes in Primary Care

1. Know your "numbers"

2. Understand how best to achieve your targeted numbers

3. Stop smoking

4. Take your prescribed medications

5. Obtain medical care from people well trained in diabetes and the chronic disease state model

("Diabetes top 5 goals" provided courtesy of Bill Polonsky, CDE, PhD.)

The goals of therapy for managing T2DM include controlling hyperglycemia, helping patients achieve treatment goals, preventing disease progression, preserving β-cell function and mass, avoiding hypoglycemia, and minimizing patients' risk for developing long-term complications. Lifestyle interventions, including dietary counseling, physical activity, and self–blood glucose monitoring, remain the foundation of diabetes care. Pharmacotherapy plays an essential role in slowing disease progression, minimizing symptomatology, and improving quality of life. The ADA suggests that the A1C target for *most* individuals with diabetes is ≤ 7%. Clinicians should not delay initiating or intensifying drug therapy in patients who demonstrate deterioration in A1C levels. Drugs should be chosen based on their proven durability as well as their likelihood of inducing hypoglycemia and weight gain. Knowledge about the pathophysiology of the disease process should always guide our prescribing of appropriate medications.

Patients with T2DM have a risk of death from cardiovascular disease that is two to six times higher than euglycemic individuals.[305] Failure to address and correct modifiable risk factors such as hyperglycemia, hypertension and dyslipidemia will increase the risk of poor outcomes in patients with T2DM.[306] The Steno-2 Study compared the effect of an intensified, multifactorial intervention to that of conventional treatment on hyperglycemia, hypertension and dyslipidemia in patients with T2DM and microalbuminuria over 7.8 years.[307] Eighty patients were assigned to receive conventional care based on recommendations established in 1988 by the Danish Medical Association. These recommendations were subsequently revised in 2000 requiring revision of the initial protocol (see Table10-29). Eighty patients were randomized to undergo intensive multifactorial intervention

TABLE 10-29 STENO Treatment Goals for the Conventional and Intensive Therapy Cohorts

Conventional Cohort			Intensive Cohort	
Variable	1993–1999	2000–2001	1993–1999	2000–2001
Systolic BP (mm Hg)	<160	<135	<140	<130
Diastolic BP (mm Hg)	<95	<85	<85	<80
A1C (%)	<7.5	<6.5	<6.5	<6.5
Fasting total cholesterol (mg/dL)	<250	<190	<190	<175
Fasting triglycerides mg/dL	<195	<180	<150	<150
Aspirin therapy for patients with known ischemia	Yes	Yes	Yes	Yes
Aspirin therapy for patients with peripheral vascular disease	No	No	Yes	Yes
Aspirin therapy for patients with CAD or peripheral vascular disease	No	No	No	Yes
Treatment with ACE irrespective of blood pressure	No	Yes	Yes	Yes

Adapted from Gaede P, et al. *N Engl J Med.* 2003;348:383–393.

targeting strict treatment goals as noted in Table 10-29. Lifestyle intervention as well as intensive stepwise pharmacologic therapy was introduced and titrated as needed to guide patients toward their desired metabolic goals. Intensive modification of all risk factors resulted in an absolute reduction of all microvascular and macrovascular events by 50% over 8 years.

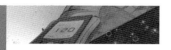

SUMMARY

Effective treatment of T2DM requires early initiation of appropriate therapies, frequent monitoring, and reassessment to make certain that therapeutic goals are being attained. T2DM is a progressive disease. Exposure to chronic hyperglycemia can cause macrovascular and microvascular complications, many of which may already be apparent when a patient is initially diagnosed as having T2DM. Multiple defective metabolic pathways work to overcome the body's defensive mechanisms, resulting in loss of β-cell function and mass. One by one other hormonal infrastructures fail resulting in significant fasting and postprandial hyperglycemia.

PCPs, as a group, manage over 90% of all patients who have T2DM. As such, we must have a better understanding of our role as patient educators, advocates, and medical providers for patients suffering from this complex metabolic disease state. We must never forget that simply achieving an A1C of "close to 7%" is not considered acceptable. Care should be individualized and must incorporate therapies that are safe and efficacious. The risks of hypoglycemia and weight gain should be addressed prior to prescribing any agents to patients with T2DM. With 11 different approved classes of agents at our disposal for use in patients with T2DM, PCPs have the tools they need to guide their patients toward successful diabetes management.

Specialists and PCPs intensify diabetes management in different ways.[308] Although PCPs are not afraid to add a second or third oral agent to a patient's treatment regimen, diabetes specialists are aggressive with insulin management. Patients with an A1C greater than 8.5% are five times more likely to be placed on insulin by a specialist than by a PCP. Patients who consult specialists for poorly controlled diabetes are more likely to be successfully managed to a targeted A1C by the specialist than by the primary care provider.[309] However, fewer than 50% of patients with poor glycemic control receive intensification of their glucose-lowering regimen by either specialists or a PCP. By familiarizing themselves with the ADA and AACE clinical practice guidelines, PCPs may also become more successful in treating patients to target, rather than having them struggle through long periods of failure.

Management of patients with T2DM should combine lifestyle intervention with pharmacotherapy. Intervention should be aggressive to minimize β-cell apoptosis in the short term and reduce the long-term risk of diabetes-related complications. As most patients with T2DM will eventually require insulin therapy, physicians should not hesitate to discuss this possibility during the early stages of the disease. Doing so will likely make the transition from oral agents to injectable therapy more acceptable to the patient.

While most guidelines agree that lifestyle modifications and metformin are first line in the management of T2DM, there is widespread disagreement about subsequent steps in the escalation of medical therapy. Although sulfonylureas are less expensive than other agents, they tend to favor weight gain, hypoglycemia, and have limited durability. Sulfonylureas are not β-cell friendly by any means and may have a negative effect on cardiovascular outcomes. Therefore, one should consider using drugs such as GLP-1 agonists for patients who are overweight and have baseline A1C levels greater than 1.2% above their recommended target. DPP-4 inhibitors are weight neutral and like the GLP-1 agonists favor β-cell preservation. The DPP-4 inhibitors allow a physiologic rise in the endogenous level of native GLP-1, whereas the more powerful pharmacologic actions associated with injectable GLP-agonists provide more potent effects such as weight and A1C reduction. However, because the GLP-1 agonists result in greater receptor site binding than DPP-4 inhibition, their side effect profile might be problematic in some patients.

Pioglitazone has been shown to preserve β-cell cell function, reduce vascular inflammation, and improve lipid parameters. However, recent postmarketing data suggest that long-term use of pioglitazone in women may result in an increased risk of bone fractures. The FDA has also warned of a potential increased risk of bladder cancer in patients using pioglitazone for more than one year. Thus, prolonged use of this class of drug is suspect at this time.

T2DM patients with elevated triglycerides and multiple cardiovascular risks may consider using the bromocriptine D2 agonist. To date cycloset is the only drug that has received FDA approval for cardiovascular risk reduction in patients with T2DM.

Patients with significant hyperglycemia at the time of diagnosis (A1C greater than 9%) should be initiated on intensive insulin therapy as will be discussed in Chapter 12 in order to eliminate glucose toxicity and restore any endogenous β-cell insulin production and peripheral insulin sensitivity. On occasion, sustained remission of T2DM will be attainable for several months following the termination of intensive insulin therapy.[21,22]

Patients suspected of having monogenetic diabetes should be tested for the specific defect that may be responsible for their metabolic dysfunction. Many patients with monogenetic diabetes may be managed with sulfonylureas and lifestyle interventions.

Metabolic surgery is offered to less than 1% of all patients who suffer from clinically severe obesity. Gastric bypass and lap-banding surgical intervention offered to the appropriate patients may result in remission of diabetes.

REFERENCES

1. CDC National Diabetes Fact Sheet, 2011. http://www.cdc.gov/diabetes/pubs/pdf/ndfs_2011.pdf. Accessed February 17, 2012.
2. Unger J. Intensive management of type 2 diabetes. *Emerg Med.* 2001;33:28–43.
3. American Diabetes Association. Standards of medical care in diabetes—2012. *Diabetes Care.* 2012;35(suppl 1):S13–S14.
4. Kahn R, Alpern P, Borch-Johnsen K, et al. Age at initiation and frequency of screening to detect T2DM: a cost-effectiveness analysis. *Lancet.* 2010;375:1365–1374.
5. Trogdon JG, Hylands T. Nationally representative medical costs of diabetes b time since diagnosis. *Diabetes Care.* 2008;31(12):2307–2311.
6. Medco Health Solutions, Inc. Drug Trend Report. http://www.medcohealth.com/art/drug_ trend/pdf/DT_Report_2008.pdf. Accessed March 9, 2012.
7. Piette JD, Heisler M, Wagner TH. Problems paying out-of-pocket medication costs among older adults with diabetes. *Diabetes Care.* 2004;27:384–391.
8. Cramer JA. A systematic review of adherence with medications for diabetes. *Diabetes Care.* 2004;27:1218–1224.
9. American Heart Association. Statistics you need to know: statistics on medication. http://www. americanheart.org/presenter.jhtml?identifier= 107. Accessed March 9, 2012.
10. Osterberg L, Blaschke T. Adherence to medication. *N Engl J Med.* 2005;353:487–497.
11. International Expert Committee: International Expert Committee report on the role of the A1C assay in the diagnosis of diabetes. *Diabetes Care.* 2009;32:1327–1334.
12. Hu FB, Manson JE, Stampfer MJ. Diet, lifestyle, and the risk of type 2 diabetes in women. *N Engl J Med.* 2001;345:790–797.
13. Hedley AA, Ogden CI, Johnson CL. Prevalence of overweight and obesity among U.S. children, adolescents, and adults, 1999–2002. *JAMA.* 2004;291:2847–2850.

14. Tuomilehto J, Linstrom J, Eriksson JG. Prevention of type 2 diabetes mellitus by changes in lifestyle among subjects with impaired glucose tolerance. *N Engl J Med.* 2001;344:1343–1350.

15. Pan XR, Li GW, Hu YH. Effects of diet and exercise in preventing NIDDM in people with impaired glucose tolerance: the Da Qing IGT and Diabetes Study. *Diabetes Care.* 1997;20:537–544.

16. Knowler WC, Barrett-Connor E, Fowler SE, et al.; and the Diabetes Prevention Program Research Group. Reduction in the incidence of type 2 diabetes with lifestyle intervention or metformin. *N Engl J Med.* 2002;346:393–403.

17. Diabetes Prevention Program Research Group. 10-year follow-up of diabetes incidence and weight loss in the Diabetes Prefvention Program Outcomes Study. *Lancet.* 2009;374(9702):1677–1686.

18. Kahn SE, Haffner SM, Heise MA, et al.; ADOPT Study Group. Glycemic durability of rosiglitazone, metformin or glyburide monotherapy. *N Engl J Med.* 2006;355:2427–2443.

19. Ivy JL, Zderic TW, Fogt DL. Prevention and treatment of non-insulin dependent diabetes mellitus. *Exerc Sport Sci Rev.* 1999;27:1–35.

20. Kriska AM, Saremi A, Hanson RL. Physical activity, obesity, and the incidence of type 2 diabetes in a high risk population. *Am J Epidemiol.* 2003;158:669–675.

21. Weng J, Li Y, Xu W, et al. Effect of intensive insulin therapy on beta cell function and glycaemic control in patients with newly diagnosed T2DM: a multicentre randomised parallel-group trial. *Lancet.* 2008;371:1753–1760.

22. Li Y, Xu W, Liao Z, et al. Induction of long-term glycemic control in newly diagnosed type 2 diabetic patients is associated with improvement of beta cell function. *Diabetes Care.* 2004;27:2597–2602.

23. Mykkanen L, Haffner SM, Kuusisto J, et al. Serum proinsulin levels are disproportionately increased in elderly prediabetic subjects. *Diabetologia.* 1995;38(10):1176–1182.

24. Schernthaner G, Morton JM. Bariatric surgery in patients with morbid obesity and type 2 diabetetes. *Diabetes Care.* 2008;31(suppl 2):S297–S302.

25. Rubino F, Gagner M. Potential of surgery for curing T2DM. *Ann Surg.* 2002;236:554–559.

26. McTigue K, Larson JC, Valoski A, et al. Mortality and cardiac and vascular outcomes in extremely obese women. *JAMA.* 2006;296:79–86.

27. Leibson CL, Williamson DF, Melton LJ III, et al: Temporal trends in BMI among adults with diabetes. *Diabetes Care.* 2001;24:1584–1589.

28. Chan JM, Rimm EB, Colditz GA et al. Obesity, fat distribution, and weight gain as risk factors for clinical diabetes in men. *Diabetes Care.* 1994;17:961–969.

29. Perreault L, Kahn SE, Christophi CA, et al. Regression from pre-diabetes to normal glucose regulation in the diabetes prevention program. *Diabetes Care.* 2009;32(9):1583–1588.

30. O'Brien PE, Dixon JB, Laurie C, et al. Treatment of mild to moderate obesity with laparoscopic adjustable gastric banding or an intensive medical program: a randomized trial. *Ann Intern Med.* 2006;144:625–633.

31. Anderson JW, Grant L, Gotthelf L, et al. Weight loss and long-term follow-up of severely obese individuals treated with an intense behavioral program. *Int J Obes.* 2006;31:488–493.

32. Schernthaner G, Brix J, Kopp Hans-Peter, et al. Cure of T2DM by metabolic surgery? A critical analysis of the evidence in 2010. *Diabetes Care.* 2011;34(suppl 2):S355–S360.

33. Rosa G, Mingrone G, Manco M, et al. Molecular mechanisms of diabetes reversibility after bariatric surgery. *Int J Obes (Lond).* 2007;31:1429–1436.

34. Pories WJ, Swanson MS, MacDonald KG, et al. Who would have thought it? An operation proves to be the most effective therapy for adult-onset diabetes mellitus. *Ann Surg.* 1995;222:339–350.

35. Camastra S, Manco M, Mari A, et al. Beta cell function in morbidly obese subjects during free living: long-term effects of weight loss. *Diabetes* 2005;54:2382–2389. NOW 32 SCHERN.

36. Mechanick JI, Kushner RF, Sugerman HJ, et al. American Association of Clinical Endocrinologists,the Obesity Society and American Society for Metabolic and Metabolic surgery Medical Guidelines for Clinical Practice for the Perioperative, Nutritional, Metabolic and Nonsurgical support of the Metabolic surgery Patient. *Endocr Pract.* 2008;14(suppl 1):1–83.

37. Buchwald H, Estok R, Fahrbach K, et al. Weight and T2DM after metabolic surgery: systematic review and meta-analysis. *Am J Med.* 2009;122:248–256.

38. Tice JA, Karliner L, Walsh J, et al. Gastric banding or bypass? A systematic review comparing the two most popular bariatric procedures. *Am J Med.* 2008;121:885–893.

39. Chapman AE, Kiroff G, Game P, et al. Laparoscopic adjustable gastric banding in the treatment of obesity: a systematic literature review. *Surgery.* 2004;135(3):326–351.

40. Keidar A. Metabolic surgery for T2DM reversal: the risks. *Diabetes Care.* 2011;34(suppl 2):S361–S366.

41. Pories WJ, MacDonald KG Jr, Morgan EJ, et al. Surgical treatment of obesity and its effect on diabetes: 10-y follow-up. *Am J Clin Nutr.* 1992;55(2 suppl):582S–585S

42. Vigneri P, Frasca F, Sciacca L, et al. Diabetes and cancer. *Endocr Relat Cancer.* 2009;16:1103–1123.

43. Sjöström L, Gummesson A, Sjöström CD, et al. Swedish Obese Subjects Study. Effects of metabolic surgery on cancer incidence in obese patients in Sweden (Swedish Obese Subjects Study): a prospective, controlled intervention trial. *Lancet Oncol.* 2009;10:653–662.

44. Hoerger TJ, Zhang P, Segel JE, et al. Cost-effectiveness of metabolic surgery for severely obese adults with diabetes diabetes care. *Diabetes Care* 2010;33:1933–1939.

45. Bult MJ, van Dalen T, Muller AF. Surgical treatment of obesity. *Eur J Endocrinol.* 2008;158(2):135–145.

46. Schauer P, Ikramuddin S, Hamad G, et al. The learning curve for laparoscopic Roux-en-Y gastric bypass is 100 cases. *Surg Endosc.* 2003;17:212–215.

47. Flum DR, Belle SH, King WC, et al. Perioperative safety in the longitudinal assessment of metabolic surgery. *N Engl J Med.* 2009;361(5):445–454.

48. Nguyen NT, Paya M, Stevens CM, et al. The relationship between hospital volume and outcome in metabolic surgery at academic medical centers. *Ann Surg.* 2004;240:586–593.

49. Weller WE, Hannan EL. Relationship between provider volume and postoperative complications for bariatric procedures in New York State. *J Am Coll Surg.* 2006;202:753–761.

50. Parikh MS, Laker S, Weiner M, et al. Objective comparison of complications resulting from laparoscopic bariatric procedures. *J Am Coll Surg.* 2006;202(2):252–261.

50a. Flum DR, Belle SH, King WC, et al. Longitudinal Assessment of Metabolic surgery (LAMS) Consortium. Perioperative safety in the longitudinal assessment of bariatric. *N Engl J Med.* 2009;361(5):445–454.

51. Laferre're B, Teixeira J, McGinty J, et al. Effect of weight loss by gastric bypass surgery versus hypocaloric diet on glucose and incretin levels in patients with T2DM. *J Clin Endocrinol Metab.* 2008;93:2479–2485.

52. Service GJ, Thompson GB, Service FJ, et al. Hyperinsulinemic hypoglycemia with nesidioblastosis after gastric-bypass surgery. *N Engl J Med.* 2005;353:249–254.

53. le Roux CW., Aylwin SJ, Batterham RL, et al. Gut hormone profiles following metabolic surgery favour an anorectic state, facilitate weight loss, and improve metabolic parameters. *Ann Surg.* 2006;243 108–114.

54. Dixon JB, O'Brien PE. Health outcomes of severely obese type 2 diabetic subjects 1 year after laparoscopic adjustable gastric banding. *Diabetes Care.* 2002;25:358–363.

55. Dixon JB, Dixon AF, O'Brien PE. Improvements in insulin sensitivity and beta cell function (HOMA) with weight loss in the severely obese: homeostatic model assessment. *Diabet Med.* 2003;20:127–34.

55a. Mingrone G, Panunzi S, De Gaetano A, et al. Bariatric surgery versus conventional medical therapy for type 2 diabetes. *N Engl J Med.* 2012;366:1577–1585.

55b. Schauer PR, Sangeeta R, Kashyap MD, et al. Bariatric surgery versus intensive medical therapy in obese patients with diabetes. *N Engl J Med.* 2012;366:1567–1576.

55c. Dixon JB, Zimmet P, Alberti KG, et al. Bariatric surgery: an IDF statement for obese type 2 diabetes. *Diabet Med.* 2011;28:628–642.

56. UK Prospective Diabetes Study (UKPDS) Group. Intensive blood-glucose control with sulphonylureas or insulin compared with conventional treatment and risk of complications in patients with type 2 diabetes (UKPDS 33). *Lancet.* 1998;352:837–853. Erratum in: *Lancet* 1999;14;354:602.

57. Abdul-Ghani M, Tripathy D, DeFronzo RA. Contributions of beta cell dysfunction and insulin resistance to the pathogenesis of impaired glucose tolerance and impaired fasting glucose. *Diabetes Care.* 2006;29:1130–1139.

58. Butler AE, Janson J, Bonner-Weir S, et al. Beta cell deficit and increased beta cell apoptosis in humans with T2DM. *Diabetes.* 2003;52(1):102–110.

59. Diabetes Prevention Program Research Group. The prevalence of retinopathy in impaired glucoe tolerance and recent-onset diabetes I the Diabetes Prevention Program. *Diabet Med.* 2007;24:137–144.

60. DeFronzo RA. From the triumvirate to the ominous octet: a new paradigm for the treatment of type 2 diabetes mellitus. *Diabetes.* 2009;773-795.

61. Chang AM, Halter JB. Aging and insulin secretion. *Am J Physiol Endocrinol Metab.* 2003;284: E7–E12.

62. Holick MF. Vitamin D deficiency. *N Engl J Med.* 2007;357:266–281.

63. Bland R, Markovic D, et al. Expression of 25-hydroxyvitamin D3-1 alpha hydroxylase in pancreatic islets. *J Steroid Biochem Mol Biol.* 2004;89–90:121–125.

64. Hewison M, Zehnder D, Bland R, et al. 1 Alpha-hydroxylase and the action of vitamin D. *J Mol Endocrinol.* 2000;25:141–148.

65. Barengolts E. Vitamin D role and use in prediabetes. *Endocr Pract.* 2010;16(3):476–485.

66. Pittas AG, Dawson-Hughes B, Li T, et al. Vitamin D and calcium intake in relation to T2DM in women. *Diabetes Care.* 2006;29(3):650–656.

67. Malecki MT, Klupa T, Wolkow P, et al. Association study of the vitamin D: 1 Alpha-hydroxylase (CYP1alpha) gene and type 2 diabetes mellitus in a Polish population. *Diabetes Metab.* 2003;29:119–124.

68. Thomas GN, Scragg R, Jiang CQ, et al. Hyperglycaemia and vitamin D: a systematic overview. *Curr Diabetes Rev.* 2012;8(1):18–31.

69. Unger J. Reducing oxidative stress in patients with T2DM mellitus: a primary care call to action. *Insulin.* 2008;3:176–184.

70. Leahy JL, Cooper HE, Weir GC. Impaired insulin secretion associated with near normoglycemia: study in normal rats with 96-h in vivo glucose infusions. Diabetes 1987;36:459–464.

71. Kosaka K, Kuzuya T, Hagura R, et al. Insulin response to oral glucose load is consistently decreased in established non-insulin-dependent diabetes mellitus: the usefulness of decreased early insulin response as a predictor of non-insulin-dependent diabetes mellitus. *Diabetes Med.* 1996;13:S109–S119.

72. Leahy JL, Bonner-Weir S, Weir GC. Beta-cell dysfunction induced by chronic hyperglycemia: current ideas on mechanism of impaired glucose-induced insulin secretion. *Diabetes Care.* 1992;15:442–455.

73. Del Prato S, Leoanetti F, Simonson DC, et al. Effect of sustained physiologic hyperinsulinaemia and hyperglycaemia on insulin secretion and insulin sensitivity in man. *Diabetologia.* 1994;37:1025–1035.

74. Arner P. Insulin resistance in T2DM: role of fatty acids. *Diabetes Metab Res Rev.* 2002;18(suppl 2):S5–S9.

75. Saltiel AR, Kahn CR. Insulin signaling and the regulation of glucose and lipid metabolism. *Nature.* 2001;414:799–806.

76. Lee Y, Hirosel T, Ohneda M, et al. Beta cell lipotoxicity of non-insulin dependent diabetes mellitus of obese rats: impairment in adipocyte-beta cell relationships. *Proc Natl Acad Sci U S A.* 1994;91:10878–10882.

77. Shimabukuro M, Ohneda M, Lee Y, et al. Role of nitric oxide in obesity-induced beta cell disease. *J Clin Invest.* 1991;100:290–295.

78. Gremlich S, Bonny C, Waeber G, et al. Fatty acids decrease IDX-1 expression in rat pancreatic islets and reduce GLUT2, glucokinase insulin and somatostatin levels. *J Biol Chem.* 1997;272:30261–30269.

79. Paolisso G, Tataranni PA, Foley JE, et al. A high concentration of fasting plasma non-esterified fatty acids is a risk factor for the development of T2DM. *Diabetologia.* 1995.38:1213–1217.

80. Charles MA, Eschwege E, Thibult N, et al. The role of non-esterified fatty acids in the deterioration of glucose tolerance in caucasian subjects: results of the Paris Prospective study. *Diabetologia* 1997;40:1101–1106.

81. Arner P: Free fatty acids: do they play a central role in T2DM? *Diabetes Obes Metab.* 2001;3(suppl 1)11–19.

82. Després J-P. Abdominal obesity as an important component of insulin resistance syndrome. *Nutrition.* 1993;9:452–459.

83. Ruderman N, Chrisholm D, Pi-Sunnyer FX, et al. The metabolically obese, normal-weight-weight individual revisited. *Diabetes.* 1998;47:699–713.

84. Oseid K, Cotrell DA, Orabella MM. Insulin sensitivity, glucose effectiveness and body fat distribution pattern un nondiabetic offspring of patients with NIDDM. *Diabetes Care.* 1991;14:890–896.

85. Ross R. Effects of diet-and exercise-induced weight loss on visceral adipose tissue in men and women. *Sports Med.* 1997;24:55–64.

86. Groop LC, Bonadonna RC, Del Prato S, et al. Glucose and free fatty acid metabolism in non-insulin dependent diabetes mellitus: evidence for multiple sites of insulin resistance. *J Clin Invest.* 1989;84: 205–215.

87. DeFronzo RA, Ferrannini E, Simonson DC. Fasting hyperglycemia in non-insulin-dependent diabetes mellitus: contributions of excessive hepatic glucose production and impaired tissue glucose uptake. *Metabolism.* 1989;38(4):387–395.

88. Caro JF, Sinha MK, Raju SM, et al. IR kinase in human skeletal muscle from obese subjects with and without noninsulin dependent diabetes. *J Clin Invest.* 1987;79:1330–1337.

89. Paz K, Hemi R, LeRoith D, et al. A molecular basis for insulin resistance: elevated serine/threonine phosphorylation of IRS-1 and IRS-2 inhibits their binding to the juxtamembrane region of the insulin receptor and impairs their ability to undergo insulin-induced tyrosine phosphorylation. *J Biol Chem.* 1997;272:29911–29918.

90. Laws A, Reaven GM. Evidence for an independent relationship between insulin resistance and fasting plasma HDL-cholesterol, triglyceride and insulin concentrations. *J Intern Med.* 1992;231:25–30.

91. Matsuda M, DeFronzo RA, Glass L, et al. Glucagon dose response curve for hepatic glucose production and glucose disposal in type 2 diabetic patients and normal individuals. *Metabolism.* 2002;51:1111–1119.

92. Guyton JR, Hall JE. Insulin, glucagon, and diabetes mellitus. In: Guyton JR, Hall JE, eds. *Textbook of Medical Physiology.* Philadelphia, PA: Elsevier Saunders; 2006:961–977.

93. Triplitt C, DeFronzo RA. Exenatide: first in class incretin mimetic for the treatment of T2DM mellitus. *Expert Rev Endocrinol Metab.* 2006;1:329–341.

94. Unger J. Incretins: Clinical perspectives, relevance, and applications for the primary care physician in the treatment of patients with T2DM. *Mayo Clin Proc.* 2010;85(12 suppl):S38–S49.

95. Kielgast U, Holst JJ, Madsbad S. Treatment of type 1 diabetic patients with glucagon-like peptide-1(GLP-1) and GLP-1R agonists. *Curr Diabetes Rev.* 2009;5:266–275.

96. Weiss R, D'Adamo E, Santoro N, et al. Basal alpha-cell up-regulation in obese insulin-resistant adolescents. *J Clin Endocrinol Metab.* 2011;96(1):91–97.

97. Nauck M, Stockmann F, Ebert R, et al. Reduced incretin effect in type 2 (non-insulin-dependent) diabetes. *Diabetologia.* 1986;29(1):46–52.

98. Drucker DJ, Sherman SI, Gorelick FS, et al. Incretin-based therapies for the treatment of T2DM: evaluation of the risks and benefits. *Diabetes Care.* 2010;33:428–433.

99. Pratley R. GIP: An inconsequential incretin or not? *Diabetes Care.* 2010;33(7):1691–1692.

100. Russell-Jones D. Molecular, pharmacological and clinical aspects of liraglutide, a once-daily human GLP-1 analogue. *Mol Cell Endocrinol.* 2009;297:137–140.

101. Sathananthan A, Man CD, Micheletto F, et al. Common genetic variation in GLPIR and insulin secretion in response to exogenous GLP-1 in nondiabetic subjects: a pilot study. *Diabetes Care.* 2010;33(9):2123–2125.

102. Tahrani AA, Barnett AH. Dapagliflozin: a sodium glucose cotransporter 2 inhibitor in development for T2DM. *Diabetes Ther.* 2010;1(2):45–56.

103. Wright EM. Renal Na(+)-glucose cotransporters. *Am J Physiol Renal Physiol.* 2001;280:F10–F18.

104. Sandoval DA, Bagnol D, Woods SC, et al. Arcuate glucagon-like peptide 1 receptors regulate glucose homeostasis but not food intake. *Diabetes.* 2008;57:2046–2054.

105. Sandoval DA, Bagnol D, Woods SC, et al. Arcuate glucagon-like peptide 1 receptors regulate glucose homeostasis but not food intake. Diabetes 2008:57:2046–2054.

106. Sandoval DA, Bagnol D, Woods SC, et al. Arcuate glucagon-like peptide 1 receptors regulate glucose homeostasis but not food intake. Diabetes 2008:57:2046–2054.

107. Matsuda M, Liu Y, Mahankali S, et al. Altered hypothalamic function in response to glucose ingestion in obese humans. *Diabetes* 1999;48:1801–1806.

108. Saltiel AR, Kahn CR. Insulin signaling and the regulation of glucose and lipid metabolism. *Nature.* 2001;414:799–806.

109. Barnett AH, Eff C, Leslie RD, et al. Diabetes in identical twins: a study of 200 pairs. *Diabetologia.* 1981;20:87.

110. Bennett PH. Epidemiology of diabetes mellitus. In: Rifkin H, Porte D Jr, eds. *Ellenberg and Rifkin's Diabetes Mellitus.* New York: Elsevier;1990:363.

111. Eriksson J, Franssila-Kallunki A, Ekstrand A, et al. Early metabolic defects in persons at increased risk for non-insulin-dependent diabetes mellitus. *N Engl J Med.* 1989;321:337.

112. Knowles NG, Landchild MA, Fujimoto WY, et al. Insulin and amylin release are both diminished in first-degree relatives of subjects with type 2 diabetes. *Diabetes Care.* 2002;25:292.

113. http://projects.exeter.ac.uk/diabetesgenes/rarediabetes/index.htm. Accessed May 30, 2011.

114. Fajans SS, Bell GI, Polonsky KS. Molecular mechanisms and clinical pathophysiology of maturity-onset diabetes of the young. *N Engl J Med* 2001;345:971–980.

115. Fajans SS, Bell GI. MODY. History, genetics, pathophysiology and clinical decision making. *Diabetes Care.* 2011;34;1878–1884.

116. Froguel P, Zouali H, Vionnet N, et al. Familial hyperglycemia due to mutations in glucokinase: definition of a subtype of diabetes mellitus. *N Engl J Med.* 1993 328:697–702.

117. Polonsky K, Sturis J, Bell G. Noninsulin-dependent diabetes mellitus: a genetically programmed failure of the beta cell to compensate for insulin resistance. *N Engl J Med.* 1996.334:777–783.

118. Unger RH. Reinventing T2DM: pathogenesis, treatment, and prevention. *JAMA.* 2008;299:1185–1187.

119. Pearson ER, Liddell WG, Shepherd M, et al. Sensitivity to sulphonylureas in patients with hepatocyte nuclear factor-1alpha gene mutations: evidence for pharmacogenetics in diabetes. *Diabet Med.* 2000;17:543–545.

120. Tuomi T, Honkanen EH, Isomaa B, et al. Improved prandial glucose control with lower risk of hypoglycemia with nateglinide than glibenclamide in patients with maturity–onset diabetes of the young. *Diabetes Care.* 2006;29:189–194.

121. Matschinsky FM, Zelent B, Doliba N, et al. Glucokinase activators for diabetes therapy. May 2010 status report. *Diabetes Care.* 2011;34(suppl 2):S236–S243.

122. Doliba N, Qin W, Najafi H, et al. Piragliatin, an allosteric activator of glucokinase, increases glucose-induced respiration and insulin release of pancreatic islets from type 2 diabetics. *Poster presented at University of Pennsylvania IDOM/DERC Spring Symposium*, March 10, 2010.

123. Grimsby J, Sarabu R, Corbett WL, et al. Allosteric activators of glucokinase: potential role in diabetes therapy. *Science*. 2003;301:370–373.

124. Lumb AN, Gallen IW. Treatment of HNF1-alpha MODY with the DPP-4 inhibitor Sitagliptin. *Diabet Med*. 2009;26:189–190.

125. Ahluwalia R, Perkins K, Ewins D, et al. Exenatide: a potential role in treatment of HNF1-alpha MODY in obese patients? *Diabet Med*. 2009;26, 827–835. *Letter to the Editor*. 835.

126. Turner RC. The U.K. prospective diabetes study: a review. *Diabetes Care*. 1998;21(suppl 3):C35–C38.

127. Alexander GC, Sehgal NL, Maloney RM, et al. National trends in treatment of type 2 diabetes mellitus, 1994–2007. *Arch Intern Med*. 2008;168(19):2088–2094.

128. Diabetes Control and Complications Trial Research Group. The effect of intensive diabetes treatment on the development and progression of long-term complications in insulin-dependent diabetes mellitus: the Diabetes Control and Complications Trial. *N Engl J Med*. 1993;329:978–986.

129. Ohkubo Y, Kishikawa H, Araki E, et al. Intensive insulin therapy prevents the progression of diabetic microvascular complications in Japanese patients with NIDDM: a randomized prospective 6-year study. *Diabetes Res Clin Pract*. 1995;28:103–117.

130. The Action to Control Cardiovascular Risk in Diabetes Study Group: Effects of intensive glucose lowering in T2DM. *N Engl J Med*. 2008;358:2545–2559.

131. Nathan DM, Buse JB, Davidson MB, et al. Diabetes: A Consensus Algorithm for the Initiation Medical Management of Hyperglycemia in Type 2 and Adjustment of Therapy: a consensus statement of the American Diabetes Association and the European Association for the Study of Diabetes. *Diabetes Care*. 2009;32:193–203.

132. Hirsch IB, Brownlee M. Beyond hemoglobin A1c: need for additional markers of risk for diabetic microvascular complications. *JAMA*. 2010;303 (22). 2291–2292.

132a. Inzucchi SE, Bergenstal RM, Buse JB, et al. Management of hyperglycaemia in type 2 diabetes: a patient-centered approach. Position statement of the American Diabetes Association (ADA) and the European Association for the Study of Diabetes (EASD). *Diabetologia*. 2012. DOI 10.1007/s00125-012-2534-0.

133. Hellman R, Regan J, Rosen F. Effect of intensive treatment of diabetes on the risk of death or renal failure in NIDDM and IDDM. *Diabetes Care*. 1997;20:258–264.

134. Nathan DM, Buse JB, Davidson MB, et al. Management of hyperglycemia in type 2 diabetes: a consensus algorithm for the initiation and adjustment of therapy. *Diabetes Care*. 2006;29:1963–1972.

134a. Riddle MC. The Treat-to-Target Trial and related studies. *Endocr Pract*. 2006;12(suppl 1):71–79.

134b. Ismail-Beigi F, Moghissi E, Tiktin M, et al. Individualizing glycemic targets in type 2 diabtes mellitus: implications of recent clinical trials. *Ann Intern Med*. 2011;154:554–559.

135. Rodbard HW, Jellinger PS, Davidson JA, et al. Statement by an American Association of Clinical Endocrinologist/American College of Endocrinology Consensus Panel on T2DM Mellitus: an algorithm for glycemic control. *Endocrine Pract*. 2009;15(6):541–559.

136. American Diabetes Association. Economic costs of diabetes in the U.S. in 2007. *Diabetes Care*. 2008;31(3):596–615.

137. Unger J, Marcus AO. Glucose control in the hospitalized patient. *Emerg Med*. 2004;12–18.

138. Wysowski DK, Armstrong G, Governale L. Rapid increase in the use of oral antidiabetic drugs in the United States, 1990–2001. *Diabetes Care*. 2003;26:1852–1855.

139. Kennedy DL, Piper JM, Baum C. Trends in use of oral hypoglycemic agents 1964–1986. *Diabetes Care*. 1988;1:558–562.

140. Doar JW, Thompson ME, Wilde CE, et al. Diet and oral antidiabetic drugs and plasma sugar and insulin levels in patients with maturity-onset diabetes mellitus. *Br Med J*. 1976;1:498–500.

141. Korytkowski M, Thomas A, Reid L, et al. Glimepiride improves both first and second phases of insulin secretion in type 2 diabetes. *Diabetes Care*. 2002;25:1607–1611.

142. Holstein A, Plaschke A, Egberts E-H. Lower incidence of severe hypoglycaemia in type 2 diabetic patients treated with glimepiride versus glibenclamide [abstract]. *Diabetologia*. 2000;43(suppl 1):A40.

143. Bugos C, Austin M, Viereck C, et al. Long-term treatment of type 2 diabetes mellitus with glimepiride is weight neutral: a meta-analysis. *Diabetes Res Clin Pract*. 2000;50(suppl 1):29–31.

144. Schade DS, Jovanovic L, Schneider J. A placebo-controlled, randomized study of glimepiride in patients with type 2 diabetes mellitus for whom diet therapy is unsuccessful. *J Clin Pharmacol*. 1998;38:636–641.

145. Simonson DC, Kourides IA, Feinglos M, et al. Efficacy, safety, and dose-response characteristics of glipizide gastrointestinal therapeutic system on glycemic control and insulin secretion in NIDDM: results of two multicenter, randomized, placebo-controlled clinical trials. *Diabetes Care*. 1997;20:597–606.

146. Kimmel B, Inzucchi SE. Oral agents for type 2 diabetes: an update. *Clin Diabetes.* 2005;23:64–76.
147. Zimmerman BR. Sulfonylureas. *Endocrinol Metab Clin North Am.* 1997;26:511–521.
158. van Staa T, Abenhaim L, Monette J. Rates of hypoglycemia in users of sulfonylureas. *J Clin Epidemiol.* 1997;50:735–741.
159. Bodmer M, Meier C, Krähenbühl S, et al. Metformin, sulfonylureas, or other antidiabetes drugs and the risk of lactic acidosis or hypoglycemia: a nested case-control analysis. *Diabetes Care.* 2008;31(11): 2086–2091.
150. Gangji AS, Cukierman T, Gerstein HC, et al. A systematic review and meta-analysis of hypoglycemia and cardiovascular events: a comparison of glyburide with other secretagogues and with insulin. *Diabetes Care.* 2007;30:389–339.
151. American Diabetes Association. Gestational diabetes mellitus. *Diabetes Care.* 2004;27(suppl 1):S88–S90.
152. Langer O, Conway DL, Berkus MD, et al. A comparison of glyburide and insulin in women with gestational diabetes mellitus. *N Engl J Med.* 2000;343:1134–1138.
153. Garratt KN, Brady PA, Hassinger NL, et al. Sulfonylurea drugs increase early mortality in patients with diabetes mellitus after direct angioplasty for acute myocardial infarction. *J Am Coll Cardiol.* 1999;33:119–124.
154. Riddle M. Editorial: sulfonylureas differ in effects on ischemic preconditioning: is it time to retire glyburide? *J Clin Endocrinol Metab.* 2003;88(2):528–530.
155. Zeller M, Danchin N, Simon D, et al. Impact of type of preadmission sulfonylureas on mortality and cardiovascular outcomes in diabetic patients with acute myocardial infarction. *J Clin Endocrinol Metab.* 2010;95:4993–5002.
156. Zoungas S, Patel A, Chalmers J, et al. Severe hypoglycemia and risks of vascular events and death. *N Engl J Med.* 2010;363;15:1410–1418.
157. The ADVANCE Collaborative Group. Intensive blood glucose control and vascular outcomes in patients with T2DM. *N Engl J Med.* 2008;358(24):2560–2570.
158. Unger J, Parkin C. Hypoglycemia in insulin-treated diabetes: a case for increased vigilance. *Postgr Med.* 2011;123(4):81–91.
159. Gerich JE, Langlois M, Noacco C, et al. Lack of glucagon response to hypoglycemia in diabetes: evidence for an intrinsic pancreatic alpha cell defect. *Science.* 1973;182(108):171–173.
160. U.K. Prospective Diabetes Study Group. Effect of intensive blood-glucose control with metformin on complications in overweight patients with T2DM (UKPDS 34). *Lancet.* 1998;352:854–865.
161. Giovannucci E, Harlan DM, Archer MC, et al. Diabetes and cancer. *Diabetes Care.* 2010;33:1674–1685.
162. Bowker SL, Yasui U, Veugelers P, et al. Glucose-lowering agents and cancer mortality rates in T2DM: assessing effects of time-varying exposure. *Diabetologia.* 2010;53:1631–1637.
163. Bowker SL, Majumdar SR, Veugelers P, et al. Increased cancer-related mortality for patients with T2DM who use sulfonylureas or insulin. *Diabetes Care.* 2006;29:254–258.
164. Yang S, So YW, Maa RCW, et al. Use of sulphonylurea and cancer in T2DM: The Hong Kong Diabetes Registry. *Diabetes Res Clin Pract.* 2010;9:343–351.
165. Hollander PA, Schwartz SL, Gatlin MR, et al. Nateglinide, but not glyburide, selectively enhances early insulin release and more effectively controls post-meal glucose excursions with less total insulin exposure [abstract]. *Diabetes.* 2000;49(suppl 1):447P.
166. Haffner SM, Stern MP, Hazuda HP, et al. Cardiovascular risk factors in confirmed prediabetic individuals: does the clock for coronary heart disease start ticking before the onset of clinical diabetes? *JAMA.* 1990;263:2893–2898.
167. Hanefeld M, Koehler C, Henkel E, et al. Post-challenge hyperglycaemia relates more strongly than fasting hyperglycaemia with carotid intima-media thickness: the RIAD Study: risk factors in impaired glucose tolerance for atherosclerosis and diabetes. *Diabetes Med.* 2000;17:835–840.
168. DECODE Study Group. Glucose tolerance and mortality: comparison of WHO and American Diabetic Association diagnostic criteria. *Lancet.* 1999;354:617–621.
169. Jovanovic L, Dailey G III, Huang WC, et al. Repaglinide in type 2 diabetes: a 24-week, fixed-dose efficacy and safety study. *J Clin Pharm.* 2000;40:49–57.
170. Horton ES, Clinkingbeard C, Gatlin M, et al. Nateglinide alone and in combination with metformin improves glycemic control by reducing mealtime glucose levels in type 2 diabetes. *Diabetes Care.* 2000;23:1660–1665.
171. Hollander PA, Schwartz SL, Gatlin MR, et al. Importance of early insulin secretion: comparison of nateglinide and glyburide in previously diet-treated patients with type 2 diabetes. *Diabetes Care.* 2001;24:983–988.

172. Hu S, Wang S, Dunning BE. Glucose-dependent and glucose-sensitizing insulinotropic effects of nateglinide: comparison to sulphonylureas and repaglinide. *Int J Exp Diabetes Res*. 2001;2:63–72.

173. Saloranta C, Guitard C, Pecher E, et al. Nateglinide improves early insulin secretion and controls postprandial glucose excursions in a prediabetic population. *Diabetes Care*. 2002;25:2141–2146.

174. Goke B, Herrmann-Rinke C. The evolving role of alpha-glucosidase inhibitors. *Diabetes Metab Rev*. 1998;14(suppl 1):S31–S38.

175. Hanefeld M, Fischer S, Schulze J, et al. Therapeutic potentials of acarbose as first-line drug in NIDDM insufficiently treated with diet alone. *Diabetes Care*. 1991;14:732–737.

176. Hotta N, Kabuta H, Sano T, et al. Long-term effect of acarbose on glycaemic control in noninsulin-dependent diabetes mellitus: a placebo-controlled double-blind study. *Diabetes Med*. 1993;10:134–138.

177. Scott R, Lintott CJ, Zimmet R, et al. Will acarbose improve the metabolic abnormalities of insulin-resistant type 2 diabetes mellitus? *Diabetes Res Clin Pract*. 1999;43:179–185.

178. van de Laar FA, Lucassen PL, Kemp J, et al. Is acarbose equivalent to tolbutamide as first treatment for newly diagnosed type 2 diabetes in general practice? A randomised controlled trial. *Diabetes Res Clin Pract*. 2004;63:57–65.

179. Chiasson JL, Josse RG, Leiter LA. The effect of acarbose on insulin sensitivity in subjects with impaired glucose tolerance. *Diabetes Care*. 1996;19:1191–1194.

180. Chiasson JL, Josse RG, Gomis R, et al. The STOP-NIDDM Trial Research Group: acarbose treatment and the risk of cardiovascular disease and hypertension in patients with impaired glucose tolerance: the STOP-NIDDM trial. *JAMA*. 2003;290:486–494.

181. Inzucchi SE, Maggs DG, Spollett GR, et al. Efficacy and metabolic effects of metformin and troglitazone in type II diabetes mellitus. *N Engl J Med*. 1998;338:867–872.

182. Iozzo P, Hallsten K, Oikonen V, et al. Effects of metformin and rosiglitazone monotherapy on insulin-mediated hepatic glucose uptake and their relation to visceral fat in type 2 diabetes. *Diabetes Care*. 2003;26:2069–2074.

183. Klip A, Leiter LA. Cellular mechanism of action of metformin. *Diabetes Care*. 1990;13:696–704.

184. Nagi D, Yudkin J. Effects of metformin on insulin resistance, risk factors for cardiovascular disease, and plasminogen activator inhibitor in NIDDM subjects. *Diabetes Care*. 1993;16:621–629.

185. DeFronzo R, Goodman A. The multicenter study group: efficacy of metformin in patients with non-insulin dependent diabetes mellitus. *N Engl J Med*. 1995;333:541–549.

186. Grant P. The effects of high- and medium-dose metformin therapy on cardiovascular risk factors in patients with type II diabetes. *Diabetes Care*. 1996;19:64–66.

187. Grant PJ. The effects of metformin on the fibrinolytic system in diabetic and non-diabetic subjects. *Diabetes Metab*. 1991;17:168–173.

188. Chu NV, Kong APS, Kim DD, et al. Differential effects of metformin and troglitazone on cardiovascular risk factors in patients with type 2 diabetes. *Diabetes Care*. 2002;25:542–549.

189. Johnson JA, Majumdar SR, Simpson SH, Toth EL. Decreased mortality associated with the use of metformin compared with sulfonylurea monotherapy in type 2 diabetes. *Diabetes Care*. 2002;25:2244–2248.

190. Nathan DM. Some answers, more controversy, from UKPDS. *Lancet*. 1998;352:832–833.

191. Garber AJ, Larsen J, Schneider SH, et al. Simultaneous glyburide/metformin therapy is superior to component monotherapy as an initial pharmacological treatment for type 2 diabetes. *Diabetes Obes Metab*. 2002;4:201–208.

192. DeFronzo RA, Goodman AM. Efficacy of metformin in patients with non-insulin-dependent diabetes mellitus. *N Engl J Med*. 1995;333:541–549.

193. Garber AJ, Duncan TG, Goodman AM, et al. Efficacy of metformin in type II diabetes: results of a double-blind, placebo-controlled, dose-response trial. *Am J Med*. 1997;103:491–497.

194. Lord JM, Flight IH, Norman RJ. Metformin in polycystic ovary syndrome: systematic review and meta-analysis. *Br Med J*. 2003;327:951–953.

195. Fujioka K, Ledger G, Stevens J, et al. Once-daily dosing of a metformin extended release (Met-XR) formulation: effects on glycemic control in patients with type 2 diabetes currently treated with metformin [abstract]. *Diabetes*. 2000;49(suppl 1):431P.

196. Misbin RI, Green L, Stadel BV, et al. Lactic acidosis in patients with diabetes treated with metformin. *N Engl J Med*. 1998;338:265–266.

197. Lalau JD, Vermersch A, Hary L, et al. T2DM in the elderly: an assessment of metformin (metformin in the elderly). *Int J Clin Pharmacol Ther Toxicol* 1990;28:329–332.

198. Lipska KJ, Bailey CJ. Use of metformin in the setting of mild-to-moderate renal insufficiency. *Diabetes Care*. 2011;34:1431–1437.

199. Landman GWE, Kleefstra N, Van Hateren KJJ, et al. Metformin associated with lower cancer mortality in T2DM. ZODIAC-16. *Diabetes Care.* 2010;33:322–326.
200. Horlen C, Malone R, Bryant B, et al. Frequency of inappropriate metformin prescriptions. *JAMA.* 2002;287:2504–2505.
201. Calabrese A, Coley K, DaPos S, et al. Evaluation of prescribing practices: risk of lactic acidosis with metformin therapy. *Arch Intern Med.* 2002;162:434–437.
202. Masoudi FA, Wang Y, Inzucchi SE, et al. Metformin and thiazolidinedione use in Medicare patients with heart failure. *JAMA.* 2003;290:81–85.
203. Bailey CJ, Turner RC. Metformin. *N Engl J Med.* 1996;334:574–579.
204. Ting RZ, Szeto CC, Chan MH, et al. Risk factors of vitamin B_{12} deficiency in patients receiving metformin. *Arch Intern Med.* 2006;166:1975–1979.
205. Spiegelman BM: PPAR-γ: adipogenic regulator and thiazolidinedione receptor. *Diabetes.* 1998;47:507–514.
206. Miyazaki Y, Mahankali A, Matsuda M, et al. Improved glycemic control and enhanced insulin sensitivity in type 2 diabetic subjects treated with pioglitazone. *Diabetes Care.* 2001;24:710–719.
207. Ikeda M, Nakahara I, Shiba Y, et al. High plasma free fatty acids decrease splanchnic glucose uptake in patients with non-insulin-dependent diabetes mellitus. *Endocr J.* 1998;45:165–173.
208. Arita Y, Kihara S, Ouchi N, et al. Paradoxical decrease of an adipose-specific protein, adiponectin, in obesity. *Biochem Biophys Res Commun.* 1999;257:79–83.
209. Yamauchi T, Kamon J, Waki H, et al. The fat derived hormone adiponectin reverses insulin resistance associated with both lipoatrophy and obesity. *Nat Med.* 2001;7:941–946.
210. Weyer C, Funahashi T, Tanaka S, et al. Hypoadiponectimia in obesity and type 2 diabetes: close association with insulin resistance and hyperinsulinemia. *J Clin Endocrinol Metab.* 2001;86:1930–1935.
211. Hotta K, Funahashi T, Arita Y, et al. Plasma concentration of a novel adipose specific protein adiponectin in type 2 diabetic patients. *Arterioscler Thromb Vasc Biol.* 2000;20:1595–1599.
212. Adams M, Montague CT, Prins JB, et al. Activators of peroxisome proliferator-activated receptor gamma have depot-specific effects on human preadipocyte differentiation. *J Clin Invest.* 1997;100:3149–3153.
213. Kruszynska YT, Mukherjee R, Jow L, et al. Skeletal muscle peroxisome proliferator-activated receptor-gamma expression in obesity and non-insulin-dependent diabetes mellitus. *J Clin Invest.* 1998;101:543–548.
214. Howard G, O'Leary DH, Zaccaro D, et al. The Insulin Resistance Atherosclerosis Study (IRAS) Investigators: insulin sensitivity and atherosclerosis. *Circulation.* 1996;93:1809–1817.
215. Ovalle F, Bell DSH. Lipoprotein effects of different thiazolidinediones in clinical practice. *Endocr Pract.* 2002;8:406–410.
216. American Diabetes Association. Standards of medical care for patients with diabetes mellitus. *Diabetes Care.* 2005;25(suppl 1):S15–S16.
217. ACTOS (pioglitazone) prescribing information. Takeda Pharmaceuticals America, Inc. Deerfield, IL. 60015. January, 2012.
218. Greenberg AS, Pittas AG. Thiazolidinediones in the treatment of type 2 diabetes. *Expert Opin Pharmacother.* 2002;3:529–540.
219. Nesto RW, Bell D, Bonow RO, et al. Thiazolidinedione use, fluid retention, and congestive heart failure: a consensus statement from the American Heart Association and American Diabetes Association. *Circulation.* 2003;108:2941–2948.
220. Simonson DC. Etiology and prevalence of hypertension in diabetic patients. *Diabetes Care.* 1988;11:821–827.
221. Füllert S, Schneider F, Haak E, et al. Effects of pioglitazone in non-diabetic patients with arterial hypertension: a double-blind, placebo-controlled study. *J Clin Endocrinol Metab.* 2002;87:5503–5506.
222. Bruno G, Cavallo-Perin P, Bargero G, et al. Association of fibrinogen with glycemic control and albumin excretion rate in patients with non-insulin dependent diabetes mellitus. *Ann Intern Med.* 1996;125:653–657.
223. Freed M, Fuell D, Menci L, et al. Effect of combination therapy with rosiglitazone and glibenclamide on PAI-1 antigen, PAI-1 activity and tPA in patients with type 2 diabetes (abstract). *Diabetoliogia.* 2000;43(suppl 1):A267.
224. Mohanty P, Aljada A, Ghanim H, et al. Rosiglitazone imporves vascular reactivity, inhibits reactive oxygen species (ROS)f generation, reduces p47phox subunit expression in mononuclear cells (MNC) and reduces C-reactive protein (CRP) and monocyte chemotactic protein-1 (MCP-1): evidence of a potent anti-inflammatory evvect (abstract). *Diabetes.* 2001;50(suppl 2):A68.
225. Nash DT. Insulin resistance, ADMA levels, and cardiovascular disease. *JAMA.* 2002;287:1451–1452.
226. Defronzo R. Pharmacological therapy for type 2 diabetes mellitus. *Ann Intern Med.* 1999; 131:281–303.

227. Buchanan TA, Xiang AH, Peters RK. Preservation of pancreatic beta-cell function and prevention of type 2 diabetes by pharmacological treatment of insulin resistance in high-risk Hispanic women. *Diabetes.* 2002;46:701–710.

228. Schwartz AV. TZDs and bone: a review of the recent clinical evidence. *PPAR Res.* Vol. 2008. doi:10.1155/2008/297893. Article ID 297893, 6 pages.

229. Schwartz AV. Diabetes, TZDs, and bone: a review of the PPAR clinical evidence Research. *PPAR Res.* Vol. 2006, Article ID 24502. 6 pages.

230. Takeda, Observation of an increased incidence of fractures in female patients who received long-term treatment with ACTOS (pioglitazone HCl) tablets for T2DM mellitus. (Letter to Health Care Providers), March 2007, http:// www.fda.gov/medwatch/safety/2007/Actosmar0807.pdf

231. Grey A, Bolland M, Gamble G, et al. The peroxisome proliferator-activated receptor-γ agonist rosiglitazone decreases bone formation and bone mineral density in healthy postmenopausal women: a randomized, controlled trial. *J Clin Endocrinol Metab.* 2007;92(4):1305–1310.

232. Glintborg D, Andersen M, Hagen C, et al. Association of pioglitazone treatment with decreased bone mineral density in obese premenopausal patients with polycystic ovary syndrome: a randomized, placebo-controlled trial. *J Clin Endocrinol Metab.* 2008;93(5):1696–1701.

233. Dormandy J, Bhattacharya M, van Troostenburg de Bruyn AR. Safety and tolerability of pioglitazone in high-risk patients with T2DM: an overview of data from PROactive. *Drug Saf.* 2009;32:187–202.

234. U.S. Food and Drug Administration. FDA drug safety communication: ongoing safety review of actos (pioglitazone) and potential increased risk of bladder cancer after two years exposure [Internet], 2010. Silver Spring, MD, U.S. Food and Drug Administration. Available from http://www.fda. gov/Drugs/DrugSafety/ucm226214.htm. Accessed June 11, 2011.

235. Agence française de sécurité sanitaire des produits de santé. Suspension de l'utilisation des médicaments contenant de la pioglitazone (Actos, Competact) [communiqué]. June 9, 2011. Available at: http://www. afssaps.fr/Infos-de-securite/Communiques-Points-presse/Suspension-de-l-utilisation-des-medicaments-contenant-de-la-pioglitazone-Actos-R-Competact-R-Communique. Accessed March 9, 2012.

236. Piccinni C, Motola D, Marchesini G, et al. Assessing the association of pioglitazone use and bladder cancer through drug adverse event reporting. *Diabetes Care.* 2011;34:1369–1371.

237. http://www.fda.gov/Drugs/DrugSafety/ucm259150.htm Accessed June 15, 2011.

238. Gaziano JM, Cincotta AH, O'Connor CM, et al. Randomized clinical trial of quickrelease bromocriptine among patients with T2DM on overall safety and cardiovascular outcomes. *Diabetes Care.* 2010;33:1503–1508.

239. DeFronzo RA. Bromocriptine: a sympatholytic, D2-dopamine agonist for the treatment of T2DM. *Diabetes Care.* 2011;34:789–794.

240. Borg MA, Sherwin RS, Borg WP, et al. Local ventromedial hypothalamus glucose perfusion blocks counterregulation during systemic hypoglycemia in awake rats. *J Clin Invest.* 1997;99:361–365.

241. Oltmans GA. Norepinephrine and dopamine levels in hypothalamic nuclei of the genetically obese mouse (ob/ob). *Brain Res.* 1983;273:369–373.

242. Luo S, Luo J, Cincotta AH, et al. Suprachiasmatic nuclei monoamine metabolism of glucose tolerant versus intolerant hamsters. *Neuroreport.* 1999;10:2073–2077.

243. Luo S, Luo J, Meier AH, et al. Dopaminergic neurotoxin administration to the area of the suprachiasmatic nuclei induces insulin resistance. *Neuroreport.* 1997;8:3495–3499.

244. Luo S, Luo J, Cincotta AH. Chronic ventromedial hypothalamic infusion of norepinephrine and serotonin promotes insulin resistance and glucose intolerance. *Neuroendocrinology.* 1999;70:460–465.

245. Bays HE, Cohen DE. Rationale and design of a prospective clinical trial program to evaluate the glucose-lowering effects of colesevelam HCl in patients with T2DM mellitus. *Curr Med Res Opin.* 2007;23: 1673–1684.

246. Suzuki T, Oba K, Igari Y, et al. Colestimide lowers plasma glucose levels and increases plasma glucagon-like PEPTIDE-1 (7-36) levels in patients with T2DM mellitus complicated by hypercholesterolemia. *J Nippon Med Sch.* 2007;74:338–343.

247. Beysen C, Deines KC, Tsang EL, et al. Colesevelam HCl improves glucose metabolism and increases plasma glucagon-like peptide 1 and glucose-dependent insulinotropic polypeptide concentrations in subjects with T2DM. *Presented at the Annual Meeting of the European Association for the Study of Diabetes.* Vienna, Austria, September 29–October 2, 2009.

248. Bays HE, Goldberg RB, Truitt KE, et al. Colesevelam hydrochloride therapy in patients with T2DM mellitus treated with metformin: glucose and lipid effects. *Arch Intern Med.* 2008;168:1975–1983.

249. Fonseca VA, Rosenstock J, Wang AC, et al. Colesevelam HCl improves glycemic control and reduces LDL cholesterol in patients with inadequately controlled T2DM on sulfonylurea-based therapy. *Diabetes Care*. 2008;31:1479–1484.

250. Goldberg RB, Fonseca VA, Truitt KE, et al. Efficacy and safety of colesevelam in patients with T2DM mellitus and inadequate glycemic control receiving insulin-based therapy. *Arch Intern Med*. 2008;168:1531–1540.

251. Welchol prescribing information. http://www.welchol.com/pdf/Welchol_PI.pdf. Accessed June 17, 2011.

252. Handelsman Y. The role of colesevelam HCl in T2DM mellitus therapy. *Postgrad Med*. 2009;121(suppl 1):19–24.

253. Handelsman Y, Abby SL, Jin X, et al. Colesevelam HCl improves fasting plasma glucose and lipid levels in patients with prediabetes. *Postgrad Med*. 2009;121:62–69.

254. Bayliss WM, Starling EH. On the causation of the so-called 'peripheral reflex secretion' of the pancreas. *Proc Royal Soc Lond[Biol]*. 1902;69:352–353.

255. Moore B, Edie ES, Abram JH. On the treatment of diabetes mellitus by acid extract of duodenal mucous membrane. *Biochem J*. 1906;1:28–38.

256. McIntyre N, Holdsworth CD, Turner DS. Intestinal factors in the control of insulin secretion. *J Clin Endocrinol Metab*. 1965;25(10):1317–1324.

257. Drucker DJ, Nauck MA. The incretin system: glucagon-like peptide-1 receptor agonists and dipeptidyl peptidase-4 inhibitors in T2DM. *Lancet*. 2006;368(9548):1696–1705.

258. Holst JJ, Vilsboll T, Deacon CF. The incretin system and its role in type 2 diabetes mellitus. *Mol Cell Endocrinol*. 2009;297:127–136.

259. Toft-Nielsen MB, Damholt MB, Madsbad S, et al. Determinants of the impaired secretion of glucagon-like peptide-1 in type 2 diabetic patients. *J Clin Endocrinol Metab*. 2001;86:3717–3723.

260. Drucker DJ. The biology of incretin hormones. *Cell Metab*. 2006;3:153–165.

261. Ahren B. DPP-4 inhibitors. *Best Pract Res Clin Endocrinol Metab*. 2007;21:517–533.

262. Davidson, JA. Incorporating incretin-based therapies into clinical practice: differences between glucagon-like peptide 1 receptor agonists and dipeptidyl peptidase 4 inhibitors. *Mayo Clin Proc*. 2010;85(12 suppl):S27–S37.

263. Unger J. Clinical efficacy of GLP-1 agonists and their place in the diabetes treatment algorithm. *J Am Osteopath Assoc*. 2011;111 (2 suppl 1):eS2–eS9.

264. Garber AJ. Incretin effects on beta cell function, replication and mass: the human perspective. *Diabetes Care*. 2011;34(suppl 2):S258–S263.

265. DeFronzo RA, Okerson T, Viswanathan P, et al. Effects of exenatide versus sitagliptin on postprandial glucose, insulin and glucagon secretion, gastric emptying, and caloric intake: a randomized, cross-over study. *Curr Med Res Opin*. 2008;(10):2943–2952.

266. DeFronzo RA, Ratner RE, Han J, et al. Effects of exenatide (exendin-4) on glycemic control and weight over 30 weeks in metformin-treated patients with T2DM. *Diabetes Care*. 2005;28(5):1092–1100.

267. Zinman B, Hoogwerf BJ, Durán García S, et al. The effect of adding exenatide to a thiazolidinedione in suboptimally controlled T2DM: a randomized trial [published correction appears in *Ann Intern Med*. 2007;146(12):896]. *Ann Intern Med*. 2007;146(7):477–485.

268. Buysschaert M, Preumont V, Oriot PR, et al; UCL Study Group for Exenatide: one-year metabolic outcomes in patients with T2DM treated with exenatide in routine practice. *Diabetes Metab*. 2010;36(5):381–388.

269. Pinelli NR, Cha R, Brown MB, et al. Addition of thiazolidinedione or exenatide to oral agents in T2DM: a meta-analysis. *Ann Pharmacother*. 2008;42(11):1541–1551. doi:10.1345/aph.1L198.

270. Byetta prescribing information. San Diego, CA: Amylin Pharmaceuticals, Inc.; 2011.

270a. Buse JB, Bergenstal RM, Glass LC, et al. Use of twice-daily exenatide in Basal insulin-treated patients with type 2 diabetes: a randomized, controlled trial. *Ann Intern Med*. 2011;18;154(2):103–112.

271. Tracy MA, Ward KL, Firouzabadian L, et al. Factors affecting the degradation rate of poly(lactide-co-glycolide) microspheres in vivo and in vitro. *Biomaterials*. 1999;20(11):1057–1062.

272. Bydureon prescribing information. Amylin Pharmaceuticals. 2012. http://www.bydureon.com

273. Drucker DJ, Buse JB, Taylor K, et al. Exenatide once weekly versus twice daily for the treatment of type 2 diabetes: a randomised, open-label, non-inferiority study. *Lancet*. 2008;372(9645):1240–1250.

274. Bergenstal RM, Wysham C, Macconell L, et al. Efficacy and safety of exenatide once weekly versus sitagliptin or pioglitazone as an adjunct to metformin for treatment of type 2 diabetes (DURATION-2): a randomised trial. *Lancet*. 2008;376(9739):431–439.

275. Diamant M, Van Gaal L, Stranks S, et al. Once weekly exenatide compared with insulin glargine titrated to target in patients with type 2 diabetes (DURATION-3): an open-label randomised trial. *Lancet*; 375(9733):2234–2243.

276. Russell-Jones D, cuddihy RM, Hanefeld M, et al. Efficacy and safety of exenatide once weekly versus metformin, pioglitazone, and sitagliptin used as monotherapy in drug-naïve patients with type 2 diabetes [DURATION-4]: a 26-week double-blind study. *Diabetes Care*. 2012;35(2):252–258.

277. Blevins T, Pullman J, Malloy J, et al. DURATION-5: Exenatide once weekly resulted in greater improvements in glycemic control compared with exenatide twice daily in patients with type 2 diabetes. *J Clin Endocrinol Metab*. 2011;96(5):1301–1310.

278. https://investor.lilly.com/releasedetail2.cfm?ReleaseID=554248 Accessed March 10, 2012.

279. Buse JB, Henry RR, Han J, et al. Effects of exenatide (exendin-4) on glycemic control over 30 weeks in sulfonylurea-treated patients with type 2 diabetes. *Diabetes Care*. 2004;27(11):2628–2635.

280. Bjerre Knudsen L, Madsen LW, Andersen S, et al. Glucagon-like Peptide-1 receptor agonists activate rodent thyroid C-cells causing calcitonin release and C-cell proliferation. *Endocrinology*. 2010;151(4):1473–1486.

281. Buse JB, Rosenstock J, Sesti G, et al.; LEAD-6 Study Group. Liraglutide once a day versus exenatide twice a day for T2DM: a 26-week randomised, parallel-group, multinational, open label trial (LEAD-6). *Lancet*. 2009;374(9683):39–47.

282. Buse JB, Sesti G, Schmidt WE, et al. Liraglutide Effect Action in Diabetes-6 Study Group. Switching to once-daily liraglutide from twice-daily exenatide further improves glycemic control in patients with T2DM using oral agents. *Diabetes Care*. 2010;33(6):1300–1303.

282a. Victoza prescribing information. http://www.novo-pi.com/victoza.pdf

282b. DeVries JH, Bain SC, Rodbard HW, et al. Sequential intensification of metformin treatment in type 2 diabetes with liraglutide followed by randomized addition of basal insulin prompted by A1C targets. *Diabetes Care*. 2012. (Accepted for publication-NN Trial 1842.)

283. Dore DD, Seeger JD, Arnold CK. Use of a claims-based active drug safety surveillance system to assess the risk of acute pancreatitis with exenatide or sitagliptin compared to metformin or glyburide. *Curr Med Res Opin*. 2009;25(4):1019–1027.

284. Monami M, Marchionni N, Mannucci E. Glucagon-like peptide-1 receptor agonists in T2DM: a meta-analysis of randomized clinical trials. *Eur J Endocrinol*. 2009;160(6):909–917.

285. Parkes D, Jodka C, Smith P, et al. Pharmacokinetic actions of exendin-4 in the rat: comparison with glucagon-like peptide-1. *Drug Dev Res*. 2001;53:260–267.

286. Dicker D. DPP-4 inhibitors: impact on glycemic control and cardiovascular risk factors. *Diabetes Care*. 2011;(suppl 2):S276–S278.

287. Dave DJ. Saxagliptin: a dipeptidyl peptidase-4 inhibitor in the treatment of type 2 diabetes mellitus. *J Pharmacol Pharmacotherap*. 2011;2(4):230–235.

288. Onglyza prescribing information. Princeton, NJ: Bristol-Myers Squibb; 2011.

289. Fura A, Knanna A, Vyas V, et al. Pharmacokinetics of the dipeptidyl peptidse 4 inhibitor saxagliptin in rats, dogs, and monkeys and clinical projections. *Drug Metab Dispos*. 2009;37:1164–1171.

290. Dhillon S, Weber J. Saxagliptin. *Drugs*. 2009;69:2103–2114.

291. Jadzinsky M, Pfutzner A, Paz-Pacheco E, et al. Saxagliptin given in combination with metformin as initial therapy improves glycaemic control in patients with type 2 diabetes compared with either monotherapy: a randomized controlled trial. *Diabetes Obes Metab*. 2009;11:611–622.

292. Hollander P, Li J, Allen E, et al.; DV 181-013 Investigators. Saxagliption added to a thiazolidinedione improves glycemic control in patients with type 2 diabetes and inadequate control on thiazolidinedione alone. *J Clin Endocrinol Metab*. 2009;94:4810–4819.

293. Cooper M, von Eynatten M, Emser A, et al. Efficacy and safety of linagliptin in patients with T2DM with or without renal impairment: results from a global phase 3 program. *71th Scientific Sessions of the American Diabetes Association*, San Diego, California. 2011;1068-P.

294. U.S. Food and Drug Administration. Information for healthcare professionals: acute pancreatitis and sitagliptin -marketed as Januvia and Janumet- [Internet], 2009. Available from http://www.fda.gov/Drugs/DrugSafety/PostmarketDrugSafety InformationforPatientsanProviders/Drug Safety InformationforHeathcareProfessionals/ ucm183764. Accessed July 1, 2011.

295. Tradjenta prescribing information. Ridgefield, CT: Boehringer Ingelheim Pharmaceuticals, Inc.; Accessed April 2, 2012.

295a. Zinman B, Schmidt WE, Moses A, et al. Achieving a clinically relevant composite outcome of an HbA1c of 7% without weight gain or hypoglycaemia in type 2 diabetes: a meta-analysis of the liraglutide clinical trial programme. *Diabetes Obes Metab*. 2012;14(1):77–82.

296. Guidance for industry. Diabetes Mellitus-Evaluating cardiovascular risk in new antidiabetic therapies to treat type 2 diabetes. http://www.fda.gov/downloads/Drugs/GuidanceComplianceRegulatoryInformation/Guidances/ucm071627.pdf. Accessed March 10, 2012.

297. National Heart, Lung and Blood Institute. http://www.nhlbi.nih.gov/health/prof/heart/other/accord/q_a.htm. Accessed March 1, 2012.

298. Einhorn D, Rendell M, Rosenzweig J, et al. Pioglitazone hydrochloride in combination with metformin in the treatment of type 2 diabetes mellitus: a randomized, placebo-controlled study: the Pioglitazone 027 Study Group. *Clin Ther*. 2000;22:1395–1409.

299. Fonseca V, Rosenstock J, Patwardhan R, et al. Effect of metformin and rosiglitazone combination therapy in patients with type 2 diabetes mellitus. *JAMA*. 2000;283:1695–1702.

300. Jonas D, Van Scoyoc E, Gerrald K, et al. Drug class review: newer diabetes medications, TZDs, and combinations: final original report [Internet]. *Drug Class Reviews* February 2011. http://www.ncbi.nlm.nih.gov/pubmed/21595121).

301. http://www.diabetesmonitor.com/b446.htm. Accessed July 1, 2011.

302. Straton IM, Adler AI, Neil AW, et al. Association of glycaemia with macrovascular and microvascular complications of T2DM (UKPDS 35): prospective observational study. *BMJ*. 2000;321(7258):405–412.

303. National Diabetes Information Clearinghouse NDIC. http://www.diabetes.niddk.nih.gov/dm/pubs/statistics/#Amputations. Accessed July 5, 2011.

304. Reiber GE, Boyko EJ, Smith DG. Lower extremity foot ulcers and amputations in diabetes. NIH Publication available online: http://diabetes.niddk.nih.gov/dm/pubs/america/pdf/chapter18.pdf. Accessed March 10, 2012.

305. Gu K, Cowie CC, Harris MI. Diabetes and decline in heart disease mortality in U.S. adults. *JAMA*. 1999;281:1291–1297.

306. Stamler J, Vaccaro O, Neaton JD, et al. Diabetes, other risk factors, and 12-yr cardiovascular mortality for men screened in the Multiple Risk Factor Intervention Trial. *Diabetes Care*. 1993;16:434–444.

307. Gaede P, Vedel P, Larsen N, et al. Multifactorial intervention and cardiovascular disease in patients with T2DM. *N Engl J Med*. 2003;348:383–389.

308. Shah BR, Hux JE, Laupacis A, et al. Clinical inertia in response to inadequate glycemic control. *Diabetes Care*. 2005;28:600–606.

309. Aschner P, Kipnes MS, Lunceford JK. Effect of the dipeptidyl peptidase-R inhibitor sitagliptin as monotherapy on glycemic control in patients with type 2 diabetes. *Diabetes Care*. 2006;29:2632–2637.

Type 1 Diabetes in Adults

The patient who knows the most lives longest.
—*Eliot Joslin, MD, Student, educator, patient advocate, innovator, author, diabetes pioneer. 1869–1962.*

■ Historical Perspective: The Discovery of Insulin

The discovery of insulin in 1922 by Frederick Banting and Charles Best remains one of the most dramatic achievements in the history of medicine. Before the availability of insulin, a child newly diagnosed with type 1 diabetes (T1DM) survived on average 1 year.[1] Patients were treated with caloric-restricted diets averaging 500 to 700 calories per day. So strict were these dietary restrictions that patients were forced to count out the exact number of berries that they could eat per day and would be labeled as "noncompliant" if they added any extra food to their daily dietary intake. Surviving patients with diabetes would lose an extraordinary amount of weight and yet would remain under the threshold for developing diabetic ketoacidosis (DKA) as long as they could maintain their starvation diets.

Leonard Thompson, 14 years old, was the first patient ever to receive an injection of insulin. Weighing only 65 lb on admission to Toronto General Hospital 2 years after being diagnosed with diabetes, Leonard appeared pale, with a distended abdomen and breath that smelled of acetone. "All of us knew that he was doomed," wrote a senior medical student in attendance.[2] The boy had survived on a caloric intake of only 450 calories daily, just enough to keep him from becoming ketotic. Anxious to try out his unpurified pancreatic extract on human subjects rather than dogs, Dr. Banting, a general surgeon by training, injected Leonard with 15 mL of a "thick brown muck" on January 11, 1922. (The dose chosen was 50% of the dose thought to be appropriate for a dog of equal weight.) Leonard's blood glucose dropped from 440 to 320 mg per dL and he continued to have ketonuria. Unfortunately, Leonard developed multiple sterile abscesses from the injections. Banting thought that his experiment was a failure, despite the 25% improvement in glycemic response to the extract.

A biochemist, James Collip (who shared the Nobel Prize for Medicine with Banting and Best in 1923), was able to purify the extract in his own laboratory. On January 23, 1922, Leonard Thompson received 5 mL of the purified drug, followed by a second dose of 20 mL 6 hours later. The next day he received two 10-mL injections. His initial blood glucose level of 520 mg per dL fell to 120 mg per dL within 24 hours and his ketonuria disappeared. The patient's condition continued to improve with the insulin extract.

413

TABLE 11-1. Currently Marketed Insulin Analogue Preparations

Name of Insulin	Brand Name
Insulin glargine	Lantus (Aventis)
Insulin aspart	NovoLog (Novo Nordisk)
Insulin lispro	Humalog (Lilly)
Insulin detemir	Levemir (Novo Nordisk)
Insulin glulisine	Apidra (Aventis)
75% insulin lispro protamine suspension, 25% insulin lispro	Humalog Mix 75/25 (Lilly)
50% insulin lispro protamine suspension, 50% insulin lispro	Humalog Mix 50/50 (Lilly)
70% insulin aspart protamine suspension, 30% insulin aspart (BIAsp 30)	NovoLog Mix 70/30 (Novo Nordisk)

Compliance was one of Leonard's weaker points. During a celebration marking the 10th anniversary of the discovery of insulin, the world's poster boy for diabetes became comatose after consuming an excessive amount of alcohol and party pastries. Fortune again prevailed, allowing Leonard to survive another hospitalization until finally succumbing to pneumonia at age 27.

The first commercial insulin preparations contained numerous impurities and varied in potency by up to 25% per lot. In the 1930s, the first long-acting preparation, protamine zinc insulin (PZI), was marketed, which reduced the number of injections required for adequate insulin replacement.[3] PZI was used once daily without adding any short-acting insulin, setting a trend that lasted until the 1950s when NPH and zinc insulin (Lente) were marketed. For the next 25 years, diabetes was treated using two injections of NPH and regular insulin featuring the famous 2/3:1/3 ratio, in which higher doses of insulins were given with breakfast. In the 1980s, the introduction of human insulin eliminated commonly observed insulin allergies and the cosmetically disfiguring immune-mediated lipoatrophy requiring patients to "rotate" the sites of their injections to prevent areas of skin atrophy.[4] In the 1990s, the relationship between improving glycemic control and reducing diabetes-related complications was confirmed.[5,6]

The absorption patterns and pharmacologic actions of the standard insulins did not match the physiologic nature of endogenous insulin. Patients experienced wide daily glycemic changes, including hypoglycemia, while maintaining acceptable A1C levels. In an attempt to mimic normal pancreatic endogenous insulin action, insulin analogues were developed. The first insulin analogue, lispro, was introduced in 1996 followed shortly thereafter by insulin aspart. The newest fast-acting analogue, insulin glulisine, became available in 2005. Table 11-1 lists the currently marketed insulin analogue preparations. Insulin analogues are more physiologic than NPH and regular insulin, thereby allowing patients to experience more flexibility and safety with their treatment regimens.

▮ T1DM Disease Classification

T1DM accounts for 5% to 10% of all individuals diagnosed with diabetes and results from a cellular-mediated autoimmune destruction of the pancreatic β-cells. Markers of the immune destruction of β-cell include islet cell autoantibodies (ICAs), autoantibodies to insulin (IAA), autoantibodies to GAD (GAD65), an antibody to an insulinoma-associated antigen-2 (ICA512), and autoantibodies to the tyrosine phosphatases (IA-2 and IA-2β).[7] One and usually more of the autoantibodies are present in 85% to 90% of individuals when fasting hyperglycemia is initially detected.

In T1DM, the rate of β-cell destruction varies. Whereas infants and children tend to demonstrate rapid β-cell death, adults typically present with a lengthy prodromal phase leading to latent autoimmune diabetes of adulthood (LADA).[8] Some patients, particularly children and adolescents, may present with ketoacidosis as the first manifestation of the disease. Others have modest fasting hyperglycemia that can rapidly change to severe hyperglycemia and/or ketoacidosis in the presence of infection or other sources of physiologic stress. Still others, particularly adults, may retain residual β-cell function (remaining C-peptide positive) sufficient to prevent ketoacidosis for many years; such individuals eventually become dependent on insulin for survival and are at risk for ketoacidosis. At this latter stage of the disease, there is little or no insulin secretion, as manifested by low or undetectable levels of plasma C-peptide. Immune-mediated diabetes commonly occurs in childhood and adolescence, but may occur at any age, even in the eighth and ninth decades of life.

Patients with T1DM are prone to other autoimmune disorders such as autoimmune thyroid disease (15% to 30%), celiac disease (4% to 9%), and Addison disease (0.5%). Assays for thyroid peroxidase autoantibodies (TPOAb) in autoimmune thyroid disease, tissue transglutaminase autoantibodies (TTGAb) in celiac disease, and 21-hydroxylase autoantibodies (21OHAb) in Addison disease may be used to screen for asymptomatic patients to identify one's risk of clinical progression. Thirty-three percent of patients with T1DM screen positive for at least one additional organ-specific autoantibody when initially diagnosed with diabetes, and 19% have evidence of clinical disease. Given the high preponderance of these antibodies at the onset of T1DM, screening for coexisting autoimmune disorders appears to be warranted.[9]

Nearly 50% of African-American, nonwhite Hispanic, and other minority ethnic group patients with newly diagnosed ketoacidosis may appear to have T1DM when in fact their diagnosis is one of "Flatbush diabetes." These patients are typically obese, have a strong family history of T2DM, and lack autoantibodies. Their initial clinical symptoms include acute onset of polyuria, polydipsia, weight loss, fatigue, and metabolic decompensation. However, upon initiation of insulin, β-cell function and insulin sensitivity are restored and they begin to secrete measurable and predictable amounts of endogenous insulin. Increased susceptibility to glucose desensitization could be one cause of Flatbush diabetes.[10]

Patients with near-complete insulin deficiency who remain antibody-negative are classified as having "type 1B diabetes."[11] Most type 1B patients are of African or Asian ancestry. Table 11-2 lists the facts and figures related to T1DM in the United States and worldwide.

Pathogenesis of T1DM: From Cause to Cure

Two questions are always asked by patients with T1DM and their family members: "How did I get this disease?" and "When will you find a cure?" Affecting a cure or preventing any disease demands that one understand its pathogenesis, determine the risk factors that heighten one's susceptibility to the condition, and develop a model that allows one to accurately predict the likely course of disease progression. For diabetes, this assignment is akin to assembling a jigsaw puzzle where the manufacturer forgot to include several important anchoring pieces. Successful completion of the puzzle requires the "players" to initially locate the four anchoring corners. Work then centers on precisely filling in as many pieces of the puzzle as possible as each placement is challenged by other players in the scientific community. Just when one thinks the puzzle is nearing completion, an anchoring corner morphs. The broad picture that was once viewed with anxious anticipation is now just a distant memory. Although we have become better assemblers of jigsaw puzzles for our efforts, the search begins anew for those all-important anchoring corners. For scientists, locating these important four corners of the puzzle is proving to be an elusive task. What are the four anchoring corners of T1DM disease prevention and cure?

- Question #1: What is the triggering mechanism for autoimmune β-cell destruction?

Our first puzzle corner identifies the specific origin of T1DM. Does T1DM result from genetic susceptibility in individuals who perhaps lack a protective mechanism that permits an aggressive

TABLE 11-2. Facts and Figures for T1DM

- Prevalence of T1DM in United States is 0.15% of population (2001)

- In U.S. adolescents, incidence most common in youth aged 10–14 (25.9/100,000) and lowest among youth aged 15–19 (13.1 per 100,000)

- Incidence rates are similar between males and females

- Across all ages, non-Hispanic whites had the highest prevalence of T1DM (1.03 and 2.88 cases per 1,000 youth in younger and older youth, respectively)

- The age-adjusted incidence of T1DM ranged between 0.1 per 100,000/y in China and Venezuela and 40.9 per 100,000/y in Finland

- Annual increase in incidence worldwide was 2.8%/y between 1990 and 1999

- All continents showed statistically significant increases during this time (4.0% in Asia, 3.2% in Europe, 5.3% in North America), except Central America and the West Indies where incidence decreased to 3.6%

- Environmental risk factors early in life are cited as possibly contributing to the increasing incidence of T1DM: enteroviral infections in pregnant women, older maternal age (39–42 y), preeclampsia, cesarean section delivery, increased birth weight, early introduction of cow's milk proteins, and an increased rate of postnatal growth (weight and height). Vitamin D supplementation may be protective. Viruses may initiate autoimmunity toward the β-cell, while other exposures may overload a β-cell and accelerate diabetes development

- In general, incidence increases with age, peaking at puberty. After puberty, incidence rate significantly drops in young women but remains relatively high in males up to age 29–35 y. In Finland, the overall boy-to-girl ratio of incidence was 1.1; at the age of 13 y, it was 1.7 (1.4–2.0)

References
1. American Diabetes Association. Standards of medical care in diabetes—2010. *Diabetes Care*. 2010;33(suppl 1): S11–S61.
2. Palta M, LeCaire T. Managing T1DM: trends and outcomes over 20 years in the Wisconsin Diabetes Registry cohort. *WMJ*. 2009;108:231–235;
3. Patterson CC, Dahlquist GG, Gyürüs E, et al. Incidence trends for childhood T1DM in Europe during 1989–2003 and predicted new cases 2005–20: a multicentre prospective registration study. *Lancet*. 2009;373:2027–2033.
4. Harjutsalo V, Sjöberg L, Tuomilehto J. Time trends in the incidence of T1DM in Finnish children: a cohort study. *Lancet*. 2008;371:1777–1782.
5. Soltesz G, Patterson CC, Dahlquist G, et al. Worldwide childhood T1DM incidence: what can we learn from epidemiology? *Pediatr Diabetes*. 2007;8(suppl 6):6–14.
6. Writing Group for the SEARCH for Diabetes in Youth Study Group, Dabelea D, Bell RA, et al. Incidence of diabetes in youth in the United States. *JAMA*. 2007;297:2716–2724.
7. Liese AD, D'Agostino RB, et al.; SEARCH for Diabetes in Youth Study Group. The burden of diabetes mellitus among U.S. youth: prevalence estimates from the SEARCH for Diabetes in Youth Study. *Pediatrics*. 2006;118:1510–1518; ISSN: 1098-4275.
8. DIAMOND Project Group; Incidence and trends of childhood T1DM worldwide 1990-1999. *Diabet Med*. 2006;23:857–866.

and sustained autoimmune destruction process within the pancreatic islets? To what extent do environmental factors play in triggering the pathogenesis of autoimmune dysfunction in genetically prone patients? Finding genetically prone individuals would allow us to vaccinate against T1DM. Moreover, patients who are noted to have an autoimmune response within their islets can undergo therapeutic interventions to "reboot" their immune system. Therefore, finding this piece of the puzzle is of utmost importance.

Studying the genetics of T1DM has been very time intensive. Over 100 candidate genes (a gene suspected to be involved with a particular disease) on 14 different chromosomes have been detected that influence one's likelihood of either developing T1DM or preventing the disease.[12,13] Candidate genes do not appear to have any effect on disease pathogenesis or progression, only on disease protection and susceptibility.

Two combinations of HLA genes (or haplotypes) are of particular importance: DR4-DQ8 and DR3-DQ2 are present in 90% of children with T1DM and are considered susceptibility genes.[14] A third haplotype, DR15-DQ6, is found in less than 1% of children with T1DM, compared with more than 20% of the general population, and is considered to be protective against the development of T1DM.[15] The genotype combining the two susceptibility haplotypes (DR4-DQ8/DR3-DQ2) contributes the greatest risk of the disease and is most common in children in whom the disease develops very early in life.[16] First-degree relatives of these children are themselves at greater risk of T1DM than are the relatives of children in whom the disease develops later.[17] The overall risk of an offspring of a mother with T1DM developing T1DM is 3%.[18]

Can environmental factors trigger T1DM within different ethnic populations? One of the most striking characteristics of T1DM is the large geographic variability in the incidence. Scandinavia and the Mediterranean island of Sardinia have the highest incidence rates of T1DM in the world, whereas Asian populations have the lowest rates.[19] For example, a child in Finland is 400 times more likely to develop diabetes than one in China.[20] While there is a strong south–north gradient in the incidence, "hot spots" in warm climates have also been reported (Sardinia, Puerto Rico, Kuwait).

Does the geographic and ethnic variability observed within T1DM "hot spots" suggest that an environmental "trigger" activates T1DM in genetically susceptible patients who populate that region? Identification of such environmental factors has proved frustratingly difficult. The most popular candidates are viruses, with enteroviruses, rotavirus, and rubella being suspects. The strongest data to date have supported a role for rubella.[21,22] Infants infected with congenital rubella syndrome are said to be at increased risk of T1DM.[23] Yet Finland, where vaccination has effectively eradicated rubella, still has the highest incidences of T1DM.[24] There is also evidence that some enteroviruses (e.g., Coxsackie B viruses) are less prevalent in countries with high incidences of T1DM (e.g., Finland) than in countries with low incidences but geographically similar populations (e.g., Russian Karelia).[25] This observation may be in keeping with the concept of the hygiene hypothesis, which proposes that environmental exposure to microbes, other pathogens, and their products early in life promotes innate immune responses that suppress atopy and perhaps autoimmunity.[26] In Western cultures, the developing immune system of the infant is no longer exposed to widespread infection, which may contribute to the current increases in incidence observed in atopic and autoimmune diseases.

Other environmental risk factors that have been linked to T1DM pathogenesis include the frequency and duration of breastfeeding[27] and the consumption of cow's milk.[28,29]

A study published by Mohr et al.[30] suggested an association in the incidence of T1DM and low ultraviolet light radiation. This could support a contributing role of vitamin D in reducing the risk of developing the risk of T1DM. Mohr suggested that a 350-fold range of age-standardized incidence rates of T1DM, from an average of 0.1 per 100,000 in boys less than 14 years of age in China to 37 per 100,000 in boys less than 14 years in Finland.[19] Exposure of the skin to sunlight is the source of 80% to 95% of circulating vitamin D and its metabolites. Thus, availability and intensity of sunlight, which are highly related to latitude, are strong correlates of the principal circulating vitamin D metabolite in the serum, 25-hydroxyvitamin D [25(OH)D]. The authors suggest that children aged ≥ 1 year who live more than 30 degrees from the equator should consume 1,000 to 2,000 IU per day of vitamin D_3, especially during winter, to substantially reduce their risk of developing T1DM.

A population-based study by Gorham et al.[31] examined electronic medical records of military personnel in the San Diego area from 1990 through 2005. During this time, the age-adjusted incidence rate of new-onset T1DM in military personnel aged 18 to 44 was 17.5 per 100,000 person years (for men), with rates being twice as high in blacks as in whites (31.5 vs. 14.5 per 100,000, $p < 0.001$). In women, the age-adjusted incidence rate was 13.6 per 100,000 with rates being twice as high in black as for white women (21.8 vs. 9.7% per 100,000, $p < 0.001$). The incidence of insulin requiring diabetes peaked annually in the winter–spring season. The authors concluded that winter season and black skin pigmentation substantially reduced the photosynthesis of vitamin D_3 in the skin of black soldiers, creating a higher prevalence of vitamin D deficiency. This vitamin deficiency, in turn, was thought to be an environmental contributing factor to the initiation of pathways that could trigger autoimmune destruction of β-cells.

The most recent evidence suggest that compromises in proper regulation of self-reactive and protective immune responses may be the result of abnormal activities of a population of T-regulatory (T-reg) cells. Loss of the "T-reg" cells promotes the initiation and progression of the autoimmune process.[32] Other studies have implicated stressful lifestyles and dietary practices such as the consumption of artificial sweeteners, caffeine, and even smoked fish.

In summary, one should perhaps consider a multitude of individual environmental triggers that have an effect of dysregulation of normal immune protection over the course of several months or years during one's prediabetes stage. Hence, many "environmental criminals" have been implicated in T1DM pathogenesis, but none has been convicted by a jury of peer reviewers.[26]

- Question #2: What are the natural history and progression of T1DM?

The second anchoring piece of the puzzle for T1DM cure and prevention must accurately depict the natural history of T1DM allowing scientists to establish effective points of intervention. In 1986, George Eisenbarth proposed that patients born with a genetic susceptibility to T1DM encounter a disease-inciting environmental agent that elicits an autoimmune reaction within the pancreatic islets resulting in the appearance of autoantibodies.[33] Patients with detectable autoantibodies may exhibit loss of β-cell function and first-phase insulin response at different rates. A faster rate of progression to diabetes was observed in subjects with abnormal baseline glucose tolerance than among those with normal baseline glucose tolerance but low first-phase insulin response to an intravenous glucose challenge.[40] A recently published study suggests that a combination of metabolic markers derived from oral glucose tolerance tests performed on ICA-positive patients with low first-phase insulin response improves the accuracy of predicting the 5-year progression to T1DM.[33a]

Still to be explained is why some patients who possess a histocompatibility complex haplotype that favors progression toward T1DM will not develop any signs of impaired glucose metabolism. Others possessing the same haplotypes will develop diabetes at a young age, whereas diabetes onset may be delayed until adult life in others. Forty to fifty percent of the risk for T1DM appears to be associated with the MHC complex or IDDM 1 loci. The MHC genes most associated with diabetes in white people are known as the human leukocyte antigens HLA DR3 and HLA DR4. Other racial groups are less well studied and may have different MHC gene profiles. More than 90% of European ancestry individuals with T1DM will have one or the other of these DR3 or DR4 haplotypes, but about 40% of the general population has one of these gene locations as well. The presence of high-risk haplotypes and evidence of positive antibodies, however, strongly predict the development of diabetes. Some MHC genes are protective against T1DM. Less than 1% of individuals with diabetes have these protective haplotypes.[36] Perhaps points of intervention may be based within ethnic and genetic profiling. The inciting environmental event(s) that trigger autoimmunity over time have yet to be identified beyond speculation. More likely, multiple triggers are required to induce autoimmune dysregulation in genetically susceptible individuals. Once β-cell injury occurs, is the loss of mass and function linear, and could one experience periods of remission and β-cell recovery? Unfortunately, we have yet to define the most effective measurement of β-cell mass and function in vivo. Why in some cases does β-cell injury or death progress rapidly and in others the destruction of islets is protracted as in LADA? Can β-cell regeneration occur in some patients who initially experience significant apoptosis? Remember those Flatbush diabetes patients who present with acute onset of DKA only to recover nearly complete β-cell insulin secretion.[37]

- Question #3: What are the best predictable risk factors for developing T1DM?

Predicting who is likely to develop T1DM and how this information may be clinically applicable provides the next puzzle cornerstone piece. In one study, adult patients who tested positive for GAD65 antibodies, thyroid peroxidase antibodies, and IA-2AB showed a faster disease progression than patients who were positive only for GAD65 antibody. Thus, the number, rather than the specific autoantibody, appears to predict disease progression over a 4-year period.[38]

Ethical and financial barriers may limit the utility of screening high-risk patients for T1DM. Only 1 person in 300 is diagnosed with T1DM before age 20. Assuming the cost of autoantibody screening ranges between $241 and $788 per patient, one would spend a minimum of $73,000 per single case of T1DM identified that would *possibly* progress to clinical diabetes.[39] Once screened, how could this information be used to prevent or delay the onset of T1DM?[40] From a practical standpoint, who should perform and interpret the results of autoantibody testing? Finally, once a patient tests autoantibody positive, how will this information be handled by third-party payers or by government-run health-care programs?

T1DM may be predicted in individuals based upon not only the presence of one or more autoantibodies but the titers of those antibodies obtained at the time of testing. GAD65 and ICA antibodies have the highest predictability for T1DM.[41] The combination of GADAs and IA-2As has a high sensitivity and specificity for T1DM in family members, although prospective studies from birth have shown that IAAs are usually the first or among the first antibodies to appear in young children.[42] An observational study of 3475 Finnish children who were initially recruited in 1980 for a population-based study on cardiovascular risk collected GAD and IA-2A antibodies. Sera were again collected in 1986 and 2007.[43] One-time screening for GAD-65 antibodies and IA-2As was capable of identifying 60% of patients who developed T1DM over 27 years. The highest predictive value was seen in those testing initially positive for both GAD-65 and IA-2As, but the sensitivity dropped from 50% for either test alone to 39%.

- Question #4: How can T1DM be prevented?

The final keystone piece of the T1DM puzzle identifies means by which the disease can be prevented. T1DM occurs in individuals in whom genetic susceptibility outweighs genetic protection. Distinctive environmental triggers play a supporting role in provoking a cellular-mediated autoimmune process to one or more β-cell proteins (autoantigens). As islet cell destruction occurs, autoantibodies are delivered into the pancreatic lymph nodes where destructive T-effector cells are produced that outnumber the stabilizing T-reg cells. Initially, the decline in β-cell function and loss of β-cell mass presents clinically as loss of first-phase insulin response to an intravenous glucose challenge. Over time, patients progress through stages of "dysglycemia" [glucose values greater than 200 mg per dL at 30, 60, or 90 minutes during an oral glucose tolerance test (OGTT)]. Ultimately, the clinical syndrome of T1DM becomes evident when the majority of β-cell function has been lost and most β-cells have been destroyed. At this juncture, frank hyperglycemia supervenes.

In one study, the metabolic profiles of 54 patients from the Diabetes Prevention Trial-1 were evaluated over time to obtain a clinical profile of metabolic progression to T1DM over a period of 2.5 years before diagnosis.[44] All subjects had OGTTs at 6-month intervals beginning 30 months prior to being diagnosed with T1DM. Most had OGTTs at diagnosis. Changes in OGTT glucose and C-peptides (an indicator of one's endogenous insulin production) were examined and paired between time points. The data indicate that hyperglycemia begins to develop at least 2 years prior to the time of diagnosis after which glucose levels continue to increase gradually until 6 months prior to diagnosis. OGGT levels rise sharply within 6 months of the diagnosis. As hyperglycemia worsens, fasting C-peptide levels remain constant. The consistency of the fasting C-peptide-to-fasting glucose ration indicates that fasting endogenous insulin levels are maintained to a large extent until one is diagnosed with T1DM. Stimulated C-peptide levels tend to fall rapidly beginning 6 months prior to the diagnosis. Thus, with progression to T1DM, fasting insulin secretion is preserved to a greater extent than postprandial glucose.

At what point in this disease progression can T1DM be prevented? To date, no intervention has been developed that can unequivocally prevent the development of T1DM or arrest the progression of immune system destruction of β-cells after diagnosis, although some promising studies have given the field much encouragement. One novel technique uses monoclonal antibodies to "reboot" dysregulated immune functioning in patients newly diagnosed with T1DM. Monoclonal antibodies are produced in a laboratory and target a specific predetermined antigen. Immune destruction of islet cells is mediated by T-lymphocytes that express CD3, CD4, and CD8 receptors on their cell surface. If one binds a monoclonal antibody (otelixizumab) to a CD3 receptor in newly diagnosed patients with T1DM, endogenous insulin production improves for 4 years. However, disease remission does not occur.[45]

Rituximab, an anti-CD20 chimeric antibody that depletes B-lymphocytes, has shown encouraging initial clinical results. A recent TrialNet-funded study demonstrated that a four-dose course of rituximab could preserve β-cell function over a 1-year period in patients with newly diagnosed T1DM.[46] Vaccination with an alum-formulated GAD65 autoantigen failed to slow the loss of stimulated C-peptide, improve A1C, daily insulin doses, or rates of hypoglycemia in newly diagnosed patients with T1DM when compared with a placebo vaccine.[47]

Systemic anti-inflammatory agents such as IL-1 receptor antagonists[48] and agents that stimulate β-cell proliferation are also being studied as potential components of a multidrug prevention of β-cell destruction.[49]

Therapies directed at preventing or reversing immune destruction of β-cells appear to have positive effects that are only transient. Attempts to reboot the immune system may be countered by a surge of islet autoantibody production that overwhelm the very protective mechanisms they are designed to protect. Future preventive therapies for T1DM will need to offer combination interventions in order to fully mitigate one's dysregulated immune.

Another area of research interest involves β-cell regeneration and replacement. This complex restorative process will require a more comprehensive insight into the mechanics of β-cell differentiation and proliferation. Potential sources of β-cells include existing β-cells, stem cells, progenitor cells, and pancreatic ductal cells. Stem cells can proliferate indefinitely and differentiate into any cell type including normal β-cells. However, stem cells have yet to be used in clinical trials, so their efficacy and potential risks, particularly of tumorigenecity, are not known. In addition, stem cell-derived β-cells may be more susceptible to immunologic attack.

Although there are inspiring opportunities in diabetes prevention and reversal, most of these efforts are unfolding at large academic or research-focused medical centers. Nonetheless, there is a vital role for family physicians who work with individuals at high risk for developing T1DM.

In families with established T1DM, all first-degree relatives, including the parents of the patient (if they are less than 45 years of age), are at increased risk for T1DM and should be counseled regarding this risk. Identical twins are at the greatest risk. Second- and third-degree relatives of a patient with T1DM are also at heightened risk if they are less than 21 years of age.

Once apprised of their diabetes risk, individuals should be made aware of T1DM screening and intervention studies such as T1DM TrialNet through the National Institutes of Health (http://www.diabetestrialnet.org/). The advantages of screening for T1DM risk through such research-oriented programs include state-of-the-art antibody determinations in specialized research laboratories, a superb follow-up and support network of T1DM specialists, protection of laboratory data from insurance carriers, and the opportunity to participate in further clinical research studies aimed at diabetes prevention. Participating in a research study incurs no cost to patients or their insurance companies.

Family physicians may also provide effective education that may prevent T1DM. Early use of vitamin D supplementation may protect against T1DM progression, although the exact mechanism is uncertain. Vitamin D is a potent modulator of the immune system and is involved in regulating cell proliferation and differentiation.[50] A meta-analysis of data from five observational studies recently indicated that children supplemented with vitamin D had a 29% reduction in T1DM risk compared to their unsupplemented peers.[51] Nevertheless, firm conclusions that can be drawn from these data in terms of appropriate recommendations are limited by the lack of specification of dosage, duration, and particular vitamin D preparations. Thus, data from adequately powered, randomized, controlled trials are still needed. Infants should receive 400 IU daily of vitamin D supplementation until supplementation until they are ingesting equivalent amounts of vitamin D through formula milk and other nutrient sources. Infants who have limited sunlight exposure should continue the supplements indefinitely.[52]

Pathogenesis of T1DM

The term "diabetes" represents a syndrome of disorders all characterized by an impairment of pancreatic β-cell ability to secrete insulin. The American Diabetes Association (ADA) and the World Health Organization (WHO) recognize two forms of diabetes. T1DM results from pancreatic β-cell destruction secondary to an autoimmune process or an uncertain (idiopathic) etiology. These patients are prone to ketoacidosis. Diseases that secondarily result in pancreatic β-cell destruction (cystic fibrosis) are not classified as T1DM. Patients with T2DM have deficient insulin secretion from the pancreatic β-cell in association with peripheral insulin resistance. There is no evidence of autoimmunity in patients with T2DM whose pathophysiology appears to be genetically and environmentally predetermined.

Epidemiologic studies have suggested two distinct peak occurrences of T1DM: during puberty and near age 40.[53] Ten to thirty percent of patients with T2DM also develop autoantibodies similar to patients with T1DM. These patients are referred to as having LADA.

Initially, patients with T1DM have a protracted preclinical phase during which autoantibodies can be detected against their pancreatic β-cells in genetically susceptible individuals.[54] At least 80% to 90% of the β-cell mass must be lost before the patient develops hyperglycemia. Both a reduction in β-cell mass and the direct inhibition of insulin secretion by cytokines appear to result in a hyperglycemic state.[55]

Patients who are likely to progress to T1DM develop IAAs, glutamic acid decarboxylase antibodies (GADAbs), ICAs, and insulinoma-associated protein-2 autoantibodies (IA-2Abs). Interestingly, some patients who do *not* develop diabetes also produce these autoimmune markers. However, unlike patients with T1DM, their autoantibody levels tend to wax and wane over time. Patients who are more at risk for developing T1DM often have two or more autoantibodies present at any given time.[56] The presence of IAAs appears to place patients most at risk for developing childhood T1DM.[57]

LADA is a slowly progressive form of autoimmune diabetes characterized by adult age at diagnosis, the presence of diabetes-associated autoantibodies, and the lack of insulin requirement at the time of diagnosis. The fact that insulin is not required for treatment at the time of diagnosis is intended to distinguish LADA from adult-onset T1DM and T2DM.

Some have referred to this disorder as being type 1.5 diabetes mellitus.[58] Patients with LADA tend to have a more aggressive disease than T2DM, characterized by a shorter time to failure of oral hypoglycemic agents and progressive β-cell failure leading to insulin deficiency. Eighty to ninety percent of patients with LADA will require insulin within the first few years after diagnosis.[59] Therefore, physicians should differentiate LADA from T2DM whenever possible. LADA has also been diagnosed with increasing frequency in children who appeared to have T2DM.[60]

Several clinical phenotypes are useful in differentiating LADA from T2DM. When compared with T2DM patients, individuals with LADA at the time of their initial diagnosis of diabetes appear to have many of the following clinical and laboratory characteristics[61]:

- Lower body mass index (BMI)
- More common symptom presentation such as polyuria and polydipsia
- Lower mean waist and hip circumference
- Lower waist-to-hip ratio
- Shorter duration of diet or oral antidiabetic treatment before requiring insulin therapy
- Higher A1C levels

Our ability to classify patients as having either T1DM, LADA, or T2DM is dependent on the evaluation of autoimmune markers in patients who clinically present as having T2DM. Immunologic differences exist between T1DM and LADA. LADA patients are often positive for only a single autoantibody, whereas T1DM patients frequently have two or more autoantibodies detectable at diagnosis.[58] LADA patients are more likely to test positive for GAD or ICAs but not IAA and IA-2Ab.[58]

Because patients with LADA more rapidly lose their ability to produce endogenous insulin within the first few years after their diagnosis, they soon require exogenous insulin for treatment of their diabetes. Therefore, once a patient is suspected of having LADA, insulin should be initiated to maintain better glycemic control early during the course of the disease, to limit glycemic variability, and to prevent diabetes complications during a variable transition period of β-cell functional decline. The rationale for early insulin intervention though would be improving glycemic control while protecting β-cell function. The exact mechanisms for the apparent beneficial effects of exogenous insulin treatment appear to secondary to the induction of β-cell rest within the autoimmune inflamed islets. Insulin down-regulates β-cell metabolism releasing them from hyperglycemic stress.[62] β-cells, producing high amounts of insulin, are more susceptible to immune-mediated killing and are also associated with higher antigen expression.[63]

Studies evaluating GLP-1 usage in subjects with T1DM showed reduction of fasting hyperglycemia and glycemic excursions after a meal, accompanied by reduction in glucagon secretion.[64] Additionally, in islet transplant recipients, exendin-4 has stimulated insulin secretion and demonstrated an ability to reduce exogenous insulin requirements. Current clinical trials test the hypothesis that its use at the time of islet transplantation might be of help in preserving islet mass.[65] Although not evaluated yet in LADA, these agents have a potential therapeutic value in such a setting.

Endocrine Components of Euglycemia

Glucose homeostasis in euglycemic individuals involves a complex web of hormonal interactions. The ultimate goal in patients with T1DM is to approximate normal physiology as closely as possible through intensification of their metabolic defects. Carbohydrates in the form of glucose are the key source of energy for muscles and the brain. The two primary sources of circulating glucose are hepatic glucose production and ingested carbohydrate. In the fasting state, glucagon is secreted from the pancreatic α-cells that stimulates the hepatic production of glucose through glycogenolysis (the breakdown of glycogen) and gluconeogenesis (the formation of glucose from noncarbohydrate molecules, e.g., amino acids and lactic acidosis). This "basal glucose" prevents hypoglycemia while supplying sufficient energy sources for the brain in the fasting state.

Following a meal, the postprandial glucose peak occurs between 1 and 2 hours with a mean peak time of 75 minutes.[66] Rapid-acting insulin analogues display a maximum effect at approximately 100 minutes following subcutaneous injection. Thus, injections or bolusing of these analogues should be initiated 15 minutes prior to the start of a meal in order to synchronize the peak insulin action with the rise in the glycemic excursion in the postabsorptive state.[67]

Insulin is normally secreted into the portal circulation in two phases. In the fasting state, basal insulin is secreted at the approximate rate of 1 U per hour in order to minimized hepatic glucose production.[68] Basal insulin also limits lipolysis and excess flux of free fatty acids to the liver, which can result in a state of postabsorptive insulin resistance. The circulating glucose levels are maintained at a level that allows for the extraction of this energy source by obligate glucose consumers such as the central nervous system. The lack of adequate basal insulin stimulates hormone-sensitive lipase and free fatty acid release from fat stores, which, in turn, stimulates hepatic production and release of ketone bodies, leading to ketogenesis and DKA.

Eating prompts a 5- to 10-fold increase in prandial insulin release from the pancreatic β-cells in euglycemic individuals. With each meal, a rapid first-phase insulin response occurs, limiting the rise in ambient plasma glucose levels. First-phase insulin response terminates quickly so that hypoglycemia does not occur. The second-phase insulin release follows limiting glycemic excursions as carbohydrates are absorbed from the gastrointestinal tract. This postabsorptive state may last between 4 and 6 hours and is dependent upon the food content of each meal. High-fat meals (such as pizza) prolong the postabsorptive state.[69]

Fat is stored in the body as triglycerides and converted to free fatty acids plus glycerol by lipolysis. Following ingestion of a fatty meal, the fat is stored in adipose tissue or may be transported to the muscle where it becomes oxidized and used as an energy source. Excessive levels of triglycerides and circulating free fatty acids can inhibit insulin signaling resulting in postprandial insulin resistance.[70]

Glucagon is a counterregulatory hormone, which, when released from the pancreatic α-cell, promotes hepatic gluconeogenesis and reversal of hypoglycemia. A euglycemic individual would signal glucagon secretion via a reduction in insulin release by the pancreatic β-cell coupled with low glucose stimulation of the α-cell.[10] However, in patients with T1DM, a signaling defect between the β- and α-cells may account for failure to mount an acceptable counterregulatory response in a hypoglycemic state. With the autoimmune loss of glucose-dependent β-cell insulin secretion, signaling pathways between the α- and β-cells appear to be disrupted.[71]

Amylin is a peptide hormone that is cosecreted from pancreatic β-cells with insulin and is thus deficient in patients with diabetes. Amylin inhibits glucagon secretion, delays gastric emptying, and acts to improve satiety. Amylin also suppresses postprandial triglyceride concentrations and is known to reduce markers of oxidative stress as well as endothelial cell dysfunction.[72]

Catecholamines, cortisol, and growth hormone also assist in the prevention and reversal of hypoglycemia. Fasting hyperglycemia often occurs in patients with diabetes as physiologic basal insulin secretion is not sufficient to overcome the proglycemic effects of variable growth hormone secretion.[73]

• Physiologic Insulin Replacement Therapy

The ultimate goal of insulin replacement therapy is to mimic the normal insulin response to hyperglycemia in both the fasting and postprandial states. Euglycemic individuals produce enough insulin to maintain blood glucose values in a very narrow range (85 to 140 mg per dL). The concentration of glucose in plasma of healthy individuals remains within this normal range despite large fluctuations in nutritional intake and physical activity.

Physiologic insulin replacement regimens include the use of basal-bolus insulin preparations and continuous subcutaneous insulin infusion (insulin pump therapy—see Chapter 13).[74] Nonphysiologic regimens include NPH with or without a rapid-acting insulin, the use of premixed insulin analogues, and a single dose of analogue basal insulin given once or twice daily because these interventions fail to mimic normal β-cell production and secretion of insulin observed in euglycemia. Physiologic insulin therapies should be individualized and titrated based upon the factors shown in Table 11-3.

Patients can increase the likelihood of success with a given prescribed insulin regimen by understanding the pharmacokinetic and glucodynamic profiles of the prescribed insulins. Once insulin is initiated, self–blood glucose monitoring and paired glucose testing (see Chapter 12) can be used to identify patterns reflective of hypoglycemia, fasting hyperglycemia, and postprandial hyperglycemia. Pattern recognition is the first step in allowing patients to safely and efficiently achieve their targeted glycemic goals.[75,76]

The insulins that have been used *historically* to manage diabetes have pharmacodynamic effects (variability of absorption from injection site, time to peak effect, duration of action) and glycodynamic effects (ability to reduce hyperglycemia) that are often not physiologic. The glucodynamics and pharmacodynamics of insulin analogues are *more* predictable when compared with NPH and regular human insulin (RHI).[77–79] In general, studies have shown that rapid-acting analogues are also superior to RHI for lowering glycosylated hemoglobin levels in patients who receive insulin by continuous subcutaneous infusion.[80]

▌ Insulin Analogue Formulations

• Basal Insulin Analogues

The two available basal analogue insulins glargine (lantus) and detemir (levemir) are described in detail in Chapter 12. Because insulin glargine is clear and NPH insulin is cloudy, clinical trials comparing these two insulins in patients with T1DM have been open label. In general, the trials have shown no differences or occasional improvements in glycemic control with insulin glargine,

TABLE 11-3. Factors That Should Be Considered When Prescribing Physiologic Insulin Replacement Therapy

Patient Parameter to Be Considered	Comment
Meal consumption	• Does the patient skip meals? • Are meals consumed on a scheduled basis? • What are the approximate size and carbohydrate content of meals?
Work schedule	• Does the patient work irregular shifts? • Does irregular work schedule have an effect on sleep? • Does the patient frequently travel? • Does travel schedule require flexible meal and insulin injection scheduling?
Adherence history	• Does the patient have a history of omitting insulin doses? • Is the patient willing to perform frequent self–blood glucose testing? • Does the patient eat three scheduled meals each day?
Activity	• Does the patient exercise? • What type of exercise does the patient do? • What time of day does exercise occur? • Does exercise time vary? • Is the patient a professional athlete? • Is the patient planning to initiate an exercise program for the first time? • What are the patient's glucose targets before, during, and after exercise? • Is the patient knowledgeable about predicting and treating hypoglycemia?
History of hypoglycemia	• Does the patient have a history of HAAF? • Does the patient live alone? • Does the patient know how to predict and manage hypoglycemia? • Are there comorbidities (heart disease, chronic kidney disease, seizures, HAAF) that could preclude the patient from being intensively managed and increasing their risk of hypoglycemia? • Does the patient have access to a continuous glucose sensor? • Does the patient know to check blood glucose before driving? • What is the patient's target A1C?
Comorbidities of concern	• Coronary artery disease/cardiac arrhythmias • Preconception planning/pregnancy • Cancer • End-stage renal disease • Mental illness • Diabetic neuropathy • Diabetic retinopathy • Advanced age
Ethnic/financial concerns	• Does the patient fast for religious reasons? • Will the patient be able to afford the added costs of intensive insulin therapy? • Would the patient prefer using mixed insulin analogue and paying a single copay for two insulins?
Patient characteristics for more stringent intensification of insulin therapy	• Highly motivated adherent, excellent self-care capacities • Patient can perceive hypoglycemia • Long life expectancy • Few comorbidities • Access to diabetes support services and diabetes educators • Low cardiovascular risk • Relatively short disease duration

TABLE 11-3. Factors That Should Be Considered When Prescribing Physiologic Insulin Replacement Therapy (*Continued*)

Patient Parameter to Be Considered	Comment
Patient characteristics for less stringent intensification of insulin therapy	• Less motivated, nonadherent, poor self-care capacities • History of hypoglycemia awareness autonomic failure, especially if patient lives alone • Short life expectancy • Multiple comorbidities • Studies in patients with T2DM having a serum creatinine >2.5 mg/dL will not slow renal disease progression with intensive therapy • Cardiovascular complications (coronary artery disease, stroke, peripheral arterial disease) • Long-standing diabetes duration

although a reduction in the risk of hypoglycemia, especially nocturnal hypoglycemia, has been the rule with insulin glargine.

A recently published meta-analysis evaluated the safety and efficacy of insulin glargine in T1DM representing more than 10 years of clinical experience.[74] The data show that glargine provides consistent insulin delivery lasting up to 24 hours, which permits once-daily dosing. Glargine provides glycemic control that is at least comparable to NPH in adults, adolescents, and children. However, the risk of mild and severe episodes of hypoglycemia is significantly reduced with glargine when compared with NPH usage in adults. Combining glargine with a rapid-acting insulin analogue as part of an MDI regimen provides benefits over the use of NPH plus RHI.

Danne et al.[81] compared the within-subject variability of insulin detemir and glargine in children and adolescents with T1DM using a double-blind, crossover trial. Thirty-two children and adolescents with an A1C 7.9% ± 1% were randomized to a specific treatment sequence in which a dose of 0.4 U per kg of detemir and glargine was injected subcutaneously 24 hours apart at each of two dosing visits. Detemir demonstrated significantly less within-subject variability compared with glargine for children aged 8 to 12 and adolescents 13 to 17 years. No safety concerns were raised during this trial. In previous euglycemic clamp studies involving patients with T1DM by the same authors, the pharmacokinetic/pharmacodynamic properties of detemir did not differ across all age groups including adults aged 18 to 65 years.[82] However, there appeared to be a greater sensitivity for patients over the age of 65 years, suggesting that a slight lower dose of detemir in elderly patients may be as effective.

Patients with T1DM and T2DM have different pharmacokinetic profiles for both basal and rapid-acting insulin analogues. Obese patients with excessive visceral fat demonstrate increased whole-body insulin resistance that can minimize the glucodynamic effects of analogue insulins.[83] Insulin absorption is also affected by subcutaneous fat-layer thickness as capillary density in the subcutis is reduced in obese patients.[84] Therefore, data from pharmacokinetic studies must be interpreted separately for patients with T1DM and T2DM.

Insulin degludec (IDeg) is a new-generation ultra-long-acting basal insulin. The ultra-long effect of IDeg is primarily a result of the slow release of IDeg monomers from soluble multihexamers that form after subcutaneous injection, resulting in a prolonged duration of action (24 to 36 hours) and a smooth, stable pharmacokinetic profile at steady state.[85] Once injected into the subcutis, the IDeg forms stable multihexamers bridged by zinc additives. Over time, the zinc dissolves away from the multihexamers allowing for the release of insulin monomers into the subcutaneous space. The monomers are subsequently absorbed into the surrounding capillaries and carried via albumin to their target insulin receptor sites (see Chapter 12, Fig. 12-3).

In a phase 2, 16-week, randomized, open-label trial, patients with T1DM received either degludec or glargine with aspart insulin administered independently at mealtimes.[86] A1C levels at the conclusion of the study were comparable between all groups as were fasting glucose values. Degludec patients experienced 28% less confirmed hypoglycemia events than those using glargine. This study prespecified no confirmatory hypothesis, and no formal statistical testing was performed. Therefore, no *p* values were reported. IDeg has a fourfold lower degree of within-subject variability compared with glargine.[87] Lower within-subject variability would allow one to titrate the dose of insulin to lower glycemic targets (i.e., 70 mg per dL) without fearing increased risk of inducing hypoglycemia due to "rogue absorption" of the drug. Lower within-subject variability provides a mechanistic explanation for the lower rate of confirmed hypoglycemia observed in other degludec clinical trials.

Rapid-Acting Insulin Analogues

Rapid-acting insulin analogues begin to exhibit their glucose-lowering effects within 10 to 15 minutes following an injection, in comparison with 30 to 60 minutes onset of action of RHI (see Chapter 12, Table 12-7). Three rapid-acting insulin analogues are currently available: lispro–humalog, aspart–novolog, and glulisine–apidra. Aspart and glulisine have also been approved for injection immediately *following* a meal. Postprandial administration can be useful if a patient forgets to take the injection prior to eating. In active children, dosing insulin postmeal may minimize their risk of becoming hypoglycemic. For example, if one were to inject 4 U of a rapid-acting insulin assuming that the child would eat a meal with enough carbohydrates to match the rise in exogenous insulin levels only to have him or her run out of the house to play with friends after consuming half a sandwich, the child would likely become hypoglycemic. A parent could estimate the carbohydrates consumed and administer insulin accordingly following a meal.

Recombinant Human Hyaluronidase and Ultrafast Acting Insulin Analogues

Insulin delivered subcutaneously enters an intercellular matrix consisting of hyaluronan, salt solution, elastin, and plasma proteins maintained within a collagen fiber framework. This matrix slows dispersion of the injected drug away from the site of administration essentially acting as a barrier through which drugs must pass prior to entering the capillary bed. RHI as well as insulins lispro and aspart are formulated as hexamers, which must dissociate to monomers and dimers prior to being absorbed into the capillary bed. Glulisine is a nonhexameric drug, yet has absorption characteristics quite similar to lispro and aspart. The rapid-acting insulin analogues have been genetically engineered to dissociate into dimers and monomers at higher concentrations than RHI, thereby accelerating their time-action profiles. All three rapid-acting analogues are still too slow to provide physiologic control of prandial glucose excursions when bolused immediately prior to eating. These insulins require an optimum delay (lag time) of 20 minutes between injection and onset of meal to minimize postprandial excursions.[88]

Variable intrasubject absorption from the subcutis and changes in time-action profiles are also dependent on factors such as the viscosity of the gel matrix, dermal thickness, blood flow, and temperature at the injection site, as well as insulin dose and concentration.[89] Glycemic variability is frustrating for patients who experience unpredictable blood glucose responses to the same meal and insulin dose on any given day.

When used as adjunctive therapy for a patient using insulin, hyaluronidase increases its dispersion and absorption of the drug through enzymatic breakdown of hyaluronan, thereby reducing the viscosity of the gel matrix. This increases the permeability of the insulin within the subcutis permitting the drug to reach the capillary bed much more quickly[90] (Fig. 11-1). A recombinant human hyaluronidase (rHuPH20) has been developed and has been approved by the FDA as an adjuvant to improve the dispersion and absorption of other injected drugs.

Ten clinical investigations of the effect of rHuPH20 on insulin delivery have been initiated, and data are available for eight of these studies.[90] The addition of rHuPH20 appears to improve the

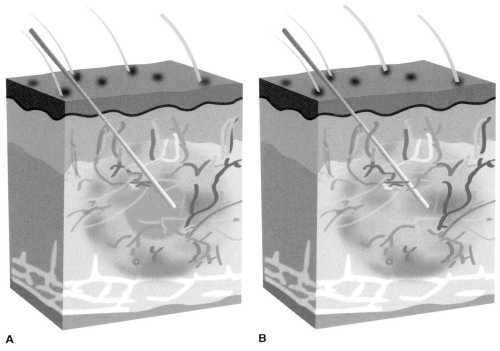

A   B

Figure 11-1 • A,B. Hyaluronidase Mechanism of Action.
Hyaluronan is a large polymer found in interstitial tissue. Any drug injected into the subcutaneous space must pass through this gel matrix prior to entering the capillary system. Drug action times are slowed by the presence of hyaluronan. Hyaluronidase catalyzes the rapid depolymerization of hyaluronan, thereby enhancing the rapid dispersion of coinjected drugs. This synergistically accelerates absorption into the capillary circulation and increases time-action profiles. The local tissue changes that occur following an injection of hyaluronidase are fully reversible and restored following each dose.

variability of responses to identical day-to-day injections, PK profile with increasing insulin doses, as well as improvements in absorption over an aging insulin pump infusion site. When compared with control rapid-acting insulin injections, assessed endpoints are approximately 50% improved with the use of rHuPH20 (Fig. 11-2). Further studies will be required to determine safety, efficacy, and appropriate patient selection for the use of recombinant human hyaluronidase.

Several other approaches are being evaluated to accelerate the time-action profiles of rapid-acting insulins. These include faster acting insulin analogue preparations, warming of infusion sites of insulin pumps, and alternative routes of drug administration (microneedle infusion sets, inhaled insulin, and intraperitoneal insulin pumps).

Prescribing the Treatment Regimen for Physiologic Insulin Replacement

Physiologic insulin replacement therapy for patients with T1DM can best be accomplished with the use of a basal-bolus insulin regimen. The ultimate goal of physiologic insulin replacement therapy is to mimic the normal basal and postmeal patterns of glucose and insulin as seen in a euglycemic individual. Findings from large randomized trials clearly demonstrate that early and aggressive management of glycemia significantly decreases the development and progression of both microvascular and macrovascular complications of diabetes.[5,91,92] Unfortunately, intensification of therapy and improved glycemic control is often associated with an increased frequency of severe hypoglycemia.[5]

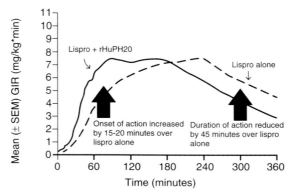

Figure 11-2 • Hyaluronidase Efficacy in Accelerating Prandial Insulin Pharmacokinetics and Pharmacodynamic Profiles in Patients with Diabetes.
The addition of rHuPH20 to insulin lispro doubles the time-action profile of the insulin and reduces the patient's exposure to the insulin by 50% after 2 hours. The onset of action of exogenous insulin is increased by approximately 15 to 20 minutes with rHuPH20, and the duration of action of the analogue is reduced by 45 minutes. (Adapted from Muchmore D, Hompesch M, Morrow L, et al. Human hyaluronidase coinjection consistently accelerates prandial insulin pharmacokinetic (PK) and glucodynamics (GD) across studies and populations. *American Diabetes Association Scientific Sessions*. San Diego, CA. June 24–28, 2011:965-P, with permission.)

Thus, the rate-limiting step to diabetes intensification remains the fear of inducing iatrogenic hypoglycemia by either the patient or the prescriber of the treatment regimen.

Insulin pump therapy using rapid-acting insulin analogues improves glycemic control, reduces the frequency and severity of hypoglycemic reactions, and is the most physiologic of all available treatment regimens for patients with T1DM.[93] Pump therapy is described in detail in Chapter 13. The goals of physiologic insulin replacement therapy are listed in Table 11-4.

Therapeutic interventions for patients with T1DM should be prescribed that are likely to allow the patient to successfully attain their targeted glycemic goals. Patients and prescribers will need to

TABLE 11-4. Goals of Physiologic Insulin Replacement Therapy

- Prescribe a protocol that will allow the patient to achieve ADA-targeted fasting blood glucose level of 90–130 mg/dL

- Target 2 h postprandial blood glucose levels <180 mg/dL

- Minimize the rise in postprandial blood glucose levels from premeal baseline levels of ≤ 50 mg/dL

- Minimize the risk of developing hypoglycemia by instructing patients on appropriate pattern glucose testing and means by which hypoglycemia may be predicted and treated proactively

- Allow patients to self-titrate their basal and prandial insulin doses based upon specified treatment targets (fasting and postprandial glucose excursions)

- Encourage use of Certified Diabetes Educators to assist patients in appropriately learning and incorporating their treatment regimens with their active lifestyle

- Stress the importance of diabetes self-management skills. Unlike other chronic illnesses (such as cancer, multiple sclerosis, arthritis, and migraine), the ultimate decision maker on disease management is the patient. In fact, decisions on insulin dosing, carbohydrate intake, activity restriction, and sick day management must be considered multiple times each day. Health-care providers must educate the patient on all aspects of diabetes self-management in order for this disease to be treated successfully

- Treatment must be customized based on cultural and personal preferences whenever possible (see Chapter 14)

work together to not only initiate the most appropriate treatments but make adjustments based on factors such as micronutrient intake, activity level, long distance travel, shift work, preconception planning, pregnancy, perioperative care, initiation of systemic steroids during cancer treatments, and even religious fasting days. Patients with T1DM need to consider many therapeutic decisions on a daily basis, most of which are made without physician guidance. Amazingly, most patients will become quite adept at adjusting their insulin doses according to their specific immediate metabolic requirements. On occasion, the patient may bolus inappropriate doses of insulin. Clinicians should *never* rebuke patients for missing their fasting or postprandial glucose targets. After all, they are doing the best they can with the insulin dosing resources provided by YOU!

A euglycemic individual has an intact and functioning islet making food consumption as simple as passing a second grade math test if you were Albert Einstein! Unfortunately, patients with T1DM have no functioning β-cells or α-cells. Their brains smell the food, quantify the carbohydrate content, and estimate the dose of insulin that must be given, before producing and secreting endogenous insulin 10 to 15 minutes before eating directly into the portal circulation. These lucky individuals even have intact glycemic counterregulatory mechanisms that minimize one's risk of becoming hypoglycemic while sleeping or following a meal.

Patients with T1DM are not so lucky. Self–blood glucose levels must be monitored before eating. Both the quantity and food groups that will be consumed should be determined. Insulin should be injected 10 to 15 minutes prior to eating, unless the blood glucose level is less than 80 mg per dL. A 2-hour postprandial glucose level may be checked to determine if supplemental insulin is needed to reverse a hyperglycemic value. If the paired test demonstrates a "negative delta" from baseline, the patient is trending toward hypoglycemia and should take appropriate action to monitor and prevent such an event. If one does become hypoglycemic, overtreatment may result in "reactive hyperglycemia" as well as a recurrent hypoglycemic event within 24 hours due to disordered glucose counterregulation.[94]

Customized prescribing allows the patient to develop the confidence required to safely and accurately administer insulin according to their prescribers suggested specifications. The skills required to initiate, titrate, and modify insulin therapy are well within the skill sets of primary care physicians.

• Step 1: Determine the total daily dose (TDD) of insulin

Intensification of insulin therapy for patients with T1DM should incorporate the use of multiple daily injections (MDIs). Adjustment in the dosing parameters would be based on home blood glucose monitoring. Patients who are able to self-titrate based on a prescribed insulin algorithm can safely and effectively achieve their glycemic targets with teaching time.[95–99,99a]

The following steps will guide the clinician toward appropriate initiation of basal-bolus insulin dosing parameters for patients with T1DM:

Establish the Total Daily Dose of Insulin

The TDD is equal to the weight in kg × 0.7.

For example, a 70-kg patient would require $70 \times 0.7 = 49$ U of insulin daily. Adolescents may require 1 to 2 U per kg per day, while older individuals may require only 0.5 to 0.6 U per kg per day. TDDs may be rounded off for easier management. In this example, the 49 U per day can be changed to 50 U per day.[100]

• Step 2: Determine the dose of basal insulin analogue (glargine or detemir) and rapid-acting insulin (aspart, lispro, or glulisine)

Basal insulin minimizes the effects of hepatic glucose production, thus keeping blood glucose levels regulated in the fasting state. The basal insulin requirement is equal to 50% of the TDD (Fig. 11-3). Thus, a patient requiring 50 U of insulin per day would require approximately 25 U of basal insulin.

Total Daily Dose of Insulin

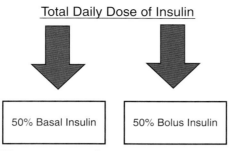

Figure 11-3 • Total Daily Dose of Insulin.

The remaining 50% would be dedicated to bolus insulin. These percentages may vary from patient to patient. Some individuals may require a 40%/60% split favoring bolus insulin. When prescribing a basal insulin, tell the patient a specific time to administer the injection, that is, 9:00 PM, as the drug lasts 22 to 24 hours. Erratic injection times will result in unpredictable fasting glucose levels. Once initiated the basal insulin can be titrated by increasing the dose by 1 U daily until their fasting blood glucose is less than 100 mg per dL.[96] If a patient becomes hypoglycemic at any time of the day, reduce the basal insulin dose by 2 U and discontinue the dose titration.

Patients may be switched from glargine to degludec using a 1:1 ratio of insulin. Thus, a patient using 30 U of glargine once daily should be transitioned to using degludec 30 U. Table 11-5 shows the suggested basal insulin dosing titration algorithm of degludec that is based upon the mean of 3 consecutive days of prebreakfast self–blood glucose measurements. Degludec has been shown to improve long-term glycemic control in patients with T1DM when given as a component of basal-bolus therapy. The first time to meet titration target was shorter with degludec versus glargine (median 5 vs. 10 weeks). Rates of nocturnal confirmed hypoglycemia (recorded glucose level less than 56 mg per dL or a severe episode requiring assistance for reversal) were 25% lower for degludec than glargine. Confirmed hypoglycemic events were similar between the two insulins as were the total daily mean insulin doses (50:50 split of basal:bolus for degludec/aspart and glargine/aspart).[101]

• Step 3: Establish prandial dosing regimen

Determining the meal time dose of insulin is the most challenging aspect of T1DM management. Appropriate insulin dosing requires calculations that take into account the patient's current blood glucose value, the target blood glucose, the insulin-to-carbohydrate ratio (which can vary according

 TABLE 11-5. Titration Algorithm of IDeg[a]

Mean of 3 Consecutive Days of Prebreakfast Self–Blood Glucose Values (mg/dL)	Degludec Adjustment (U)
<56	−4
	(If dose is >45 U, reduce by 10%)
57–70	−2
	(If dose >45 U, reduce by 5%)
71–90	0
91–180	+2
181–270	+4
≥270	+6

[a]Note that in this clinical trial the target blood glucose range was 71 to 90 mg per dL.
From Heller S, Francisco AMO, Pei H, et al. Insulin degludec improves long-term glycemic control with less nocturnal hypoglycemia compared with insulin glargine: 1-year results from randomized basal-bolus trial in type 1 diabetes. *American Diabetes Association 71st Scientific Sessions*. San Diego, CA. 70-OR. June 25, 2011.

to the time of day or meal consumed), the total carbohydrate content of a meal, and the anticipated activity level following a meal. The key elements of successful insulin therapy are optimizing glycemic control while minimizing hypoglycemia. This may be accomplished by using a simple prandial insulin dosing algorithm or using insulin-to-carbohydrate ratios. Insulin-to-carbohydrate ratios allow flexibility in food choices and enable relatively precise matching of mealtime insulin needs.

Most primary care physicians do not have access to registered dietitians (RDs) or Certified Diabetic Educators in their practice. There is also limited time in our schedules to teach patients about insulin:carbohydrate ratios. "carb counting" does have many *disadvantages*, especially within a primary care setting. (1) carb counting works best if one's glycemic control is ideal. Attempting to carbohydrate count when glucose levels are averaging 250 mg per dL will fail. (2) Insulin:carbohydrate ratios may vary based on the time of the day. Insulin sensitivity is highest in afternoon, while patients are more insulin resistant upon awakening due to the secretion of cortisol and other counterregluatory hormones. (3) Carbohydrate absorption is influenced by fat content in food. The rate of appearance of exogenous glucose in the circulation is altered by consuming greater than 42 g of fat with a meal. High-fat meals cause glucose absorption to become biphasic with a second peak elevation appearing 3 hours after the meal is consumed. Dietary carbohydrate absorption remains incomplete even up to 7 hours following the consumption of a high-fat meal.[102] Meals containing less than 17 g of fat reduce glucose absorption within 3 hours of the meal consumption and do not result in hyperglycemia rebound thereafter.[103] Absorption patterns of carbohydrates and fats demonstrate cultural and ethnic variance. Southern Europeans tend to exhibit a more rapid peak of postprandial lipemia compared with Northern Europeans.[104] Thus, correctly counting carbohydrate when one is consuming more than 17 g of fat for a given meal may be an exercise in futility unless, of course, the patient is Italian! (4) Dietary fiber is not usually digested. If a patient is carbohydrate counting and a meal contains ≥5 g of fiber per serving, the total amount of fiber must be subtracted from the total amount of carbohydrates consumed prior to calculating an insulin dose. For example, if a meal contains 25 g of carbohydrates and 5 g of fiber, the insulin dose should be calculated based on the consumption of only 20 g of carbs.[105] (5) Patients may notice a unique response to certain carbohydrate containing foods that will require adjustments of their mealtime insulin doses based more on experience rather than a mathematical calculation.

A simplified approach to prescribing prandial insulin for patients with T1DM that the author has found particularly efficient and useful in clinical practice is based on a study published by Bergenstal et al.[106] in *Diabetes Care*. This randomized controlled study in obese patients with T2DM demonstrated that a simple algorithm to adjust mealtime insulin glulisine was as effective as adjusting mealtime insulin using insulin-to-carbohydrate ratios.

Table 11-6 shows a simplified algorithm for initiating and adjusting prandial insulin for patients with T1DM.

Once a patient incorporates physiologic insulin replacement therapy into their daily routine, adjustments in doses of either basal or prandial insulin may be safely determined via structured glucose testing.[107] Patients with T1DM require frequent blood glucose testing. Ideally, testing should be performed prior to eating as well as 90 to 120 minutes after finishing the meal in order to minimize postprandial glycemic excursions beyond 180 mg per dL. Paired (structured) glucose testing similar to that displayed in Table 11-7 should be provided to all patients using insulin. Patients should test before and after a designated meal at least 3 days each week. The 2-hour postprandial blood glucose level should not rise greater than 50 mg per dL. The table lists specific reasons that a patient would experience postprandial hyperglycemia and also predict the onset of hypoglycemia. If 2-hour postprandial, "delta" is a negative value, one is at risk for developing hypoglycemia. Rapid-acting insulin absorption occurs predictably over a period of 4 hours. If 10 U is injected at noon, 6 U remains at the site of the insulin depot at 2 PM. Assuming the premeal glucose level is 150 and the blood glucose value at 2:00 PM is 90, the delta would be 150-90 or –60 mg per dL. The patient still has 6 U of insulin on board implying the glucose level is falling, placing the patient at risk of becoming hypoglycemic. This patient should monitor their blood glucose level again within 30 to 60 minutes. Any blood glucose patterns demonstrating fasting or nocturnal hypoglycemia would

TABLE 11-6. Simplified Algorithm for Prandial Insulin Administration in Patients with T1DM

- Step 1: Determine baseline prandial insulin dosage
  Dose of prandial insulin = 0.1 U/kg/meal (e.g., a 70-kg patient would require 70 × 0.1 U = 7 U rapid-acting insulin per meal)

- Establish the "lag time" for insulin injection
  Insulin should be injected 15 min before a meal unless the blood glucose level prior to eating is <80 mg/dL

- Allow patient to adjust insulin dosage based on size of the meal
  Dose of prandial insulin is adjusted as follows:

Meal Size	Prandial Insulin Dose Adjustment
Standard meal	No change
Very large meal with dessert	+ 3 U from baseline
Large meal without dessert	+1–2 U from baseline
Smaller than usual meal	−1 to 2 U from baseline

  For example, a patient with a baseline prescribed prandial insulin dose of 7 U plans to eat a Thanksgiving size feast. The dose of insulin would be 7 + 3 = 10 U injected 15 min before eating.

- Adjust initial baseline dose of insulin periodically based on the results of "structured glucose testing"

necessitate a reduction in basal insulin dosing. Consistent patterned postprandial elevations should be countered with an increase in premeal rapid-acting insulin dosing. Bedtime basal insulin doses may need to be titrated in response to persistent fasting hyperglycemia.

• Step 4: Applying a correction dose to normalize premeal hyperglycemia

Insulin adjustments are made when individualized blood glucose targets are not met either acutely or chronically. Any dosing adjustment of insulin should be based on one's self–blood glucose values. Unfortunately, insulin dosing adjustments are easier taught than performed by the patient. Although patients will acknowledge the need to adjust their insulin boluses, fear of inducing hypoglycemia by overcorrecting has been cited as the primary reason for not applying the proper corrective dose.[108] Patients also tend to misjudge their own glucose level prior to dosing insulin believing that they are in the "target range," when in fact they are either hypo- or hyperglycemic. Unfortunately, patients may also become lax and simply bolus based on how their perception of their current glucose value rather than on documented self-monitored plasma glucose. One should counsel patients that bolusing 10 U of rapid-acting insulin for an unchecked glucose value of 50 mg per dL could have disastrous consequences, whereas that same 10 U given 15 minutes before eating with a blood glucose of 120 mg per dL would be very appropriate.

In cases where the premeal baseline glucose levels are elevated (greater than 180 mg per dL), one could apply an "insulin correction factor" to the mealtime bolus in order to achieve a targeted baseline value of 150 mg per dL. The "1800 Rule" is most often used for this purpose as shown in Figure 11-4.[100] To minimize the risk of inducing hypoglycemia, one should be cautious not to correct a blood glucose value lower than 150 mg per dL.

• Carbohydrate Counting for Patients with T1DM

A variety of methods can be used to estimate the nutrient content of meals, including carbohydrate counting, the exchange system, and experience-based estimation. By testing pre- and postprandial

TABLE 11-7. Example of Paired Glucose Testing for Patients with T1DM

Date	Premeal Glucose	2-H Postmeal Glucose	Delta (Difference between Baseline Glucose and 2-h Postmeal Glucose)	Reasons for Delta Being <50 mg/dL (This Could Indicate Impending Hypoglycemia) List Actions Taken for Hypoglycemia	Reasons for Delta Being >50 mg/dL List Corrective Actions
2/13	125	225	+100		Bolus given at meal time rather than 15 min prior to eating. Mismatch of insulin to carbs (ate dessert). Will give 2 U for dessert next time
2/14	110	154	44 (At target)	—	
2/15	227	117	−110	Overcorrected on premeal insulin dose. Did become hypoglycemic 3 h after eating, but consumed 15 g of carbs	
2/16	153	169	16	Perfect	No need for adjustments for this type of food

Instructions for paired glucose testing:

- Check blood glucose levels before breakfast, lunch, dinner, as well as 2 h after that meal 3 d/wk.
- Write down the numbers on this form and consider the possible reasons why the postmeal glucose would be <50 or >50 mg/dL from baseline.
- Write down corrective action plan. We will discuss this next visit.
- Possible reasons for delta being ≥50 mg/dL (resulting in postmeal hyperglycemia)
- Mismatch of insulin: carbs. Too little insulin given and too many carbs consumed

(Continued)

TABLE 11-7. Example of Paired Glucose Testing for Patients with T1DM (Continued)

- Delay in lag time (time insulin bolus is given in relation to meal. Insulin should normally be bolused 15–30 min *before* beginning a meal unless the premeal glucose is <80 mg/dL)
- Insulin pump malfunction
- Snacking between end of meal and the time test is taken
- Excessive use of caffeine in the AM
- Using an improper type of insulin pump bolus (square wave only, not dual wave)
- Improper technique for self–blood glucose testing. (Handling foods such as fruit or sugar before testing will result in a false reading of the blood glucose strip. Wash your hands before testing)
- Possible reasons for delta being ≤50 (predictive of postmeal hypoglycemia)
- Too much insulin
- Not enough carbs
- Too much activity that lowers glucose levels
- Consumption of alcohol without eating carbs
- Possible reasons for delta > 100
- Omission of insulin dose
- Mismatch of insulin:carbs. Ate a very large meal and gave too little insulin
- Illness (such as the flu)
- Medication (corticosteroids)
- Insulin has gone bad (this can occur if insulin is exposed to excessive heat or if insulin is being used beyond its expiration date)
- Formulas to remember that will help minimize risk of hypoglycemia:
  - After 1 h, 90% of that bolus remains in the skin ready to be absorbed
  - After 2 h, 60% of that bolus remains in the skin ready to be absorbed
  - After 3 h, 40% of that bolus remains in the skin ready to be absorbed
  - After 4 h, 10% of that bolus remains in the skin ready to be absorbed

For example: 10 U given at 10 AM when blood glucose is 100 mg per dL. At noon, the blood glucose is 80 mg per dL. However, 60% of that 10 U dose remains to be absorbed, meaning 6 U remain in the insulin depot. Blood glucose level is therefore trending downward and one should be vigilant for hypoglycemia.

1800/Total daily dose of insulin = Expected drop in blood glucose/1 U of insulin

For example: If the TDD of insulin is 70 U, the correction factor would be:

1800/70 = 25.7 (round off to 25)

- Thus, if the premeal blood glucose is 200 mg per dL, and the target blood glucose is 150 mg per dL, one would give a correction factor of 2 U in addition to base insulin dose at that particular meal. If a patient normally would bolus 7 U prior to eating, a 200 mg per dL premeal glucose value would allow the patient to add 2 U to baseline dose. The total dose now becomes 7 + 2 = 9 U.
- Patients who plan to eat a large meal may also further adjust the insulin dose according to the options mentioned in Table 11-6.
- Blood glucose testing should be performed 2 hours after eating to make certain that one has not trended toward hypoglycemia.

Figure 11-4 • The Rule of 1800 (Insulin Correction Factor).

glucose, many individuals use experience to evaluate and achieve postprandial glucose goals with a variety of foods. To date, research has not demonstrated that one method of assessing the relationship between carbohydrate intake and blood glucose response is better than other methods.[109]

Carbohydrate counting has become the preferred method of matching insulin requirements with meal content for many patients using insulin pumps and MDIs. However, carbohydrate counting takes practice, patience, and education. The process can be quite challenging even for the most dedicated patients for several reasons. The amount of carbohydrate ingested is usually the primary determinant of postprandial response, but the type of carbohydrate also affects this response. Blood glucose response to carbohydrate intake may be influenced by the type of carbohydrate ingested, style of preparation, ripeness, degree of processing, fat content of the meal, and degree of insulin resistance. The recommended daily minimum requirement of carbohydrates for any individual is 130 g per day.[110]

Some patients may insist on learning to count carbohydrates as part of their diabetes self-management skill set. Basic carbohydrate counting helps patients get started with the carbohydrate counting system. Carbohydrate foods are identified as starches, fruit, milk, and desserts. Emphasis is placed on consistency in the timing, type, and amount of carbohydrate-containing foods consumed. Early on, discussion of portion sizes is also key to understanding the concept of what a serving of carbohydrate is. Carbohydrates are measured in grams and may be referred to in grams or servings. One carbohydrate serving is equal to 15 g of carbohydrate. Table 11-8 lists some examples of 15-g carbohydrate servings. Advanced carbohydrate counting includes understanding pattern management and how to use insulin-to-carbohydrate ratios.

Once one understands the "meaning of the carbohydrate," patients become official "carb sharks" analogous to a "card shark" who gets thrown out of the Las Vegas casinos for counting cards (not carbs). Carb sharks learn to read food labels that list the number of carbohydrates per serving and then must calculate the total amount of carbs they will be consuming for a given meal. For example, if a label reads "20 grams of carbohydrates per serving" yet contains 2 servings per can, the carbohydrate counter would dose insulin differently based on whether they will be eating half the carbohydrates content (20 g) or the total amount of carbs in the food (40 g). Carb sharks should be encouraged to make a simple carbohydrate "budget" for meals and snacks as shown in Figure 11-5.

Patients must also be provided with an insulin:carbohydrates ratio allowing them to adjust the dose of their insulin based on the carbohydrate content of their meals. In general, the more the

TABLE 11-8. Examples of 15-G Carbohydrate Servings

- Starches: 1 slice of bread, 1/3 cup of cooked pasta, 3/4 cup of dry cereal
- Fruit: 1 small piece of fruit or 8 oz of fruit juice
- Milk: 1 cup of skim milk or 3/4 cup of yogurt
- Desserts: 2 small cookies or 1/2 cup of ice cream

Meal	Number of Carbohydrate Servings[a]	Total Carbohydrate (grams)
Breakfast	4	60
Lunch	3	45
Dinner	4	60
Snack	1	15
Daily Total	11	170

[a]Each carbohydrate serving contains 15 g of carbs

Grams Carbohydrates	Servings
0–5	Do not count
6–10	Half
11–20	1
21–25	1.5
26–35	2

Figure 11-5 • A "Carb Shark's" Basic Carbohydrate Budget Plan for a Day Based on Packaged Food Labels.

carbohydrates consumed, the larger the dose of insulin that will be needed to minimize postprandial excursions. To estimate how many grams of carbohydrates are covered by 1 U of rapid-acting insulin analogue, the "rule of 500" is employed as shown in Figure 11-6.[111]

The insulin:carbohydrates ratio may also be determined by using the following formula:
Alternative Method for Determining the Insulin:carbohydrate Ratio
Insulin:carbohydrate Ratio = Insulin Sensitivity Factor (ISF) × 0.33

- For example: TDD of Insulin =3 70 U

1,800/70 = 25.7 (The ISF is derived from dividing 1,800 by the TDD of insulin)
Now, 25.7 × 0.33 = 8.48 (round off to 8).
The insulin:carb ratio is 1:8. This means that 1 U of rapid-acting insulin covers 8 g of carbohydrates. If one is consuming a bag of chips (35 g of carbohydrates), the appropriate dose of insulin is 35/8 = 4 U.

Patients may have different insulin:carbohydrate ratios for each meal. The ratio may also change with body weight, variations in physical activity, menstruation, travel, level of glycemic control, and illness. Frequent adjustment in the insulin:carb ratio may be necessary and are best determined with the assistance of a Certified Diabetic Educator or an RD.

Remember, high-fat meals slow carbohydrate absorption requiring adjustment of prandial insulin doses. Deduct foods containing less than 5 g of fiber from the total carb content of the meal as well as before counting the remaining carbohydrates.

500/TDD of Insulin = Grams of carbohydrates covered by 1 U of rapid-acting insulin analogue
- For example: Total daily dose of insulin = 70 U
- 500/70 U= 7
- 1 U of rapid-acting insulin covers 7 g of carbs
- If one is consuming 45 g of carbohydrates for breakfast, they must inject 45/7 U = 6 U bolused 15 minutes before eating (assuming the blood glucose level is greater than 80 mg per dL.)

Figure 11-6 • Rule of 500 for Determining Insulin: Carb Ratio. (Walsh J, Roberts R, Bailey T, et al. *Using Insulin: Everything you Need for Success with Insulin.* San Diego, CA: Torrey Pines Press; 2003.)

• Exercising with T1DM

During the transition from rest to exercise, skeletal muscles shift from using predominantly free fatty acids released from adipose tissue to a mixture of muscle triglycerides, muscle glycogen, and glucose derived from the breakdown of liver glycogen (glycogenolysis). During the initial stages of moderate exercise, muscle glycogen is the primary energy source. However, as exercise becomes more prolonged, glycogen stores become depleted requiring the body to rely on circulating free fatty acids and plasma glucose as a fuel source. During heavy exercise (30 to 60 minutes at 80% of VO_2 max), peripheral glucose utilization may be as high as 1 to 1.5 g per minute.[112] This source of energy must be continuously replaced at an equal rate to prevent the onset of exercise-induced hypoglycemia. In euglycemic individuals, plasma glucose levels are sustained during exercise because pancreatic insulin secretion decreases while levels of glucagon, growth hormone, cortisol, and catecholamines increase.

Patients with T1DM lack the ability to regulate both endogenous insulin secretion and counter-regulatory hormones in response to exercise making maintenance of physiologic fuel regulation nearly impossible. Thus, patients must adjust carbohydrate consumption, insulin dosing, as well as exercise intensity, mode, and duration in order to minimize the risk of hypoglycemia and exercise-induced DKA.

The risk of hypoglycemia is greatest in any patient who is intensively managed using either MDI or insulin pump therapy. Exercise will acutely increase peripheral glucose utilization within skeletal muscles, thus making circulating exogenous insulin "turbo charged." Several factors (Table 11-9) contribute to this acute over-insulinization and hypoglycemia commonly observed in patients exercising with T1DM.

An individual with poor metabolic control is at risk for inducing ketoacidosis in response to vigorous exercise.[113] Prolonged exercise will trigger hepatic glucose production. A patient with a baseline blood glucose level of 240 mg per dL who is insulinopenic and has relative peripheral insulin resistance will note a rise in plasma glucose levels as exercise intensifies. Hyperglycemia and ketosis can result in dehydration and acidosis. Exercise increases plasma concentrations of catecholamines and glucocorticoids resulting in further augmenting hyperglycemia and ketone production.[114] Clinically, patients may note impairment in their overall exercise performance.

Table 11-10 lists suggested practical guidelines to minimize blood glucose excursions before, during, and after exercise for patients with T1DM.

During exercise, patients with T1DM should maintain an adequate level of hydration. Dehydration may result in impaired performance, muscle cramps, hyperglycemia, heat stroke, and rhabdomyolysis. Patients with rhabdomyolysis will present with severe muscle cramps, fatigue, and

TABLE 11-9. Factors That Favor Induction of Exercise-Induced Hypoglycemia in Patients with T1DM

- The rate of absorption of subcutaneously injected insulin is increased with exercise.
- Blood flow through the peripheral muscles is increased during exercise. Delivery of insulin to receptor sites in the skeletal muscles is therefore increased resulting in more rapid glucose disposal within the myocytes. Skeletal muscles become highly insulin sensitive. (Wasserman DH, Davis SN, Zinman B. Fuel metabolism during exercise in health and diabetics. In: Ruderman NB, Devlin JT, Schneider S, et al., eds. *Handbook of Exercise in Diabetes*. Alexandria, VA. American Diabetes Association; 2002:63–100.)
- Exogenous plasma insulin levels do not decrease during exercise. The inability to suppress insulin levels during exercise following an injection results in hyperinsulinemia. Hepatic glucose production is suppressed favoring the onset of hypoglycemia within 20–60 min after the onset of exercise. (Schiffrin A, Parikh S. Accommodating planned exercise in T1DM patients on intensive treatment. *Diabetes Care*. 1985;8:337–342.)
- Hypoglycemia during exercise may result from impaired glucose counterregulation caused by previous exposure to hypoglycemic events. Hypoglycemia induced during exercise will often reoccur throughout and during sleep. (Cryer PE, Davis SN, Shamoon H. Hypoglycemia in diabetes. *Diabetes Care*. 2003;26(6):1902–1912.)

TABLE 11-10. Suggestions for Minimizing Blood Glucose Excursions Before, During, and After Exercise for Patients with T1DM

Before exercise	• Determine the timing, mode (aerobic vs. resistance training), and intensity of exercise to be performed • Perform blood glucose monitoring prior to exercise • "Safe" target blood glucose prior to initiating moderate exercise should be 120–180 mg/dL • If blood glucose level is <120 mg/dL, consumption of 15 g of carbohydrates is appropriate to provide an energy source for exercise • Do *not* exercise if blood glucose levels are ≥250 mg/dL and ketosis is present or if glucose levels are ≥300 mg/dL and no ketones are present • If activity is moderate or strenuous, lasts < 90 min and begins within 90 min of a meal, prandial doses of lispro, aspart, and glulisine are warranted • Insulin doses may need to be increased and monitored more frequently during periods of prolonged resistance training or when training occurs in a warm environment • Consume 250 mL of fluids 20 min prior to exercise in order to maintain hydration
During exercise	• Monitor blood glucose level every 30 min • Continue fluid intake of 250 mL every 20 min during vigorous exercise • If blood glucose drops < 100 mg/dL during periods of moderate or intense exercise, consume 15 g of carbohydrates every 20–30 min • Consider use of a continuous glucose sensor that would indicate direction of blood glucose values during exercise
After exercise	• Monitor blood glucose level overnight if exercise is atypical • Consider consuming additional slow-acting carbohydrates to protect against exercise-induced nocturnal hypoglycemia • Patients with hypoglycemia awareness autonomic failure (HAAF) should wear a continuous glucose sensor that will alert them to the onset of nocturnal hypoglycemia

occasional fevers following a session of vigorous exercise often without having had appropriate fluid rehydration. The most useful confirmatory laboratory test is serum creatine kinase (CK), which is often found to be 5 to 10 times above the upper limits of normal in patients with rhabdomyolysis. Levels should be repeated every 6 to 12 hours until a peak level is established. Once CK levels have peaked (usually at values of several hundred to hundreds of thousands of units per liter), levels will decrease by 30% to 40% per day. Urine analysis may show the presence of hemoglobin or myoglobin. Acute renal failure develops in 30% to 40% of patients and is the most serious complication in the days after the initial presentation. A serum creatinine greater than 1.7 mg per dL in the presence of hyperkalemia and myoglobinuria warrants an immediate nephrology consult for the management of acute renal failure due to rhabdomyolysis.[115]

Patients with T1DM should remain hydrated by consuming 250 mL every 20 minutes of exercise with the first drink preceding exercise by 20 minutes.[116] Carbohydrate-electrolyte beverages (e.g., Gatorade-light) may be best for activities lasting greater than 60 minutes as these drinks contain both carbohydrate and fluids.

Insulin pump patients may easily adjust their insulin delivery in anticipation of their exercise time, duration, and intensity. Patients using basal insulin detemir or glargine are not able to make simple changes in their dosing regimens to accommodate their acute exercise schedules. A recently published study compared plasma glucose levels and hypoglycemia incidence following exercise in patients with T1DM using NPH, detemir, and glargine.[117] Patients exercised 5 hours following their last rapid-acting meal-time injection of insulin while using either NPH, detemir, or glargine basal insulin. During 30 minutes of exercise, 5 (11%) participants on insulin detemir developed minor hypoglycemia, 6 (12%) for NPH, and 18 (38%) for glargine. From the end of exercise to 150 minutes following the conclusion of activity, 5 (11%) on insulin detemir, 7 (14%) on NPH, and 9 (19%) on insulin glargine developed minor hypoglycemia. Overall, glargine patients experience 50% more episodes of minor hypoglycemia than patients taking detemir from the start of exercise to 150 minutes after exercise. Therefore, based on this study, one might consider using insulin detemir over glargine for patients who are proactively engaging in moderate-to-heavy exercise on a routine basis.

Assessing asymptomatic patients with T1DM for silent ischemia prior to initiating an exercise program remains controversial and is not recommended by the ADA.[118] Cardiac autonomic neuropathy (CAN) can increase one's risk of postural hypotension, impaired thermoregulation, impaired night vision (due to abnormal pupillary reaction to light and accommodation), and unpredictable carbohydrate delivery to the gut predisposing to hypoglycemia. Autonomic cardiomyopathy is strongly associated with sudden death in patients with diabetes.[119] Any patient with CAN should undergo extensive cardiac evaluation prior to initiating any type of planned moderate exercise activity.[118] Clinical judgment should be used to determine individual risk and advise patients on ways by which they can safely and effectively exercise considering their current level of metabolic control.

All patients with peripheral neuropathy should wear proper footwear and inspect their feet daily for presence of ulceration and calluses. Studies have shown that moderate-intensity walking may not lead to increased risk of foot ulcers or ulcerations in patients with this microvascular complication.[120]

A reduction in prandial doses of rapid-acting insulin is warranted when exercise is moderate or strenuous, lasts less than 90 minutes, and begins within 90 minutes of the previous meal. When strenuous exercise lasts greater than 60 minutes or moderate exercise is prolonged greater than 90 minutes, the basal insulin dose may need to be reduced 2 to 4 hours prior to that activity. Patients who exercise on a daily basis should consider using an insulin pump as programmable basal rates can be established based upon anticipated exercise time. In addition, patients may set a temporary basal rate to reduce insulin delivery if exercise is prolonged or one has an erratic schedule. Obviously, one cannot adjust the dose of basal insulin glargine or detemir to adjust for the onset of exercise once the drug is injected. One should target a preexercise blood glucose value of 120 to 160 mg per dL. Fifteen grams of carbohydrates may be consumed if the blood glucose level is ≤100 mg per dL. Blood glucose values should be monitored every 30 to 60 minutes to make certain that one is not becoming hypoglycemic.

Hypoglycemia may be difficult to detect during strenuous exercise as the sweating, palpitations, fatigue, blurry vision, or weakness may occur with exhaustion and low blood glucose values. Continuous glucose sensors may also be useful in monitoring for hypoglycemia during exercise. Glucose tablets or liquids should be carried at all times for rapid correction of hypoglycemia.

Pramlintide

Pramlintide (Symlin) is an analogue possessing pharmacodynamic properties similar to those of the native amylin. The addition of pramlintide to exogenous insulin therapy improves long-term glycemic control beyond that obtained with insulin therapy alone without weight gain or an increased risk of hypoglycemia.[121]

In clinical trials, the addition of pramlintide to patients with insulin-requiring T1DM and T2DM has been shown to reduce the A1C approximately 0.5% to 1.0% from baseline when compared with placebo.[122] The percentage of patients who are able to achieve the ADA glycemic target (A1C less than 7%) was two to three times greater when pramlintide was added to an established insulin regimen.

One of the most frustrating adverse events associated with overall glycemic improvement in patients using insulin therapy is weight gain. Insulin is a natural growth hormone. Exogenous insulin doses are often substantially higher than the amount of insulin produced by a normally functioning pancreas. Theoretically, exogenous insulin may down-regulate β-cell function, further reducing one's ability to produce and secrete amylin hormone. Amylin is a neuroendocrine hormone that binds to the postrema area of the brain and reduces satiety. Patients with T1DM with a BMI greater than 27 kg per m² lost an average of 1.6 kg over a 26-week period when compared with those taking placebo.[122]

The glucose-lowering effects of pramlintide are related to the drug's ability to improve gastric emptying and reduce postmeal glucagon levels. Pramlintide has minimal effect on fasting glucose levels.

Oxidative stress, the imbalance between free radical production and antioxidant consumption, is a significant pathogenic factor in the development of microvascular and macrovascular complications.[72] Hyperglycemia, both acute and chronic, increases oxidative stress and endothelial cell dysfunction in patients with both T1DM and T2DM.[123] The addition of pramlintide to regular insulin in T1DM has been demonstrated to reduce both postprandial glycemic excursions and biomarkers of oxidative stress.[124]

Pramlintide is generally well tolerated, the most common side effect being nausea, which occurs in up to 40% of patients using the drug. However, GI symptoms tend to resolve over the first 2 to 4 weeks of therapy. Advising patients to limit their fatty food intake when initiating pramlintide therapy will lessen their nausea considerably. High-fat foods trigger the release of cholestokinin, an intestinal hormone that tends to intensify nausea. Doses must be titrated slowly to minimize nausea.

Pramlintide alone does not cause hypoglycemia. However, when the drug is used as adjunct therapy in patients using mealtime insulin, hypoglycemia can occur, particularly in patients with T1DM. The following steps may be taken to limit treatment-emergent hypoglycemia in patients with T1DM using pramlintide:

1. Reduce the dose of mealtime insulin by 50%.
2. Patients with insulin pumps using a combined immediate and extended-wave bolus might consider reducing their initial bolus by 75% while increasing the extended-wave bolus insulin dose by 25% delivered over a 3-hour period.
3. Patients must be vigilant regarding the possibility of hypoglycemia. Monitoring blood glucose levels 1 to 2 hours after using pramlintide is essential. Patients with hypoglycemic unawareness who are reluctant to perform frequent home blood glucose monitoring may not be acceptable candidates for using pramlintide.

Pramlintide should be initiated in patients with T1DM at 15 µg and increased every 3 to 7 days by an additional 15 µg until reaching a well-tolerated maintenance dose of 60 µg. At this dose, patients should experience no nausea and some degree of appetite suppression. If significant nausea persists at the 45- or 60-µg dose level, reduce the dose to 30 µg. Patients who are intolerant of pramlintide at 30 µg should consider stopping the drug. T2DM patients can initiate therapy at 60 µg with an increase to 120 µg within 3 to 7 days, depending on their ability to tolerate the drug. Oral agents may be continued at the pre-pramlintide doses.

Table 11-11 summarizes the treatment protocol for using pramlintide.

Patients who are using insulin pump therapy should adjust only their mealtime boluses while taking pramlintide. Basal insulin rates need not be altered. Patients can correct preprandial hyperglycemia, but the ISF should be reduced initially by 50%. For example, if 1 U of analogue insulin normally reduces glucose levels by 25 mg per dL; with pramlintide, that same dose of insulin may reduce glucose levels by 50 mg per dL.

▌ Management of Severe Insulin Resistance Using U-500 Insulin

A euglycemic individual consuming a standard diet secretes approximately 45 U of endogenous insulin per 24 hours, including 10 U for breakfast, 13 U for lunch, 14 U for dinner, and 8 basal U

TABLE 11-11. Administration of Pramlintide to Patients with T1DM and T2DM

Notes on Pramlintide Dosing for Patients with T2DM
1. Initiate pramlintide at 60 g immediately before major meals.
2. Reduce preprandial rapid-acting insulin, including fixed-mix insulins, by 50%.
3. Monitor blood glucose levels before meals, 2 h after meals, and at bedtime.
4. Increase dose to 120 g when no nausea has occurred for 3 to 7 d. If nausea occurs at 120 g, reduce dose to 60 g.
5. Adjust dose of insulin to optimize glycemic control once the target dose of pramlintide (Symlin) is achieved and nausea has stopped. The dose of Symlin may actually be pushed beyond that recommended in the package insert if the patient is not experiencing satiety or nausea. Over time, slowly increase the dose until the patient develops satiety or nausea or has other adverse events such as postprandial hypoglycemia. If doses are gingerly increased to the point of satiety, weight loss will be more prominent.
6. The physician should be contacted weekly until a target dose of pramlintide (Symlin) is achieved, pramlintide is well tolerated, and blood glucose levels are stable.

Notes on Pramlintide Dosing for Patients with T1DM
1. Initiate pramlintide at 15 g immediately before major meals.
2. Reduce preprandial rapid-acting insulin, including fixed-mix insulins, by 50%.
   Injecting insulin immediately after the meal may reduce the incidence of postprandial hypoglycemia in some patients.
3. Monitor blood glucose levels before meals, 2 h after meals, and at bedtime.
4. Increase pramlintide dose to the next increment (30, 45, 60 g) when no nausea has occurred for 3 d. If significant nausea persists at the 45- to 60-g dose, pramlintide should be decreased to 30 g. If the 30-g dose is not tolerated, Symlin should be discontinued.
5. Adjust dose of insulin to optimize glycemic control once the target dose of pramlintide (Symlin) is achieved and nausea has stopped. The dose of Symlin may actually be pushed beyond that recommended in the package insert if the patient is not experiencing satiety or nausea. Over time, slowly increase the dose until the patient develops satiety, nausea, or has other adverse events such as postprandial hypoglycemia. If doses are gingerly increased to the point of satiety, weight loss will be more prominent.
6. Doctor should be contacted weekly until a target dose of pramlintide is achieved, pramlintide is well tolerated, and blood glucose levels are stable.

Administration of Pramlintide
1. Inject pramlintide into the thigh or abdomen at least 2 inches from the insulin depot site. Clicking should be audible as the dial moves downward during the administration of the dose. Hold the pen in place against the skin for 10 sec following the injection to confirm delivery of the entire dose.
2. Use a new needle for each injection.
3. If dose is missed at a given meal, simply give the prescribed dose at the following meal. Do not double up or attempt to "catch up" by increasing the dose at another meal.

to suppress hepatic glucose production in the fasting state. At least 50% of the endogenous insulin released by the pancreas is extracted by the liver during the initial transhepatic passage so that the total peripheral delivery of insulin is approximately 22 U per day.[125] Insulin resistance occurs when the hormone's action to lower blood glucose levels is severely impaired. In order for insulin action to occur, insulin must bind with receptors on the cell surfaces of skeletal muscles and adipose tissue. If insulin receptors are down-regulated or absent, cells become unresponsive to insulin action. In response to prolonged and persistent hyperglycemia, the pancreas will produce an excessive amount of insulin in an attempt to restore ambient glucose levels to normal. However, the high levels of circulating endogenous insulin results in down-regulation of insulin receptors and impairment of insulin action. Inflammatory cytokines may inhibit the expression of peroxisome proliferator-activated receptor genes leading to a state of insulin resistance.[126] Some individuals may be insulin resistant despite having normal numbers of insulin receptors on their cell surfaces.[127] Thus, the exact pathogenesis of insulin resistance is uncertain.

Patients in whom glycemic control deteriorates despite using more than 200 U of exogenous insulin daily are considered to be insulin resistant.[128] As a result of having prolonged and significant hyperglycemia, these patients may become symptomatic and frustrated over the lack of efficacy of different treatment protocols. One treatment option for treating insulin resistance is the use of human regular U-500 insulin, which by design is five times more concentrated (500 U per mL) than the standard U-100 insulin (100 U per mL). Because U-500 insulin is highly concentrated, lower volumes of the drug can be injected, resulting in a smaller and more efficiently absorbed insulin depot. A patient who normally injects 50 U of U-100 prior to a meal needs to administer only 10 U of U-500.

Advantages of U-500 usage include improved insulin absorption, fewer (and lower volume) injections to enhance comfort and compliance, and, importantly, cost savings, with U-500 insulin costing approximately $0.02 per U, less than one-fifth of the cost of insulin analogues. Potential candidates include insulin-resistant patients receiving multiple daily doses of insulin, particularly after transplant, or steroid treatment. Patients with systemic infection or gestational diabetes causing severe insulin resistance or patients with genetic and autoimmune defects of insulin action also may benefit from such treatment.[129]

A study by Neal showed that 20 insulin-resistant patients who were converted to U-500 insulin were able to lower their A1C from baseline (9.6%) by 1.1% over 3 to 6 months.[130] There was no reported significant hypoglycemia in any of the patients.

Knee et al.[131] described a series of four patients treated off label with U-500 insulin by means of insulin pump therapy. Three months after conversion to U-500 therapy, the average A1C decreased from 10.8% to 7.6%, and within 6 months, the average A1C was 7.3%. With use of U-500, the absolute volume of pumped insulin infused per day decreased by at least fourfold, leading to a cost saving for insulin of up to $2,600 per year, while the cost of pump supplies was reduced by up to $3,400 annually. All patients had subjective improvement in quality of life.

The most clinically significant distinguishing factors between rapid-acting insulins and U-500 include onset of action, time to peak effect, and duration of action. Rapid-acting insulin analogues demonstrate a peak effect within 90 minutes of administration and a 4-hour duration of action. This compares with U-500 having an onset of action and peak effect within 2 to 4 hours after administration with a duration of up to 24 hours.[132]

Table 11-12 displays a practical guide to dosing U-500 insulin for highly insulin-resistant patients. U-500 insulin can be injected subcutaneously or administered via an insulin pump.

Tables 11-13 and 11-14 discuss additional tips on using U-500 insulin.

▌ Thinking "Outside the Box"

On frequent occasions, patients will present with unique problems requiring therapeutic interventions that are controversial, not evidence based, or published in expert opinion guidelines. If one understands the pathogenesis of the disease state that they are attempting to manage and desires to customize targeted glycemic goals for patients, unique, off-label, therapeutic options may be considered.

Patients with T1DM often have difficulty controlling both fasting and postprandial blood glucose excursions secondary to their inability to block the untimely and excessive secretion of glucagon. Furthermore, the preferred glucagon response to hypoglycemia is inappropriate or absent in patients with T1DM.[71] Despite the fact that nonphysiologic secretion of both insulin and glucagon contributes to hyperglycemia, the accepted pharmacologic management of T1DM consists solely of either MDI or insulin pump therapy. Practical therapies that, in combination with insulin can reduce insulin requirements, minimize postprandial excursions, reduce the risk of hypoglycemia, and are weight neutral would be of special interest in the management of T1DM.

In fasting subjects with T1DM, Creutzfeldt et al. found that a continuous infusion of GLP-1 reduced fasting hyperglycemia from 241 to 180 mg per dL and glucagon concentrations by 50%.

TABLE 11-12. Practical Dosing Guide to U-500 Insulin

Total Daily Dose of Insulin (U/d)[a]	Injection Frequency/ Delivery Schedule	Total Daily U-500 Dose Given at Each Meal	U-500 Dose Titration
200–299	2 injections/d (breakfast and dinner)	Breakfast: 60% Dinner: 40%	• Blood glucose <50 mg/dL above or below target range: increase or decrease U-500 by 5 U (0.01 mL) per dose/bolus. Changes made weekly
	3 injections/d (breakfast, lunch, and dinner)	Breakfast: 40% Lunch: 30% Dinner: 40%	• Blood glucose ≥50 mg/dL above or below target range: increase or decrease U-500 by 10 U (0.02 mL) per dose/bolus. Changes made weekly
	Via insulin pump	1 U = 0.01 mL; 0.01 mL of U-500 insulin = 5 U	• Changes made weekly as above
300–599	3 injections/d (breakfast, lunch, and dinner)	Breakfast: 40% Lunch: 30% Dinner: 40%	• Blood glucose level within 100 mg/dL above or below target range: Increase or decrease U-500 in increments of 25 U (0.05 mL) per dose/bolus • Blood glucose level >100 mg/dL above or below target range: increase or decrease U-500 in increments of 50 U (0.1 mL) per dose/bolus
	4 injections/d (breakfast, lunch, dinner, and bedtime	Breakfast: 30% Lunch: 30% Dinner: 30% Bedtime: 10%	• Blood glucose level within 100 mg/dL above or below target range: Increase or decrease U-500 in increments of 25 U (0.05 mL) per dose/bolus • Blood glucose level >100 mg/dL above or below target range: increase or decrease U-500
	Via insulin pump	1 U = 0.01 mL; 0.01 mL of U-500 insulin = 5 U	• As above

[a]To calculate the dose of U-500 insulin, divide the TDD by 5. Thus, a person requiring an estimated 300 U of U-100 units daily would inject 300/5 = 60 U of U-500 daily.
Note: Consider placing patients on exenatide or liraglutide plus metformin while they use U-500 to minimize weight gain.

TABLE 11-13. U-500 Tips of the Trade

- U-500 insulin should be injected using tuberculin syringes.

- When writing a prescription for U-500 insulin, note the actual insulin units to be injected and the volume to be injected to minimize prescribing errors. Thus, a typical prescription should read, "Insulin U-500 Regular, 150 U," inject 0.3 mL subcutaneously TID 15–30 min prior to meals. Table 11-12 shows the pharmacologic equivalence and proper injection volume to be administered using tuberculin syringes in patients using U-500 insulin.

- Although hypoglycemia is unlikely to occur in patients who are highly insulin resistant, family members should be fully instructed on the proper use of emergency glucagon for severe hypoglycemic events.

- Patients who are successful at weight loss may be switched to U-100 as their insulin requirements decline.

- If patients are hospitalized, make certain that their U-500 accompanies them to the hospital as most hospital pharmacies do not stock highly concentrated insulin.

- Instruct patients to notify their pharmacies to keep additional U-500 insulin in stock for them.

- The injection of U-500 should be given in the abdomen before breakfast because insulin depots are absorbed fastest from the abdomen. Absorption from the arm is faster than from the leg. The doses of insulin can be altered based on the patient's ability to attain the targeted blood glucose levels. Three months after starting A1C therapy, an A1C should be repeated to determine if the patient is moving toward the selected target.

Endogenous insulin levels were only slightly increased. The patients had their normal dose of intermediate acting insulin reduced by 50% the night before the study, resulting in fasting hyperglycemia and hyperglucagonemia.[133] In another study in which T1DM patients were well insulinized and euglycemic, GLP-1 infusion had no effect on either glucagon secretion or insulin concentrations suggesting that GLP-1 action may be glucose dependent.[134] Thus, GLP-1 will have a glucose-lowering effect only in patients who are addressing safety concerns about inducing hypoglycemia when combining a GLP-1 agonist with exogenous insulin in patients with T1DM. Other studies have demonstrated that GLP-1 can control postprandial excursions by normalizing gastric emptying and inhibiting glucagon secretion in the fed state.[135,136]

Kielgast et al.[137] treated 19 patients with T1DM (10 with residual β-cell function who were C-peptide positive and 9 without β-cell function who were C-peptide negative) to determine the effect of 4 weeks of liraglutide treatment on glycemic control. Insulin doses were optimized prior to entry into the experimental protocol (which could partially account for the reduction in A1C during this short study). Insulin doses were reduced significantly in both cohorts, and patients experienced less time spent at glycemic levels less than 70 mg per dL on continuous glucose monitoring. The

 TABLE 11-14. Pharmacologic Equivalence and Injection Volume for Tuberculin Syringe Administration for Patients Using U-500 Insulin

U-500 Dose (U)	U-100 Equivalent Dose (U)	Volume Administered Via Tuberculin Syringe (mL)
40	200	0.4
30	150	0.3
20	100	0.2
15	75	0.15
10	50	0.1

C-peptide-positive patients decreased their A1C from 6.6% to 6.4% over 4 weeks compared with a decline from 7.5% to 7.0% in the C-peptide-negative group. Eighteen of 19 patients lost weight during the study. The most common adverse event was nausea and vomiting that occurred within the first 2 to 3 days of dosing and resolved spontaneously or subsequent to dose reduction. During the 4th week of the study, postprandial glucagon levels were significantly reduced, yet increased appropriately during exercise when glucose levels began to fall. This suggests that liraglutide works in a glucose-dependent manner even in patients with T1DM.

Figure 11-7A,B shows the continuous glucose monitor download of a 35-year-old patient diagnosed with T1DM at age 16. He is using an insulin pump and has a history of hypoglycemia awareness autonomic failure (HAAF). The patient was started on liraglutide 0.6 mg per day for 2 weeks after which his dose was increased to 1.2 mg per day. He did experience nausea, but no vomiting during the first 7 days of therapy. Figure 11-7B shows near complete resolution of his hypoglycemia after 4 weeks on combination therapy. His TDD of pumped rapid-acting insulin was reduced by 20%.

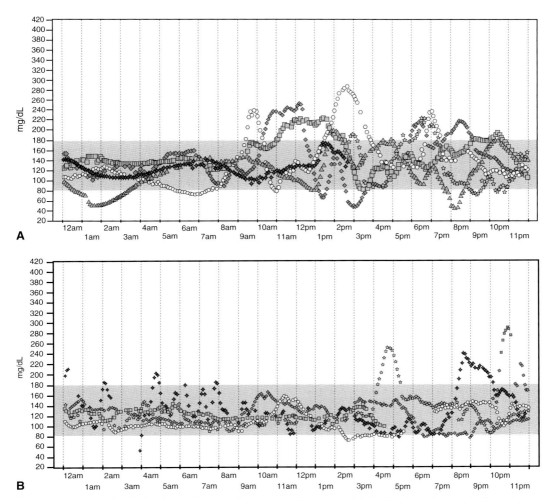

Figure 11-7 • A. Patient's continuous glucose monitoring model day tracings demonstrating glycemic variability at baseline trending toward hypoglycemia. **B.** While using liraglutide 1.2 mg per day in addition to rapid-acting insulin via continuous subcutaneous insulin infusion, the patient's glycemic variability appears to have improved with absence of hypoglycemic events. Note: the use of liraglutide in patients with T1DM is **NOT** approved by the FDA. Insulin should never be discontinued when using liraglutide in patients with T1DM. (Case presented courtesy of Jeff Unger, MD.)

What might be the optimal time to consider introducing a GLP-1 agonist into the treatment regimen of a patient with T1DM? One could consider that the optimal time for GLP-1 intervention would be immediately after a patient is diagnosed with T1DM. At this time, the patient still has some residual pancreatic β-cell mass and function that can be protected with the use of a GLP-1 agonist.[138] GLP-1 introduction shortly after diagnosis could induce a faster and longer remission (honeymoon period) than with the use of insulin alone, explained solely by the glucoregulatory effects of the GLP-1 receptor agonist and delayed gastric emptying. During this phase of T1DM, more patients might be able to discontinue insulin, reduce their risk of hypoglycemia, minimize postprandial oxidative stress, and lessen the likelihood of developing long-term diabetes-related complications.

Liraglutide is not approved for use with insulin, yet coadministration of liraglutide 1.8 mg and insulin detemir produces additive glucose-lowering effects without affecting the pharmacokinetice profile of either therapeutic agent.[139] When used concurrently, neither the dose of detemir nor liraglutide requires titration algorithm adjustments based upon this PK study that was performed in patients with T2DM.

In our clinical practice, liraglutide has been used frequently to improve glycemic control in patients with T1DM (Fig. 11-7A,B). When liraglutide at doses of 0.6, 1.2, or 1.8 mg daily are injected once daily in either MDIs of insulin or patients using insulin pumps, patients note reduction in their appetite, weight loss, improvement in postprandial and fasting glucose levels, and a reduced glycemic variability. Patients must be informed that the use of liraglutide in T1DM is strictly off-label and under no circumstances should they ever discontinue use of their insulin therapy. Immediately after initiating liraglutide, patients may experience a feeling of satiety. Some patients reduce their caloric intake by as much as 30% to 50%. If a patient attempts to eat despite experiencing satiety they are likely to become nauseated. In our experience, approximately 5% of patients with T1DM are unable to tolerate liraglutide in combination with insulin, most often secondary to the GI side effects. A patient with a personal history or family history of medullary thyroid carcinoma should not receive liraglutide. Liraglutide should never be used in a patient with a history of pancreatitis. Any patient who experiences abdominal pain associated with nausea and vomiting while on liraglutide should undergo a workup for acute pancreatitis. The drug should be discontinued if pancreatitis is suspected and not reinitiated if the diagnosis is confirmed.

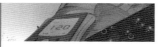

SUMMARY

T1DM is a chronic and progressive illness that requires constant vigilance on the part of the patient. Unlike other chronic diseases such as cancer, diabetes requires that multiple and complex decisions be made each day in order to prevent both acute (hypoglycemia) and long-term complications. Although diabetes self-management may appear to be overwhelming, the tools that are available today are much more effective at restoring one's normal quality of life in comparison to the painful and unpredictable insulins that we read about in the historical pages. When insulin was first discovered by Banting, Best, McCleod, and Collip in 1922, patients receiving the drug often injected in secrecy, even refusing to inform their spouses that they had diabetes. Preparing an injection of insulin took up to 20 minutes, because the glass syringes and needles had to be washed and sterilized at home. The glucodynamics of the original animal insulin was unpredictable, with each vial containing over 80,000 parts per million of impurities. The standard dose was "4 cc twice daily." Patients would often become hypoglycemic, and self–blood glucose monitoring did not become available commercially until 1972.[140]

Today patients have the luxury of using insulin pens, insulin pumps, real-time continuous glucose sensors, and blood glucose meters that can be downloaded, computer analyzed, and transmitted over the Internet for immediate interpretation. Clinical trials are evaluating methods by which T1DM may be predicted, prevented, or reversed by perhaps rebooting one's immune system. The path toward finding a cure for T1DM becomes more meaningful to each of the 13,000 newly diagnosed Americans each year who are forced to initiate exogenous insulin therapy. Yet, for all of the woe and distress that insulin therapy conjures in our minds, we should think back to the days just before World War I. At that time, being diagnosed with diabetes was a death sentence. In 1920, diabetes was simple to diagnose yet impossible to treat. Patients suffered from malnutrition, cataracts, blindness, gangrene, impotence, and immune-resistant, often fatal diseases, such as pneumonia, tuberculosis, boils, and carbuncles. Surgeons recognized the futility of operating on patients with gangrenous limbs who were likely to die from surgical complications. Women who were lucky enough to conceive miscarried, unable to carry their babies to term. The life span of a newly diagnosed patient with T1DM was 6 to 12 months. Acetonemia was prevalent in hospital wards that bore the "sickish sweet smell of rotten apples" signifying the presence of patients dying from DKA.

The discoverers of insulin gave our world not only the gifts of life and longevity. Physicians were able to offer something other than snake oil and prayer to their most vulnerable patients. The proof of the drug efficacy was observed in the patients who were near death when they received their first injections only to regain their strength, their weight, and their health within a matter of weeks.

Of course, we see patients each day who complain about glucose self-monitoring and are fearful about dying of diabetes-related complications. Yet, each day we offer new means by which each patient may gain self-confidence in managing his or her own disease. Each day that we are able to assist a patient successfully achieve their glycemic targets is a tribute to all of the scientists, patients, volunteers, and clinicians who have dedicated their lives to helping patients with T1DM to live a full and complication-free life.

REFERENCES

1. Bliss M. *The Discovery of Insulin.* Chicago, IL: University of Chicago Press; 1984:11–20.
2. Best CH. The first clinical use of insulin. *Diabetes.* 1956;5:65–67.
3. Joslin EP. *A Diabetic Manual for the Mutual Use of Doctor and Patient.* 7th ed. Philadelphia, PA: Lea & Febiger; 1941.
4. Kumar O, Miller L, Mehtalia S. Use of dexamethasone in treatment of insulin lipoatrophy. *Diabetes.* 1977;26:296–299.
5. Diabetes Control and Complications Trial Research Group. The effect of intensive treatment of diabetes on the development and progression of long-term complications in insulin-dependent diabetes mellitus. *N Engl J Med.* 1993;329:977–986.
6. UK Prospective Diabetes Study (UKPDS) Group. Intensive blood glucose control with sulphonylureas or insulin compared with conventional treatment and risk of complications in patients with type 2 diabetes (UKPDS 33). *Lancet.* 1998;352:837–853.
7. American Diabetes Association. Definition and description of diabetes mellitus. *Diabetes Care.* 2012;34 (suppl 1):S64–S65.
8. Unger J. Diagnosing and managing latent autoimmune diabetes in adults. *Practical Diabetology.* 2008;21(1):32–37.
9. Triolo TM, Armstrong TK, McFann K, et al. Additional autoimmune disease found in 33% of patients at T1DM onset. *Diabetes Care.* 2011;34(5):1211–1213.
10. Umpierrez GE, Smiley D, Kitabchi AE. Narrative review: Ketosis-prone type 2 diabetes mellitus. *Ann Int Med.* 2006;144(5):350–357.
11. Notkins AL, Lernarmk A. Autoimmune T1DM: resolved and unresolved issues. *J Clin Invest.* 2001;108:1247–1252.
12. T1DBase: a bioinformatics resource for T1DM researchers. Available at http://t1dbase.org/cgi-bin/welcome.cgi. Accessed February 19, 2011.
13. Wallace C, Smyth DJ, Maisuria-Amer M, et al. The imprinted DLK1-MEG3 gene region on chromosome 14q32.2 alters susceptibility to T1DM. *Nat Genet.* 2010;42(1):68–71.

14. Devendra D, Eisenbarth GS. Immunologic endocrine disorders. *J Allergy Clin Immunol.* 2003;111: S624–S636.

15. Eisenbarth GS, Gottlieb PA. Autoimmune polyendocrine syndromes. *N Engl J Med.* 2004;350:2068–2079.

16. Caillat-Zucman S, Garchon HJ, Timsit J, et al. Age-dependent HLA genetic heterogeneity of type 1 insulin-dependent diabetes mellitus. *J Clin Invest.* 1992;90:2242–2250.

17. Gillespie KM, Gale EAM, Bingley PJ. High familial risk and genetic susceptibility in early onset childhood diabetes. *Diabetes.* 2002;51:210–214.

18. Masharani U, German MS. In: Gardner G, Shoback D, ed. *Greenspan's Basic Clinical Endocrinology,* 9th ed. McGraw-Hill; 2011:587, Chapter 17.

19. Karvonen M, Viik-Kajander M, Moltchanova E, et al. Incidence of childhood T1DM worldwide. Diabetes Mondiale (DiaMond) Project Group. *Diabetes Care.* 2000;23:1516–1526.

20. Diabetes Epidemiology Research International Group. Geographic patterns of childhood insulin-dependent diabetes mellitus. *Diabetes.* 1988;37:1113–1119.

21. Honeyman MC, Coulson BS, Stone NL, et al. Association between rotavirus infection and pancreatic islet autoimmunity in children at risk of developing T1DM. *Diabetes.* 2000;49:1319–1324.

22. Hyoty H. Enterovirus infections and T1DM. *Ann Med.* 2002;34:138–147.

23. Ginsberg-Fellner F, Witt ME, Fedun B, et al. Diabetes mellitus and autoimmunity in patients with the congenital rubella syndrome. *Rev Infect Dis.* 1985;7(suppl 1):S170–S176.

24. Peltola H, Davidkin I, Paunio M, et al. Mumps and rubella eliminated from Finland. *JAMA.* 2000;284:2643–2647.

25. Viskari H, Ludvigsson J, Uibo R, et al. Relationship between the incidence of T1DM and maternal enterovirus antibodies: time trends and geographical variation. *Diabetologia.* 2005;48:1280–1287.

26. Gale EA. A missing link in the hygiene hypothesis? *Diabetologia.* 2002;45:588–594.

27. Borch-Johnsen K, Joner G, Mandrup-Poulsen T, et al. Relation between breast-feeding and incidence rates of insulin-dependent diabetes mellitus: a hypothesis. *Lancet.* 1984;2:1083–1086.

28. Dahl-Jorgensen K, Joner G, Hanssen KF. Relationship between cow's milk consumption and incidence of IDDM in childhood. *Diabetes Care.* 1991;14:1081–1083.

29. Martin JM, Trink B, Daneman D, et al. Milk proteins in the etiology of insulin-dependent diabetes mellitus (IDDM). *Ann Med.* 1991;23:447–452.

30. Mohr SB, Garland CF, Gorham ED, et al. The association between ultraviolet B irradiance, vitamin D status and incidence rates of T1DM in 51 regions worldwide. *Diabetologia.* 2008;51:1391–1398.

31. Gorham ED, Barrett-Conner E, Highfill-Mcroy RM, et al. Incidence of insulin-requiring diabetes in the U.S. military. *Diabetologia.* 2009;52:2087–2091.

32. Bisikirska BC, Herold KC. Regulatory T cells and T1DM. *Curr Diab Rep.* 2005;5(2):104–109.

33. Eisenbarth GS. Type I diabetes mellitus: a chronic autoimmune disease. *N Engl J Med.* 1986;314: 1360–1368.

33a. Xu P, Beam CA, Cuthbertson D, et al. Prognostic accuracy of immunologic and metabolic markers for type 1 diabetes in a high-risk population. *Diabetes Care.* 2012;DOI: 10.2337/dc12-0183.

34. Atkinson M, Gale EA: Infant diets and T1DM: too early, too late, or just too complicated? *JAMA.* 2003;290:1771–1772.

35. Pugliese A. Genetics of T1DM. *Endocrinol Metab Clin North Am* 2004;33:1–16, vii.

36. Savola K, Ebeling T, et al. Genetic, autoimmune and clinical characteristics of childhood and adult-onset T1DM. *Diabetes Care.* 2000;23:1326–1332.

37. Holland AM, Gonez LJ, Harrison LC. Progenitor cells in the adult pancreas. *Diabetes Metab Res Rev.* 2004;20:13–27.

38. Maioli M, Pes GM, Delitala G, et al. Number of autoantibodies and HLA genotype, more than high titers of glutamic acid decarboxylase autoantibodies, predict insulin dependence in latent autoimmune diabetes of adults. *Eur J Endocrinol.* 2010;163(4):541–549.

39. Hahl J, Simell T, Ilonen J, et al. Costs of predicting IDDM. *Diabetologia.* 1998;41:79–85.

40. Diabetes Prevention Trial–T1DM Study Group. Effects of insulin in relatives of patients with T1DM mellitus. *N Engl J Med.* 2002;346:1685–1691.

41. Orban T, Sosenko JM, Cuthbertson D, et al. Pancreatic islet autoantibodies as predictors of T1DM in the diabetes prevention trial-type 1. *Diabetes Care.* 2009;32(12):2269–2274.

42. Ziegler AG, Hummel M, Schenker M, et al. Autoantibody appearance and risk for development of childhood diabetes in offspring of parents with T1DM: the 2-year analysis of the German BABYDIAB Study. *Diabetes.* 1999;48:460–468.

43. Knip M, Korhonen S, Kulmala P, et al. Prediction of T1DM in the general population. *Diabetes Care*. 2010;33(6):1206–1212.

44. Sosenko JM, Palmer JP, Greenbaum CJ, et al. Patterns of metabolic progression to type 1 diabetes in the Diabetes Prevention Trial-Type 1. *Diabetes Care*. 2006;29(3):643–649.

45. Keymeulen B, Vandemeulebroucke E, Ziegler AG, et al. Insulin needs after CD3-antibody therapy in new-onset T1DM. *N Engl J Med*. 2005;362:2598–2608.

46. Pescovitz MD, Greenbaum CJ, Krause-Steinraug H, et al. T1DM trialNet Anti-CD20 Study Group. Rituximab, B-lymphocyte depletion and preservation of beta-cell function. *N Engl J Med*. 2009;361: 2143–2152.

47. Ludvigsson JH, Krisky D, Casas R, et al. GAD65 antigen therapy in recently diagnosed type 1 diabetes mellitus. *N Engl J Med*. 2012;366:433–442.

48. Larsen CM, Faulenbach M, Vaag A, et al. Interleukin-1-receptor antagonist in type 2 diabetes mellitus. *N Engl J Med*. 2007;356:1517–1526.

49. Sherry NA, Chen W, Kushner JA, et al. Exendin-4 improves reversal of diabetes in NOD mice treated with anti-CD3 monoclonal antibody by enhancing recovery of beta cells. *Endocrinology*. 2007;148:5136–5144.

50. Zella JB, DeLuca HF. Vitamin D and autoimmune diabetes. *J Cell Biochem*. 2003;88;216–222.

51. Zipitis CS, Akobeng AK. Vitamin D supplementation in early childhood and risk of T1DM: a systematic review and meta-analysis. *Arch Dis Child*. 2008;93:512–517.

52. Misra M, Pacaud D, Petryk A, et al. Vitamin D deficiency in children and its management: review of current knowledge and recommendations. *Pediatrics*. 2008;122:398–417.

53. Bruno G, Runzo C, Cavallo-Perin P, et al. Incidence of type 1 and type 2 diabetes in adults aged 30–49 years: the population-based registry in the province of Turin, Italy. *Diabetes Care*. 2005;28:2613–2619.

54. Seyfert-Margolis V, Gisler TD, Asare AL. Analysis of T-cell assays to measure autoimmune responses in subjects with type 1 diabetes. *Diabetes*. 2006;55:2588–2594.

55. Han X, Sun Y, Scott S, Bleich D. Tissue inhibitor of metalloproteinase-1 prevents cytokine-mediated dysfunction and cytotoxicity in pancreatic islets and beta-cells. *Diabetes*. 2001;50:1047–1055.

56. Greenbaum CJ, Brooks-Worrell BM, Palmer JP, et al. Autoimmunity and prediction of insulin dependent diabetes mellitus. In: Marshall SM, Home PD, eds. *The Diabetes Annual*, 8th ed. Philadelphia, PA: Elsevier; 1994:18–35.

57. Hoppu S, Ronkainen MS, Kimpimaki T, et al. Insulin autoantibody isotypes during the pre-diabetic process in young children with increased genetic risk of type 1 diabetes. *Pediatr Res*. 2004;55:236–242.

58. Juneja R, Palmer JP. Type 1½ diabetes: myth or reality? *Autoimmunity*. 1999;29:65–83.

59. Borg H, Gottsater A, Fernlund P, et al. A 12-year prospective study of the relationship between islet antibodies and beta-cell function at and after the diagnosis in patients with adult-onset diabetes. *Diabetes*. 2002;51:1754–1762.

60. Hathout EH, Thomas W, El-Shahawy M, et al. Diabetic autoimmune markers in children and adolescents with type 2 diabetes. *Pediatrics*. 2001;107:E102.

61. Juneja R, Hirsch IB, Naik RG, et al. Islet cell antibodies and glutamic acid decarboxylase antibodies, but not the clinical phenotype, help to identify type 1 (½) diabetes in patients presenting with type 2 diabetes. *Metabolism*. 2001;50:1008–1013.

62. Argoud GM, Schade DS, Eaton RP. Insulin suppresses its own secretion in vivo. *Diabetes*. 1987;36: 959–996.

63. Aaen K, Rygaard J, Josefsen K, et al. Dependence of antigen expression on functional state of beta-cells. *Diabetes*. 1990;39:697–701.

64. Dupre J. Glycaemic effects of incretins in type 1 diabetes mellitus: a concise review, with emphasis on studies in humans. *Regul Pept*. 2005;128:149–157.

65. Ghofaili KA, Fung M, Ao Z, et al. Effect of exenatide on β-cell function after islet transplantation in type 1 diabetes. *Transplantation*. 2007;83:24–28.

66. Slama G, Elgraby F, Sola A, et al. Postprandial glycaemia: a plea for the frequent use of delta postprandial glycaemia in the treatment of diabetic patients. *Diabetes Metab*. 2006;32:187–192.

67. LuiJf YM, van Bon AC, Hoekstra JB, et al. Premeal injection and rapid-acting insulin reduces postprandial glycemic excursions in T1DM. *Diabetes Care*. 2010;33:2152–2155.

68. Kruszynska YT, Home PD, Hanning I, et al. Basal and 24-h C-peptide and insulin secretion rate in normal man. *Diabetologia*. 1987;30:16–21.

69. Sheard NF, Clark NG, Brand-Miller JC, et al. Dietary carbohydrate (amount and type) in the prevention and management of diabetes: a statement by the American Diabetes Association. *Diabetes Care*. 2004;27(9):2266–2271.

70. Belfort R, Mandarino L, Kashyap S, et al. Dose-response effect of elevated plasma free fatty acid on insulin signaling. *Diabetes*. 2005;54(6):1640–1648.
71. Gerich JE, Langlois M, Noacco C, et al. Lack of glucagon response to hypoglycemia in diabetes: evidence for an intrinsic pancreatic alpha cell defect. *Science*. 1973;182:171–173.
72. Unger J. Reducing oxidative stress in patients with type 2 diabetes mellitus: a primary care call to action. *Insulin*. 2008;3:176–184.
73. Parker DC, Rossman LG. Sleep release of human growth hormone in treated juvenile diabetics: simliarity to normal subjects and nonsuppression by hyperglycemia. *Diabetes*. 1971;20:691–695.
74. Garg S, Moser E, Dain MP, et al. Clinical experience with insulin glargine in T1DM. *Diabetes Technol Ther*. 2011;12(11):835–846.
75. Rodbard H, Schnell O, Unger J, et al. Decision support tools dramatically improve clinicians' ability to interpret structured SMBG data. Late-Breaking Poster presentation. *ADA 71st Scientific Session*. San Diego, CA. June 24–28, 2011;24-LB.
76. Polonsky WH, Jelsovsky A, Panzera S, et al. Primary care physicians identify and act upon glycemic abnormalities found in structured, episodic blood glucose monitoring data from non-insulin-treated type 2 diabetes. *Diabetes Technol Ther*. 2009;11(5):283–291.
77. Gale EA. A randomized, controlled trial comparing insulin lispro with human soluble insulin in patients with T1DM on intensified insulin therapy. *Diabet Med*. 2000;17:209–214.
78. Heise T, Nosek L, Rønn BB, et al. Lower within-subject variability of insulin detemir in comparison to NPH insulin and insulin glargine in people with T1DM. *Diabetes*. 2004;53:1614–1620.
79. Bolli GB. Insulin treatment in T1DM. *Endocr Pract*. 2006;12(suppl 1):105–109.
80. Hirsch IB. Insulin analogues. *N Engl J Med*. 2005;352:174–183.
81. Danne T. Insulin detemir is characterized by more reproducible pharmacokinetic profile than insulin glargine in children and adolescents with T1DM: results from a randomized, double-blind, controlled trial. *Pediatr Diabetes*. 2008;9:382–387.
82. Danne T. Insulin detemir is characterized by a consistent pharmacokinetic profile across age-groups in children, adolescents, and adults with T1DM. *Diabetes Care*. 2003;26:3087–3092.
83. Gautier JF, Mourier A, de Kerviler E, et al. Evaluation of abdominal fat distribution in noninsulin-dependent diabetes mellitus: relationship to insulin resistance. *J Clin Endocrinol Metab*. 1998;83:1306–1311.
84. Sindelka G, Heinemann L, Berger M, et al. Effect of insulin concentration, subcutaneous fat thickness and skin temperature on subcutaneous insulin absorption in healthy subjects. *Diabetologia*. 1994;37:377–380.
85. Jonassen I, Havelund S, Ribel U, et al. Insulin degludec is a new generation ultra-long acting basal insulin with a unique mechanism of protraction based on multi-hexamer formation (Abstract). *Diabetes*. 2010;59(suppl 1):A11.
86. Birkeland KI, Home PD, Wendisch U, et al. Insulin degludec in T1DM: a randomized controlled trial of a new-generation ultra-long-acting insulin compared with insulin glargine. *Diabetes Care*. 2011;34(3):661–665.
87. Heise T, Hermanski L, Nosek L, et al. Insulin degludec: less pharmacodynamics variability than insulin glargine under steady state conditions (Abstract). *Diabetetolgia*. 2010;53(suppl 1):S387.
88. Howey DC, Bowsher RR, Brunelle RL, et al. [Lys(B28), Pro(B29)]-human insulin: effect of injection time on postprandial glycemia. *Clin Pharmacol Ther*. 1995;58:459–446.
89. DeWitt DE, Hirsch IB. Outpatient insulin therapy in type 1 and type 2 diabetes mellitus: scientific review. *JAMA*. 2003;289:2254–2264.
90. Vaughn DE, Muchmore DB. Use of recombinant human hyaluronidase to accelerate rapid insulin analogue absorption: experience with subcutaneous and continuous infusion. *Endoc Pract*. 2011;17:914–921.
91. Nathan DM, Cleary PA, Backlund JY, et al. Intensive diabetes treatment and cardiovascular disease in patients with T1DM. *N Engl J Med*. 2005;353:2643–2653.
92. The Writing Team for the DCCT/EDIC Research Group: effect of intensive therapy on microvascular complications of T1DM mellitus. *JAMA*. 2002;287:2563–2569.
93. Skyler JS, Ponder S, Kruger D, et al. Insuln pump therapy in your practice. *Clinical Diabetes*. 2007;25(2):50–56.
94. Unger J, Parkin C. Hypoglycemia in insulin-treated diabetes: a case for increased vigilance. *Postgr Med*. 2011;123(4):81–91.
95. Blonde L, Merilainen M, Karwe V, et al. Patient-directed titration for achieving glycaemic goals using a once-daily basal insulin analogue: an assessment of two different fasting plasma glucose targets: the TITRATE study. *Diabetes Obes Metab*. 2009;11(6):623–631.

96. Harris S, Yale J-F, Dempsey E, et al. Can family physicians help patients initiate basal insulin therapy successfully? Randomized trial of patient-titrated insulin glargine compared with standard oral therapy: lessons for family practice from the Canadian INSIGHT trial. *Can Fam Physician* 2008;54:550–558.

97. Riddle MC, Rosenstock J, Gerich J. The Treat-to-Target Trial: Randomized addition of glargine or human NPH insulin to oral therapy of type 2 diabetic patients. *Diabetes Care*. 2003;26:3080–3086.

98. Meneghini L, Koenen C, Weng W, et al. The usage of a simplified self-titration dosing guideline (303 Algorithm) for insulin detemir in patients with type 2 diabetes: results of the randomized, controlled PREDICTIVE 303 study. *Diabetes Obes Metab*. 2007;9(6):902–913.

99. Liebl A. Insulin intensification: the rationale and the target. *Int J Clin Pract Suppl*. 2009;(164):1–5.

99a. Holman RR, Farmer AJ, Davies MJ, et al.; 4-T Study Group: three-year efficacy of complex insulin regimens in type 2 diabetes. *N Engl J Med*. 2009;361(18):1736–1747.

100. Unger J. Management of T1DM. *Prim Care Clin Office Pract*. 2007;34(4):791–808.

101. Heller S, Francisco AMO, Pei H, et al. Insulin degludec improves long-term glycemic control with less nocturnal hypoglycemia compared with insulin glargine: 1-year results from the randomized basal-bolus trial in type 1 diabetes. *American Diabetes Association 71st Scientific Sessions*. San Diego, CA, June 26, 2011:70-OR.

102. Normand S, Khalfallah Y, Louche-Pelissier C, et al. Influence of dietary fat on postprandial glucose metabolism (exogenous and endogenous) using intrinsically 13 C-enriched durum wheat. *Br J Nutr*. 2001;85(6):3–11.

103. Frayn KN. Effects of fat on carbohydrate absorption: more is not necessarily better. *Br J Nutr*. 2001;86:1–2.

104. Zampelas A, Roche H, Knapper JM, et al. Differences in postprandial lipaemic response between Northern and Southern Europeans. *Atherosclerosis*. 1998;139:83–89.

105. Kulkarni KD. Carbohydrate counting: a practical meal-planning option for people with diabetes. *Clin Diabetes*. 2005;23(3):120–122.

106. Bergenstal RM, Johnson M, Powers MA. Adjust to target in type 2 diabetes: comparison of a simple algorithm with carbohydrate counting for adjustment of mealtime insulin glargine. *Diabetes Care*. 2008;31(7):1305–1310.

107. Polonsky WH, Fisher L, Schikman CH. Structured self-monitoring of blood glucose significantly reduces A1C levels in poorly controlled, noninsulin-treated type 2 diabetes: Results from the structured testing program study. *Diabetes Care*. 2011;34(2):262–267.

108. Reach G, Zerrouki A, Leclercq D, et al. Adjusting insulin doses: from knowledge to decision. *Patient Educ Couns*. 2005;56 (1):98–103.

109. American Diabetes Association. Nutrition recommendations and interventions for diabetes: a position statement for the American Diabetes Association. *Diabetes Care*. 2008;31(suppl 1):S61–S78.

110. Institute of Medicine. *Dietary Reference Intakes: Energy, Carbohydrate, Fiber, Fat, Fatty Acids, Cholesterol, Protein, and Amino Acids*. Washington, DC: National Academies Press; 2002.

111. American Diabetes Association. Living with diabetes. http://www.diabetes.org/living-with-diabetes/treatment-and-care/medication/insulin/getting-started.html. Accessed February 24, 2012.

112. Wasserman DH, Davis SN, Zinman B. Fuel metabolism during exercise in health and diabetics. In: Ruderman NB, Devlin JT, Schneider S, et al., eds. *Handbook of Exercise in Diabetes*. Alexandria, VA: American Diabetes Association; 2002:63–100.

113. Riddell MC, Perkins BA. T1DM and vigorous exercise: applications of exercise physiology to patient management. *Can J Diabetes*. 2006;30(1):63–71.

114. Marliss EB, Vranic M. Intense exercise has unique effects on both insulin release and its roles in glucoregulation: implications for diabetes. *Diabetes*. 2002;51(suppl 1):S271–S283.

115. Lin AC, Lin CM, Wang TL, et al. Rhabdomyolysis in 119 students after repetitive exercise. *Br J Sports Med*. 2005;39(1) 9:e3 (http://www.bjsportmed.com/cgi/content/full/39/1/e3). doi: 10.1136/bjsm.2004.01323.

116. Petrie HJ, Stover EA, Horswill CA. Nutritional concerns for the child and adolescent competitor. *Nutrition*. 2004;20:620–631.

117. Arutchelvam V, Heise T, Dellweg S. Plasma glucose and hypoglycemia following exercise in people with T1DM: a comparison of three basal insulins. *Diabet Med*. 2009;26(10):1027–1032.

118. American Diabetes Association Clinical Practice Recommendations. *Diabetes Care*. 2011;34(suppl 1):S24.

119. Wackers FJ, Young LH, Insucchi SE, et al. Detection of ischemia in asymptomatic diabetics investigators. Detection of silent myocardial ischemia in asymptomatic diabetic subjects: the DIAD study. *Diabetes Care*. 2004;27:1954–1961.

120. Lemaster JW, Reiber GE, Smith DG, et al. Daily weight-bearing activity does not increase the risk of diabetic foot ulcers. *Med Sci Sports Exerc.* 2003;35:1093–1099.

121. Hollander PA, Levy P, Fineman MS, et al. Pramlintide as an adjunct to insulin therapy improves long-term glycemic and weight control in patients with type 2 diabetes: a 1-year randomized controlled trial. *Diabetes Care.* 2003;26:784–790.

122. Weyer C, Maggs DG, Fineman M, et al. Amylin replacement with pramlintide as an adjunct to insulin therapy facilitates a combined improvement in glycemic and weight control in T1DM [Abstract]. *Diabetologia.* 2001;44(suppl 1):A237.

123. Ceriello A: Acute hyperglycaemia and oxidative stress generation. *Diabet Med.* 1997;14(suppl 3): S45–S49.

124. Ceriello A, Piconi L, Quagliaro L, et al. Effects of pramlintide on postprandial glucose excursions and measures of oxidative stress in patients with T1DM. *Diabetes Care.* 2005;28(3):632–637.

125. Eaton RP, Allen RC, Schade DS, et al. "Normal" insulin secretion: the goal of artificial insulin delivery systems? *Diabetes Care.* 1980;3:270–273.

126. Tanaka T, Itoh H, Doi K, et al. Down regulation of peroxisome proliferator-activated receptor gamma expression by inflammatory cytokines and its reversal by thiazolidinediones. *Diabetologia.* 1999;42: 702–710.

127. Caro JF, Amatruda JM. Glucocorticoid-induced insulin resistance: the importance of post-binding events in the regulation of insulin binding, action, and degradation in freshly isolated and primary cultures of rat hepatocytes. *J Clin Invest.* 1982;69:866–875.

128. Cochran E, Gorden P. Use of U-500 insulin in the treatment of severe insulin resistance. *Insulin.* 2008;3:211–218.

129. Garg R, Johnston V, Mcnally PG, et al. U-500 insulin: why, when and how to use in clinical practice. *Diabetes Metab Res Rev.* 2007;23:265–268.

130. Neal MJ. Analysis of effectiveness of human U-500 insulin in patients unresponsive to conventional insulin therapy. *Endocr Pract.* 2005;11:305–308.

131. Knee TS, Seidensticker DF, Walton JL, et al. A novel use of U-500 insulin for continuous subcutaneous insulin infusion in patients with insulin resistance: a case series. *Endocr Pract.* 2003;9:181–186.

132. Jorgensen KH, Hansen AK, Buschard K. Five fold increases of insulin concentration delays in the absorption of subcutaneously injected human insulin suspensions in pigs. *Diabetes Res Clin Pract.* 2000;50:161–167.

133. Creutzfeldt WO, Kleine N, Willms B, et al. Glucagonostatic actions and reduction of fasting hyperglycemia by exogenous glucagon-like peptide-1 (17-36) amide in type 1 diabetic patients. *Diabetes Care.* 1996;19:580–586.

134. Meier JJ, Nauck MA. Glucagon-like peptide 1 (GLP-1) in biology and pathology. *Diabetes Metab Res Rev.* 2005;21:91–117.

135. Behme MT, Dupre J, McDonalt THJ. Glucagon-like peptide 1 improve glycemic control in T1DM. *BMC Endocr Disord.* 2003;10:1–9.

136. Dupre J, Behme MT, McDonalt TJ. Exendin-4 normalized postcibal glycemic excursions in type 1 diabetes. *J Clin Endocrinol Metab.* 2004;89(7):3469–3473.

137. Kielgast U, Krarup T, Holst JJ. Four weeks of treatment with liraglutide reduces insulin dose without loss of glycemic control in type 1 diabetic patients with and without residual beta cell. *Diabetes Care.* 2011;34:1463–1468.

138. Kielgast U, Holst JJ, Madsbad S. Treatment of type 1 diabetic patients with glucagon-like peptide-1 (GLP-1) and GLP-1R agonists. *Curr Diabetes Rev.* 2009;5:266–275.

139. Morrow L, Hompesch M, Guthrie H, et al. Coadministration of liraglutide with insulin detemir demonstrates additive pharmacodynamic effects with no pharmacokinetic interaction. *Diabetes Obesity Metab.* 2011;13(1):75–80.

140. Mendoza.com. Living with diabetes. http://www.mendosa.com/history.htm. Accessed March 12, 2011.

Insulin Initiation and Intensification for Patients with T2DM

Hard work pays off in the future; laziness pays off now.

—*Steven Wright, Comedic Philosopher*

Introduction Ninety percent of Americans with T2DM are being managed within primary care practices.[1] Historically, primary care physician (PCPs) have preferred to treat patients with oral antidiabetes medications rather than insulin.[2] Early intensification of diabetes therapies using available insulin analogues can minimize the risk of long-term complications associated with exposure to chronic hyperglycemia.[3] PCPs should take an active role in prescribing insulin therapy to patients with T2DM who have evidence of symptomatic hyperglycemia, glycemic variability, and pancreatic β-cell failure. Although there is general agreement among experts as to the necessity of incorporating insulin therapy in patients with T2DM, differences in opinion exist as to the most appropriate time and means by which insulin should be initiated. This chapter discusses how insulin therapy can be rationally, safely, and efficiently introduced to patients in a busy primary care practice.

Many primary care practices lack access to certified diabetic educators, nurse practitioners, or physician assistants. Therefore, the burden of teaching patients to inject and titrate insulin often rests with the physician or medical assistant. Yet, patients are able to acquire the skills of injecting and adjusting insulin very quickly. When provided with the skills, specific glycemic targets, and the tools to treat diabetes successfully, patients discover that diabetes self-management becomes an exciting challenge rather than a confusing burden on their daily lives.

Standard Surrogate Outcome Measures That Differentiate Insulin Products

Insulins are formulated to bind to and activate receptors located within target organs. The resultant pharmacologic action ultimately lowers plasma glucose levels to the desired range. The fact that not all insulins are created equally allows practitioners to customize their treatment protocols for

453

TABLE 12-1. Surrogate Outcome Measures That Are Considered Beneficial for Insulin Therapies

- Changes in FPG, plasma glucose level after a standard meal, plasma glucose level after oral administration of 75 g of glucose, 7-point glucose tests (within 24 h)

- Reduction in A1C.

- Superiority or noninferiority to other insulin products depending on the trial design.

- Effects on markers of insulin resistance and diabetes comorbidities (blood pressure and lipids).

- Effect on weight (approval for a treatment of a new T2DM drug or biologic whose principal mechanism of action appears to be by weight loss may be granted if the product also demonstrates clinically meaningful and statistically significant improvement in glycemia).

- Novel insulin products must demonstrate noninferiority to approved and standard regiments without being associated with undue hypoglycemia. Studies must demonstrate attempts to actually improve glycemia as opposed to simple maintenance of pretrial levels of control. Thus, treat-to-target clinical trials must be performed.

- When seeking approval of a new formulation of premixed short- and long-acting insulins, the sponsor should establish the distinctiveness and usefulness of the premixed products compared to each individual component. The bioavailability of the new premixed insulin should remain comparable to the total bioavailability of the short-acting insulin product.

From U.S. Department of Health and Human Services. Food and Drug Administration. Center for Drug Evaluation and Research. Guidance for Industry. Diabetes Mellitus: Developing drugs and therapeutic biologics for treatment and prevention. Draft Guidance. 2008. http://www.fda.gov/downloads/Drugs/GuidanceComplianceRegulatoryInformation/Guidances/UCM071624.pdf Accessed February 2, 2012.

each patient. When designing insulin clinical trials, the U.S. Food and Drug Administration (FDA) has provided guidance on drug development.[4] Table 12-1 lists the outcome measures that the FDA considers most important when evaluating the safety and efficacy of existing or novel insulin agents. This information is important when interpreting the results of clinical trials and comparing novel insulin therapies.

Despite being the most powerful and complex therapeutic option for T2DM, the FDA has approved all insulin formulations without providing guidance for specific dosing regimens. Instead, the FDA recommends that the prescriber be familiar with the patient's metabolic needs, including eating habits and lifestyle variables prior to dosing insulin. Insulin use is more complicated than swallowing a pill or even injecting a glucagon-like peptide-1 (GLP-1) agonist. Table 12-2 lists treatment emergent events commonly experienced by patients using insulin therapies.

Physiology and Pathogenesis of Insulin Secretion in Diabetes

In the fasting state, insulin is produced by the pancreatic β-cells at the rate of approximately 1 unit (U) per hour to blunt the effect of hepatic glucose production.[1] A meal-time stimulus, mediated in large part by the release of gut-derived incretin hormones, prompts a 5- to 10-fold rise in hepatic portal vein insulin concentration that mitigates postprandial hyperglycemia. Glucose-dependent insulin secretion occurs in two phases. The rapid first-phase insulin response (Fig. 12-1), which occurs over 3 to 5 minutes just prior to the onset of a meal, is genetically predetermined. An absent or blunted first-phase insulin response has been observed in subjects whose first-degree relatives also have diabetes.[5]

The second-phase insulin response begins approximately 15 minutes after carbohydrates are consumed, during which time healthy β-cells produce and secrete insulin until all carbohydrates have been absorbed from the gut and the plasma glucose levels have been normalized. Loss of β-cell

TABLE 12-2. Treatment Emergent Adverse Events of Insulin Therapies

- Reactive/iatrogenic hypoglycemia (insulin stacking)
- Glycemic variability
- Nonadherence to prescribed therapy
- Injection site discomfort
- Incorrect dosing
- Omission of dosing either by design or due to improper education (such as lack of knowledge regarding sick day regimens)
- Mistakenly confusing fast-acting analogue for basal insulin and vice versa
- Improper dosing technique resulting in nonprescribed dosing deliver
- Confusion as to how to titrate basal and prandial insulin regimen
- Insulin allergy
- Appearance of lipoatrophy or lipodystrophy
- Peripheral edema
- Rapid deterioration of diabetic neuropathic symptoms
- Rapid deterioration of diabetic proliferative retinopathy
- Weight gain
- Increased appetite
- Headache triggered by hypoglycemia

mass and function impairs second-phase insulin response over time resulting in a progression toward chronic hyperglycemia.

Islet amyloid polypeptide (IAPP), also known as amylin, is released from β-cells in response to nutrient stimuli similar to those of insulin. Amylin is cosecreted with insulin in a 1:100 amylin–insulin ratio.[6] Amylin functions include inhibition of glucagon secretion from pancreatic α-cells, inhibition of gastric emptying, and regulation of satiety.[7] Conditions such as insulin resistance, obesity,

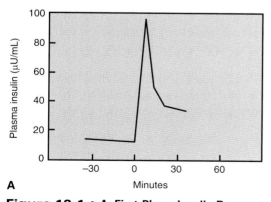

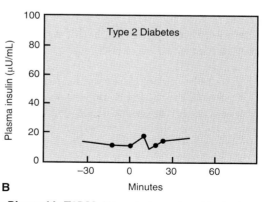

Figure 12-1 • **A. First-Phase Insulin Response is Blunted in T2DM.** Normal glycemic subject who was given an intravenous glucose challenge at time 0 after an overnight fast. The insulin levels increase quickly in response to the glucose stimulus, but decrease within 30 minutes. This is a normal first-phase insulin response. (Adapted from Robertson RP, Porte D Jr. The glucose receptor: a defective mechanism in diabetes mellitus distinct from the β-adrenergic receptor. *J Clin Invest*. 1973;52:870–876.) **B.** This patient with T2DM was given a similar intravenous glucose challenge and demonstrates an absence of first-phase insulin response.

and pregnancy tend to favor increased insulin/amylin secretion and resistance, whereas impaired glucose tolerance (IGT) and both T1DM and T2DM result in reduced secretion of both peptides in response to both oral and IV stimulation.[8] Prolonged exposure to even modestly elevated glucose has been associated with β-cell desensitization, increased apoptosis (β-cell death), delays in first-phase β-cell response to oral glucose, and attenuated second-phase insulin release.[9] First-degree relatives of individuals with T2DM manifest both decreased amylin and insulin responses when presented with an IV glucose challenge.[10]

The amino acid sequence of amylin is capable of forming amyloid fibrils within pancreatic islets. The amyloid fibrils become cytotoxic to the β-cells resulting in the apoptosis and loss of β-cell mass.[11] The injured β-cells respond by secreting a disproportionate amount of proinsulin relative to mature insulin.[12] Medications that favor the secretion of mature insulin over proinsulin are believed to promote β-cell stability or salvation.

To summarize, chronic hyperglycemia leads to amyloid deposition within the β-cells that, over time, reduces the insulin secretory function of the islet. Prolonged exposure to hyperglycemia will result in β-cell death and a reduction in β-cell mass. Clinically, patients will lose their first-phase insulin response and note a blunted second-phase response toward both oral and IV stimulation. Damaged β-cells secrete more proinsulin than mature insulin both in the basal and postprandial states.

Genetically prone individuals with progressive β-cell dysfunction and loss of β-cell mass will, in time, become unresponsive to the pharmacologic actions of oral antidiabetes drugs (OADs). Successful attainment of the American Diabetes Association (ADA)-recommended glycosylated hemoglobin (A1C) target of 7% can only be achieved with exogenous insulin therapy when β-cell mass and function have been severely compromised.[13] Although exogenous basal insulin may work initially allowing many patients with T2DM to achieve their target A1C, prandial insulin will eventually be required as adjunctive therapy.

Insulin for T2DM. Why Start Now?

Chronic hyperglycemia, even in the prediabetic state, has been demonstrated to cause microvascular and macrovascular complications. In the Diabetes Prevention Program, diabetic retinopathy was observed in 8% of patients with IGT and increased to 13% of patients who progressed to diabetes.[14] Seventy-seven percent of patients with idiopathic peripheral neuropathy demonstrated abnormal glucose metabolism when they received a 75-g glucose challenge. Fifty-six percent of patients were found to have abnormal oral glucose tolerance testing results, including 26 with IGT and 15 with clinical diabetes.[15] Other potentially harmful consequences associated with chronic hyperglycemia include oxidative stress, endothelial dysfunction, insulin resistance, hypertension, and intravascular inflammation.[16]

A number of landmark randomized clinical trials have established that insulin therapy reduces the risk of microvascular complications.[17,18] Intensified and customized targeted glycemic control is crucial for reducing the incidence of microvascular complications in patients with T2DM. Evidence supports efforts that favor the induction of "metabolic memory," a theoretical protective mechanism through which early reversal and avoidance of hyperglycemia appear likely to minimize one's risk of developing long-term complications.[19,20] The UK Prospective Diabetes Study (UKPDS) demonstrated that aggressive glycemic control with sulfonylureas or insulin in treatment-naïve patients over 10 years reduced the risk of any microvascular endpoint compared to conventional treatment (relative risk reduction 25%; $p = 0.0099$).[17]

At the conclusion of the UKPDS, the median A1C of the intensively treated cohort was 7% compared to that of the conventionally managed group's A1C of 7.9%. Over the ensuing 10 years, the A1Cs of these two groups equilibrated, as diabetes intervention was placed in the hands of patients and their treatment teams. Nevertheless, those patients who were originally intensively managed had statistically significant reductions in rates of microvascular disease, any diabetes-related endpoints,

TABLE 12-3. High-Risk Patients with T2DM whose A1C Target Should Be Greater Than 7.5%

- History of frequent hypoglycemia or hypoglycemia awareness autonomic failure (HAAF)
- History of cardiovascular disease or stroke
- Shortened life expectancy
- Multiple comorbidities
- Lives alone and would be unable to recover from an episode of severe hypoglycemia
- Suboptimally managed mental illness
- Patients with disturbed eating disorders

diabetes-related deaths, death from any cause, and risk of myocardial infarction compared with conventionally treated patients.[3] This "legacy effect" further supports the notion that early reversal of hyperglycemia and intensification of diabetes management should be the standard of care for nearly all patients with diabetes.

The greatest impact in reducing microvascular complications will occur when A1C is reduced from very poor to very good control. However, the risks of inducing hypoglycemia may outweigh the benefits of attempting to target A1C levels less than 7% in "high-risk" individuals.[21] Individualized glycemic goals should be prioritized on the basis of factors listed in Table 12-3. Patients at low risk for developing hypoglycemia or having a cardiovascular event should adopt glycemic targets as close to normal as possible. A general rule of thumb for healthy patients with T2DM is to treat as soon as possible, for as long as possible, targeting A1C levels as low as possible, using therapeutic interventions which are as safe and rational as possible.

The potential of intensive glycemic control to reduce cardiovascular disease in patients with T2DM is subject to rigorous debate. The UKPDS demonstrated a 16% reduction in cardiovascular complications (combined fatal or nonfatal MI and sudden death) in the intensive glycemic arm, although this narrowly missed being statistically significant ($p = 0.052$). However, in the 10-year UKPDS follow-up, those patients originally assigned to the intensive cohort had long-term reductions in MI (15% with sulfonylurea or insulin as initial pharmacotherapy and in all-cause mortality (13% with sulfonulurea or insulin) both statistically significant.[3]

Results of three large trials [Action to Control Cardiovascular Risk in Diabetes (ACCORD), ADVANCE, and Veterans Affairs Diabetes Trial (VADT)] suggested no significant reductions in CVD outcomes with intensive glycemic control in high-risk populations who had more advanced diabetes than those subjects who participated in the UKPDS (see Chapter 7—Macrovascular Disease). The mortality findings in ACCORD and subgroup analyses of VADT suggest that the potential risks of intensive glycemic control in high-risk patients with long-standing diabetes, a history of severe hypoglycemia, advanced atherosclerosis, and advanced age outweigh the benefits. These patients should have prescribed glycemic targets which are far less stringent and safer. The recommended glycemic targets for nonpregnant adults with diabetes are shown in Table 12-4.

Timing of Insulin Initiation

Expert opinion agrees that insulin is the most powerful tool in our diabetes pharmacologic armamentarium. For most PCPs and specialists, our biggest challenge is confronting patients regarding the necessity to use insulin and at what point the drug must be initiated. The fact that early initiation of intensive insulin therapy reduces insulin resistance and appears to induce β-cell rest suggest that one should initiate insulin sooner rather than later in a treatment-naive patient with T2DM.[22]

The bedrock of therapy for patients with T2DM remains lifestyle intervention (increasing activity levels) in combination with maximally tolerated doses of metformin. If glycemic goals

TABLE 12-4. Glycemic Targets for Adults with Diabetes Based on Guidelines Published by the American Diabetes Association (ADA) and the American Association of Clinical Endocrinologists (AACE)

Parameter	Target: ADA Guidelines	Target: AACE Guidelines
A1C <6% (individual goal)[a]	≤6.5%[a]	
	7% (general goal)[a]	
Fasting plasma glucose[b]	90–130 mg/dL	<110 mg/dL
Postprandial plasma glucose	<180 mg/dL	<140 mg/dL

[a]Upper limit of "normal" is 6% using a Diabetes Control and Complications Trial–based assay.
[b]Postprandial glucose (PPG) measurements should be obtained 1–2 h after beginning the meal. PPG levels typically peak around 90 min after starting a meal.
Notes: The AACE recommends a more rigorous A1C goal for all patients than the ADA's general recommendation of 7.0%. Instead, AACE advocates a goal of ≤6.5%, based on the epidemiologic analysis of the United Kingdom Prospective Diabetes Study (UKPDS) data, which showed that the risk for both microvascular and macrovascular complications of diabetes increased at A1C values ≥6.5%. These guidelines may be modified for individual patients whose functional state or risk for other adverse treatment effects (e.g., hypoglycemia) is thought to outweigh the benefits of optimal glucose control. In addition, AACE recommends treatment targets for FPG and 2-h PPG of 110 and 140 mg/dL, respectively. These targets are based on the increased cardiovascular risk associated with plasma glucose values above these levels. (Data from American Diabetes Association. Standards of Medical Care. *Diabetes Care*. 2012;Suppl 1:S20; and American Association of Clinical Endocrinologists. *Endocr Pract*. 2002;8(suppl):5–11.

are not achieved or sustained within 2 to 3 months, additional therapies should be introduced immediately. The ADA recommends that insulin be introduced in patients whose A1C is greater than 8.5% or if the patient is symptomatic secondary to chronic hyperglycemia (fatigue, weight loss, blurred vision, frequent urination, and paresthesias in extremities).[13] Each patient's success in improving fasting and postprandial glucose values as well as minimizing their incidence of hypoglycemia should be regularly assessed by both the clinician and the patient. Rational behavioral and pharmacologic interventions should be employed daily in order to achieve one's targeted glycemic goals while minimizing the risk of hypoglycemia. Glycemic control reduces the risk of microvascular complications related to diabetes. "Glycemic burden" is defined as the time that a patient spends at an A1C level greater than 8%.[23] A prospective, population-based study using retrospective observational data from over 7,000 patients demonstrated that patients accumulated 5 years of glycemic burden with A1C greater than 8% from their time of diagnosis until insulin was initiated and 10 years of burden from the time their baseline A1C exceeded 7%.[23] Clinicians should become more ambitious in treating patients with T2DM to their targets and use therapies that are less likely to fail.

The American Association of Clinical Endocrinologists recommends using insulin when the endogenous insulin-secreting capacity of the β-cells has been exceeded. Insulin should be initiated in any patient with symptoms suggestive of chronic hyperglycemia (thirst, weight loss, blurry vision, paresthesias in hands and feet, weight loss, frequent urination) and an A1C ≥ 8.5% as well as for any asymptomatic patient whose A1C exceeds 9%.[24] Basal insulin therapy is simple to initiate and may be self-titrated successfully by patients who are insulin naive. Prandial insulin may be added to regimens if targeted A1C levels are not achieved with basal insulin plus OADs. Figure 12-2 summarizes the recommendations of the American Association of Clinical Endocrinologists for insulin initiation.

Barriers to Insulin Initiation

Even modest reductions in A1C translate into meaningful improvements in economic and medical endpoints.[25] A family physician (FP) who does not have access to certified diabetes educators, nurse practitioners, or physician assistants becomes the sole pharmacotherapeutic designer and educator for insulin initiation and intensification. To some busy practitioners this may present a daunting

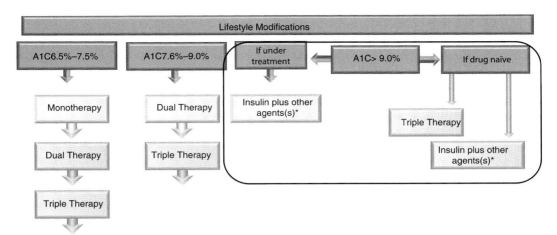

Figure 12-2 • **American Association of Clinical Endocrinologists Recommendations for Management of Hyperglycemia in Patients with T2DM.*** Patients with A1C levels ranging from 6.5% to 7.5% may be treated with monotherapy initially. However, dual- and triple-drug therapy may be considered as well. Those with A1C levels of 7.6% to 9.0% require combination therapy either dual or triple therapy. Incretin agents may be used at any point in the continuum. Patients with A1C levels greater than 9% who are not responding to incretins or OADs and are symptomatic should be placed on insulin immediately. Those patients who are treatment-naive are presumed to have some remaining β-cell function and may respond to either combination therapy with incretins + OADs or insulin + OADs. (Adapted from Rodbard HW, Jellinger PS, Davidson JA, et al. AACE/ACE consensus statement. Statement by an American Association of Clinical Endocrinologists/American College of Endocrinology consensus panel on type 2 diabetes mellitus: an algorithm for glycemic control. *Endocr Pract.* 2009;15(1):540–559.) *Safety and efficacy of therapeutic selection trump drug cost.

task. As is frequently the case in clinical practice, insulin initiation is delayed simply because physicians and patients alike are susceptible to misconceptions and fear about disease progression and the role insulin plays.[26]

Recent randomized controlled clinical trials demonstrate that insulin treatment can be readily initiated and successfully intensified for many insulin-naive patients within the primary care setting using simple treat-to-target protocols.[27,28,29] In fact, insulin-naive patients have been found to be as adept at intensifying their own insulin regimens as are physicians, and PCPs just as proficient as endocrinologists at titrating basal insulin therapies. The keys to insulin initiation in primary care are outlined in Table 12-5.

Patient fears present a substantial barrier to insulin initiation and are commonly based on the perception that insulin therapy is a sign of failure.[30] This concern can be addressed by reassuring patients that the need for insulin arises as a natural consequence of loss of β-cell function and diabetes progression. Patients who receive education about their individual glycemic goals [A1C less than 7%; fasting plasma glucose (FPG) 70 to 130 mg per dL; 2-hour postprandial glucose (PPG) less than 180 mg per dL] are more likely to accept insulin therapy as a necessary intervention.[31]

Fear of developing hypoglycemia as well as lack of understanding about how to minimize one's risk and effectively manage this potentially life-threatening adverse event must be addressed prior to initiating insulin therapy. The reported incidence rates for hypoglycemia in T2DM range from 0 to 7.3 episodes per patient-year, depending on the treatment, duration of the disease, and the cutpoints used to define severe hypoglycemia; however, when matched for duration of insulin therapy, the frequency of severe hypoglycemia in T2DM is similar to that seen in T1DM.[32] Population-based data suggest that the incidence of severe hypoglycemia necessitating emergency medical treatment in insulin-treated T2DM approaches that in T1DM.[32] Notably, because the prevalence of T2DM is approximately 20 times greater than that of T1DM, and because most T2DM patients will eventually require insulin treatment, these data suggest that most hypoglycemic episodes, including those of severe hypoglycemia, occur in patients with T2DM.

TABLE 12-5. Keys to Successful Initiation of Insulin in Primary Care

- Suggest that insulin will help patients achieve glycemic targets and minimize the risk of long-term complications
- Allow patients to actively participate in their insulin regimen and dose titration (basal-bolus, mixed insulin, basal-plus, basal only, concentrated insulin, addition of adjunctive therapies such as pramlintide or a GLP-1 agonist)
- Always praise patients on insulin for their efforts at achieving their glycemic targets at their visits
  - Remember, patients who are using insulin do not have normally functioning pancreases
  - They are performing their own insulin dose calculations, perhaps multiple times each day
  - Insulin prescribers should do everything possible to help patients become successful users of insulin
- Individualize therapy to meet the needs of each patient
  - Determine which treatment algorithm might work best for each patient
- Emphasize the importance of lifestyle intervention
  - This should minimize weight gain and reduce postprandial glucose excursions
- Consider group office visits to have patients meet with a certified diabetes educator
  - Often 8–20 patients can be seen at group visits; they are time efficient and reimbursable by third-party payers
- Provide each patient with an individualized, written insulin protocol to which they can refer
- Prescribe insulin pen devices whenever possible
  - Dose titration of insulin is much more accurate with pens than with vials and syringes
  - Patient acceptance and ease of use are much greater with pen devices
- Teach patients how to identify and *appropriately* manage hypoglycemic events
- The initial dose of basal insulin is 10 U. Many insulin-resistant patients may require 0.4–0.6 U/kg/d. The dose will need to be titrated based on prescribed algorithms
  - Continue metformin if possible
  - Discontinue pioglitazone (weight gain) and sulfonylureas (hypoglycemia risk and weight gain)
- If patient requires >60 U of basal insulin per day and his or her A1C is >7%, add a rapid-acting insulin analogue to the largest meal of the day
  - The dose for rapid-acting insulin is 0.1 U/kg/meal
- If A1C is not reduced to target after 3 months of basal plus bolus, add a second injection at the next largest meal of the day
  - Repeat the A1C at 3 mo and if still above target, add a third meal-time injection
- Patients on basal-bolus insulin therapy should consider structured glucose testing in order to identify and correct hypoglycemia, fasting hyperglycemia, and postprandial hyperperglycemia
- Define the patient's glycemic targets (A1C, fasting, and postprandial)
- Use insulin analogues preferentially over human insulins to minimize glycemic variability and risk of hypoglycemia
- Use simplified insulin titration schedules for both basal and prandial insulins
- Inform the patient that their dose will gradually need to increase to reach targets, so they are not surprised and upset each time a titration is needed and they don't blame themselves for needing to increase

Physician barriers to initiation of insulin include concerns about risks to patients and their competence for self-management of their disease. Time restraints exist within busy practices for teaching patients how to use insulin as well as how to effectively titrate their doses. Insulin can be safely and efficiently initiated within the primary care setting by a designated nursing assistant. Pharmaceutical companies will gladly provide certified diabetic educators who will demonstrate injection techniques to office staff employees and explain various insulin protocols which can be passed on to patients. The ADA provides extensive educational material regarding insulin and other medications available at no charge in both written and auditory formats on their Web site (http://www.diabetes. org/living-with-diabetes/treatment-and-care/medication/insulin/). Group office visits offer another cost-effective means by which patients can learn to initiate and titrate insulin.[33] With appropriate educational efforts, patients with T2DM can be successfully transitioned from oral agents to basal bolus therapy within the primary care setting.

Before initiating an insulin regimen, consider the individual's eating, sleeping, exercise patterns, and motivation for diabetes self-management. Availability of different formulations of insulin and delivery systems permits a great deal of flexibility toward tailoring regimens to a patient's specific needs. Optimally, insulin replacement therapy replicates physiologic insulin secretion in the fasting and postprandial states. Healthy, euglycemic individuals produce sufficient insulin to maintain a plasma glucose level between 85 and 140 mg per dL. Thanks to exquisite and complex regulatory mechanisms, plasma glucose levels in healthy people remain within a narrow range throughout wide fluctuations in activity level and food intake. Coordination between pancreatic β-cell insulin secretion, α-cell glucagon secretion, and peripheral insulin action at liver, skeletal muscle, and fat maintains euglycemia, the balance associated with the normal physiologic state.

The Molecular Pharmacology of Basal Insulins

Euglycemic individuals secrete basal insulin into the portal circulation in the fasting state at the rate of 1 U per hour in order to suppress hepatic glucose production.[34] The complex interactions between basal insulin, hepatic glucose output, and glucagon secretion (from the pancreatic α-cells) will maintain FPG in the range of 80 to 90 mg per dL. Exogenous basal insulin delivery attempts to simulate the constant low levels of insulin produced by the pancreas in the fasting state. Ideal basal insulins must have specific characteristics that will closely match the glucodynamic (glucose lowering) and pharmacokinetic (absorption, metabolism, distribution, and excretion) profile of endogenous insulin as shown in Table 12-6.

TABLE 12-6. Characteristics of the Ideal Exogenous Basal Insulin

- Usage results in effective fasting glycemic control
- Low risk of nocturnal and confirmed hypoglycemia associated with initiation and maintenance of therapy
- Drug allows for flexible dosing schedule to accommodate patients with active or irregular lifestyles
- Precise dosing that can be administered in a pen device
- Ability of a patient to give large doses (>80 U) in a single injection
- A duration of action long enough to be given in a single injection in all doses for all patients
- Painless administration
- Basal insulin has a predictable duration of action
- Basal insulin has low intra- and intersubject variability

Patients who are prescribed the older formulations of human insulins [neutral protamine Hagedorn (NPH) and Lente] find themselves being transformed from observers of the X Games to unsigned participants in these exhilarating events! Because these dare devil NPH patients experience daily highs and lows, twists and turns, pharmacists should provide each "Diabetes game athlete" with a helmet to minimize brain injury. These "D-gamers" continually strike their foreheads with the palms of their hands trying to determine the cause of their day-to-day glycemic variability. NPH demonstrates significant intrasubject variability of absorption, which may reach up to 35%.[35] Absorption of NPH can be influenced by the patient's age, body weight, site of injection, and the number of units injected into the subcutaneous depot.[36] Clinically, this would imply that a patient's fasting blood glucose values would likely vary considerably each day. If the NPH is injected twice daily or given at bedtime, one would be at high risk for developing hypoglycemia. The only advantage of using NPH today in patients with T2DM might be the cost; approximately $50 cheaper per vial than a basal insulin analogue.

Two long-acting insulin analogues are currently commercially available [insulin glargine (IGlar) and insulin detemir], while a third, insulin degludec (IDeg), has been submitted to the FDA and European Medicines Agency (EMA) for approval. Other novel basal insulin analogues such as LY2605541 (Lilly, Boehringer Ingelheim) are in phase 3 clinical trials.[37] Sanofi-Aventis is studying a U-300 formulation of insulin glargine (HOE901).[38] While glargine, detemir, and degludec differ only slightly in molecular structure, they demonstrate improved pharmacodynamic characteristics, reduced risk of nocturnal hypoglycemia, and reduced intrasubject variability compared with human NPH.[39]

By modifying human insulin at two sites, the isoelectric point is raised from pH 5.4 to 6.7 making the molecule less soluble at the physiologic pH of subcutaneous tissue and delays the absorption of the drug. The prolonged absorption of this insulin glargine is due to the slow dissolution of the insulin microprecipitate that forms within the skin's neutral pH.[39]

Insulin detemir's prolonged action is accomplished by attaching a 14-carbon fatty acid chain (myristic acid) to the lysine residue at position B29. The side chain contributes to enhanced self-association of insulin detemir and reversible albumin binding in the subcutaneous depot. Insulin absorption is normally dependent upon the movement of the drug across capillary membranes which is, in turn, determined by capillary flow rate. A high flow rate will decrease capillary concentration and increase absorption from the interstitial space, while a low flow rate will delay absorption from the interstitium. Insulin detemir is 98% albumin bound once injected into the subcutaneous tissue. When bound to albumin, the insulin forms a rather large complex that does not easily traverse capillary membranes. Thus, the plasma concentration of detemir is relatively constant and independent of capillary flow rate that explains the insulin's decreased variability in absorption compared with glargine and NPH.[40]

Insulin degludec is an ultra–long acting novel insulin preparation with an action profile attributable to the formation of soluble multiheximers at the injection site (Fig. 12-3). Inside the pen injector, the insulin diheximers are bound by phenol. Following an injection into the subcutaneous depot, phenol rapidly disperses, allowing multihexamer formation around zinc molecules. Zinc is gradually dispersed allowing the insulin monomers to disassociate from the ends of the multiheximers. The insulin monomers are absorbed into the interstitial space and surrounding capillaries where they are reversibly bound to albumin and transported to target receptors. Figure 12-4 shows the different molecular structures of the basal insulins that account for their protracted pharmacokinetic profiles. Table 12-7 shows the pharmacokinetic profiles of all insulin preparations.

▎ Clinical Implications of Insulin Pharmacokinetics

Glargine and detemir are characterized by a relatively flat time–action profile. Both basal insulins have onsets of action within 1 to 4 hours and steady states within 2 to 3 days. In a once-daily dosing double-blind, randomized, crossover, investigator-initiated study in patients with T2DM, the pharmacokinetic and pharmacodynamics actions of basal insulin analogues were found to be equivalent (Fig. 12-5).[41] The mean dose of detemir was similar to that of glargine (26 U per day). The absence

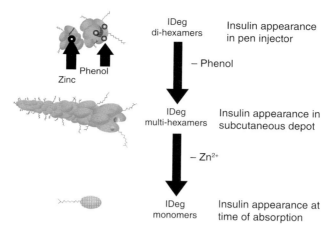

Figure 12-3 • Novel Mechanism of Dissolution, Absorption, and Capillary Transport of Insulin Degludec. The ultra-long effect of insulin degludec (IDeg) results from the slow release of insulin monomers from soluble multi-hexamers that form after subcutaneous injection. As zinc dissolves away from the degludec multihexamers, the monomers released into the subcutaneous space are absorbed into surrounding capillaries and carried via albumin binding to their target insulin receptor sites. (Adapted from Ciba: Investigator's Brochure, 4th ed. Novo Nordisk A/S. 23-Mar-2009; Niswender KD. Basal insulin: physiology, pharmacology, and clinical implications. *Postgrad Med.* 2011;123(4):17–26; and King AB, Poon K. Glargine and detemir: Safety and efficacy profiles of the long-acting basal insulin analogues. *Drug Healthc Patient Saf.* 2010;2:213–223.)

of clear peaks in the time–action profiles of glargine and detemir contributes to the lower risk of hypoglycemia with both these analogues versus NPH. In addition, the analogues demonstrate less variability in absorption compared with NPH in Figure 12-6, suggesting that the analogues have a more predictable glucose-lowering effect than NPH.[42]

One question, which is open to speculation is why some exogenous insulin preparations are associated with weight gain, whereas others tend to favor weight loss or weight neutrality. Insulin therapy is commonly associated with weight gain.[43] However, weight changes have been noted to be somewhat dependent upon the type of insulin used to treat patients with T2DM.[44] Weight gain may be due in part to improved glycemic control, resulting in decreased glycosuria. The kidneys require calories to excrete glucose in the urine. As hyperglycemia improves, caloric expenditure decreases and weight tends to increase. Defensive eating driven by fears of hypoglycemia may also contribute to weight gain. Insulin also has anabolic effects as reflected by the fact that patients with diabetes gain lean as well as fat mass.[45]

Treatment with NPH has been consistently associated with weight gain.[46] A meta-analysis of clinical trial results indicate that insulin detemir is associated with less weight gain than NPH. There was not statistical difference noted in weight between patients using detemir and those using glargine (-0.37 kg detemir vs. glargine; $p = 0.048$).[47] Other large-scale clinical trials demonstrated significantly superior effects of insulin detemir on weight gain versus NPH and glargine.[48–51]

Practical Initiation and Titration of Basal Insulins

Successful initiation of basal insulin requires patients to (1) understand their glycemic targets and (2) know how to safely achieve these targets. In clinical trials, patients who are provided with a specific titration algorithm as well as fasting glucose targets are most always able to lower their A1Cs from baseline toward their prescribed target. The following basal insulin titration intensification protocols may be quickly and successfully implemented with any primary care patient. Clinicians may choose the algorithm that is most likely to be relevant for each of their patients requiring insulin intensification.

Molecular Structures of Basal Insulin Analogues

Insulin Glargine

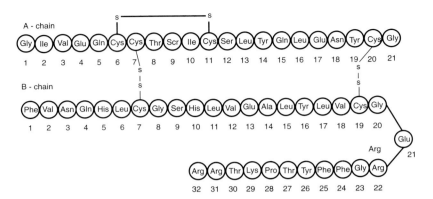

Insulin Detemir

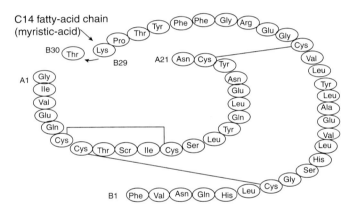

Insulin Degludec

• Canadian Insight Trial Protocol

The Canadian Insight Trial's objective was to determine whether FPs could effectively implement bedtime basal insulin therapy as successfully as could endocrinologists using a simplified titration schedule.[28] Four hundred and five patients with T2DM were randomized to receive either insulin glargine via a self-titration algorithm or conventional therapy with physician-based doses of oral agents for 24 weeks. The baseline A1C of the study cohort was 7.5% to 11% and all patients were either treatment naive or taking a single oral agent. The primary outcome was the time to achieve two consecutive A1C values less than 6.5%. Post-hoc analysis sought to determine whether patients' outcomes differed in terms of the above measures depending on whether they had been treated by diabetes experts or FPs. Patients randomized to the insulin glargine group were initiated on 10 U of insulin to be taken at a consistent time each evening before bedtime. Fasting glucose levels were checked daily. The dose of insulin glargine was subsequently increased 1 U each evening until patients achieved a fasting glucose level of 99 mg per dL. Mean reductions in A1C and FPG levels and rates of hypoglycemia were comparable in the two groups. The PCPs achieved a greater reduction in FPG with insulin glargine than with oral agents (FPG: –74.5 mg per dL vs. –44.1 mg per dL, $p = 0.0001$; specialists: –62.4 mg per dL vs. –39.4 mg per dL, $p = 0.0013$). The PCPs reduction in A1C was also superior to that achieved by the specialists when insulin use was compared with that of oral agent dose titration (–1.64% vs. –1.26%, $p = 0.0058$; specialists –1.41% vs. –1.24%, $p = 0.3331$). PCPs were more aggressive in their use of insulin, whereas the specialists used more oral agents. No differences in the rates of hypoglycemia were noted between the cohorts. The Canadian Insight Trial suggests that PCPs could easily and safely implement a patient-driven, single-unit, basal dosing-adjustment protocol within their private practices.

• PREDICTIVE 303 Protocol

The Predictable Results and Experience in Diabetes through Intensification and Control to Target: An International Variability Evaluation 303 (PREDICTIVE 303 Study) is a patient-driven algorithm tested within the primary care setting.[27] The primary endpoint of this safety and efficacy study was to determine whether treatment-naive patients could be "empowered" to adjust their insulin dose every 3 days simply by monitoring their fasting glucose levels. In addition, could their dosing adjustments result in improved glycemic targets and less hypoglycemia compared with that of a standardized clinic-based dosing protocol? A total of 5,619 patients with T2DM having an A1C less than 12% were randomized to receive insulin detemir via a predetermined, self-adjusted protocol (Table 12-8) or one that was physician directed. After 26 weeks, both cohorts demonstrated equal A1C reductions of approximately 0.6% from the mean baseline of 8.5%. Although the incidence of overall hypoglycemia

---

Figure 12-4 • Molecular Structures of Basal Insulin Analogues. Glargine: The amino acid asparagine at position A21 in human insulin is replaced with glycine, and two arginines are added to the C-terminus of the β-chain. These modifications cause a shift in the isoelectric point toward neutrality. At a pH of 4 in acidic solution, glargine is not soluble at the physiologic neutral pH of subcutaneous tissue. Once injected, glargine forms a microprecipitate that is slowly absorbed over 24 hours through the interstitial space and into the capillaries. Detemir: Differs from human insulin in that the amino acid threonine in position B30 is omitted and a carbon 14 fatty acid chain (myristic acid) is attached to lysine at B29. The myristic acid side chain allows for protracted duration of action by reversibly binding to albumin and permitting self-association or binding to its own structure creating a larger, more stable hexameric structure, which will slowly be converted into a more active monomeric form. Degludec: Differs from human insulin in that the threonine in position B30 has been omitted, and a side chain consisting of glutamic acid spacer along with a fatty acid side chain has been attached. The protracted action of degludec is related to its ability to self-assemble into soluble multi hexamers at the injection site and, to a lesser degree, through the ability to bind to albumin via the fatty-acid side chain. The formation of multi hexamers result in a slow release of degludec into the bloodstream, resulting in a stable action profile extending up to 42 hours.

TABLE 12-7. Characteristics of Human Insulin Preparations

Insulin Preparations	Onset of Action	Peak Action (h)	Duration of Action (h)
Human insulins			
Prandial insulin			
Regular human insulin	30–60 min	2–4	6–8
Intermediate-acting			
NPH	1–4 h	6–10	10–16
Mixed insulins			
70/30 (70% NPH, 30% regular)	0.5–1	first peak in 2–3 h, second peak several hours later	10–16
50/50 0.5–1		first peak in 2–3 h, second peak several hours later	10–16
(50% NPH, 50% regular)			
Insulin analogues			
Basal insulin analogues			
Glargine	1–4 h	No pronounced peak	24
			(Terminal half-life = 12.5 h)
Detemir	1–4 h	No pronounced peak	20–24
Degludec[a]	NA	No peak	>24 h
			Terminal half-life = 25 h
IDegAsp[a]	10 min[b]	No peak	>24 h
(Insulin Degludec + Aspart)			Equal to Degludec
Rapid-acting prandial analogues			
Lispro/aspart/glulisine	5–15 min	1–2	3–4
Premixed analogues			
Lispro mix 75/25	15 min	0.5–1.2	10–16
(75% protamine lispro/			
25% lispro)			
BiAsp 70/30	15 min	0.5–1.2	10–16
70% protamine aspart/			
30% aspart			
Lispro mix 50/50	15 min	0.5–1.2	10–16

[a]These insulins are in phase 3b clinical trials and have been submitted for review to the FDA.
[b]Notes on degludec and IDegAsp: Degludec has a flat profile under steady-state conditions. There is no peak. Therefore, "time to peak action" and onset of action become irrelevant. Steady state for degludec is achieved on the third day of treatment. The effect of the previous injection will cover the time between injection and onset of action of the subsequent injection. Duration of action is dose-dependent. Higher doses increase the duration of action for any insulin. The terminal half-life of insulin degludec is 25 h compared with 12.5 h for insulin glargine. There are no published data regarding the duration of action of insulin degludec. However, the end of action (end of action is defined as blood glucose levels exceeding 150 mg/dL) was not reached by 42 h after the conclusion of glucose clamping for subjects receiving either 0.6 U/kg or 0.8 U/kg. The duration of action of IDegAsp is determined by the IDeg component. The onset of action of IDegAsp is based upon the aspart component. BiAsp has an onset of action of 10 min and a duration of action of 1–3 h. (http://www.novonordisk.ca/PDF_Files/NovoMix30PM022505_En.pdf)

TABLE 12-7. Characteristics of Human Insulin Preparations *(Continued)*

Aventis, Inc., Kansas City, MO; 2000. DeWitt DE, Hirsch IB. Outpatient insulin therapy in type 1 and type 2 diabetes mellitus: scientific review. *JAMA.* 2003;289(17):2254–2264. Heise T, Hovelmann U, Nosek L, et al. Insulin degludec has a two-fold longer half-life and a more consistent pharmacokinetic profile than insulin glargine. American Diabetes Association 71st Scientific Sessions. San Diego, CA: 2011:37-LB. Nosek L, Heise T, Bottcher S, et al. Ultra-long acting insulin degludec has a flat and stable glucose lowering effect. American Diabetes Association 71st Scientific Sessions. San Diego, CA: 2011:49-LB.

Insulin aspart 70/30, 70% insulin aspart protamine/30% insulin aspart; insulin lispro 75/25, 75% insulin lispro protamine/25% insulin lispro; NPH, neutral protamine Hagedorn; INH, inhaled insulin.

From Garg SK, Ulrich H. Achieving goal glycosylated hemoglobin levels in type 2 diabetes mellitus: practical strategies for success with insulin therapy. *Insulin.* 2006;1:109–121; Lepore M, Pampanelli S, Fanelli C, et al. Pharmacokinetics and pharmacodynamics of subcutaneous injection of long-acting human insulin analogue glargine, NPH insulin, and ultralente human insulin and continuous subcutaneous infusion of insulin lispro. *Diabetes Care.* 2000;49:2142–2148; Hirsch IB. Insulin analogues. *N Engl J Med.* 2005;352:174–183; Levemir package insert. Novo Nordisk, Inc., Princeton, NJ; 2005; Glargine package insert.

was not statistically significant between the two groups, the patient-directed cohort demonstrated slightly higher rates of nocturnal hypoglycemia. Like the Canadian Insulin Glargine for Hyperglycemia Treatment (INSIGHT) Trial, PREDICTIVE 303 concludes that patients who are insulin naive can safely adjust their insulin doses when instructed on a specific glycemic goal-directed algorithm.

The PREDICTIVE 303 study was powered to evaluate only the safety and efficacy of self-dose adjustment empowerment within a primary care setting. The TITRATE study was subsequently designed to compare the efficacy and safety of two FPG titration targets 80 to 110 mg per dL and a more "ambitious" target of 70 to 90 mg per dL using a patient-directed treat-to-target algorithm for once-daily basal insulin in insulin-naive patients with T2DM.[52] Patients with A1Cs between 7% and 9% were randomized to either the 80 to 110 mg per dL or the 70 to 90 mg per dL treatment arms. The dose titration for both arms of the study is shown in Table 12-9. Overall, both treatment groups achieved a mean A1C level of 6.9% at the end of the 20-week study. The majority of subjects in both titration groups also achieved the ADA-recommended A1C level of less than 7%. At the

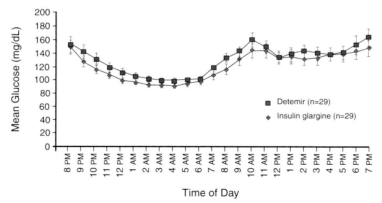

Figure 12-5 • Comparable Continuous Glucose Monitor Sensor Profiles with Insulin Detemir and Insulin Glargine. Twenty-nine patients with T2DM were placed on a continuous glucose sensor. Their previous insulin therapy was discontinued but use of any concurrent oral agents was permitted. Either insulin glargine or detemir was injected at 20:00, 2 hours after dinner. Insulin doses were adjusted during the "titration phase," lasting 3 to 4 days, to achieve fasting glucose levels of 70 to 120 mg per dL with less than 5% of the sensor readings less than 70 mg per dL. Once the subject achieved two consecutive days at goal, the insulin treatment was switched to the other blinded insulin therapy and the process was repeated. Each point on the graph represents the treatment groups' mean glucose for each hour of the day for patients while on glargine and while on detemir. It is interesting to note that in all cases, glucose levels tend to fall from 8 PM to 6 AM, then rise thereafter with either insulin. (Adapted from King AB. Once-daily insulin detemir is comparable to once-daily insulin glargine in providing glycaemic control over 24 hours in patients with type 2 diabetes: a double-blind, randomized, crossover study. *Diabetes Obes Metab.* 2009;11:69–71, with permission.)

Variability in Time Action Profile of Basal Insulins

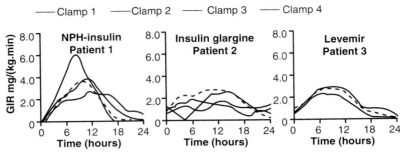

Figure 12-6 • Variability in Time Action Profile of Basal Insulins. Fifty-four patients with T1DM received four single subcutaneous doses of 0.4 U per kg of either insulin detemir, glargine, or NPH under euglycemic glucose clamp conditions on four study days. The pharmacodynamics (glucose infusion rates) and pharmacokinetic (serum insulin concentrations of the basal insulin preparations) were recorded for 24 hours after dosing. Insulin detemir was associated with less variability than other basal insulins. The coefficients of variation for three insulins were 27% detemir versus 59% NPH versus 46% glargine. This implies that detemir has a more predictable glucose-lowering effect than both NPH and glargine. (Adapted from Heise T, Nosek L, Ronn BB, et al. Lower within-subject variability of insulin detemir in comparison to NPH insulin and insulin glargine in people with type 1 diabetes. *Diabetes*. 2004;53(6):1614–1620.

end of the study period, 64.3% of subjects in the 70 to 90 mg per dL cohort achieved A1C levels less than 7% compared with 54.5% of subjects in the 80 to 110 mg per dL group (95% CI: 1.03 to 3.37, odds ratio 1.86, $p = 0.04$). The overall rates of hypoglycemia episodes were low and were comparable between treatment groups. Almost all hypoglycemic events were considered minor or symptomatic only. One subject in the 70 to 90 mg per dL titration cohort did experience a single episode of major hypoglycemia. TITRATE demonstrated that lowering the fasting glucose level to an ambitious target (70 to 90 mg per dL) using a self-directing algorithm with once-daily insulin detemir in insulin-naive patients increases the probability of safely achieving an A1C of less than or equal to 7% within 20 weeks.

• Calculating Basal Insulin Dose for a Patient Who is Unwilling or Incapable of Self-titration

Some patients with T2DM may be unable, unwilling, or incapable of titrating any doses of basal insulin for a variety of reasons. For these individuals, how should the dose of basal insulin be determined?

 TABLE 12-8. 303 Predictive Protocol[a]

Average Fasting Glucose over Previous 3 Days (mg/dL)	Basal Insulin Adjustment Based on Glucose Average
<80	–3 U
80–110	No adjustment
>110	+3

[a]Patients continued their oral antidiabetic doses during the trial. Dose reductions or discontinuation of sulfonylureas were permitted if patients were experiencing hypoglycemia. The initial dose of insulin detemir was 0.1–0.2 U/kg or 10 U/d taken at dinner or bedtime.
From Meneghini L, Koenen C, Weng W, et al. The usage of a simplified self-titration dosing guideline (303 Algorithm) for insulin detemir in patients with type 2 diabetes: results of the randomized, controlled PREDICTIVE 303 study. *Diabetes Obes Metab*. 2007;9:902–913.

TABLE 12-9. The TITRATE Insulin Adjustment Protocol[a]

Average Fasting Glucose over Previous 3 Days (mg/dL)	Basal Insulin Adjustment Based on Glucose Average
Using 70–90 mg/dL target	−3 U
<70	No adjustment
70–90	+3 U
>90	
Using 80–110 mg/dL target	−3 U
<80	No adjustment
80–110	+3 U
>110	

[a]Patients continued their oral antidiabetic doses during the trial. Dose reductions or discontinuation of sulfonylureas was permitted if patients experienced hypoglycemia. The initial dose of insulin detemir was 0.1–0.2 U/kg or 10 U daily taken at dinner or bedtime.
From Blonde L, Merilainen M, Karwe V, et al. Patient directed titration for achieving glycaemic goals using a once-daily basal insulin analogue: an assessment of two different fasting plasma glucose targets—the TITRATE study. *Diabetes Obes Metab.* 2009;11:623–631.

From Figure 12-7, one may safely calculate the initial basal insulin dose for a patient with T2DM. Both insulin glargine and detemir should be administered at a consistent time each day. "Flexible dosing" or omitting doses is likely to result in a rise in fasting blood glucose values of 18 to 36 mg per dL over 1 to 2 days for insulin glargine.[53]

Treat-to-target studies performed in patients with T2DM using a single injection of basal insulin successfully achieve A1C levels of less than 7% in approximately 60% of all subjects.[27,28,54] Over time, as β-cell function deteriorates, targeted glycemic control becomes more difficult to maintain using a single injection of basal insulin. Fasting glucose levels may be acceptable, yet postprandial hyperglycemia will result in a rise in A1C.

Estimation Of Initial Basal Insulin Dose For A Patient With Type 2 Diabetes

- Total daily insulin dose= 0.7 unit per kg/day

- Basal insulin requirements= 0.35 units per kg/day

(Example: A 100-kg patient would require approximately 100 x .35 u/kg/d= 35 units per day)

- Alternatively, patients may be initiated on 10 units at bedtime. The dosage is titrated slowly upward by the clinician 1-3 units every 2-3 days until the fasting glucose level reaches the desired target. The dosage may also be reduced by 10%–20% if the patient experiences hypoglycemia.

Figure 12-7 • **Estimation of Initial Basal Insulin Dose for a Patient with T2DM**

Timely and Appropriate Prandial Insulin Initiation and Intensification

Basal insulin therapy may help patients achieve glycemic goals for a time, but predictable and progressive pancreatic β-cell dysfunction necessitates the eventual addition of mealtime insulin to minimize postprandial hyperglycemia excursions. Postprandial glycemic variability elicits more oxidative stress than chronic, sustained hyperglycemia leading to endothelial dysfunction, vascular inflammation, atherosclerosis, and microvascular complications.[55–58] Pharmacologic interventions with insulin analogues reduce oxidative stress and vascular inflammation while improving endothelial function. Insulin intensification in patients with T2DM is cost-effective by reducing health-care costs related to OAD usage and significantly lowering the frequency and duration of inpatient hospitalizations.

The Treating To Target in T2DM Study (the 4-T Study), provides some insight into when insulin should be initiated in patients and at what time during the course of their disease prandial insulin might be initiated.[59] Over 700 patients with T2DM who were on dual OAD therapy were randomized into this study. One group was randomized to biphasic insulin aspart 70/30 twice daily. The second group was randomized to prandial insulin aspart three times daily, while the third cohort was managed with basal insulin detemir once daily at bedtime. The trial used a clinically relevant titration protocol with clinic visits every 3 months. After 1 year, patients who continued to have unacceptable rates of hyperglycemia (defined as A1C greater than 10% after one measurement, two consecutive A1C measurements greater than 8% at or after 24 weeks of therapy, or an A1C greater than 6.5% at the end of year 1) were eligible for intensification of their insulin regimens. Therapy with a sulfonylurea was replaced with an additional type of rapid-acting or mixed insulin regimen as follows:

- Aspart was added t.i.d to the detemir-initiated arm, starting with 10% of the current total daily basal dose (minimum of 4 U; maximum of 6 U).
- Detemir (10 U) was added at bedtime to the aspart-initiated arm.
- Aspart was added at midday to the aspart mix 70/30 initiated arm, starting with 10% of the current total daily dose (minimum of 4 U; maximum of 6 U). (This regimen is used in Europe to manage diabetes, but not in the United States).

The primary outcome of the first 4-T Study published in 2007 was A1C.[60] Small but significant differences were noted between the three groups. The cohort with the highest A1C included those patients randomized to basal insulin at bedtime. The patients with the lowest A1C had received prandial insulin aspart. However, none of the groups achieved the target A1C of less than 6.5%. As one would expect, basal insulin resulted in optimal reduction of FPG, whereas prandial insulin improved postmeal glucose excursions better than basal or mixed insulins. Less weight gain and fewer episodes of hypoglycemia were noted in the basal insulin cohort. Thus, after 1 year, the 4-T conclusions were as follows: (1) regimens using biphasic or prandial insulin reduced A1C to a greater extent than basal but were associated with a greater risk of hypoglycemia and weight gain. (2) Most patients are likely to require more than one type of insulin to achieve target A1C levels over time, as very few individuals were able to maintain their A1C levels at less than 6.5%.

Because the investigators noted a progression in the disease process for their patients with T2DM and an inability to reduce A1C, patients were randomized to be placed on prandial insulin. After two additional years in the 4-T Study, the A1C levels were identical between all three cohorts. What did reach statistical significance was the fact that those patients initiated on basal insulin monotherapy at the end of 3 years had less severe forms of hypoglycemia and less weight gain.

The overall aggregate A1C level at the conclusion of the 3-year 4-T Study was 6.9%. Patient commencing therapy with basal or prandial insulin achieved glycemic targets more often than those initiating therapy with biphasic insulin. The lowest weight gain and lowest rate of hypoglycemia occurred in the detemir plus aspart group, with 63% of patients achieving an A1C of less than 7%. Finally, the 4-T Study supports starting insulin therapy with once-daily basal insulin and adding prandial insulin if glycemic goals are not met within 1 year. Table 12-10 summarizes the appropriate timing for initiating prandial insulin as add-on to basal insulin therapy (also known as the basal-plus intervention).

TABLE 12-10. When Should Insulin Therapy Be Intensified with Prandial Insulin?

- When the recommended A1C level of <7% is not reached despite successful basal insulin dose titration which has achieved FPG levels ≤100 mg/dL
- Basal insulin dose titration is limited by nocturnal hypoglycemia
- Basal insulin usage exceeds 60 U/d
- Add prandial insulin if glycemic goals (A1C) are not met within 1 year of starting basal insulin therapy)[a]
- "BeAM Factor" >55 mg/dL[b]
  - BeAM factor = the difference between bedtime and AM blood glucose levels
  - Patients titrating basal insulin to a fasting glucose target of ≤100 mg/dL who had a BeAM factor >55 mg/dL are less likely to achieve an A1C ≤7% (p <0.0001) without experiencing nocturnal hypoglycemia. Therefore, these patients should be placed on prandial insulin
  - BeAM factor >55 mg/dL is associated with an increased risk of nocturnal hypoglycemia (p <0.0001), but not overall hypoglycemia

[a]Holman RR, Farmer AJ, Davies MJ, et al. Three-year efficacy of complex insulin regimens in type 2 diabetes. *N Engl J Med.* 2009;361:1736–1747
[b]Zisman A, Aleksandra V, Zhou R. The BeAM Factor: An easy-to-determine, objective, clinical indicator for when to add prandial insulin vs continued basal insulin titration. ADA Scientific Sessions. San Diego, CA: Abstract; 2011:1121-P.

Rapid-acting insulin analogues exhibit a peak onset of pharmacodynamic activity at 60 minutes postinjection. Peak carbohydrate absorption following a meal occurs at approximately 75 to 90 minutes after eating begins. In order to blunt the expected rise in postabsorptive glycemic excursions, the rapid-acting insulin analogues should be injected 15 minutes prior to eating. Insulin should be injected at the onset of meal if the self-monitored glucose level is less than 80 mg per dL.[61] The delay between the injection and onset of the consumption of the meal is known as the "insulin lag time." Patients who inject just prior to a meal may experience postprandial hyperglycemia although they have calculated their insulin dose appropriately.

If one is uncertain as to which meal should be targeted for intervention, "structured" glucose testing should be performed for 3 days prior to and 2 hours after each meal. The meal with the highest "delta" (the difference in blood glucose values between premeal and 2-hour postprandial levels) becomes the initial point of intercession.

Uncertainty as to which meal should be targeted for "intervention" should prompt the initiation of *structured glucose testing*. Structured glucose testing allows patients to identify specific glycemic patterns, which may be corrected with appropriate pharmacologic or lifestyle interventions. The patterns that are easiest to identify and most often amenable to therapeutic intensification include hypoglycemia, fasting hyperglycemia, and postprandial hyperglycemia.[62] Testing should be performed before and 2 hours after each meal for 3 days prior to the patient's next scheduled appointment. The difference between the baseline premeal and the 2-hour postprandial glucose levels is known as the "delta." The meal with the highest "delta" becomes the initial point of intercession for prandial insulin.

Structured glucose testing also provides a useful means by which patients may learn to self-titrate their mealtime insulin doses. The fundamentals of insulin pharmacokinetics and pharmacodynamics may also be conceptualized by patients who are either new to insulin therapy or those who need a refresher course after years of insulin use. Table 12-11 provides some basic "tips" on interpreting delta values as well as some educational strategies that may improve glycemic control.

Choosing the most appropriate meal to initiate prandial insulin may be inconsequential. A study investigating the efficacy of injecting the rapid-acting insulin analogue glulisine at either breakfast or at the main mealtime in patients with T2DM on a background insulin glargine plus OADs resulted in significant improvement in A1C levels regardless of meal specificity.[63]

TABLE 12-11. Interpretation of Structured Glucose Testing Delta Values[a]

Delta Value (mg/dL)	Interpretation	Intervention
0–50	• Correct insulin given for amount of carbohydrates consumed • Correct lag time procedure followed	• None
51–100	• Insulin to carbohydrate mismatch • Incorrect lag time • Possible snacking in between end of meal and 2-h test	• Increase prandial insulin dose 1–2 U next time this type of food is eaten • Make sure to inject insulin at least 15 min prior to meals
100–200	• Possibly had elevated blood glucose prior to meal time and did not give a correction dose • Insulin to carb mismatch • Was insulin omitted • Errors in glucose monitoring technique	• Teach patient how to use a premeal insulin sensitivity factor (see Chapter 11 on T1DM) • If patient omitted insulin they will see the error of their ways • If postmeal delta is consistently elevated, increase baseline insulin dose by 1 U/d until delta is 0–50 or 2 h postprandial glucose is <140 mg/dL • Educate patient on proper blood glucose monitoring. Touching fruit, cakes, or ice cream after a meal may result in false elevation of blood glucose values
Any negative delta value (i.e., −25)	• Miscalculation of insulin to carb ratio. Too much insulin bolused for amount of carbs eaten. Patient is likely to become hypoglycemic in the next 1–2 h	• Educate patient regarding insulin absorption principles: 1 h after bolusing 90% of rapid-acting insulin analogue remains in depot. Two hours after bolusing 60% of insulin remains in depot. Thus, if 10 U of insulin is given at 8 AM, at 10 AM 6 U remain to be absorbed. A premeal glucose of 120 and a 2 h postmeal glucose of 90 calculate the delta as being −30 mg/dL. The patient still has 6 U remaining to be absorbed and is likely to become hypoglycemic. Appropriate surveillance and intervention should be initiated

The delta is calculated by determining the difference between the premeal and 2-h postprandial glucose values.
A physiologic rise in 2-h postprandial glucose levels from baseline in euglycemic individuals is ≤50 mg/dL.
(Basu A, Man CD, Basu R. Effects of type 2 diabetes on insulin secretion, insulin action, glucose effectiveness, and postprandial glucose metabolism. *Diabetes Care*. 2009;32:866–872.

Structured glucose testing performed before each meal, 2 hours after eating, and at bedtime beginning 3 days prior to a patient's office visit may assist the physician in recognizing and correcting unfavorable glycemic patterns such as hypoglycemia, fasting hyperglycemia, and postprandial hyperglycemia (Fig. 12-8). Patterns recognition should initially target elimination of hypoglycemic events followed by a reduction in fasting hyperglycemia and postabsorptive hyperglycemia. Patients

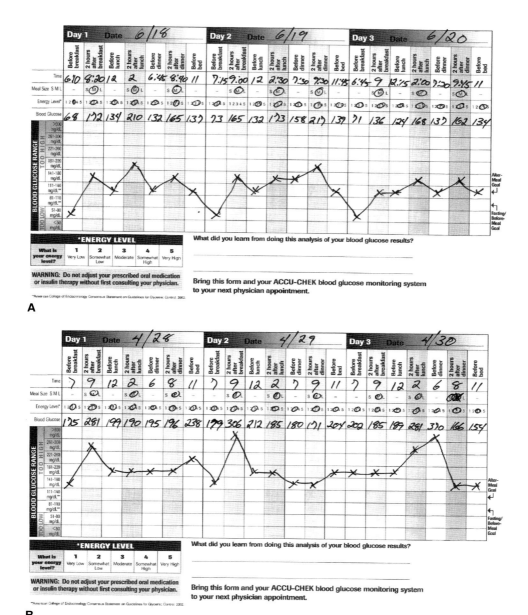

Figure 12-8 • A. Pattern glucose testing demonstrating hypoglycemia on three consecutive mornings. Patient would be instructed to reduce the dose of their basal insulin by 3 to 4 U. **B.** Paired glucose testing demonstrating persistent fasting and postprandial hyperglycemia. Treatment options would be to teach patient how to self-titrate basal insulin to a fasting target of less than 100 mg per dL, consider insulin intensification with prandial dosing, add a DPP-4 inhibitor (sitagliptin) or GLP-1 agonist, increase dose of metformin, reduce carbohydrate intake for meals, or switch to a mixed insulin analogue. Patient should also be screened for obstructive sleep apnea, which is known to cause insulin resistance (see Chapter 8).

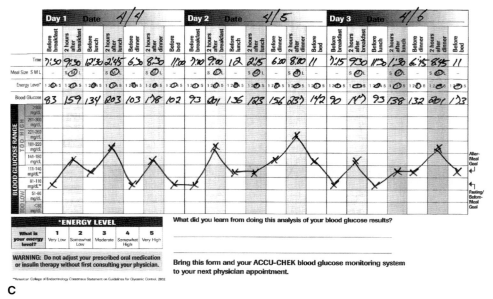

C

Figure 12-8 • *(Continued)* **C.** This patient has normal fasting glucose levels, but persistent postprandial excursions. Treatment considerations include adding a DPP-4 inhibitor (sitagliptin) to the basal insulin regimen, increasing the dose of metformin, adding bromocriptine, reducing carbohydrate intake for meals, or adding prandial insulin.

who perform structured testing have successfully reduced their A1Cs by 0.3% over 1 year.[62,64,61] Table 12-11 lists the interpretations of postprandial delta values, which patients should consider when performing structured testing.

If after 3 months the A1C does not meet the recommended target, structured glucose testing should be repeated for 3 days. First, evaluate the "delta" for the meal during which the initial intervention was initiated. The average delta should be less than 50 mg per dL, which is considered to be "physiologic."[65] If the delta is significantly greater than 50 mg per dL, consider increasing the baseline dose of prandial insulin at that meal until the 2-hour postprandial glucose level is 0 to 50 mg per dL from baseline. One could also consider adding a second mealtime injection of a rapid-acting insulin analogue at either breakfast or lunch. The initial dose of any prandial rapid-acting insulin can be approximated as 0.1 U per kg per meal. Thus, a 100-kg person would require 10 U of a rapid-acting analogue, which would be injected 15 minutes prior to eating. If the 2-hour postprandial glucose is 0 to 50 mg per dL, the correct amount of insulin was given to cover the carbohydrate content of that meal. However, if the 2-hour postprandial glucose level is consistently greater than 50 mg per dL, the patient can adjust the mealtime dose of insulin by 1 U per day until the targeted delta is achieved.[1]

Prandial insulin analogue initiation and titration are summarized in Table 12-12.

Insulin Degludec Dosing Titration Algorithm

The safety and efficacy of insulin degludec have been evaluated in several clinical trials including a 16-week randomized, open label, parallel-group, phase II study.[66] Patients were randomized to receive either once-daily insulin degludec or insulin glargine in combination with metformin. The baseline A1C levels were 7% to 11%. At the conclusion of the trial, the mean A1C levels were identical between the two groups. However, the odds ratio of confirmed hypoglycemia (defined as plasma glucose of less than 59 mg per dL or requiring assistance) was 0.44 for degludec versus 0.26 for glargine.

TABLE 12-12. Practical Approaches to Initiating and Titrating Prandial Insulin in Patients with T2DM

Option 1
• Initial dose for lispro, aspart, or glulisine is 0.1 U/kg/meal
• Insulin is injected 15 min prior to eating if blood glucose is >80 mg/dL. Inject at onset of meal if blood glucose is <80 mg/dL. If one is uncertain as to when meal will be served or how much food will be consumed, one may inject within 15 min of finishing the meal
• The dose of insulin may be adjusted based upon the anticipated size of the meal (not on the amount of carbohydrates to be consumed) 　• For very large meals with dessert, add 3 U from baseline insulin dose 　• For moderate-sized meals, add 2 U from baseline insulin dose 　• For small meals, subtract 1–2 U from baseline insulin dose
• Structured glucose testing should be performed for 3 consecutive days to determine if the premeal glucose level is consistently 90–130 mg/dL. If not, consider altering basal insulin dose. The targeted delta for the 2-h postprandial blood glucose values should be 0–50 mg/dL. If not, adjustments should be made in the baseline pre-meal insulin dose

Option 2
• The starting dose of prandial insulin is 10% of the total basal insulin dose per meal
• Reduce the dose of basal insulin by 10%
• (Thus, a patient who is injecting 40 U of basal insulin would bolus 4 U of lispro, aspart, or glulisine 15 min before a meal)
• Adjustments in dose of mealtime insulin may be made by targeting 2-h postprandial glucose values of ≤160 mg/dL

From Unger J. Diagnosis and management of type 2 diabetes and prediabetes. In: Jeff Unger MD, ed. *Primary Care Clinics in Office Practice;* 2007;34(4):731–759.

The dose titration algorithm for most degludec phase III clinical trials is shown in Table 12-13. The initial dose is 10 U daily taken within 1 hour before the start of the evening meal up until bedtime. Weekly dose titrations are based upon the patient's self-monitored blood glucose levels obtained before breakfast (lowest value from three consecutive days) targeting fasting glucose concentrations between 70 and 90 mg per dL.

TABLE 12-13. Suggested Dose Titration of Insulin Degludec[a]

Lowest Fasting Self-monitored Blood Glucose Value Obtained in 3 Consecutive Days (mg/dL)	Insulin Degludec Dose Adjustments (U)
<56	−4 (for a dose of >45 U, suggest a dose reduction of 10%)
56–70	−2 (for a dose of >45 U, suggest a dose reduction of 5%)
70<90	No adjustment
91<126	+2
127–144	+4
145–162	+6
>162	+8

[a]Although this protocol exists for clinical trial use, clinicians are encouraged to individualize care based on a patient's history of hypoglycemic unawareness or coexisting medical conditions.

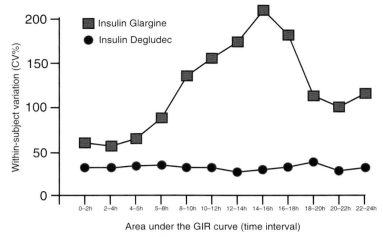

Figure 12-9 • Pharmacodynamic Variability over 24 Hours at Steady State: A Comparison of Insulin Glargine and Insulin Degludec. The within-subject variation for IDeg is consistently lower than IGlar over 24 hours, which may be due to the slow release of IDeg monomers from soluble multi hexamers that form after subcutaneous (SC) injection. IDeg's lower within-subject variability is thought to contribute to the lower risk of hypoglycemia observed in clinical studies. (Adapted from Heise T, Hermanski L, Nosek L, et al. The pharmacodynamics variability of insulin degludec is consistently lower than insulin glargine over 24 hours at steady state. ADA's 71st Annual Scientific Sessions. San Diego, CA: Abstract; 2011:0960-P).

Owing to degludec's flat pharmacokinetic profile (Fig. 12-9) and low intrasubject variability, higher doses of this insulin may be administered to patients in order to target fasting glucose levels of 70 to 90 without experiencing more frequent episodes of hypoglycemia. Several studies involving degludec have demonstrated that the cumulative incidence of hypoglycemia is comparable to insulin glargine during the initial 16-week dose titration phase, but becomes less frequent during the maintenance phase of the study.[67,68]

Intentional insulin omission occurs in up to 20% of patients with T2DM on a regular basis.[69] Risk factors for insulin omission include advancing age, lack of education, low income, perceived pain, and embarrassment from having to inject. For patients who tend to omit insulin doses, the use of a long-acting basal insulin such as degludec may prove to be their drug of choice.

A 26-week open-label, randomized trial in patients with T2DM (mean A1C 8.4%; FPG 161 and duration of diabetes 10.6 years) was performed to evaluate the noninferiority of IDeg dosed once-daily in a flexible regimen (a compulsory, rotating morning and evening schedule, creating 8- to 40-hour dosing intervals compared to insulin glargine given at the same time each day).[70] Insulin was added to existing OAD therapy and titrated to an FPG of less than 90 mg per dL. The A1C levels were identical at the conclusion of the trial, as were the safety endpoints. However, the extreme dosing protocol had no negative effects on fasting control for up to 40 hours following a prescribed omission of IDeg. Omission of the insulin for any reason for up to 40 hours is not likely to compromise glycemic control.

When approved, insulin degludec may also be marketed in a U-200 formulation that will be useful for insulin-resistant patients or those requiring more than 80 U of basal insulin in a single injection. "Low-volume degludec" (IDeg 200) contains the same amount of insulin per injected unit as IDeg 100, but in half the volume. Each pen click will contain 2 rather than 1 unit of insulin. Insulin degludec will be administered only via a prefilled disposable FlexTouch pen injector. The design includes an internal spring, which when triggered by a light touch, dispenses insulin from within the barrel of the pen rather than from force applied externally as the thumb applies pressure against a triggering mechanism. At the conclusion of the dose delivery, the pen produces an audible click that reassures the patient that drug delivery has been completed. FlexTouch pens have demonstrated consistent dosing accuracy across low-, medium-, and high-insulin boluses.[70a] This brand of pen may be particularly useful for patients with impaired manual dexterity.

Degludec can also be coformulated with the rapid-acting prandial insulin aspart, resulting in a soluble product containing two different insulin analogues. A single injection of IDegAsp will consist of 70% long-acting basal insulin and 30% rapid-acting prandial insulin.[68] Thus, IDegAsp will permit patients to target both fasting and mealtime glycemic control in a single injection. IDeg may be used for both insulin initiation and intensification for those patients who require mealtime glycemic adjust of insulin. Until now, combining a rapid-acting prandial insulin analogue with a long-acting basal analogue in one injection has not been possible.

A 16-week open label three-armed trial in poorly controlled patients with T2DM compared the use of once-daily IDegAsp + metformin to insulin degludec + aspart (AF) + metformin and insulin glargine (IGlar) + metformin.[68] The baseline A1C in these patients was 8.5%. Insulin was administered before dinner and titrated to a fasting glucose of 72 to 108 mg per dL. After 16 weeks, mean A1C decreased in all groups to comparable levels (IDegAsp: 7.0%; AF: 7.2%; IGlar: 7.1%). A similar proportion of subjects achieved A1C of 7.0% without confirmed hypoglycemia in the past 4 weeks of treatment (IDegAsp: 51%; AF: 47%; IGlar: 50%). IDegAsp provided markedly better post-dinner plasma glucose control than IGlar. However, this did not translate into improved overall glycemic control; at the end of the trial, no apparent difference in A1C was found between treatments.

Premixed Insulin Analogues

Premixed preparations combine rapid-acting (prandial) and long-duration (basal) insulins in a single vial or pen injector. The use of these fixed-dose insulins can reduce dosing errors that may occur when patients attempt to mix NPH and regular insulin in the same syringe. If one combines NPH with a rapid-acting analogue, the injection must be immediate to avoid alteration in the glucose-lowering effects of the analogue. Patients with visual impairment may have a family member preload their rapid- and intermediate-acting insulin into syringes for use later in the day. However, this may result in absorption variability and hypoglycemia. Use of these premixed preparations is simple, user friendly, and more physiologic than NPH plus regular injections.

The human premixed insulins (Humulin 50/50, Humulin 70/30, Novolin 70/30) combine regular plus NPH in a single dose. Thirty units of 50/50 insulin would consist of 15 U regular plus 15 U of NPH. The 70/30 preparations consist of 70% NPH and 30% regular insulin. When used, these insulins must be injected at least 30 minutes prior to mealtime.

Analogue premixed insulins include lispro Mix 75/25, lispro Mix 50/50, and Biaspart Mix 70/30. Unlike human mixed insulins, the analogues consist of a set percentage of rapid-acting insulin (either lispro or aspart) plus the rapid-acting insulin combined with protamine, which delays the absorption of that insulin component. By prolonging the duration of action of a percentage of aspart or lispro within the mixed insulin, protamine improves the glucodynamic effect of the insulin. A patient using a mixed insulin would receive the benefits of a basal and bolus insulin in a single injection. Thus, a 20-U dose of lispro 75/25 would contain 5 U of lispro plus 15 U of lispro plus protamine. The analogue premixed insulins should be injected 15 minutes prior to eating to minimize postprandial glycemic excursions.

Although less expensive than the analogues, the human premixed insulins are less effective at minimizing postprandial glycemic excursions than analogue premixed insulins.[71] Premixed analogues can result in hypoglycemia. However, the incidence of severe hypoglycemia appears to be slightly higher for individuals using the human premixed formulations (2% to 14% of patients) versus those using the premixed analogues (2% to 8% of patients).[72]

Premixed insulin analogues might be useful for patients having a baseline A1C between 8.5% and 10%. Candidates who might be successful users of premixed insulin analogues include those

TABLE 12-14. Dosing Protocol for the 1,2,3 Study Using BiAspart Mix 70/30 Insulin

- Begin by dosing Aspart Mix 70/30 12 U 10–15 U before dinner
- Increase dose of Aspart Mix 70/30 by 2 U every 2 d until the pre-breakfast glucose level is <110 mg/dL
- Check the A1C after 3 months. If not <6.5%, add a second injection of Aspart Mix 70/30, beginning with 6 U given 10–15 min before breakfast. Continue monitoring the AM glucose readings and adjusting the dinner dose of insulin as before
- Increase the breakfast dose 2 U every 2 d if the dinner glucose readings are averaging >110 mg/dL
- Check A1C after 3 months
- If the A1C remains >6.5%, begin using a lunchtime dose of BiAspart Mix70/30, starting with 4 U injected 10–15 min before eating. Monitor a 2-h post lunch blood glucose level. Increase the lunchtime dose of Aspart Mix every 2 d by 2 U until the post lunch glucose levels are <140 mg/dL
- Check A1C after 3 months. If not ≤7%, other treatment options should be considered

who eat three meals daily and keep a regular scheduled routine of work and physical activity. Another advantage of mixed insulin analogues is that patients receive two insulins for a single copay. The initiation and titration of premixed insulins have proven successful in allowing patients to achieve their ADA-recommended glycemic targets.

In a 48-week, multicenter, open-label trial, patients who had T2DM and who were not achieving targets on oral agents (with or without once-daily basal insulin therapy with NPH or glargine) were titrated with BiAspart Mix 70/30 to target plasma glucose levels.[73] This study included 100 patients and was conducted in three separate phases. In phase 1, patients initiated treatment with BiAspart Mix 70/30 once before supper. Dosing frequency was increased to twice-daily in phase II and to three-times daily in phase III at 16 and 32 weeks, respectively, if patients did not achieve an A1C of less than 6.5%. Patients completed end-of-study when they achieved A1C less than or equal to 6.5% or 48 weeks, whichever came first. At the end of the trial, 77% of patients achieved A1C levels of less than 7.0%, and 60% of patients attained an A1C level of less than or equal to 6.5% through once, twice, or three-times daily dosing of BiAspart Mix70/30. The dosing titration protocol for the 1,2,3 Study is shown in Table 12-14.

Whether or not treatment-naive patients should begin treatment with basal insulin or a mixed insulin analogue was the primary learning objective of the INITIATE Trial.[74] Two hundred and three patients with poorly controlled diabetes on OADs having baseline A1Cs greater than 8% were randomized to taking either insulin glargine or BiAspart Mix 70/30 for 28 weeks. At the conclusion of the study, 66% of patients taking BiAspart Mix 70/30 reached the recommended ADA target A1C of less than 7% compared with only 40% of those taking insulin glargine. As expected, the postprandial glycemic excursions for the BiAspart Mix 70/30 group were approximately 25% lower than those patients using glargine. Minor hypoglycemic events occurred more commonly in patients taking mixed insulin, but no episodes of severe hypoglycemia were recorded during the trial.

Management of Severe Insulin Resistance

Insulin resistance is a serious therapeutic dilemma despite advances in oral agents and the introduction of insulin analogues. Commensurate with the twin global epidemics of obesity and T2DM, sales of concentrated U-500 insulin in the United States increased to 71% from 2005 through 2008.[75] Common etiologies of severe insulin resistance are outlined in Table 12-15.

A normoglycemic individual consuming a standard diet secretes approximately 45 U per 24 hours, including 10 U for breakfast, 13 U for lunch, 14 U for dinner, and 8 basal U to suppress

TABLE 12-15 Causes of Severe Insulin Resistance

- Obesity
- Use of protease inhibitors for the treatment of human immunodeficiency virus and graft-versus-host disease after bone marrow transplantation, both of which may result in an acquired form of lipodystrophy
- Insulin receptor defects (type A insulin resistance syndromes)
- Insulin receptor autoantibodies (type B insulin resistance syndrome)
- Patient error in inserting insulin pump infusion sets or administration of subcutaneous insulin doses
- Hyperandrogenism in girls (hirsutism, acne, oligo/amenorrhea, and polycystic ovaries)
- Rare inherited disorders such as leprechaunism with insulin-receptor mutations
- Use of glucocorticoids
- Hypertriglyceridemia
- Coronary artery disease
- Monogenetic diabetes (MODY)

From Lane WS, Cochran EK, Jackson JA, et al. High-dose insulin therapy: is it time for U-500 insulin? *Endocr Pract.* 2009;15(1):71–79; Barb D, Mantzoros C. Diagnosing obesity, diabetes mellitus and the insulin resistance syndrome. In: Mantzoros C, eds. *Obesity and Diabetes.* Totowa, NJ: Humana Press, Inc; 2006:129.

hepatic glucose production in the fasting state. At least 50% of the endogenous insulin released by the pancreas is extracted by the liver during the initial transhepatic passage so that the total peripheral delivery of insulin is approximately 22 U per day.[76] Insulin resistance occurs when the hormone's action to lower blood glucose levels is severely impaired. In order for insulin action to occur, insulin must bind with receptors on the cell surfaces of skeletal muscles and adipose tissue. If insulin receptors are down-regulated or absent, cells become unresponsive to insulin action. In response to prolonged and persistent hyperglycemia, the pancreas will produce an excessive amount of insulin in an attempt to restore ambient glucose levels to normal. However, high levels of circulating endogenous insulin result in down-regulation of insulin receptors and impairment of insulin action. Inflammatory cytokines may inhibit the expression of peroxisome proliferator-activated receptor (PPAR) genes, leading to a state of insulin resistance.[77] Other individuals may be insulin resistant despite having normal numbers of insulin receptors on their cell surfaces. These patients may exhibit postreceptor binding defects or insulin antibodies, which preclude normal insulin action from occurring.[78]

Patients in whom glycemic control deteriorates despite using more than 200 U of exogenous insulin daily are considered to be insulin resistant.[79] As a result of having prolonged and significant hyperglycemia, these patients become frustrated over the lack of efficacy of different treatment protocols.

One option for treating insulin resistance is the use of human regular U-500 insulin. U-500 is five times more concentrated (500 U per mL) than the standard U-100 insulin (100 U per mL). Because U-500 insulin is highly concentrated, lower volumes of the drug can be injected, resulting in a smaller and more efficiently absorbed insulin depot. A patient who normally injects 50 U of U-100 prior to a meal needs to administer only 10 U of U-500.

Several treatment options have been suggested for initiating U-500, transitioning patients from U-100 to U-500 insulin regimens and using U-500 in insulin pumps.[80,81] One such algorithm that may be adapted for use in primary care is displayed in Figure 12-10.

Excessive hepatic glucose production in patients with severe insulin resistance results in sustained fasting hyperglycemia. Therefore, one may consider initiating U-500 insulin as a single injection given at bedtime (Table 12-16). The rationale for this protocol is also based upon the pharmacokinetics of U-500 insulin. Regular U-100 insulin demonstrates a peak effect within 2 to 4 hours of administration and a 5- to 7-hour duration of action compared with U-500, which has an onset and duration of action similar to those of regular insulin but a duration of action of up to 24 hours.[82]

Dosing Algorithm For U-500 Insulin

Total Daily Dose of U-100 Insulin Patient Is Taking	Injection Frequency of U-500 Insulin	Weighted Doses of U-500 Insulin Injections	Dosing Adjustments of U-500 Insulin
200–299	• 8 AM and 6 PM	• 60 TDD % in AM; 40% TDD in PM	BG level <50 mg/dL above or below target range: Increase or decrease U-500 in increments of 5 units per dose/bolus
300–600	8 AM, noon, 6 PM	40% TDD in AM, 30% TDD at noon, 30% at 6 PM	BG level within 100 mg/dL above or below target range: Increase or decrease U-500 in increments of 25 units per dose/bolus

TDD= total daily dose of insulin, BG=blood glucose

Figure 12-10 • Dosing Algorithm for U-500 Insulin. (Adapted from Cochran E, Gordon P. Use of U-500 insulin in the treatment of severe insulin resistance. *Insulin.* 2008;3:211–218.)

Because of the pharmacodynamics of U-500 insulin, dose changes are based on trends rather than on glucose levels at each dose. U-500 doses may be changed by 15% to 20% for blood glucose levels outside of an individual's targeted range. More specifically, in the dose range of 200 to 299 U per day, dose adjustments should be made in increments of 5 U per dose for blood glucose levels less than 50 mg per dL above or below the target range. For blood glucose levels greater than 50 mg per dL above or below the target range, dose adjustments should be made in increments of 10 U per dose.

The mean wholesale cost of U-500 insulin is approximately $370 per vial as compared with the $140 per vial cost of rapid-acting insulin analogues.[83] Although U-500 insulin is more expensive than other insulins on a per-milliliter basis, the actual volume of insulin used is decreased, resulting in a 50% reduction in cost per unit of insulin versus rapid-acting analogues. Recently, Medicare Part D initiated a directive to cover the cost of U-500 specifically for patients using the drug for subcutaneous injections, but not insulin pump therapy. Individual drug policies vary as to what portion of the U-500 costs must be incurred by the patient.

Weight gain is often observed with U-500 insulin use (Table 12-17). However, I have found that concomitant use of metformin (500 to 850 mg b.i.d) and liraglutide (1.8 mg per day) not only mitigates weight gain in our U-500 patients but also improves fasting and postprandial excursions.

TABLE 12-16. Bedtime Injection Protocol for Injecting U-500 Insulin

- Inject 25 U of U-500 in the abdomen at 9 PM. The target fasting blood glucose levels are <140 mg/dL

- Increase the U-500 dose every 5 d until the fasting blood glucose levels are <140 mg/dL

- For mealtime insulin, use lispro, aspart or glulisine. First target the meal that has the greatest 2-h postprandial glucose excursion. Start with 0.1 U/kg/meal. Increase dose by 1 U daily until the 2-h postprandial glucose level is "trending" toward 140–180 mg/dL for 11 w. A second meal may be targeted after 3 mon if the patient's A1C has not reached the targeted goal

TABLE 12-17. U-500 Fast Facts

- A predetermined dose of U-500 is given prior to each meal. The dose of the insulin should not normally be adjusted to compensate for preprandial hyperglycemia.

- If preprandial glucose levels are <70 mg/dL, one should inject the U-500 dose after eating.

- U-500 insulin has a slower onset of action (60 min) when compared with U-100 rapid-acting insulin analogues. The peak onset of action of U-500 is 2–4 h. Therefore, after injecting one should delay eating for at least 45–60 min. Duration of action of U-500 is 4–6 h. The duration of action of U-500 is up to 24 h. (Jørgensen KH, Hansen AK, Buschard K. Five fold increase of insulin concentration delays in the absorption of subcutaneously injected human insulin suspensions in pigs. *Diabetes Res Clin Pract.* 2000;50:161–167)

- Low-volume insulin syringes should be used for U-500 insulin injections. Dosing U-500 may be more difficult using 100-U syringes versus 30-U syringes. Although some have suggested using tuberculin syringes to draw up and inject U-500, I have found that the BD-U-100 syringes are actually much easier and practical to use for all patients. Remember that U-500 insulin is five times as concentrated as U-100. Therefore, a patient who requires 150 U of insulin would be instructed to inject 30 U of U-500 insulin (1:5) using a BD-U-100 syringe.

- Weight gain can be expected with U-500 insulin. However, improvement in A1C is usually apparent within 3 months. The risks of moderate weight gain appear to be less than the resulting effects of prolonged and uncontrolled hyperglycemia. The weight gain may be mitigated with concomitant use of metformin + liraglutide.

- Patients tend to more energetic on U-500 when compared with using high-volume U-100 insulin.

- Patients should be warned that many clinicians, nursing personnel, and pharmacists may be unfamiliar with U-500 insulin. Dosing errors may occur if someone other than the patient administers the insulin. For example, a patient receiving 10 U of U-500 insulin may develop severe hyperglycemia if given only 10 U of U-100.

- U-500 insulin often must be special ordered by pharmacies. The physician should make certain that the patient's pharmacy remains stocked with U-500 so that refills can be easily obtained.

- Patients should be instructed on how to properly use a glucagon emergency kit for severe hypoglycemia. Glucagon kits should be kept at home and in the workplace.

Proposed Individualized Insulin Initiation Algorithms for Newly Diagnosed Patients with T2DM

Nearly 3,000 cases of newly diagnosed T2DM are diagnosed in the United States daily.[84] Patients may present to PCPs as referrals from emergency departments, other specialists (such as ophthalmologists), freestanding community clinics, health screening fairs, during routine physical examinations, or while self-referred due to a family history of diabetes. A patient who presents with symptoms related to chronic hyperglycemia (thirst, weight loss, altered vision, paresthesias, and frequent urination) may be screened in the office with a random blood glucose level and venipuncture, which should be sent to a reference lab for A1C testing (see Chapter 10 on T2DM, which discusses accepted screening guidelines for T2DM).

Patients with an A1C greater than 9% who are *asymptomatic* should be given the option of being treated with triple drug therapy (insulin being one of the three pharmaceutical interventions) or initiating intensive insulin therapy to achieve β-cell rest. The American Association of Clinical Endocrinologists consensus panel guideline suggests the use of triple drug therapy initially for treatment-naive patients with A1Cs greater than 9% who are asymptomatic.[24] The triple drug therapy might include one of the following combinations:

- Metformin + GLP-1 agonist + TZD
- Metformin + GLP-1 agonist + glinide

- Metformin + GLP-1 agonist + sulfonylurea
- Metformin + DPP-4 inhibitor + glinide
- Metformin + DPP-4 inhibitor + TZD
- Metformin + DPP-4 inhibitor + sulfonylurea

Failure of a triple drug therapy to achieve one's targeted A1C or clear hyperglycemic within 3 months implies that the patient's β-cell insulin secretory capacity has been exceeded. Exogenous insulin will therefore be necessary.[24]

Based on the 2009 ADA/European Association for the Study of Diabetes (EASD) consensus algorithm, initial therapy for treatment-naive patients should consist of greater than two agents.[13] With lifestyle intervention considered as the foundation of care to which all other therapies are added, metformin, when tolerated, should be initiated immediately in combination with either basal insulin or a sulfonylurea. A1C levels should be reassessed within 3 months allowing for further therapeutic intensification to occur in a timely fashion if glycemic targets are not achieved.

More than 90% of the maximum effect of metformin is observed within 6 weeks of treatment initiation; therefore, clinicians should be able to predict when improvement in A1C will be observed. If one's A1C is not approaching the individualized target, adherence to the treatment regimen should be addressed. Perhaps the patient may be experiencing metformin intolerance (diarrhea, bloating, gastritis) and is taking the medication not *with* meals but prior to eating or at bedtime.

While patients reap the benefits of any remaining β-cell mass and function they possess, there is a strong likelihood of successfully achieving an A1C of less than 7% with the use of metformin, a basal insulin, and a dipeptidyl peptidase 4 (DPP-4) inhibitor in treatment-naive patients. Clinical trials are currently planned to access the safety and efficacy of approach.[85]

A newly diagnosed patient with T2DM should have their dietary habits addressed on the first visit. Often times, those patients who frequent guests at fast-food outlets and who consume excessive amounts of fruit drinks, regular colas, and high-calorie specialty caffeine drinks will note an immediate improvement in their blood glucose levels as they transition to healthier dietary choices.

A treatment regimen for a patient with T2DM who is insulin naive may be prescribed using the algorithm shown in Figure 12-11.

Proposed Individualized Insulin Initiation Algorithms for Patients with Advanced T2DM

The progressive decline in β-cell mass and function as reflected in deterioration in glycemic targets (A1C, fasting, and postprandial glucose levels) will necessitate insulin intensification in many patients. Basal-bolus therapy using rapid-acting insulin at mealtimes in addition to a basal insulin analogue is highly effective at improving glycemic control for patient whose A1C is greater than 9%.[86]

Insulin intensification in response to progressive insulin deficiency requires the use of rapid-acting insulin analogues prior to select meals to minimize postprandial glucose excursions. Effective control of postprandial hyperglycemia can have an important impact on improving one's A1C levels, especially those near the ADA target of 7%.[87] Basal–prandial insulin therapy emulates physiologic endogenous insulin secretion and allows separate titrations of either basal or prandial components to reflect one's individual dietary and lifestyle requirements.

A study by Davidson et al. evaluated if one or two preprandial injections before meals of greatest glycemic impact can be as effective as three premeal injections in patients with T2DM who have failed basal insulin treatment.[88] Qualified patients were permitted to continue their OAD therapy, but sulfonylureas were discontinued. Upon entering a 14-week run-in treatment phase, insulin glargine was initiated at 10 U and progressively titrated to achieve a fasting glucose target of less than 110 mg per dL. Patients whose A1C was greater than 7% at week 14 were randomized to one

Proposed Treatment Algorithm For Insulin Initiation In A Newly Diagnosed Patient With Type 2 Diabetes

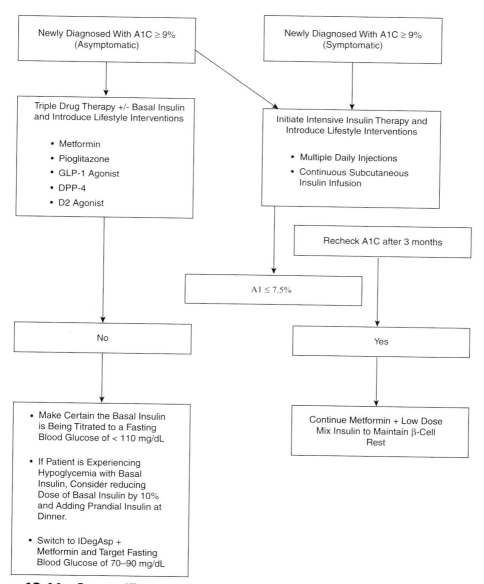

Figure 12-11 • Proposed Treatment Algorithm for Insulin Initiation in a Newly Diagnosed Patient with T2DM

of three arms: glulisine once, twice, or thrice daily prior to meals for 24 weeks. The doses of insulins were adjusted based upon self–blood glucose monitoring as shown in Table 12-18.

Although the mean decreases in A1C levels from the time of randomization of all three groups were similar, patients using more frequent mealtime injections were more successful at achieving the ADA targeted A1C goal of less than 7% (46% for the 3 per day injectors, 33% for the 2 per day injectors, and 30% for the once-daily injectors). This suggests that some patients on the basal-plus regimens would have benefitted from more frequent injections.

Table 12-18 Simultaneous Adjustments for Basal and Prandial Insulin

- **Insulin Glargine Dose Adjustment Algorithm is Based on *Fasting* Blood Glucose Values**

Mean Fasting 2-Day Blood Glucose Values (mg/dL)	Insulin Glargine Dose Adjustment Every 2 Days
>250	Increase dose at investigator discretion
110–250	+2 U
100–109	0–2 U[a]
70–99	No change
<70	−2–4[a]

[a]Specific dose adjustments based on investigator discretion

- **Insulin Glulisine Weekly Dose Adjustment is Based on Preprandial Self-monitored Blood Glucose Values and Observed Glycemic Patterns[a]**

Mealtime Dose	Pattern of Low Preprandial Blood Glucose Values (≥2 values <70 mg/dL)	Pattern of High Preprandial Blood Glucose Values (≥4 values above target)
≤10 U	−1 U	+1 U
11–20 U	−2 U	+2 U
>20 U	−3 U	+3 U

[a]The initial dose of glulisine for all patients was 10% of the total daily dose of insulin glargine at the time of randomization given with each injection 1–3 times daily. Weekly dosage targeted a preprandial blood glucose level of 70–109 mg/dL and a bedtime blood glucose value of 70–129 mg/dL while avoiding recurrent episode (≥2 events/w) of hypoglycemia. Glusine doses were titrated weekly based on pattern recognition. Adjustments for breakfast doses were based on prelunch testing. Lunch dose adjustments were based on dinner monitoring and dinner doses were adjusted based on bedtime self-monitoring values.
From Davidson MB, Raskin P, Tanenberg RJ, et al. A stepwise approach to insulin therapy in patients with type 2 diabetes mellitus and basal insulin treatment failure. *Endocr pract.* 2011;17(3):395–403.

Premixed insulin may provide another means for rapidly improving A1C in appropriately selected patients, yet provide less flexibility in use than basal bolus regimens. The INITIATE study found that twice-daily biphasic insulin aspart 70/30 was more effective than once-daily glargine at achieving A1C levels ≤7%.[74] However, patients using the mixed insulin experienced more weight gain and had a greater frequency of minor hypoglycemic events when compared with those individuals using glargine.

Figure 12-12 provides a suggested algorithm for the management of patients with advanced T2DM.

When initiating basal insulin to those with advanced T2DM, an individualized written treat-to-target algorithm should be provided to the patient. Whenever possible, insulin pen devices should be used to improve the accuracy and safety of dose self-directed dose titration. The starting dose of basal insulin can be set at 10 U given once daily or 0.4 U per kg for patients who are obese and insulin resistant. Fasting blood glucose values should be checked daily with structured testing, performed before and 2 hours after each meal for three consecutive days beginning on the week of the patient's next scheduled office appointment. Metformin, when tolerated, should be continued.

Insulin dosing errors in elderly patients are likely to result in hypoglycemia. Exogenous insulin administration with a vial and syringe will result in inconsistent dosing as well as reduced adherence to the prescribed protocol.[89,90,91] Thus, pen devices, not syringes and vials, are the preferred means by which insulin should be administered.

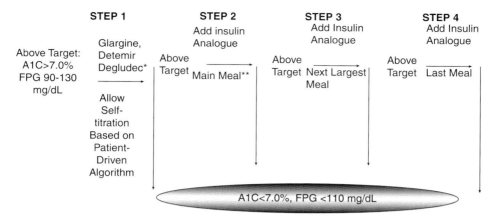

Figure 12-12 • Insulin Initiation and Intensification for Patients with Advanced T2DM***

*=Degludec may be used daily as IDeg or in combination with insulin aspart (IDegAsp) injected prior to dinner to provide both prolonged basal and a single meal's prandial insulin coverage.

**Although any meal may be targeted for rapid-acting insulin intensification, one should perform structured glucose testing before and 2 hours after each meal beginning 3 days prior to a scheduled office visit. The meal that shows the greatest 2-hour postprandial rise in glucose levels (the change in delta) should be targeted for intensification.

***Advanced T2DM implies patients who have had the disorder for greater than 5 years, those whose A1C exceeds 9%, or any patients who are no longer responding to triple-drug therapy.

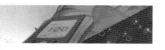

SUMMARY

Insulin should be considered an essential therapeutic intervention in patients with newly diagnosed T2DM as well as those with advanced disease. The treatment objective in those who are newly diagnosed is to establish pancreatic β-cell rest. After reversing the acute hyperglycemic state and reducing the A1C to less than 7.5%, one might consider transitioning the patient to OADs, a GLP-1 agonist, or continuing mixed insulin therapy to preserve β-cell function over time.

Patients with advanced disease have lost most of their β-cell mass and function. Their A1C levels will rise and symptoms associated with chronic hyperglycemia are likely to occur. The primary objective in these patients is to intensify their therapeutic options by targeting individualized A1C goals with insulin. Once the initial dose of insulin is prescribed, patients should be given the opportunity to self-titrate to specific fasting or postprandial glycemic levels. Randomized clinical trials have consistently proven that treat-to-target protocols are effective at lowering A1Cs in patients with poorly controlled T2DM. In addition, both treatment-naive patients and patients familiar with insulin therapy are capable of safely, effectively, and efficiently employing self-titration protocols.

Adjunctive medications such as oral agents, GLP-1 analogues (see Chapter 10), and pramlintide (see Chapter 11) may be coadministered with insulin. One should consider the risks versus benefits of using insulin with other medications, especially if they are to be used "off-label." Weight gain, hypoglycemia, complexity of therapeutic regimen, and additional costs are the primary concerns which must be addressed when intensifying therapy in patients with T2DM.

PCPs appear to be quite capable of initiating basal insulin for poorly controlled patients with T2DM. Unfortunately, controversy exists on how one should titrate the dose of basal insulin and at what point prandial insulin should be added to the regimen. Should one target dinner initially or simply prescribe a more complicated basal-prandial regimen?

Options to consider include the use of once-daily insulin degludec plus IDegAsp that combines an ultralong basal insulin analogue with a rapid-acting prandial analogue. Another option would be to use "step-therapy" initiating basal insulin first allowing patients to self-titrate, followed by a rapid-acting meal time analogue in 3 months if the targeted A1C is not achieved. Additional prandial insulin injections may be initiated, over time, until the desired A1C, fasting, and postprandial glycemic targets are attained.

Although the use of insulin in primary care may appear to be a daunting task, PCPs and their patients are well equipped for this challenge. The use of insulin pens allows for painless administration of the drug. Multiple dosing titration protocols have been published in peer-reviewed journals and can be readily adapted to a primary care practice. Patients can learn these protocols in a matter of minutes and become successful diabetes self-managers.

REFERENCES

1. Unger J. Insulin initiation and intensification in patients with T2DM for the primary care physician. *Diabetes Metab Syndr Obes.* Targets and Therapy 2011;4:253–261.
2. Hayes RP, Fitzgerald JT, Jacober SJ. Primary care physician beliefs about insulin initiation in patients with type 2 diabetes. *Int J Clin Pract.* 2008;62:860–868.
3. Holmann RR, Paul SK, Bethel MA, et al. 10-year follow-up of intensive glucose control in type 2 diabetes. *N Engl J Med.* 2008;359:1577–1589.
4. U.S. Department of Health and Human Services. Food and Drug Administration. Center for Drug Evaluation and Research. Guidance for Industry. Diabetes Mellitus: Developing drugs and therapeutic biologics for treatment and prevention. Draft Guidance. 2008. http://www.fda.gov/downloads/Drugs/Guidance-ComplianceRegulatoryInformation/Guidances/UCM071624.pdf. Accessed February 2, 2012.
5. Kosaka K, Kuzuya T, Hagura R, et al. Insulin response to oral glucose load is consistently decreased in established non-insulin-dependent diabetes mellitus: the usefulness of decreased early insulin response as a predictor of non-insulin-dependent diabetes mellitus. *Diabet Med.* 1996;13:S109–S119.
6. Adeghate E, Lalasz H. Amylin analogues in the treatment of diabetes mellitus: medicinal chemistry and structural basis of its function. *Open Med Chem J.* 2011;5(suppl 2):78–81.
7. Westermark P, Andersson A, Westermark GT. Islet amyloid polypeptide, islet amyloid, and diabetes mellitus. *Physiol Rev.* 2011;91(3):795–826.
8. Enoki S, Mitsukawa T, Takemura J, et al. Plasma islet amyloid polypeptide levels in obesity, impaired glucose-tolerance and non-insulin-dependent diabetes-mellitus. *Diabetes Res Clin Pract.* 1992;15:97–102.
9. Leahy JL, Bonner-Weir S, Weir GC. Beta-cell dysfunction induced by chronic hyperglycemia: current ideas on mechanism of impaired glucose-induced insulin secretion. *Diabetes Care.* 1992;15:442–455.
10. Knowles NG, Landchild MA, Fujimoto WY, et al. Insulin and amylin release are both diminished in first-degree relatives of subjects with type 2 diabetes. *Diabetes Care.* 2002;25:292–297.
11. Hull RL, Westermark GT, Westermark P, et al. Islet amyloid: a critical entity in the pathogenesis of type 2 diabetes. *JClin Endocrinol Metab.* 2004;89(8):3629–3643.
12. Mykkanen L, Haffner SM, Hales CN, et al. The relation of proinsulin, insulin, and proinsulin-to-insulin ratio to insulin sensitivity and acute insulin response in normoglycemic subjects. *Diabetes.* 1997;46(12):1990–1995.
13. Nathan DM, Buse JB, Davidson MB, et al. Medical management of hyperglycemia in type 2 diabetes: a consensus algorithm for the initiation and adjustment of therapy: a consensus statement of the American Diabetes Association and the European Association for the Study of Diabetes. *Diabetes Care.* 2009;32:193–203.
14. Knowler WC, Barrett-Connor E, Fowler SE, et al. Reduction in the incidence of type 2 diabetes with lifestyle intervention or metformin. *N Engl J Med.* 2002;346(6):393–403.
15. Sumner CJ, Sheth S, Griffin JW, et al. The spectrum of neuropathy in diabetes and impaired glucose tolerance. *Neurology.* 2003;60:108–111.

16. Ceriello A. New insights on oxidative stress and diabetic complications may lead to a "causal" antioxidant therapy. *Diabetes Care.* 2003;26:1589–1596.
17. UK Prospective Diabetes Study (UKPDS) Group. Intensive blood-glucose control with sulphonylureas or insulin compared with conventional treatment and risk of complications in patients with type 2 diabetes (UKPDS 33). *Lancet.* 1998;352:837–853.
18. Ohkubo Y, Kishikawa H, Araki E, et al. Intensive insulin therapy prevents the progression of diabetic microvascular complications in Japanese patients with non-insulin-dependent diabetes mellitus: a randomized prospective 6-year study. *Diabetes Res Clin Pract.* 1995;28:103–117.
19. DCCT-EDIC: Retinopathy and nephropathy in patients with type 1 diabetes four years after a trial of intensive therapy. The Diabetes Control and Complications Trial/Epidemiology of Diabetes Interventions and Complications Research Group. *N Engl J Med.* 2000;342:381–389.
20. Martin CL, Albers J, Herman WH, et al. DCCT/EDIC Research Group. Neuropathy among the diabetes control and complications trial cohort 8 years after trial completion. *Diabetes Care.* 2006;29:340–344.
21. Gerstein HC, Miller ME, Byington RP, et al. Effects of intensive glucose lowering in type 2 diabetes. Action to Control Cardiovascular Risk in Diabetes Study Group. *N Engl J Med.* 2008;358:2545–2559.
22. Weng J, Li Y, Xu W, et al. Effect of intensive insulin therapy on beta-cell function and glycaemic control in patients with newly diagnosed type 2 diabetes: a multicentre randomised parallel group trial. *Lancet.* 2008;371:1753–1760.
23. Brown JB, Nichols GA, Perry A. The burden of treatment failure in type 2 diabetes. *Diabetes Care.* 2004;27(7):1535–1540.
24. Rodbard HW, Jellilnger PS, Davidson JA, et al. AACE/ACE Consensus Statement. Statement by an American Association of Clinical Endocrinologists/American College of Endocrinology consensus panel on type 2 diabetes mellitus: an algorithm for glycemic control. *Endocr Pract.* 2009;15(1):540–559.
25. Matza LS, Boye KS, Yurgin N, et al. Utilities and disutilities for type 2 diabetes treatment-related attributes. *Qual Life Res.* 2007;16:1251–1265.
26. Riddle MC. The underuse of insulin therapy in North America. *Diabetes Metab Res Rev.* 2002;18(suppl 3):S42–S44.
27. Meneghini L, Koenen C, Weng W, et al. The usage of a simplified self-titration dosing guideline (303 Algorithm) for insulin detemir in patients with type 2 diabetes: results of the randomized, controlled PREDICTIVE™ 303 study. *Diabetes Obes Metab.* 2007;9:902–913.
28. Gerstein HC, Yale J-F, Harris SB, et al. A randomized trial of adding insulin glargine vs. avoidance of insulin in people with type 2 diabetes on either no oral glucose-lowering agents or submaximal doses of metformin and/or sulphonylureas. The Canadian INSIGHT (Implementing New Strategies with Insulin Glargine for Hyperglycaemia Treatment) Study. *Diabet Med.* 2006;23:736–742.
29. Davies M, Lavalle-Gonzalez F, Storms F, et al. Initiation of insulin glargine therapy in type 2 diabetes subjects suboptimally controlled on oral antidiabetic agents: results from the AT.LANTUS trial. *Diabetes Obes Metab.* 2008;10(suppl 2):42–49.
30. Peyrot M, Rubin RR, Lauritzen T, et al. Resistance to insulin therapy among patients and providers: results of the cross-national Diabetes Attitudes, Wishes, and Needs (DAWN) study. *Diabetes Care.* 2005;28:2673–2679.
31. Cobble ME, Peters AL. Clinical practice in type 2 diabetes: after metformin and lifestyle, then what? *J Fam Pract.* 2009;58:S7–S14.
32. Unger J, Parkin C. Hypoglycemia in insulin-treated diabetes: a case for increased vigilance. *Postgrad Med.* 2011;123(4):81–91.
33. Masley S, Sokoloff J, Hawes C. Planning group visits for high-risk patients. *Fam Pract Manag.* 2000;7:33–37.
34. Kruszynska YT, Home PD, Hanning I, et al. Basal and 24-h C-peptide and insulin secretion rate in normal man. *Diabetologia.* 1987;30:16–21.
35. Binder c, Lauritzen T, Faber O, et al. Insulin pharmacokinetics. *Diabetes Care.* 1984;7(2):188–189.
36. Heinemann L. Variability of insulin absorption and insulin action. *Diabetes Technol Ther.* 2002;4(5):673–682.
37. Clinical Trials.gov Identifier: NCT01468987 http://www.clinicaltrials.gov/ct2/show/NCT01468987?term=BIAM&rank=1
38. Clinical Trials.gov Identifier: NCT01195454. http://clinicaltrials.gov/show/NCT01195454
39. Niswender KD. Basal insulin: physiology, pharmacology, and clinical implications. *Postgrad Med.* 2011;123(4):17–26.

40. King AB, Poon K. Glargine and detemir: safety and efficacy profiles of the long-acting basal insulin analogs. *Drug Healthc Patient Saf.* 2010;2:213–223.

41. King AB. Once-daily insulin detemir is comparable to once-daily insulin glargine in providing glycaemic control over 24 h in patients with type 2 diabetes: a double-blind, randomized, crossover study. *Diabetes Obes Metab.* 2009;11:69–71.

42. Heise T, Nosek L, Ronn BB, et al. Lower within-subject variability of insulin detemir in comparison to NPH insulin and insulin glargine in people with type 1 diabetes. *Diabetes.* 2004;53(6):1614–1620.

43. Hartman I. Insuln analogs: impact on treatment success, satisfaction, quality of life, and adherence. *Clin Med Res.* 2008;6(2):54–67.

44. Meneghini LF, Orozco-Beltran D, Khunti K, et al. Weight beneficial treatments for type 2 diabetes. *J Clin Endocrinol Metab.* 2011;96(11):3337–3353.

45. Groop L, Widen E, Franssila-Kallunki A, et al. Different effects of insulin and oral antidiabetic agents on glucose and energy metabolism in type 2 (non-insulin-dependent) diabetes mellitus. *Diabetologia.* 1989;32(8):599–605.

46. Sinha A, Formica C, Tsalamandris C, et al. Effects of insulin on body composition in patients with insulin-dependent and non-insulin-dependent diabetes. *Diabet Med.* 1996;13(1):40–46.

47. Monami M, Marchionni N, Mannucci E. Long-acting insulin analogues versus NPH human insulin in type 2 diabetes: a meta-analysis. *Diabetes Res Clin Pract.* 2008;81(2):184–189.

48. Hermansen K, Davies M, Derezinski T, et al. A 26-week, randomized, parallel, treat-to-target trial comparing insulin detemir with NPH insulin as add-on therapy to oral glucose-lowering drugs in insulin-naive people with type 2 diabetes. *Diabetes Care.* 2006;29(6):1269–1274.

49. Fajardo Montanana C, Hernandez Herrero C, Rivas Fernandez M. Less weight gain and hypoglycaemia with once-daily insulin detemir than NPH insulin in intensification of insulin therapy in overweight type 2 diabetes patients: the PREDICTIVE™ BMI clinical trial. *Diabet Med.* 2008;25(8):916–923.

50. Haak T, Tiengo A, Draeger E, et al. Lower within-subject variability of fasting blood glucose and reduced weight gain with insulin detemir compared to NPH insulin in patients with type 2 diabetes. *Diabetes Obes Metab.* 2005;7(1):56–64.

51. Raskin P, Gylvin T, Weng W, et al. Comparison of insulin detemir and insulin glargine using a basal-bolus regimen in a randomized, controlled clinical study in patients with type 2 diabetes. *Diabetes Metab Res Rev.* 2009;25(6):542–548.

52. Blonde L, Merilainen M, Karwe V, et al. Patient directed titration for achieving glycaemic goals using a once-daily basal insulin analogue: an assessment of two different fasting plasma glucose targets: the TITRATE study. *Diabetes Obes Metab.* 2009;11:623–631.

53. A 26-Week Randomised, Controlled, Open Label, Multicentre, Multinational, Three-arm, Treat-to-target Trial Comparing Efficacy and Safety of Three Different Dosing Regimens of Either NN1250 or Insulin Glargine With or Without Combination With OAD Treatment, in Subjects With Type 2 Diabetes Mellitus (BEGIN™: FLEX) Available at http://www.clinicaltrials.gov/ct2/show/NCT01006291?term=BEGIN+Flex&rank=1. Accessed July 31, 2011.

54. Riddle MC, Rosenstock J, Gerich J. The treat-to-target trial: randomized addition of glargine or human NPH insulin to oral therapy of type 2 diabetic patients. *Diabetes Care* 2003:26:3080–3086.

55. Ceriello A. Oxidative stress and diabetes-associated complications. *Endocr Pract.* 2006;12(suppl 1):60–62.

56. Unger J. Reducing oxidative stress in patients with type 2 diabetes mellitus: a primary care call to action. *Insulin.* 2008;3:176–184.

57. Scognamiglio R, Negut C, de Kreutzenberg SV, et al. Effects of different insulin regimes on postprandial myocardial perfusion defects in type 2 diabetic patients. *Diabetes Care.* 2006;29:95–100.

58. Aagren M, Luo W, Moes E. Healthcare utilization changes in relation to treatment intensification with insulin aspart in patients with type 2 diabetes: data from a large U.S. managed-care organization. *J Med Econ.* 2010;13(1):16–22.

59. Holman RR, Farmer AJ, Davies MJ, et al. Three-year efficacy of complex insulin regimens in type 2 diabetes. *N Engl J Med.* 2009;361:1736–1747.

60. Holman RR, Thorne KI, Farmer AJ, et al. Addition of biphasic, prandial, or basal insulin to oral therapy in type 2 diabetes. *N Engl J Med.* 2007;357:1716–1730.

61. Luijf YM, van Bon AC, Hoekstra JB, et al. Premeal injection of rapid-acting insulin reduces postprandial glycemic excursions in type 1 diabetes. *Diabetes Care.* 2010;33:2152–2155.

62. Rodbard H, Schnell O, Unger J, et al. Decision support tools dramatically improve clinicians' ability to interpret structured SMBG data. Late-Breaking Poster presentation. ADA 71st Scientific Sessions. San Diego,CA. June 24–28, 2011. 24-LB.

63. Lankisch MR, Ferlinz KC, Leahy JL, et al. Introducing a simplified approach to insulin therapy in type 2 diabetes: a comparison of two single-dose regimens of insulin glulisine plus insulin glargine and oral antidiabetic drugs. *Diabetes Obes Metab.* 2008;10:1178–1185.

64. Polonsky WH, Fisher L, Schikman CH, et al. Structured self-monitoring of blood glucose significantly reduces A1C levels in poorly controlled, noninsulin-treated type 2 diabetes results from the Structured Testing Program study. *Diabetes Care.* 2011;34:262–267.

65. Basu A, Man CD, Basu R. Effects of type 2 diabetes on insulin secretion, insulin action, glucose effectiveness, and postprandial glucose metabolism. *Diabetes Care.* 2009;32:866–872.

66. Zinman B, Fulcher G, Rao PV, et al. Insulin degludec, an ultra-long-acting basal insulin, once a day or three times a week versus insulin glargine once a day in patients with type 2 diabetes: a 16-week, randomised, open-label, phase 2 trial. *Lancet.* 2011;DOI:10.1016/S0140-6736(10)623057.

67. Birkeland KI, Home PD, Wendisch U, et al. Insulin degludec in type 1 diabetes: a randomized controlled trial of a new-generation ultra-long-acting insulin compared with insulin glargine. *Diabetes Care.* 2011;34:661–665.

68. Heise T, Tack CJ, Cuddihy R, et al. A new-generation ultra-long-acting basal insulin with a bolus boost compared with insulin glargine in insulin-naïve people with type 2 diabetes. *Diabetes Care.* 2011;34: 669–674.

69. Peyrot M, Rubin RR, Kruger DF, et al. Correlates of insulin injection omission. *Diabetes Care.* 2010;33:240–245.

70. Meneghini L, Atkin SL, Bain S, et al. Flexible once-daily dosing of insulin degludec does not compromise glycemic control or safety compared to insulin glargine given once daily at the same time each day in people with type 2 diabetes. American Diabetes Association 71st Annual Scientific Sessions. San Diego, CA: Abstract; 2011:0035-LB.

70a. Wielandt JO, Niemeyer M, Hansen MR, et al. FlexTouch: a prefilled insulin pen with a novel injection mechanism with consistent high accuracy at low (1 U), medium (40 U), and high (80 U) dose settings. *J Diabetes Sci Technol.* 2011;5(5):1195–1199.

71. McSorley PT, Bell PM, Jacobsen LV, et al. Twice-daily biphasic insulin aspart 30 versus biphasic human insulin 30: a double-blind crossover study in adults with type 2 diabetes mellitus. *Clin Ther.* 2002;24:530–539.

72. Davidson J, Vexiau P, Cucinotta D, et al. Biphasic insulin aspart 30: literature review of adverse events associated with treatment. *Clin Ther.* 2005;27(suppl B):S75–S88.

73. Garber AJ, Wahlen J, Wahl T, et al. Attainment of glycaemic goals in type 2 diabetes with once-, twice-, or thrice-daily dosing with biphasic insulin aspart 70/30 (the 1-2-3 study). *Diabetes Obes Metab.* 2006;8(1):58–66.

74. Raskin P, Allen E, Hollander P, et al. Initiating insulin therapy in type 2 diabetes: a comparison of biphasic and basal insulin analogs. *Diabetes Care.* 2004;28:260–265.

75. Lane WS, Cochran EK, Jackson JA, et al. High-dose insulin therapy: is it time for U-500 insulin? *Endocr Pract.* 2009;15(1):71–79.

76. Eaton RP, Allen RC, Schade DS, et al. "Normal" insulin secretion: the goal of artificial insulin delivery systems? *Diabetes Care.* 1980;3:270–273.

77. Tanaka T, Itoh H, Doi K, et al. Down regulation of peroxisome proliferator-activated receptor gamma expression by inflammatory cytokines and its reversal by thiazolidinediones. *Diabetologia.* 1999;42: 702–710.

78. Caro JF, Amatruda JM. Glucocorticoid-induced insulin resistance: the importance of post-binding events in the regulation of insulin binding, action, and degradation in freshly isolated and primary cultures of rat hepatocytes. *J Clin Invest.* 1982;69:866–875.

79. Cochran E, Musso C, Gorden P. The use of U-500 in patients with extreme insulin resistance. *Diabetes Care.* 2005;28:1240–1244.

80. Neal MJ. Analysis of effectiveness of human U-500 insulin in patients unresponsive to conventional insulin therapy. *Endocr Pract.* 2005;11:305–308.

81. Quinn SL, Lansang MC, Mina D. Safety and effectiveness of U-500 insulin therapy in patients with insulin-resistant type 2 diabetes mellitus. *Pharmacotherapy.* 2011;31(7):695–702.

82. Jørgensen KH, Hansen AK, Buschard K. Five fold increase of insulin concentration delays in the absorption of subcutaneously injected human insulin suspensions in pigs. *Diabetes Res Clin Pract.* 2000;50: 161–167.

83. www.drugstore.com. Accessed August 7, 2011.

84. 2011 National Diabetes Fact Sheet. http://www.cdc.gov/diabetes/pubs/estimates11.htm#5. Accessed August 12, 2011.

85. Janumet Before Insulin Lantus In Eastern Population Evaluation Program (JUBILEE) In Type 2 Diabetic Patients. http://clinicaltrialsfeeds.org/clinical-trials/results/term=JUBILEE+Study. Accessed August 12, 2011.

86. Niswender K. Early and aggressive initiation of insulin therapy for type 2 diabetes: what is the evidence? *Clin Diabetes.* 2009;27(2):60–68.

87. Monnier L, Lapinski H, Colette C. Contributions of fasting and postprandial plasma glucose increments to the overall diurnal hyperglycemia of type 2 diabetic patients: variations with increasing levels of HbA(1c). *Diabetes Care.* 2003;26:881–885.

88. Davidson MB, Raskin P, Tanenberg RJ, et al. A stepwise approach to insulin therapy in patients with type 2 diabetes mellitus and basal insulin treatment failure. *Endocr pract.* 2011;17(3):395–403.

89. Korytowski M, Bell D, Jacobsen C, et al. A multicenter, randomized open-label, comparative two-period crossover trial of preference, efficacy, and safety profiles of a prefilled disposable pen and conventional vial/syringe for insulin injection in patients with type 1 or 2 diabetes mellitus. *Clin Ther.* 2003;25(11):2836–2848.

90. McCoy EK, Wright BM. A review of insulin pen devices. *Postgrad Med.* 2010;122(3):81–88.

91. Lee WC, Balu S, Cobden D, et al. Medication adherence and the associate health-economic impact a month patients with type 2 diabetes mellitus converting to insulin pen therapy: an analysis of third-party managed care claims data. *Clin Ther.* 2006;28(10):1712–1725.

Insulin Pumping and Use of Continuous Glucose Sensors in Primary Care

13

You miss 100 percent of the shots you never take.
—*Wayne Gretzky, Hall of Fame hockey player*

Introduction The use of continuous subcutaneous insulin infusion (CSII), also known as insulin pump therapy, allows patients with diabetes to achieve improved glycemic control (lower A1Cs) while using less daily insulin, reducing the likelihood of weight gain, and limiting diurnal glycemic variability compared with syringes, vials, and pen-injected insulin.[1] Because of the lifestyle flexibility that insulin pumpers enjoy, quality-of-life scores consistently favor CSII over multiple daily injections (MDIs).[2] Switching from MDIs to CSII will limit the number of short-term complications such as hypoglycemia and diabetic ketoacidosis (DKA), as well as long-term microvascular disease.[1,3,4] Although CSII is certainly the most sophisticated and precise insulin-delivery method currently available, patients who initiate pump therapy must become solidly committed to diabetes self-management. Blood glucose levels must be checked six to eight times daily, unless patients use concomitant continuous real-time glucose sensors. Patients must understand insulin pharmacokinetics, carbohydrate counting, and some exercise physiology. Because a pump is a mechanical device that may, on occasion, malfunction, patients must be adept at troubleshooting potential causes of acute hyperglycemia and worrisome "malglycemia." Insulin pumpers rarely panic unless they are told to "remove their pump" in the emergency department or prior to an outpatient surgical procedure by a poorly trained medical provider who views the device as being nothing more than a fancy cell phone.

Pumpers are the most knowledgeable, dedicated, and determined individuals that primary care physicians (PCPs) will come to know within their diabetes patient population. Many of these patients are self-sufficient, confident, and totally committed to improving their own outcomes. PCPs who feel comfortable managing patients with diabetes should also commit themselves to learning the dynamics and benefits of insulin pump therapy.

Insulin pump therapy is designed to simulate normal pancreatic β-cell function by physiologically delivering both basal and bolus insulin to patients with T1DM and T2DM. The basal insulin limits the hepatic glucose production that occurs in the fasting state. Prandial (bolus insulin) is normally secreted from the pancreatic β-cells in first- and second-phase responses to meals. The first-phase insulin response occurs as one prepares to eat, whereas the second-phase insulin response continues as long as necessary to prevent postprandial hyperglycemia occurring as nutrients are absorbed from the gut. The tightly controlled glycemic range (70 to 140 mg per dL) is reflective of the normal relation between basal insulin and glucose, as well as the response of the β-cells to a mealtime carbohydrate challenge, as shown in Figure 13-1.

Ideally, exogenous insulin replacement should mimic the normal glucose and insulin response to the fasting and prandial states. However, prandial injection therapy, whether given by a syringe or a pen device, cannot provide both first- and second-phase physiologic insulin dosages. The dosing of basal insulin, provided as glargine, detemir, or degludec, assumes that one's basal insulin requirements remain unchanged throughout a 24-hour period. However, if one exercises, basal insulin requirements are reduced. Before getting up in the morning, basal insulin requirements increase in response to physiologic insulin resistance caused by increased production of cortisol and growth hormone. In the afternoon hours, insulin requirements are typically lower than during the morning and evening hours. Unfortunately, once the injection of basal insulin is given, the drug's influence on basal insulin levels cannot be altered. That is, one cannot "turn up or down" the level of glargine, NPH, degludec or detemir injected the evening before in response to exercise or varying degrees of insulin resistance.

By having the ability to program changes in basal and bolus insulin-delivery rates, pump users can simulate endogenous β-cell insulin secretion. One can program higher basal rates in anticipation of periods of heightened insulin resistance (i.e., dawn phenomenon) and lower basal rates in the afternoon hours when insulin resistance is minimal. Different mealtime bolus patterns may be used to control postprandial glucose (PPG) excursions better. Basal rate profiles may also be programmed

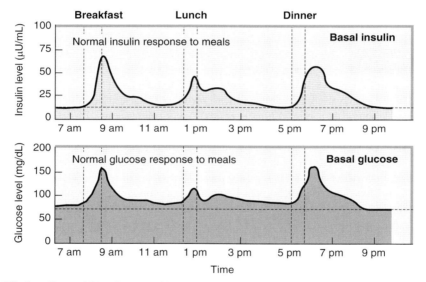

Figure 13-1 • Normal Physiology of Insulin and Glucose Response to Meals. In a nondiabetic individual, basal glucose levels range between 70 and 100 mg per dL while fasting. Basal glucose supplies the heart and central nervous system with an immediate and constant source of energy. Basal insulin levels prevent the liver from accelerating its release of glucose into the plasma via glycogenolysis and gluconeogenesis. If the patient is in the fed state, glucose levels will increase, triggering the pancreatic β-cells to release enough insulin to maintain PPG levels less than 140 mg per dL. Note that the basal and prandial glucose levels vary according to the time of day as well as the quantity and quality of consumed nutrients at any given meal. In the early morning hours, levels of circulating counterregulatory hormones (growth hormone and cortisol) are increased, resulting in a state of insulin resistance. A normally functioning pancreas overcomes this state of insulin resistance by secreting more insulin in response to these counterregulatory hormones. Therefore, insulin requirements are normally elevated in the morning. In the afternoon hours, insulin resistance is minimized, and insulin requirements decrease. Suppers tend to be the largest meal of the day, during which time one consumes the most calories, carbohydrates, and fats. The higher fat content in food will delay gastric emptying as well as the absorption of carbohydrates from the gut. Patients who must use exogenous insulin should attempt to replicate this complex interactive scheme to maintain blood glucose levels as near to normal as possible. Different basal and bolus-delivery patterns must be used to match this physiologic endogenous insulin milieu. One can see why even seasoned insulin pump patients have difficulty achieving normalcy by using exogenous insulin.

based on changes in insulin requirements that may occur around the onset of menstruation and ovulation. Patients may alter their basal insulin flow rates when using corticosteroids, chemothera-peutic agents, or protease inhibitor drugs.

Available since the 1980s, over 400,000 insulin pumps are sold worldwide annually.[5] Although 24 million Americans have diabetes, approximately 1% (280,000) of these patients are registered pump users.[6] In the United States, up to 20% of patients with T1DM are using insulin pumps. Insu-lin pumps are now reimbursed by most third-party payers who qualify for the devices.

As pumps and technologies become more user-friendly and clinically advanced, the number of patients inquiring about insulin pumps will undoubtedly increase. PCPs who are familiar with inten-sive insulin replacement therapy can successfully manage pump patients. Determinations of the basal rates, mealtime boluses, and supplemental insulin requirements are similar to the formulas used to calculate the different components of MDIs. Certified pump trainers, provided by the pump-manufac-turing companies, can be invaluable assistants when pump therapy is initiated. Nearly all pump train-ers are certified diabetic educators (CDEs) and are qualified to teach patients every aspect of insulin pump use, including safety issues, proper pump-insertion techniques, infusion-site monitoring, basal and bolus delivery patterns, and sick-day management, as well as troubleshoot acute hyperglycemia and pump malfunctions. Sales personnel can help direct interested personnel toward insulin pump education programs while serving as liaisons between the insurance companies, pump manufacturer, physician office staff, and the patient. The physician is responsible for determining and prescribing the pump parameters (basal rates, anticipated mealtime boluses, insulin-sensitivity factor (ISF), insulin-to-carbohydrate ratio, personal lag time, and type of insulin to be pumped). Insulin pump initiation can be performed in the physician's office by a certified insulin pump trainer within 60 to 90 minutes. The approach of having patients initiate pumps on saline prior to transitioning to insulin is like asking a person to live in a cave for a few weeks prior to moving into a mansion. When parameters are estab-lished in a safe manner in order to avoid hypoglycemia, adaption of pump therapy is simple and enthu-siastic. An example of a personalized insulin pump parameter form can be found in Appendix 13-1.

Some perspective pumpers may fear the high-tech gadgetry, which they associate with CSII. In reality, rookie pumpers need only know how to self-insert the pump's infusion set every 3 days and how to safely administer a physiologic mealtime bolus. The other "bells and whistles" can be adapted over time when one becomes more confident in one's ability to self-manage one's diabetes while wear-ing the pump.

Pumps do not "cure" diabetes, but offer an opportunity to manage diabetes physiologically. By improving one's overall control, the risk of diabetes-related complications—both short and long term—will be minimized. Pumpers do need to become experts in diabetes self-management. For many patients committed to insulin pump therapy, managing diabetes becomes both challenging and exciting!

For some patients with diabetes, pumping insulin becomes a family affair. Those with visual impairment or patients who have challenging dexterity issues due to arthritis may safely pump insulin with the assistance of a caregiver. In my experience, "team pumpers" are by far the most knowledgeable, enthusiastic, and ambitious diabetes managers that one will ever see in a primary care practice setting.

▌ Evolution of Modern Pump Technology

In the 1960s, a pediatrician named Arnold Kadesh developed the first "insulin pump." Worn on a backpack (Fig. 13-2A), the pump delivered insulin and glucagon intravenously. Although initially intended as a research instrument in the 1970s, pumps were found to be effective in improving gly-cemic control in patients with "brittle type 1 diabetes" (Fig. 13-2B).[7] After the MiniMed 502 pump was introduced and marketed in 1983, pump use began to grow in popularity. By 1990, the United States was home to 6,600 registered pump users.[8]

The Diabetes Control and Complications Trial (DCCT) was published in 1993.[9] At the conclu-sion of the DCCT, 42% of the intensively managed patients were using insulin pump therapy, and 56% were on MDIs. Patients in the DCCT who were on insulin pump therapy had a 0.3% lower A1C

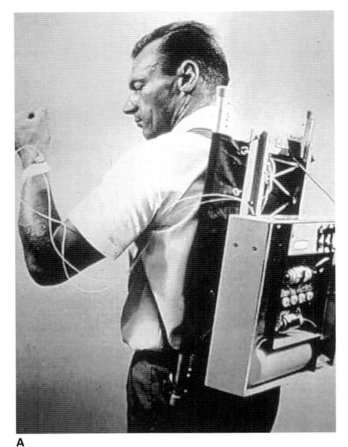

A

INSULIN PUMPS: 1978 - 1987

B

Figure 13-2 • **A.** In 1963, Arnold Kadesh, MD, developed the first insulin pump prototype designed to provide his daughter, who had T1DM, with improved glycemic control. This backpack pump delivered both intravenous insulin and glucagons. **B.** From 1978 to 1987, pumps became miniaturized.

compared with the intensively managed individuals who used MDIs. As CSII gained global popularity, the size, quality, reliability, mechanics, comfort, efficiency, and software of the pumps continued to improve. Insulin pumping now provides patients with diabetes their best hope of achieving physiologic glycemic control while reducing their incidence of short- and long-term complications.

From a primary care prospective, more patients are becoming proactive and inquiring about the benefits of using CSII to treat their own diabetes. These concerns should be addressed in an intelligent and supportive manner, remembering that any patient who requires insulin may be considered a candidate for an insulin pump. Patients are also appearing in emergency departments or operating room suites wearing their insulin pumps. Not infrequently, pumpers have been asked to "remove their cell phones while in the emergency department," or "you won't be needing that machine in the hospital." In reality, patients who use insulin pumps are extremely motivated, knowledgeable, and well versed in diabetes self-management skills. Physicians who choose to care for pump patients will need to advance their own insights into and knowledge regarding diabetes management. In so doing, these physicians will be able to provide a higher level of care to all of their diabetes patients whether or not they are using pump therapy. PCPs should sympathize with patients who might benefit from pump therapy, yet may need to wait months before seeing a diabetes specialist and even longer before actually receiving their insulin pumps. By becoming pump prescribers, PCPs will allow patients to benefit more rapidly from intensification of their diabetes regimen.

The "antique pump" infusion sets were anchored into the abdominal skin by a metal needle. The "bent needle" infusion sets tended to be uncomfortable, became easily dislodged from the subcutis, and were painfully reinserted every 2 days. The newer pumps use a spring-loaded self-inserter device (Fig. 13-3), which implants the Silastic infusion catheter painlessly into the skin. The self-inserter is necessary to drive the infusion set catheter to a uniformed subcutaneous insertion depth. Those individuals who prefer to insert the infusion set by hand will likely notice erratic glycemic control. Patients now have multiple infusion set styles from which to choose, all of which vary in regard to length of tubing, insulin delivery angle, cannula length, and method of insertion. Infusion sets have an easy point of disconnect from the site of insertion, allowing patients to be apart from their pump at any time for showering, swimming, exercising, or engaging in intimate activities. Pumps can be placed in pajamas or under a pillow while sleeping. Custom-made pump pouches are available to hide the devices virtually anywhere on the body. Wireless (tubeless) pumps are also available, which attach directly to the skin providing direct infusion of insulin from the pump to the subcutaneous depot.

Some pumps allow "discrete bolusing" by using a remote control. A woman who wears the pump under a dress could use the remote control device to signal a mealtime bolus rather than struggle with trying to remove the pump from her clothing during a boardroom meeting. An insulin reservoir within the insulin pump provides a preprogrammed individualized basal rate to each patient. Before mealtimes, the patient simply determines the blood glucose level and provides a physiologic bolus over a specified time through the infusion set. This same type of remote bolusing may be used for pediatric patients and controlled by a parent who may administer a prandial bolus

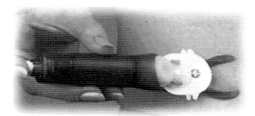

Figure 13-3 • One of Several Available Spring-loaded Insulin Pump Infusion Set Insertion Devices. After the skin is cleaned with an alcohol-based adhesive pad, the Silastic infusion-set tip is placed in the cocked inserter. As the inserter is positioned in parallel with the skin surface, light pressure is applied to the distal end of the device, which quickly and painlessly projects the catheter tip through the skin. Removing the white adhesive strips from around the catheter tips will prevent the catheter from dislodging from the infusion site for up to 72 hours.

to the child as he is running outdoors to grab his skateboard oblivious to the meal he had just consumed. Wireless pumps provide basal insulin delivery at prespecified rates. Prandial or correction boluses are administered via a hand-held remote device.

Continuous Glucose Sensors

The ultimate challenge in treating insulin-requiring diabetes is to design a reliable "closed-loop" sensor-augmented insulin pump. These insulin delivery devices incorporate the data transmitted from real-time continuous interstitial glucose sensors directly to the insulin pump. The patient will receive an infusion of insulin commensurate with the ambient interstitial glucose readings.

The safety and efficacy of the sensor-augmented pump (SAP) were evaluated in the 1-year randomized phase of the STAR 3 study for patients with T1DM.[10] Compared with subjects using MDI, those using SAP experienced greater reductions in A1C levels by 3 months, which persisted for the length of the study. A group of MDI patients within STAR 3 were allowed to switch to SAP therapy for 6 months at the conclusion of the 1-year trial.[11] The SAP patients were also allowed to remain on their therapy for an additional 6 months, extending the STAR 3 to 18 months. Of the 443 patients who completed the 1 year study, 420 elected to continue for an additional 6 months; 204 (94%) of the SAP patients continued their initial augmented pump therapy, while 190 (93%) of the MDI subjects decided to cross over to the SAP group (Fig. 13-4).

During the study phase of STAR 3, the A1C levels were reduced by 0.5% to 0.6% more with SAP treatment compared to MDI. Patients switching from MDI to SAP during the continuation phase reduced their A1Cs by a similar percentage. Patients who wore the sensor at least 60% of the time demonstrated maximal lowering of A1C.

The SAP technology has also demonstrated efficacy in automatically suspending basal insulin delivery for up to 2 hours in response to sensor-detected hypoglycemia in patients with T1DM.[12] The ability of the sensor to suspend insulin delivery automatically without patient intervention is an important step in closing the loop.

Figure 13-5 shows the first FDA approved pump-sensor device marketed: the Medtronic Real time Paradigm 722 pump. Users of the Paradigm 722 self-insert both the infusion set and a sensor-transmitting device into two separate areas in the abdomen.

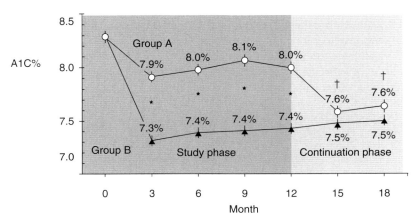

Figure 13-4 • Results of STAR 3 Trial. Group A used MDI and home blood glucose monitoring for 12 months after which they were given the option to cross over and continue on to the SAP phase of the study for an additional 6 months. Group B were maintained on SAP therapy for the entire 12-month study period before being given the option of extending their participation with SAP for an additional 6 months. (Adapted from Bergenstal RM, Tamborlane WV, Ahmann A, et al. Sensor-Augmented Pump Therapy for A1C Reduction (STAR 3) Study. Results from the 6-month continuation phase. *Diabetes Care.* 2011;34:2403–2405).

Continuous glucose monitoring (CGM) systems operate by measuring the glucose levels in interstitial fluid. The devices consist of three components: a disposable sensor that measures glucose levels, a transmitter that is attached to the sensor, and a receiver that displays and stores glucose information. The information stored in the receiver is then converted into estimated mean values of glucose standardized to capillary blood glucose levels measured during calibration.

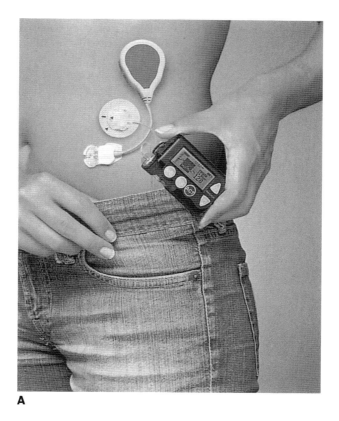

A

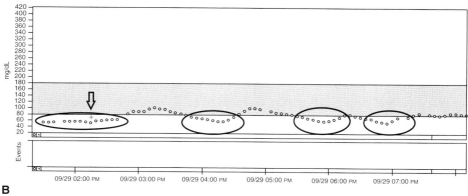

B

Figure 13-5 • **A. Medtronic 722 Sensor-augmented Pump System. B. Picture of Repeated Episodes of Hypoglycemia.** Patient on an insulin pump with multiple episodes of hypoglycemia from 1:00 PM through 7:00 PM (*circles*). The first episode of hypoglycemia last 75 minutes, as each dot represents a 5-minute interval of interstitial glucose readings. At 2:15 PM, the patient checks his blood glucose level with a finger stick (*diamond shape marker/arrow*) that corresponds well with the interstitial glucose value. An attempt is made to correct the hypoglycemic event, yet the patient continues the pattern of hypoglycemia for another 5 hours. (Case courtesy of Jeff Unger, MD)

Using a self-insertion device, a thin plastic sensor is placed into the interstitial space of the abdomen or upper arm. The microtrauma induced by the sensor insertion provokes an inflammatory reaction that consumes glucose followed by a repair process. This "calibration time" or waiting period allows the sensor signal from the interstitial fluid to stabilize. Calibration times are dependent upon the type of sensor that is inserted. The sensors display real-time glucose values and glucose trends. Some sensors sound alarms or vibrate in response to interstitial hyperglycemia or hypoglycemia exposure. Receivers can store information that may be downloaded and analyzed by computer software programs. Patients and clinicians may then analyze data related to glycemic trends, physical activity, meals, insulin usage, menstruation, illness, and concomitant medications.

Because continuous glucose sensor manufacturing has not progressed to the accuracy and precision of blood glucose meter strips, sensor glucose signals must be calibrated against corresponding blood glucose meter levels. Such calibrations transform the sensor signal into a glucose value and assume that the plasma-to-interstitial fluid glucose gradient remains relatively constant. Sensors should be calibrated when blood glucose levels are fairly constant as opposed to during the postprandial state when glucose levels are in flux. Recalibration at fixed intervals is required to prevent "sensor signal drift." Sensor levels typically trail blood glucose values by 5 to 10 minutes during periods of rapid change. From a clinical perspective, a patient may "feel hypoglycemic" with a blood glucose value of 80 mg/dL, yet the interstitial glucose reading is 90 mg/dL. Within 5 minutes, the alarm sounds as the ISF reading now reads 65 mg/dL as confirmed by the blood glucose monitor. CNS glucose levels may correlate better with ISF values than blood glucose levels.[13]

The sensor reads interstitial glucose levels every 5 minutes and transmits the data to the insulin pump surface panel for viewing and interpretation. Although the transmitting sensor data **do not** drive pump insulin delivery, the pump can be programmed to alarm for both high and low glucose values. On hearing the alarm, the patient acquires a confirmatory fingerstick glucose level and corrects the abnormality.

The FDA lists the following indications for CGM: *detecting trends and tracking patterns of glucose values; serving as an adjunct to, but not a replacement for, information obtained from standard home blood glucose monitoring; aiding in the detection of episodes of hyperglycemia and hypoglycemia and minimizing glucose excursions; and facilitating acute and long-term therapy adjustments.* All devices are indicated for patients ≥18 years of age, but only the MiniMed Guardian and Paradigm REAL-Time systems are approved for use in children aged 7 to 17 years.[14] Real-time CGM provides important feedback regarding glycemic trends in response to meals, exercise, and insulin in patients with T1DM and T2DM using prandial insulin.[15,16]

The accuracy of present day sensors is generally good, but remains imperfect. For this reason, the FDA does not allow sensor data to be used as a replacement for blood glucose values. Numerous factors may adversely affect sensor accuracy, including calibration error, sensor delay, and sensor drift. Glucose sensors require the periodic input of a blood glucose value. This calibration procedure allows for the electrical current detected by a sensor to be equated into a sensed glucose level. An inaccurate blood glucose value, due to operator error or an inaccurate glucose meter, will cause a calibration error. Sensor drift is not as well understood and is likely due to a host of factors, among them the foreign body response that attracts leukocytes, including macrophages, which consume glucose and oxygen and produce peroxide and thus interfere with the accurate measurement of glucose. Therefore, treatment decisions based on CGM results should be confirmed by a traditional blood glucose meter, especially if the sensor readings are on either end of the extreme scale, that is, severe hyperglycemia or hypoglycemia.

Sensor accuracy appears to be improved when multiple sensors are used in close proximity to one another simultaneously. Multiple sensor usage is impractical for most patients, except those who intend to use automated pump-augmented sensors. Interstitial glucose readings become more accurate when sensors are placed close together, allowing feedback for more precise subcutaneous insulin delivery.[17]

TABLE 13-1. Evidence-based Endocrine Society Clinical Practice Guideline for Use of Continuous Glucose Monitoring

Clinical Setting	Strength of Evidence
CGMS is a useful tool for glucose management in the intensive care unit or operating room	● ○ ○ ○
CGMS should be used in children and adolescents with T1DM who have achieved A1C levels <7%. CGMS will assist in maintaining the targeted A1C and limit risk of hypoglycemia	● ● ● ●
CGMS should be used in children and adolescents with T1DM who have A1C levels ≥7% who are able to use these devices on a daily basis	● ● ● ○
Intermittent use of CGMS for short-term retrospective analysis of pediatric and adult patients with diabetes in whom clinicians worry about nocturnal hypoglycemia, dawn phenomenon, and post-prandial hyperglycemia as well as in patients with hypoglycemic unawareness, those changing insulin regimens (i.e., progressing to MDI or insulin pump therapy) would be beneficial	● ○ ○ ○
CGMS should be prescribed for adults with T1DM who agree to use them on a near daily basis	● ● ● ●

Strength of recommendations: The number of filled circles represent the quality of the evidence. One filled circle denotes very low quality of evidence, whereas four filled circles indicate the highest quality.
Adapted from: Klonoff DC, Buckingham B, Christiansen JS, et al. Continuous glucose monitoring: an endocrine society clinical practice guideline. *J Clin Endocrinol Metab.* 2011;96:2968–2979.

The Endocrine Society Clinical Practice evidence-based guidelines for the use of CGM are listed in Table 13-1.

Because CGM insertion requires manual dexterity, the procedure may be difficult for patients with hand deformities or peripheral neuropathy. CGM requires that patients or caregivers respond appropriately to high- and low-alarm alerts. Any patient may benefit from CGM whether or not he or she is using intensive insulin therapy. The initial startup cost of CGM is over $1,200, with sensor costs averaging $75 apiece.

Table 13-2 lists the properties of the two commercially available continuous glucose sensors.

Improved Overall Glycemic Control and Glycemic Variability

Insulin pump therapy improves glycemic control and reduces hypoglycemia. Findings from large randomized trials clearly demonstrate that early and aggressive management of glycemia significantly decreases the development and progression of the microvascular and macrovascular complications of diabetes.[9,18,19] However, improvement in glycemic control as measured by A1C is often associated with increased frequency of severe hypoglycemia.[9] (DCCT as above) As a result, patients' and clinicians' fear of hypoglycemia has become a significant obstacle to intensified diabetes management.[20]

Insulin pump therapy with rapid-acting insulin analogues not only improves glucose control, but also reduces the rate of severe hypoglycemia compared with MDI insulin therapy in patients with T1DM and T2DM.[21–23]

A study by Downie et al. examined the trends in the prevalence of microvascular complications of 1,604 adolescents with T1DM over the course of 10 years treated with either MDI or CSII.[24] From 1990 to 1994, no patients used insulin pumps. However, 22% of adolescents in this population-based study were using CSII from 2005 to 2009. Looking at the subgroup analysis of patients intensively treated during this 5-year interval, the A1C levels were similar between those using MDI

TABLE 13-2. Comparison of Current Continuous Glucose
Monitoring Systems

Feature	Dexcom 7 Plus	Guardian Real-Time System
	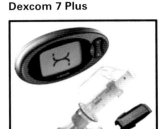	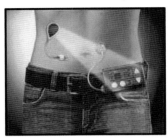
Approximate cash price for receiver, charger, and transmitter	$1,250	$1,248
Approximate cash price for each sensor	$100	$35
Sensor Life (Per FDA)	7 d	3 d
Start-up initialization time after insertion	2 h	2 h
Calibration frequency	Once 2 h after initial insertion then every 12 h of sensor life	2 h after insertion, within next 6 h after first calibration, then every 12 h for life of sensor. Will alarm if calibration value is not entered
Frequency of glucose value display	Every 5 min. Value displayed on receiver that is worn remotely	Every 5 min. Value displayed on patient's insulin pump screen
Alarms for rate of change	One each for high and low (either 2 or 3 mg/dL/min)	Can be customized to rate changes from 1.1 to 5.5 mg/dL/min for increasing or decreasing values
Display of directional trends	Displays a 1-, 3-, 6-, 12-, or 24-h graph on receiver	Displays a 3-, 6-, 12-, and 24-h graph on insulin pump screen
Sensor waterproof?	Yes	Yes
Software available for downloading?	DexCom DM Data Manager 3	Medtronic CareLink Personal
Additional information available at:	www.dexcom.com	http://www.medtronic.com/your-health/diabetes/living-with/index.htm

Adapted from Unger J, Parkin C. Recognition, prevention and proactive management of hypoglycemia in patients with type 1 diabetes. *Postgrad Med.* 2011;123(4):71–80.

versus CSII. The frequency of retinopathy was lower in the pumping patients, suggesting a positive role pumps play in minimizing glycemic variability.

In addition to improvement in A1C levels, glycemic variability can be reduced in patients using pumps. A strong correlation exists between glycemic variability and the likelihood of developing long-term complications.[25] Glycemic variability is minimized in pump patients. Because a single rapid-acting analogue is absorbed from a single insulin depot, day-to-day glycemic variability averages 3% versus 52% with NPH.[26] Improved glycemic variability is accompanied by a 15% to 20% reduction in total daily insulin requirements when compared with that in patients using MDI.[26]

Gastroparesis is a syndrome characterized by delayed gastric emptying in the absence of mechanical obstruction of the stomach. The cardinal symptoms include postprandial fullness (early satiety), nausea, vomiting, and bloating. Patients with diabetes in whom gastroparesis develops often have had diabetes for at least 10 years and typically have retinopathy, neuropathy, and nephropathy. Diabetic gastroparesis may cause severe symptoms and result in nutritional compromise, impaired glucose control, and a poor quality of life, independently of other factors such as age, tobacco use, alcohol use, or type of diabetes. Symptoms attributable to gastroparesis are reported by 5% to 12% of patients with T1DM.[27] Acute hyperglycemia (blood glucose values greater than 180 mg per dL) delays gastric emptying 15 minutes longer than euglycemic individuals.[28] Chronic hyperglycemia reduces the frequency of gastric contractions that move solid nutrients through the stomach, although liquids pass with ease.[29] Rapid-acting insulin analogues exhibit a peak onset of pharmacodynamic activity at 60 minutes after injection. Peak carbohydrate absorption following a meal occurs at approximately 75 to 90 minutes after eating begins. When the absorption of nutrients from the gut is delayed or unpredictable, determining the appropriate timing of insulin dosing becomes problematic. Glycemic control will demonstrate wide ranging variability. Patients with T1DM and symptomatic gastroparesis have demonstrated improvement in glycemic control and reduction in in-patient admission hospital days with the use of CSII versus MDI.[30]

Insulin pumps have been shown to reduce and even reverse diabetic retinopathy. An Italian study[31] of 20 patients with T1DM with an average age of 37 years and average duration of diabetes of 18 years who were followed up for 2 years showed an overall pump-driven reduction in A1C from 9.1% to 7.5%. Of 10 patients with nonproliferative diabetic retinopathy (4 mild, 5 moderate, and 1 severe), 6 showed regression to a lower grade of diabetic retinopathy. Two of four patients with proliferative retinopathy showed a reduction in retinal lesions. The enhancement in glycemic control achieved via insulin pump therapy resulted in significant improvement in diabetic retinopathy.

Insulin pump therapy with rapid-acting insulin analogues not only improves glucose control, but also reduces the rate of severe hypoglycemia compared with MDI insulin therapy in patients with T1DM and T2DM.[21–23]

In patients with T2DM, glucose control is often difficult, despite full doses of oral agents and extremely large doses of insulin. In a study involving four patients with poorly controlled T2DM, Nielsen et al. found that insulin pump therapy yielded a marked improvement in glucose concentrations with a corresponding decrease in A1C levels.[22] This improvement was associated with a significant reduction in insulin dosages, suggesting that patients with T2DM that remains uncontrolled on extremely high doses of insulin may benefit from insulin pump therapy. Wainstein et al. showed similar benefits in a larger study of 40 obese T2DM subjects.[32]

The improved A1C values associated with CSII reflect the beneficial pharmacokinetics associated with pump therapy. Insulin pumps use only a single short-acting insulin analogue for both basal and bolus insulin delivery. Multiple basal insulin rates can be programmed into the pump to match the metabolic requirements of individual patients. Neither CSII nor MDIs result in complete normalization of glucose concentrations throughout the day. However, if the A1C is reduced safely to as near normal as possible, long- and short-term diabetic complication rates will be reduced. The DCCT has demonstrated superiority of CSII versus MDIs to reduce A1C levels. CSII is superior to MDIs using NPH in reducing A1C levels[33] and has been found to be superior to MDIs when fast-acting bolus insulin is used for meals.[34] A1C levels are lower in pump patients than in those using MDIs with glargine insulin.[35]

Insulin pumps provide patients with basal, bolus, and supplemental insulin in a physiologic, programmable format, providing patients with more predictable and reproducible glycemic control (Fig. 13-6). This physiologic insulin delivery ensures conscientious pump patients of achieving near-normal basal and PPG control while minimizing glycemic variability. Most patients require one or two different basal rates, including one that reduces hyperglycemia in the early morning hours before a patient awakens. When this "dawn phenomenon" is better controlled, patients will awaken with near-normal blood glucose levels. However, if fasting blood glucose levels are consistently elevated, patients will be working to correct hyperglycemia throughout the day.

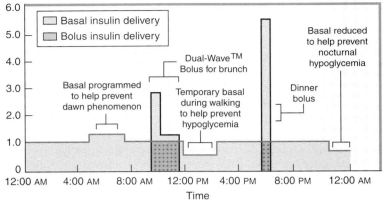

Figure 13-6 • Programmable Insulin Delivery with Pump Therapy. Patients with diabetes can receive individualized, programmable insulin delivery via pump therapy. By using only a single type of rapid-acting insulin analogue (lispro, aspart, or glulisine), the day-to-day absorption of insulin varies by less than 3%, meaning that the patient's glycemic control will be more predictable and reliable than by using other forms of basal/bolus insulin therapy. Basal rates can be programmed to match the patient's individual basal glucose requirements. For example, a higher basal rate can be programmed for the early morning hours to limit the hyperglycemia caused by "the dawn phenomenon." As insulin resistance begins to decrease in the early afternoon hours, the basal rates can be reduced. If a patient exercises consistently during a certain time of day, the basal rate can be programmed at a lower rate, beginning at the antici- pated onset of activity, and increased 1 to 2 hours after the exercise session ends. Patients can set a "temporary basal rate" in anticipation of activities that may induce hypoglycemia (such as intense exer- cise) or in response to mild hypoglycemia, so that the blood glucose level will increase by hepatic glucose production rather than by the patients having to "eat their way" out of hypoglycemia. Bolus insulin may be provided for meals in several forms. An immediate bolus may be given all at one time to correct hypergly- cemia or to prevent an increase in blood glucose levels, which will occur in response to a between-meal snack. The square-wave (extended-wave) bolus provides the patient with mealtime insulin delivery over several hours and mimics the physiologic second-phase insulin response of euglycemic individuals. A dual- wave bolus combines an immediate and extended-wave bolus, so that a percentage of the total mealtime dose of insulin is provided at the onset of the meal, and the remainder is given over a 2- to 5-hour period.

The pump's basal insulin delivery maintains ambient plasma glucose readings in the fasting state by limiting hepatic glucose production. The programmable basal rates are calculated based on the patient's size, age, gender, activity level, degree of insulin resistance, and other parameters, as shown in Table 13-3.

Patients may choose to bypass the prescribed basal delivery rate by placing themselves on a tem- porary basal rate (TBR) to either slow or increase the rate of insulin delivery. For example, mild hypo- glycemia may be treated by setting a TBR and slowing insulin delivery. By allowing the plasma glucose level to increase spontaneously, patients will not gain weight by "eating their way out of hypoglycemia."

Bolus insulin delivered by the pump simulates physiologic first- and second-phase insulin responses (Fig. 13-6). The amount of insulin to be delivered as a bolus as well as the time over which the bolus is administered is based on preprandial glucose levels, the amount of carbohydrates and fats that will be consumed during a meal, and the anticipated activity level after a meal. The three types of pumped boluses include the following:

- **Immediate (now) bolus:** If one miscalculates the mealtime bolus and records an elevated glucose level 2 to 4 hours after eating, a supplemental (correction bolus) may be admin- istered through the pump to correct the hyperglycemia. An immediate bolus may also be given for small snacks, before exercise in patients who are hyperglycemic, and after the insertion of a new infusion set.
- **Extended (square-wave) bolus:** Insulin is infused over time, typically 30 minutes to 4 hours. The extended bolus is useful for managing patients with gastroparesis and may also be administered for snacks with high fat content, such as ice cream.
- **Combination (dual-wave) bolus:** By combining the immediate and the extended-wave bolus, this becomes the most physiologic means by which prandial insulin can be delivered. After

TABLE 13-3. Approximate Total Daily Insulin Dose Requirements for Patients with T1DM

Dose (U/kg/d)	Patient's Condition
0.5	Conditioned or trained athlete
0.6	Motivated exerciser, woman in first phase (follicular) of menstrual cycle
0.7	Woman in last week (luteal phase) of menstrual cycle or in first trimester of pregnancy, adult mildly ill with a virus, child starting puberty
0.8	Woman in second trimester of pregnancy, child in midpuberty, adult with a severe or localized viral infection
0.9	Woman in third trimester of pregnancy, child at the peak of puberty, adult ill with bacterial infection
1.0	Woman at term of pregnancy, pubescent child who is ill, adult with a severe bacterial infection or illness
1.5–2.0	Severely ill man or woman, child at peak pubescence who is ill

determining the premeal glucose, the patient calculates how much additional insulin should be added or subtracted to the prescribed dose of insulin in the immediate portion of the bolus that will allow the patient to attain the targeted glucose level. Carbohydrate counting or a predetermined dose of insulin may then be administered by using the combination bolus. The extended bolus continues to deliver insulin for 2 to 4 hours, depending on the quantity and fat content of the meal. Fat tends to delay carbohydrate absorption, requiring longer extended-bolus times.

Reduction in Frequency and Severity of Hypoglycemia

Severe hypoglycemia is less frequent with CSII than with MDIs, yet the ability to perceive low blood glucose levels is less apparent to pump patients. The key to minimizing the risk of inducing hypoglycemia is to teach patients to understand the concept of "insulin on board" in order to avoid insulin stacking (Fig. 13-7).

Current generation pumps employ a feature known as "insulin on board" that can lower one's risk of insulin stacking. Using an algorithm that directs the flow of insulin to be delivered in the right amount over a specific period of time, both hyperglycemic and hypoglycemic events may be minimized. Clinical trials of autonomously functioning closed loop system pumps are planned.[36]

The most serious adverse effect of intensive insulin therapy is severe hypoglycemia, which requires the assistance of another person for reversal. In the DCCT, the incidence of severe hypoglycemia was three times greater in the group receiving MDIs than in conventional therapy (twice-daily injection) patients. In a study by Bode et al.,[21] patients switched from MDIs to CSII had a reduction in severe hypoglycemia events from 138 episodes per 100 patient-years, with MDIs, to 22 per 100 patient-years in the first year of CSII use. Hypoglycemic events remained lower in pump patients through years 2 to 4, with no increase in A1C levels. Multiple studies have confirmed a reduction in frequency of hypoglycemia associated with CSII.[37]

A study in adolescent patients with T1DM who used insulin pumps demonstrated a 64% reduction in the incidence of severe hypoglycemia ($p = 0.048$) over a 10-year period.[38] Although the data suggest that progress is being made to reduce the risk of hypoglycemia in high-risk patients, anyone who is subject to intensified diabetes control remains a target for risk modification.

Patients who are extremely sensitive to small changes in circulating exogenous insulin levels are less likely to become hypoglycemic by using pump therapy.[39] The basal and bolus delivery rates of

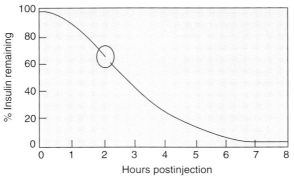

Figure 13-7 • **Insulin Stacking: Rapid-Acting Analogue "Insulin Action" Disappearance Curves.**
This graph demonstrates the amount of insulin remaining in the subcutaneous depot over time following a subcutaneous injection. After 2 hours (*circle*), 64% of the original dose remains in the depot and waiting to act. Thus, if 10 U of insulin is given at 10:00 AM, 6 U remains as active drug at noon. The glucose-lowering effects of rapid-acting analogues persist for up to 6 hours following a subcutaneous injection. If one gives a correction bolus prior to the time the insulin is completely absorbed, hypoglycemia is likely to occur. For example, if the blood glucose level is 200 mg per dL at noon and the patient injects an additional 6 U at lunchtime, the subcutaneous depot has now been increased to 12 U. Patients should always calculate how much insulin remains in the original subcutaneous depot before injecting supplemental insulin. Insulin stacking is a major cause of hypoglycemia and can easily be avoided.

insulin pumps can be adjusted by tenths of units, allowing precision dosing of the insulin during both the fasting and prandial states.

In patients who have had T1DM for more than 5 years, autonomic dysfunction develops, which precludes them from recognizing the symptoms of hypoglycemia (fatigue, sweating, blurred vision, dizziness, palpitations, and impaired cognition). Patients with *hypoglycemic unawareness* also lose their ability to produce enough counterregulatory hormones (cortisol, growth hormone, epinephrine, and glucagon) to protect them from and reverse the hypoglycemia. Activities such as driving, exercising, and caring for children may be challenging and dangerous for patients with hypoglycemic unawareness. Insulin pump therapy can restore one's ability to perceive hypoglycemia. Simply reducing the pump's basal rates and mealtime boluses will allow patients to maintain a higher target blood glucose level while minimizing the frequency and severity of hypoglycemia. For example, a target of 150 to 220 mg per dL in a patient with frequent hypoglycemia might be preferable to the standard glycemic target of 80 to 120 mg per dL. After 6 to 8 weeks of hypoglycemic avoidance, the basal rate of the insulin pump can be increased, allowing the physician to reduce the target glucose range safely toward normal.[12] As glucose levels improve, hypoglycemic awareness returns.

Paired (structured) glucose testing may be used to predict postprandial hypoglycemia.[40] Blood glucose levels are checked prior to eating and 2 hours postprandial. A delta ≤50 mg per dL is expected to occur if a patient has given an appropriate mealtime bolus based upon the amount of carbohydrates consumed. However, if the blood glucose 2 hours following a meal is less than baseline, that is, a negative delta, then the patient would expect that his or her blood glucose would be dropping.[41] For example, a premeal blood glucose is 120 mg per dL. The patient administers a dual-wave bolus consisting of 3 U "now" and 6 U extended over 3 hours to cover 140 g of carbohydrates. Two hours after eating, the patient's blood glucose has dropped from 120 to 70 mg per dL, resulting in a delta of −50. According to the insulin disappearance curve in Figure 13-7, 60% of the bolused insulin remains to be absorbed. Thus approximately 60% of 4 U is still active with the infusion site. This patient's blood glucose is dropping rapidly and appropriate steps must be taken to minimize the progression toward hypoglycemia. The square wave bolus should be stopped and glucose tablets administered. Glucose monitoring should be performed again in 1 hour to make certain that the glycemic trend is upward rather than toward worsening hypoglycemia.

Pump Therapy Reduces Total Daily Insulin Requirements and Limits Weight Gain

Reduced insulin requirements and greater flexibility in food intake may result in minimal weight gain for pump users when compared with MDI patients.[9,21] Patients intensively managed in the DCCT gained on average 10 lb more over a 6-year period than did those using conventional therapy. Because pumps infuse insulin efficiently, using only a single subcutaneous depot and one rapid-acting insulin analogue, one's total daily dose (TDD) of insulin can be reduced in many cases by 10% to 15% when compared with MDIs. Less insulin use limits weight gain.

Equally important is how pumpers can physiologically manage episodes of mild hypoglycemia. Instead of "eating their way out of hypoglycemia," pump patients may either suspend the pump or place the pump on a TBR until the blood glucose levels increase in response to increased hepatic glucose production. When one eats to correct hypoglycemia, extra calories are consumed, and the corrected blood glucose levels tend to surpass the intended target of 70 to 100 mg per dL. Faced with a postcorrection glucose of 280 after the consumption of a bowl of ice cream to correct a glucose level of 54 mg per dL, the patient may decide to give a supplemental bolus to correct the hyperglycemia. This may result in insulin stacking and a return to hypoglycemia, followed by even greater food consumption. Because pump patients tend to have less frequent episodes of hypoglycemia that they can manage with glucose tablets rather than with candy bars and ice cream, weight gain is minimized.

Lifestyle Flexibility Afforded by Insulin Pumps

CSII allows patients to have a more flexible lifestyle. Pumping simplifies irregular meal schedules, exercise, traveling, and other unplanned activities. These advantages may explain why 50% of health-care professionals with T1DM who are members of the American Diabetes Association and American Association of Diabetes Educators use insulin pumps. Patient acceptance of pump therapy is extremely high. Of patients using pumps, 97% show long-term continuation rates.[42]

Continuous Subcutaneous Insulin Infusion is More Expensive than Multiple Daily Injections

Insulin pump therapy is more expensive than traditional insulin delivery devices such as vials, syringes, and pen injectors (Table 13-4). Initial start-up costs for pump therapy average $6,100. Infusion sets, reservoirs, and catheters cost $2,500 to $2,800 per year. Pump patients are usually more willing to perform home blood glucose monitoring, adding to the expense of this necessary procedure. Pregnant patients with T1DM who are intensively managed on pump therapy will spend on average $140 per month more on all diabetes-related supplies than will patients using MDIs.[43]

Kanakis et al.[44] reviewed the relative costs of insulin pumping in 2002. Excluding the initial start-up costs of pump therapy, CSII costs approximately $2,000 more per year than syringes and vials, and $1,500 more than pen injectors.

Insulin pumps are covered by Medicare Part B if patients have evidence of T1DM based on the presence of autoantibodies or specific C-peptide criteria as shown in Table 13-5 and further explained in Appendix 13-2.[45]

C-Peptide as a Determinant of Endogenous Insulin

Endogenous insulin consists of a 21-amino acid A chain and a 30-amino acid B chain joined by the connecting peptide (C-peptide) and two disulfide bridges (Fig. 13-8).

TABLE 13-4. Insulin Pump Comparison

Feature	Roche-Disetronic Spirit	Insulet OmniPod	Medtronic Revel (Paradigm 523/723)	Animas Johnson and Johnson One Touch Ping
Retail cost[a]	$6,195 (Includes a backup pump)	$945 (Includes a PDM and 1 mo of disposable pods. Each additional pod costs $35)	$6,195 (Continuous glucose sensor is additional cost)	$6,345
Empty weight	2.8 oz	1.2 oz (Functioning Personal diabetes manager-PDM: 4 oz)	3.5 oz	3.25 oz
Basal increments	0.5–5 U/h	0.05–30 U/h	0.025 U/h	0.025 U/h
Temporary basal increments	In 10% increments from 0% to 200% and 15 min to 24 h	% or U/h (1–12 h, in 30 min increments)	+ 0.1 U increment as single basal rate for 0.5–24 h or as a % of current basal	–90% to 200% in increments of 10% for 0.5–24 h (30 min increments)
Bolus increments	0.1, 0.2, 0.5, 1.0, 2.0 U	0.05, 0.1, 0.5, 1.0 U	0.1 visual, 0.5, or 1.0 visual or audio. Remote bolusing option available	0.05 visual or audio, 0.1, 1.0, 5.0 audio. Remote option available
Bolus Wizard feature for Carb Counting?	Manual carb calculator from Accu-Chek blood glucose monitor	Manual carb counter contained in PDM	Direct from brand name meter or via manual entry into "Bolus Wizard" prior to giving meal time dose of insulin	Carb and blood glucose values entered remotely into pump remotely via Ping calculator. Pump then determines appropriate meal time bolus
Duration of 1 U insulin bolus	5 s	40 s	30 s	1 or 3 s

	Accu-Chek	OmniPod	Medtronic	Animas
Types of boluses delivered	• Standard • Quick • Extended • Multiwave	• Meal • Correction • Mean and correction • Normal	• Normal • Square wave • Correction • Extended • Dual wave	• Carb smart • EZ bolus • Dual wave • Correction
Available basal patterns	5	7	3	4
"Insulin on board" calculation to minimize stacking	Present	Present	Present	Present
Insulin reservoir size	315 U	200 U	180 or 300 U	200 U
Pumping software programs	Accu-Chek 360 Diabetes Management System automatically detects the Accu-Chek blood glucose meter or pump downloading the data with a click. Data can be printed, e-mailed, or faxed. 17 different reports are available. Accu-Chek Smart Pix device reader allows for "plug and play" technology. Reports can be uploaded to most EMR systems. 20 different reports with 29 language options	PathFinder software to download PDM	CareLink Software allows patients to upload data from pump and glucose monitor to a secure online database. Physician can view that data in advance of a visit to optimize therapy in a time efficient manner	EZ Manager Max software to download pump and blood glucose meter
Unique lousin of interest	• Personal digital assistant with Diabetes Management Tool • Patient receives a second pump as a backup	• Wireless • PDM integrates FreeStyle test strips *(Not FDA approved, however)* • Food database in PDM	• Paradigm links to continuous glucose sensor with real-time glucose readings displayed on face of pump • Bolus wizard calculator • Remote bolusing • Insulin on board displayed on home screen	• Multiple insulin to carb ratios • 500-food database in Ping meter that interacts with pump • Remote bolusing
Interacts with continuous glucose sensors?	Navigator	Dexcom	Medtronic	None
Web site	www.accu-check.com	www.myomnipod.com	www.medtronic.com/your-health/diabetes/device/index.htm	www.animas.com

*Data obtained from American Diabetes Wholesale website: http://www.americandiabeteswholesale.com/catalog/insulin-pumps_70.htm. Accessed March 18, 2011.

TABLE 13-5. Criteria for Medicare Coverage of Continuous Subcutaneous Insulin Infusion

Criteria A	Patient has completed a comprehensive diabetes education program
	Patient has used MDI (at least three injections daily for at least 6 mo)
	Patient has documented self-blood glucose monitoring at least four times daily for 2 mo prior to initiating an insulin pump
	Patient meets one or more of the following criteria while on MDI:
	• A1C > 7%
	• History of recurring hypoglycemia
	• Wide fluctuations in blood glucose before mealtime
	• Dawn phenomenon with fasting glucose frequently exceeding 200 mg/dL
	• History of severe glycemic excursions
Criteria B	Patient with diabetes has been on a pump prior to enrollment in Medicare and has documented frequency of glucose self-monitoring an average of at least four times daily during the month prior to Medicare enrollment
	In addition to meeting Criteria A and B, the following general requirements must be met:
	• Patient must be β-cell autoantibody positive (demonstrate evidence of autoimmune T1DM)
	• Patient must have evidence of being insulinopenic as defined as a fasting C-peptide that is < or 110% of the lower limit of the normal for the laboratory's measurement method. (e.g., *if the lab reports the lower limit of normal for a C-peptide as being 0.5 nmol/l, a patient would qualify for an insulin pump if the fasting C-peptide level were <0.55 nmol/l*)
	Patients with renal insufficiency have an elevation in C-peptide due to reduced renal clearance of insulin. Therefore, any individual with a creatinine clearance <50 mL/min will be defined as having insulinopenia if his or her fasting C-peptide level is <200% of the lower limit of normal of the laboratory's measurement method
	Fasting C-peptide levels will only be considered valid with a concurrently obtained fasting glucose <225 mg/dL
	All insulin pump patients must be evaluated by their treating physician at least every 3 mo
	The pump must be ordered by and the patient must be followed by a physician who manages multiple patients with CSII and who works closely with a team who is knowledgeable in the use of CSII

Medicare national coverage determinations manual. Chapter 1, Part 4 (Sections 200–310.1). Rev. 135, 09-22-11. http://www.cms.gov/manuals/downloads/ncd103c1_Part4.pdf. p. 126–127. Accessed November 21, 2011.

Potential Complications of Insulin Pumping

According to a 2010 report published by an FDA panel established to examine insulin pump complications, the agency received 16,849 adverse event reports from October 1, 2006 to September 20, 2009, including 310 mortalities (1.8%).[46] The most commonly reported patient-related problems were:

- hospitalization (21%)
- hyperglycemia (25%)
- DKA (8%)
- hypoglycemia (5%)

The most frequently identified device-related problems included:

- "unknown" (20%)
- "replace" (9%)

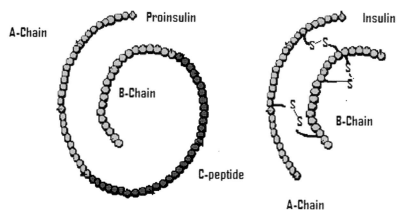

Figure 13-8 • The Precursor of Insulin, Proinsulin, is Produced Within the Endoplasmic Reticulum of the Pancreatic β-Cells. Proinsulin consists of both the A and B chains of insulin, which are connected by the connecting peptide (C-peptide) chain. Proinsulin is transported to the Golgi apparatus and packaged into secretory vesicles. The C-peptide chain is released from the center of the proinsulin sequence while the two disulfide bonds remain intact. 1 C-peptide molecule is formed with each insulin molecule. Therefore, C-peptide levels can serve as an accurate measure of endogenous insulin production. C-peptide levels in euglycemic individuals range from 0.5-2.0 ng/mL.

Human insulin consists of 51 amino acids, 30 of which constitute the B-chain and 21 comprise the A-chain. The 2 chains are linked by disulfide bonds.

- "audible alarm" (6%)
- "use of device issue" (5%)
- "device displays error message" (5%)
- "failure to deliver" (3%)

Event reports for the mortalities were often incomplete but included diabetic coma, hypoglycemia, hyperglycemia, DKA, unresponsiveness, respiratory infection, alcohol consumption, and motor vehicle accident. Adverse events cases in which a device malfunction could clearly be identified included infusion set failure or unexplained disconnection, pump alarming, overinfusion, bent cannulas, failure to deliver, suspected electromagnetic interference, display failures, and occlusions of infusion sets.

From a clinical perspective, pump occlusions, leaking infusion sets, and infusion site infections are most often observed. Pump alarms will respond to an obstructed infusion set, but not one that leaks. Insulin analogues have a very rapid half-life. If one experiences a no-delivery over 4 hours while sleeping, metabolic deterioration is likely to occur. Fortunately, over 85% of DKA events result from occlusive events rather than infusion set leakage.[47]

Skin Infections and Irritations

Subcutaneous skin infections at the infusion site are likely to occur if the patient does not change the infusion site at least every 72 hours (Fig. 13-9). Patients must be trained to recognize signs of early abscesses, which include persistent itching, pain, or redness around the infusion site, or a gradual increase in blood glucose levels as insulin absorption is reduced from an infected site. Most subcutaneous abscesses can be treated empirically with antibiotics directed at *Staphylococcus aureus* infections. Larger abscesses will require surgical drainage. Patients should use a mechanical inserter rather than attempt to place new infusion sets by hand in order to minimize glycemic variability and infection risk.

On rare occasions, the author has noted recurring localized skin irritation occurring at the insulin infusion site within 24 to 48 hours after initiating the new infusion set. Initially, patients experience mild itching around the site, which prompts them to change their infusion sets and

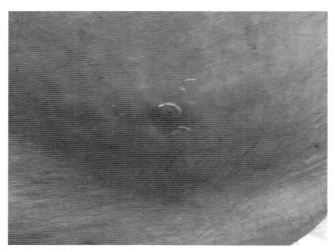

Figure 13-9 • Localized Abscess from Prolonged Use of an Insulin Pump Infusion Set. A 5-cm superficial fluctuant abscess on the abdominal wall of a patient who did not change his infusion site for 6 days. Abscess cultured positive for staph aureus. (Photo courtesy of Jeff Unger, MD)

reinsert them in a different area. However, the irritation recurs within 48 hours in association with an increase in blood glucose levels. Some patients may attempt to use supplemental insulin boluses to normalize their glucose levels, which only worsens the localized skin reaction. Being forced to change the infusion sets every 2 days increases the cost of pump therapy. Patients become frustrated by the fact that they are forced to make frequent site changes, while their glucose levels fail to normalize. Some may decide to stop pumping altogether and return to MDIs. However, by switching to a different insulin formulation (i.e., from lispro to glulisine or aspart), the patient will notice significant and rapid improvement in the suspected localized insulin allergy.[48,49]

Local reactions to exogenous insulin are associated with circulating IgE antibodies to the injected insulin.[50] The incidence of insulin resistance of an immunologic nature is quite rare, occurring in less than 0.1% of all insulin recipients.[51] Since the late 1970s, insulin manufacturers have taken additional steps to produce highly purified insulins that decreased but have not eliminated the development of insulin antibodies, dermal reactions, systemic hypersensitivity, and insulin resistance.[52,53] The rapid-acting insulin analogues, when given subcutaneously, result in development of insulin antibodies, with no significant differences shown between the analogues and unmodified human insulin. In all the clinical trials cited, insulin antibodies have no demonstrable effects on insulin dose, hypoglycemic events, or glycemic control.[54]

In a small, 12-month study, 45 patients with T1DM were randomized to conventional therapy, multiple dose, or insulin pumping with highly purified porcine insulins.[55] Researchers found an increase in insulin antibodies in the multiple dose and pump groups but not in the conventional group, suggesting that differences in methods of subcutaneous insulin administration affect antibody development. However, this study has not been repeated with contemporary human insulins. From a clinical perspective, any patient experiencing an abrupt change in glucose control, evidence of insulin resistance to both injected and pumped insulin and irritation around the site of the insulin depot should be advised to switch to an alternative type of analogue insulin. The patient will often notice an immediate return to normal glucose values. Patients can switch back to their original insulin after 6 to 8 weeks, once their presumed insulin antibodies have cleared. There is currently no commercial test available for evaluating the presence of insulin antibodies in clinical practice.

Some Physical Activities May Damage the Pump

Pumps cannot be worn during certain types of sports activities, such as playing football or rugby, or scuba diving. Although some pumps may be detailed as being "waterproof," patients should be aware that pumps exposed to water pressures below 10 feet may not maintain their protective status. Patients are therefore strongly encouraged to disconnect their pumps while participating in water sports.

Diabetic Ketoacidosis May Occur Rapidly and Without Warning in Pump Patients

DKA may occur rapidly in pump patients under the following situations: (a) an underlying infection develops, such as a viral illness or appendicitis; (b) the infusion set becomes disconnected or is improperly inserted; (c) the infusion set becomes obstructed, clogged, or filled with a large air bubble (in which case the patient's insulin dose is substituted with air); (d) the patient simply miscalculates the proper dose of insulin to administer to cover the amount of carbohydrates consumed during a meal; (e) the patient omits a mealtime dose of insulin; (f) the patient runs out of insulin in the pump reservoir; or (g) the pump has a major malfunction and fails to deliver insulin. DKA may occur in even the most compliant of patients, which emphasizes the importance of careful pump education and follow-up.

Frequent blood glucose self-monitoring should alert patients to increasing blood glucose levels, which would prompt them to institute their "emergency protocol." Patients must be informed that when faced with increasing blood glucose levels, they must always "fix the diabetes first" before troubleshooting the insulin pump to determine the cause of the interruption in insulin delivery. Subcutaneous insulin injections may be administered until the pump malfunctions are determined and corrected.

Indications for Insulin Pump Therapy

Although anyone with diabetes may be a potential pump candidate, some patients deserve special consideration for pump initiation.

Failure to Achieve Targeted A1C with Multiple Daily Injections

Failure to achieve treatment targets with elevated plasma glucose levels and A1C levels is an indication for a more aggressive yet physiologic treatment approach. One of the most common reasons certain patients do not achieve glucose treatment targets is the fear of hypoglycemia. Many patients consciously overeat to prevent hypoglycemia. By selecting insulin pump therapy, the patient can better match medical nutritional therapy and exercise with insulin administration. Precise and predictable insulin dosing is provided through the insulin pump. For example, 0.9 U might be excessive, but 0.4 U would be appropriate. A dose of 0.5 U would be difficult to administer via a syringe or even a pen injector. The basal insulin infusion via CSII is more predictable and reliable, yet adjustable. Because the basal insulin infusion is "peakless," the risk for hypoglycemia is decreased.

Whether CSII is superior to MDI in achieving A1C targets is controversial. A randomized open-label parallel multicenter study compared the safety and efficacy of using insulin lispro via

CSII with glargine-based MDI in previously treated NPH patients with T1DM.[56] The 43 patients who were randomized and completed the trial after 24 weeks demonstrated similar total daily insulin requirements, changes in A1C, fasting blood glucose levels and measures of plasma glucose variability. The total hypoglycemic events between the two groups were equivalent in numbers. Treatment satisfaction scores were higher for CSII pumpers as were the costs of therapy. This study evaluated patients using older pump technology. The authors admit that with newly marketed pumps offering the use of the bolus-wizard, which aids patients in administering more accurate prandial doses of insulin based on carbohydrate content, the statistical analysis would now favor CSII.

Two very recently published Cochrane reviews compared the use of CSII with MDI. The first review included 23 randomized studies (duration 6 days to 4 years) involving 976 participants with T1DM. A significant difference was documented in A1C response favoring CSII (weighted mean difference 0.3% vs. MDI). In addition, CSII users demonstrated greater improvements in quality-of-life measures. No differences were observed between the two treatments' effects on body weight. Severe hypoglycemia appeared to be reduced within the pumping cohorts, although no difference in the frequency of nonsevere hypoglycemia between the two regimens.[57]

The American Association of Clinical Endocrinologists suggests that CSII "appears to be justified for basal-bolus insulin therapy in patients with T1DM that is inadequately controlled with MDI."[58]

Few clinical trials have examined CSII use in patients with T2DM. In one analysis of four randomized controlled trials in patients with T2DM, no significant A1C improvement or differences in hypoglycemic risk reduction were noted with CSII versus MDI therapy over 12 weeks.[59]

▍ Hypoglycemia and Hypoglycemic Unawareness

The fear of becoming hypoglycemic is the "rate-limiting" factor in successfully achieving glucose-treatment targets. With other forms of insulin delivery, the patient with diabetes may strive for prescribed treatment targets, have hypoglycemia, and then overeat to compensate with resultant hyperglycemia. The patient is then on a "roller-coaster" glycemic curve. With CSII, a closer carbohydrate-to-insulin ratio is maintained by administering minute amounts of insulin when necessary. If the plasma glucose should decrease below the treatment target range, the patient may suspend or cease insulin infusion for a time. Weight gain is avoided through immediate insulin suspension rather than supplemental carbohydrates. In this fashion, the roller-coaster effect is minimized, hypoglycemia is less common, and the glucose level approximates treatment targets. In addition, excessive weight gain is avoided in those patients who "eat their way out of hypoglycemia."

▍ Athletes and Patients Who Incorporate Exercise into Their Daily Routines

Exercise poses a special problem for patients receiving insulin. Ideally, patients have been instructed to exercise at those times when injected subcutaneous insulin is not peaking. Each subcutaneous injection of insulin establishes a different subcutaneous depot from which insulin may be absorbed over time. As one exercises, insulin absorbed from multiple depots is more likely to result in hypoglycemia than is insulin absorbed from a single infusion site. With CSII, the patient can safely either suspend insulin infusion for a short time (less than 1 hour) or modify the basal infusion to a very low rate. If suspending infusion, the patient can determine whether to cease infusion abruptly or to administer a bolus (usually no more than 50% of the planned infusion during the exercise period) before ceasing infusion.

Although the pump should not be worn by patients who participate in contact or water sports, glycemic control is much more predictable while exercising with pumps than when using MDIs of insulin.

Persistent Fasting Hyperglycemia on Rising (Dawn Phenomenon)

In some patients, a dawn phenomenon corresponds to an increase in plasma glucose levels during the early morning hours (4:00 to 9:00 AM).[60] Insulin resistance intensifies in direct proportion to the physiologic increases in cortisol and growth hormone levels. A patient who does not have diabetes simply produces more endogenous insulin in response to these counterregulatory hormones. Patients with diabetes who inject insulin at bedtime cannot automatically increase the circulating dose of that insulin in response to an increase in glucose levels. However, programming a 100% to 150% increase in basal insulin delivery on an insulin pump for 4 to 5 hours, beginning 1 hour before the anticipated onset of the dawn phenomenon, allows the patient to waken with near-normal glycemic levels.

Pregnancy

CSII is an excellent method to achieve and maintain the meticulous glucose control required during pregnancy for the prevention of fetal malformations and obstetric complications. Unfortunately, the literature does not suggest clear evidence that insulin pumps are necessary for optimal treatment of women with T1DM during pregnancy. Nevertheless, frequent basal rates can be set during the 24-hour period, and one can administer a bolus immediately with food intake to control postprandial plasma glucose. Programmed basal-rate changes are needed, as insulin requirements are different during each of the pregnancy trimesters. Patients contemplating pregnancy will also find that using CSII simplifies their management of hyperglycemia.[61]

Use of insulin pumps in pregnant patients with T2DM or gestational diabetes appears to be safe and effective for maintaining glycemic control throughout pregnancy although doses of insulin required for such patients are usually quite high.[62]

DKA during pregnancy is associated with fetal demise. Therefore, pumpers must be adept at inspecting their infusion sites for signs of infection or accidental disconnection of insulin flow.[58] As a safety feature, and because no long-acting insulin is being pumped, NPH, 0.2 U per kg taken at bedtime given SQ is advisable.[60] Pregnant patients may choose to use alternative infusion sites such as arms or legs, as their abdomens expand in the third trimester. The morning basal rate may also be lowered to minimize the risk of hypoglycemia.

Shift Workers

Shift workers tend to have a very difficult time with glycemic control.[8] The physiologic stress caused by chronic sleep deprivation and altered work schedules results in increasing serum cortisol levels. Insulin resistance is exacerbated in response to the higher cortisol levels.[63] Patients who work altered shifts can adjust their basal rate profiles to correspond to their schedules. For example, a registered nurse who works the "graveyard shift" Monday through Friday can use a designated pump pattern on those days that would provide less basal insulin from midnight through 7:00 AM. On her days off, the pump pattern may be altered automatically by the patient so that additional insulin is provided as she sleeps from midnight through 7:00 AM. Many women also find this pattern tool useful, as their insulin requirements may jump 10% to 15% during the 3 to 5 days prior to the onset of menstruation.[64] When the patient recognizes an increase in her insulin requirements, she simply switches her pump setting from pattern A to pattern B. Pattern A can be resumed once again after 5 to 7 days as progesterone levels fall and insulin resistance wanes.

Continuation of Insulin Pump Therapy in Hospitalized Patients

As CSII usage is becoming more popular, personnel are faced with the challenge of caring for pump patients within the hospital environment. Although pumpers are often highly educated and knowledgeable regarding their diabetes self-management, the opposite can be said for staff members who may ask them to "surrender their device" on admission. Many hospitals are now developing protocols that promote a collaborative relationship between staff members and pumpers, which allows patient-directed diabetes self-management when appropriate. A study by Bailon et al. determined that continued use of insulin pumps in hospitals in select cases is safe and can minimize the effects of hyperglycemia.[65]

Pediatric Patients, Highly Insulin-Sensitive Individuals, and Poorly Compliant Adolescents

Pediatric patients may require minute amounts of insulin, which can be delivered via CSII in variations of 0.1 U of insulin for bolus and 0.05 U for basal alterations. CSII allows minute variations in the amounts of insulin infused to accommodate these specific requirements. This accuracy surpasses the dilution of U-100 insulin then injected subcutaneously.

In a review of 80 adolescent patients transferred from MDIs to either CSII or MDIs using glargine and fast-acting insulin, those switched to pumps had a significant A1C decrease from 8.4% to 7.8%, whereas MDI patients did not have a significant decrease in A1C (8.5% to 8.2%). The risk of both moderate and severe hypoglycemia declined in both groups.[66]

In 65 very young children with a mean age of 4.5 years at pump initiation (range, 1.4 to 6.9 years), mean A1C decreased significantly from 7.4% to 6.9% at 12 months, with further reductions by 2 years.[4] Severe hypoglycemia was reduced by 53%. In a randomized trial of CSII versus MDIs[67] in a group of young children with a mean age of 3.6 years, no difference in A1C or hypoglycemia was defined, although pump therapy was found to be safe and effective in young children.

Teenagers who require frequent hospitalization for DKA or find little pleasure in following an insulin regimen by using traditional pen-injector devices have been shown to reduce their incidence of hospitalizations and DKA by using CSII.[60]

Technical expertise is needed for patients using insulin pumps. To be successful pumpers, patients should become proficient at the skills listed in Table 13-6. Children and adolescents who use insulin pumps must have the assistance and encouragement of their parent(s) to manage pump therapy effectively and safely. Parents must supervise adolescents to make certain that they are not taking dangerous "short cuts." For example, some adolescents may "forget" to give a mealtime bolus when they are among friends because they do not want to attract attention to their disease state. Others may simply administer a bolus of insulin without first checking a blood glucose level, preferring to "go by how they feel" rather than by what they know is best for them. Occasionally, teenagers may delay changing their infusion set on schedule, because they have more pressing issues to which they must attend, or they may inadvertently allow their reservoirs to run out of insulin.

Disturbed eating behavior is very common in young women with T1DM. Between 45% and 80% of teenage girls are binge eaters, and up to 40% will eat while omitting insulin in an attempt to control their weight.[29] Eating disorders are associated with many negative medical outcomes, including poor metabolic control, increased frequency of diabetes-related hospitalizations, and higher rates of diabetes-related complications, particularly retinopathy and perhaps neuropathy.[68] Patients with clinically significant eating disorders should not be placed on insulin pump therapy.

TABLE 13-6. Responsibilities of the Physician, Sales Personnel, Pump Trainer, and Patients Who Are Involved in Pump Therapy

Physician Prescriber	Pump Sales Person	Certified Pump Trainer	Pump Patient
Identify and qualify the patient as a potential pump candidate	Explain the benefits of CSII to physicians and patients	The pump trainer will teach pump patients all aspects of CSII based on the parameters provided by the physician. Although the pump trainer may suggest appropriate pump parameters, the ultimate prescribing of the parameters is the responsibility of the physician	View the educational material that is delivered with the pump before the date of the pump initiation
Assist in preparing a letter of medical necessity for insulin pump therapy	Promote pump education and awareness for physicians and patients	Aspects of CSII that the pump trainers teach: Proper infusion-site insertion; How to provide a bolus; Sick-day parameters; Troubleshooting mechanical malfunctions and acute hyperglycemia; Bolus Wizard mechanics; Pump-alarm interpretation; How to change pump batteries; Exercise with the pump; Temporary suspension of the pump; Showering with the pump; Mechanics and interpretation of the sensor-augmented pump; Management of hypoglycemia; Initiation of a temporary basal rate; Using different basal profiles (i.e., one profile while menstruating and another while not); How to obtain pump supplies	Read the instruction manual before initiating the insulin pump

(Continued)

TABLE 13-6. Responsibilities of the Physician, Sales Personnel, Pump Trainer, and Patients Who Are Involved in Pump Therapy *(Continued)*

Physician Prescriber	Pump Sales Person	Certified Pump Trainer	Pump Patient
Determine pump parameters: Basal rate(s) Mealtime boluses Type of bolus patient should use at meals (normal, extended or combination) Personal lag time Insulin sensitivity factor Insulin/carbohydrate ratio Target blood glucose levels (fasting, preprandial, postprandial, bedtime, nocturnal) Type of insulin to be used in the pump (lispro, aspart, glulisine, U-500) Which, if any, pump alarms should be programmed For patients using the Medtronic 722 pumps, alarms must be programmed for hyperglycemia and hypoglycemia recognition	Assist physicians in completing the necessary paperwork for third-party payers		Perform home blood glucose monitoring before and after meals, at bedtime, and in the early AM hours Understand how to troubleshoot mechanical malfunctions and hyperglycemia Know how to manage diabetic ketoacidosis and sick days Understand the principles of exercising while on the pump Understand how to manage hypoglycemia efficiently while on a pump Understand how to perform basic pump functions including insertion of the infusion set, providing a mealtime and supplemental (correction) bolus Carry emergency supplies at all times in case of a pump malfunction
	Locate certified pump trainers for physicians who require initiation of CSII in the office setting		Understand intensive insulin therapy before beginning CSII Carb counting Proper dosing of meal-time insulin Committing to proper mealtime blood glucose monitoring and insulin administration Keeping follow-up appointments with the medical staff

Serve as a liaison between the pump manufacturer, physician, office staff, insurance company, and patient

Facilitate delivery and training of the sensor device to the patient

Determine which patient would benefit from using a pump-augmented sensor

Set sensor parameters for hyperglycemia and hypoglycemia alarms

Establish an on-site pump download station to adjust the pump parameters

Notify physician if blood glucose levels remain consistently high or low, despite following all of the prescribed treatment parameters

Learns to use the sensor to optimize their pump parameters

Train the patient in the proper technique of sensor insertion, calibration, troubleshooting, and online data management

CSII, continuous subcutaneous insulin infusion.

Special Situations that may Affect Glycemic Control: Menstruation and Traveling

Shortly before and during menstruation, some women face higher insulin requirements. Increasing the basal infusion rate in anticipation of and during menses often results in improved glucose control. A separate basal-rate profile may be initiated as glycemic control begins to worsen before the onset of menstruation. Resumption of the original basal rates can begin on days 5 to 7 of the menstrual cycle.

Traveling between time zones is simplified with the use of an insulin pump. If one normally injects the prescribed basal insulin at 10 PM while at home in Los Angeles, and then flies to New York, the basal insulin should be injected at 1:00 AM. This may require the patient to wake up from sleep to administer the injection. An insulin pump provides basal insulin 24 hours a day, so one does not have to be concerned about consistency. The flexibility provided by the insulin pump allows patients to travel safely and confidently.

Table 13-7 provides a summary of the characteristics for the most appropriate insulin pump candidates based upon the American Association of Clinical Endocrinologist Insulin Pump Task Force expert consenses.[58]

Discussing Pump Therapy with Prospective Patients

The role of PCPs in pump therapy is to identify appropriate patients for insulin intensification using CSII and provide each patient with a customized set of basal/bolus parameters. Although multiple pumps are commercially available (Table 13-4), physicians do not necessarily have to be experts in pump mechanics. Each manufacturer provides a team of support personnel (CDEs, pump trainers, and emergency telephone operators) who assist patients and physicians with any questions related to pump therapy.

Once a patient is identified as a perspective pump candidate, the pump manufacturer will work with the third party payers and coordinate training with the patient. The device company

TABLE 13-7. Appropriate Insulin Pump Candidates for Patients with T1DM and T2DM

T1DM Pump Candidates	T2DM Pump Candidates
Patients who are unable to reach glycemic goals despite adherence to MDI, especially if they exhibit: • Significant glycemic variability • Recurrent episodes of DKA • Hypoglycemia awareness autonomic failure (HAAF) • Display evidence of elevated predawn blood glucose levels (dawn phenomenon) • Have extreme insulin sensitivity that favors hypoglycemia	Insulin requiring patients who satisfy any or all of the following criteria: • Elevated C-peptide but with suboptimal control on well-intended basal/bolus intensified therapy • Substantial "dawn phenomenon" • Erratic lifestyle; shift work, frequent long-distance travel, unpredictable schedules, etc. • Severe insulin resistance (requiring >150 U of insulin/d). Patients may be candidates for U-500 insulin infusion
Patients who demand flexible lifestyle as provided by an insulin pump	Select patients with other reasons for chronic severe hyperglycemia: • Postpancreatectomy • Patients undergoing chemotherapy and receiving systemic corticosteroids

representative will also assist physicians new to pump therapy in acquiring the appropriate education to safely prescribe the customized pump parameters.

Patients who transition from MDI to CSII have reported improvement in quality of life parameters, such as treatment satisfaction and lifestyle restrictions, life expectancy (by a mean of 0.76 years as adjusted life expectancy), when compared with conventional therapy. CSII is less painful, less burdensome, interferes less with activities of daily living, and offers greater flexibility and convenience for many patients.[69–73]

Many patients with diabetes are not considered candidates for pumps because of underlying comorbidities. A poster presentation[74] examined 13 "pump-challenged" patients, whose comorbidities included severe hypoglycemic unawareness, movement disorders, attention deficit disorder, mental retardation, schizophrenia, drug or alcohol abuse, personality disorder, depression or severe panic attacks, a history of falsifying glucose records, hypoglycemic encephalopathy, and extreme insulin resistance that required U-500 insulin. Pre-CSII education took 5 months on average, and A1C levels decreased from 9.4% to 8.4% over a 6- to 12-month period. Severe hypoglycemia was reduced by 76%. The authors concluded that "success is relative," and pointed out that when dealing with this group of patients, the skill and patience of the prescribing physician and health-care team are crucial.

Patients must be familiar with using MDIs of insulin before beginning pump therapy. All medical devices, including insulin pumps, may malfunction. Patients must be able to troubleshoot the possible mechanisms for the pump malfunction and know how to manage any resultant hyperglycemia. The rule for managing any insulin pump malfunction is to "always treat the diabetes first." This may require reverting back to using MDIs temporarily until a new pump becomes available. Although insulin dosing is similar with MDIs and CSII, their primary difference is in the physiologic means of insulin delivery and the flexibility they afford. Adult patients who have no knowledge of MDIs cannot safely be placed on pump therapy.

Not all physicians may be willing to integrate insulin pump therapy into their practice. Pump physicians must be adept at helping patients select the right pump for their patient and determining the initial pumping basal and bolus parameters. Physicians should have the data from insulin pumps, home blood glucose meters and continuous glucose sensors so that appropriate therapeutic adjustments may be provided to the patient. On occasion, pumps will fail, and the pump physician will need to address an "emergency insulin protocol" until the patient is able to obtain a new pump from the manufacturer. This author keeps 10 donated back-up pumps and personal diabetes managers (PDMs) for omnipod pumps at his office, which are provided as loaners to patients whose pumps and accessories have failed. Pump companies will work with prescribers to educate patients on carb counting, ordering supplies, and troubleshooting alarms. Clinicians must also be willing to terminate insulin pump therapy when a patient fails to use the device in a safe and effective manner. For example, an elderly patient who repeatedly stacks insulin and has multiple episodes of severe hypoglycemia, despite all educational efforts to minimize this risk, should have their pump discontinued. These patients may be transitioned to mixed insulin analogues and reassessed to determine if the benefits of pumping exceed the risks of treatment emergent hypoglycemia or other adverse events. Patients who develop frequent abdominal wall abscesses because they maintain their indwelling infusion sets repeatedly for over 7 days should also have their pump supplies suspended. Some patients will argue that they are attempting to minimize costs by "recycling" their infusion sets. Unfortunately, this practice is unsafe and will ultimately lead to an increase in the cost of care. Remember, the physician is ultimately responsible for the safety of any of his or her patients, especially those who are utilizing CSII.

▌ Initiating Pump Therapy in the Primary Care Setting

Pumps may be initiated in the practitioner's office by a certified pump trainer in about 1 hour. A patient who is new to pump therapy must understand two basic principles in his or her initial training visit: (a) how to insert the infusion set and (b) how to provide a mealtime bolus. Prior to transitioning to CSII, patients should already be well trained in self–blood glucose monitoring as well as hypoglycemia prevention, recognition, and management. Some physicians place patients on CGMS concurrently with the initiation of pump therapy. The pump, sensor, and meter are then downloaded after 1 week at which time appropriate adjustments in parameters are suggested.

Over time, patients can be instructed on carbohydrate counting, emergency management of pump malfunction, bolus wizard features, pump data management, sick-day regimens, travel procedures, pump-augmented sensor systems, use of supplemental insulin, and initiation of TBRs. During the subsequent follow-up appointments, physicians may choose to add additional basal rates, change the nature of the mealtime bolus, and monitor the patient for acute and chronic complications related to CSII.

Setting the Pump Parameters (Don't Worry—This is the Easy Part!)

The following case will illustrate the steps required to determine the initial pump parameters for a patient who is beginning CSII.

Jen, aged 20, is preparing to start insulin pump therapy today. She weighs 70 kg, and she has a habit of skipping breakfast but eating a modest lunch and large dinner. She has consistent hyperglycemia on rising each morning (6:00 AM), with her fasting blood glucose values averaging 40 mg per dL greater than her prelunch values. Jen exercises for 60 minutes, 5 days a week, between 4:00 and 8:00 PM, and eats dinner around 9:00 PM. Her blood glucose levels at bedtime before initiating pump therapy have been averaging 200 mg per dL.

The following steps will guide the physician in the initial steps required for pump programming:

1. *What is Jen's anticipated TDD of insulin requirement?* (Fig. 13-10, item 1)
   - **Determine the patient's TDD of insulin.**
     The first order of business to consider when prescribing pump parameters is to determine how much insulin a patient requires over a 24-hour period. By taking the patient's current weight in kilograms and multiplying that weight by 0.7 U, one can determine the TDD of insulin required for a 24-hour period as follows:

     TDD = Weight in kg × 0.7 U

     In Jen's case, 70 kg × 0.7 = 49 U (OK to round this off to 50 U per day). The TDD of insulin also varies, depending on the patient's level of physical conditioning, age, gender, degree of the patient's *physical* stress, and body weight. A well-conditioned athlete, for example, would have a TDD of weight in kg × 0.5 U. Table 13-3 suggests dosing strategies for calculating the TDD based on these multiple factors. Keep in mind that this allows the physician to establish the *initial* dose of insulin.
   - **Assign how much of the TDD is applied to basal and how much to bolus insulin per day.**
     Once the TDD of insulin is calculated, ½ of that TDD is assigned to basal insulin delivery, and ½, to bolus insulin delivery:
   - 50% of the TDD = basal insulin
   - 50% of the TDD = bolus insulin
     In Jen's case, 25 U is applied to the basal insulin and 25 U to the bolus insulin.
   - **Determine the patient's hourly basal insulin requirements.**
     The initial hourly basal insulin requirements are determined by dividing the total basal insulin by 24 hours.
     For Jen, 25 U per 24 hours = 1.0 U per hour. Thus the initial basal rate of insulin is 1.0 U per hour.
     Additional basal rates may be programmed at future visits based on the presence of the dawn phenomenon; timing, frequency, and severity of recorded episodes of hypoglycemia; and the patient's glycemic response to exercise. Most patients require 1 to 2 basal rates. Generally, the

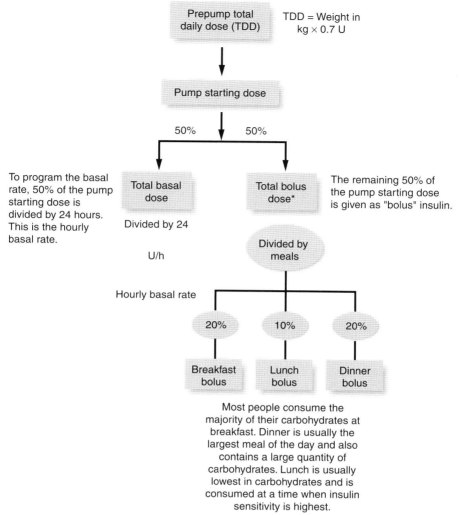

Figure 13-10 • Formulas for Programming Pump Parameters. These include total daily dose (TDD) of insulin, insulin-sensitivity factor (ISF), insulin/carbohydrate ratio (I/C), personal lag time, and rule for managing hypoglycemia. *Although many people have a 50/50 ratio of basal/bolus insulin, others may have a ratio of 40/60, meaning that more insulin is required to maintain PPG than FPG levels.

more basal rates programmed, the more complicated insulin pumping becomes for both the patient and the physician. Patients who have multiple basal rates (more than 4) programmed into their pumps, yet are unable to maintain adequate A1C levels (6.5% to 7.5%) while show-ing signs of wide glycemic variation, may improve by simply limiting them to 1 to 2 basal rates.

2. *What is Jen's insulin-sensitivity factor?* (Fig. 13-10, item 2)
The ISF allows patients to calculate the anticipated reduction in glucose level after a 1-U insulin bolus.

Patients can use the ISF to correct hyperglycemia resulting from underdosing of prandial insulin, the insulin resistance that occurs on sick days, or pre-exercise glycemic eleva-tions. Glycemic targets may vary throughout the day. Patients may be advised to maintain a daytime target of 80 to 140 mg per dL, but a nighttime target of 150 to 180 mg per dL to prevent nocturnal hypoglycemia. The "default safe target" for correcting hyperglycemia is 150 mg per dL. This allows patients to overshoot their mark slightly without becoming hypoglycemic. If the target is set too low (100 mg per dL), patients will commonly over-correct into a state of hypoglycemia.

The ISF is calculated by dividing 1,800/TDD of insulin. Jen's ISF would be 1,800/50 = 36. Thus, if the glycemic target is 150 mg per dL, and Jen's current blood glucose level is 250 mg per dL, Jen would do the following calculation to reach the target:

Step 1: 250 − 150 = 100 mg per dL
Step 2: 100/36 = 2.7 U
Step 3: Target goal = 150 during the day

Giving a 2.7-U dose at noon will allow Jen to achieve a normal glucose level within 1 to 2 hours after administering the bolus. (Note that the pumps allow patients to administer insulin by fractions of units. This cannot be done with syringes and vials or insulin pens.)

When correcting hyperglycemia, patients should be encouraged to recheck their blood glucose levels within 1 to 2 hours of the correction dose to make certain that they are approaching, yet have not exceeded, the target.

Patients who must frequently correct postprandial hyperglycemia should be provided with a revised insulin-to-carbohydrate ratio. Extending the square-wave portion of the bolus for a longer time may obviate the necessity for frequent corrections. Hyperglycemia that frequently occurs in the preprandial or fasting state requires adjustments in basal-rate insulin delivery.

3. *What is Jen's insulin/carbohydrate ratio (I/C)?* (Fig. 13-10, item 3)
   The **I/C** provides patients with an estimation of how much 1 U of insulin will cover the glycemic excursion anticipated with carbohydrate ingestion.

   Divide 450/TDD insulin to get the I/C.

   In Jen's case, 450/50 = 9. Thus, if Jen consumes 100 g of carbohydrates, she will need to administer a bolus of 100/9 = 11.1 U of insulin.

   I/Cs may vary throughout the day, often being lower in the morning and higher in the evening. Jen may actually have an I/C of 1:8 for breakfast and 1:11 for dinner. Patients who are educated on their I/C values will realize that consuming carbohydrates will necessitate a dose of insulin. For example, if Jen goes to a movie and eats popcorn, she will need to provide insulin for that carbohydrate snack. Otherwise, her blood glucose level will be very high by the time she returns home after the show.

4. *What is Jen's personal "lag time"?*
   Absorption rates differ for each patient. By calculating a **personal lag time**, postprandial glycemic excursions might be minimized.[75] The methods required to calculate the personal lag time appropriately are detailed in Figure 13-10, item 4.

   A patient with blood glucose levels greater than 180 mg per dL should increase the lag time, allowing the insulin to improve glycemic control before eating. Patients who are hypoglycemic before meals should delay the mealtime bolus until after the meal is completed to prevent a worsening of the hypoglycemic state.

5. *How should Jen's boluses be monitored and adjusted?*
   A percentage of the total amount of insulin assigned for mealtime boluses during a 24-hour period should be assigned to breakfast, lunch, and dinner. As shown in Figure 13-1, glycemic requirements are highest during the early morning hours and in the evening hours. Therefore, prandial insulin requirements are highest for breakfast and supper and lowest for lunch.

   In Jen's case a total of 25 U is assigned to prevent postprandial hyperglycemia. Jen can apply these 25 U to meals based on the amount of carbohydrates she will be consuming at each meal. However, if Jen has had trouble with carbohydrate counting, a prescribed (suggested) "baseline" dosage of insulin may be delivered at each meal. From this baseline dosage, the patient can increase or decrease the dose of prandial insulin based on several factors:

- Increase 1 to 2 U for large meals
- Decrease 1 to 2 U for smaller meals
- Calculate the ISF to determine how much insulin would be required to adjust the preprandial glucose level to 150 mg per dL and then add this total to the prescribed dose. For example, if the initial blood glucose level is 250 mg per dL, preprandial glucose target is 150 mg per dL, ISF is 1:50 mg per dL, and the suggested lunchtime dose of insulin is 4 U, the patient would take a total of 6 U for lunch (250 mg per dL – 150 mg per dL = 100/50 = 2 U. These 2 U plus the suggested lunch dose of 4 U = 6 U).

Therefore, Jen is advised to make the following decisions:

(a) If the preprandial glucose level is between 70 and 170 mg per dL, she may either count carbohydrates or plan to administer a bolus of approximately 10 U of insulin for breakfast, 4 U for lunch, and 11 U for dinner.

(b) Whenever possible, use a "dual-wave bolus" to control the anticipated hyperglycemia associated with mealtime. The dual-wave bolus consists of a rapid immediate bolus simulating normal first-phase insulin response and a square-wave bolus similar to a normal second-phase insulin release, which is administered over a 2- to 3-hour period (Fig. 13-6).

The dual-wave bolus can be administered in many different ways. Providing 50% of the total bolus immediately and 50% over a 2- to 3-hour period will work well for many patients. If the premeal glucose levels are greater than 150 mg per dL, supplemental insulin can be calculated into the initial bolus to target a 150 mg per dL glucose level. For example, if the prelunch glucose level is 250 mg per dL and the ISF is 1:25, Jen should give 4 + 2 or 6 U as an immediate bolus and 2 U as square-wave delivery over a 2-hour period. If the prelunch glucose level is less than 70 mg per dL, Jen can either reduce the immediate bolus to 1 U and give the usual square-wave bolus or begin the dual-wave bolus *after* eating to avoid hypoglycemia. Utilization of the *Bolus Wizard* available on most all manufactured insulin pumps may also be beneficial for determining the amount and timing of an individual meal bolus. The Bolus Wizard recommends insulin dosages to patients based upon glucose levels, food intake, and information preset by the user (target blood glucose, insulin sensitivity, and insulin-to-carbohydrate ratios). The pump also tracks *insulin on board,* which minimizes the risk of over bolusing and inducing hypoglycemia. With practice, patients will learn how to deliver the most physiologic dual-wave bolus for each meal consumed. Patients who use pramlintide with their insulin pumps may experience less hypoglycemia if 25% of their mealtime bolus plus their correction bolus are given with the meal and 75% of the calculated bolus is provided over a 3-hour period. Pramlintide patients who are prone to postprandial hypoglycemia may even begin their mealtime boluses *after* they complete their meal rather than just before the onset of the carbohydrate intake.

6. *What type of insulin should Jen use while pumping?*
The majority of patients use a rapid-acting insulin analogue (lispro, aspart, or glulisine) as their pumped insulin. A study published by Bode determined that the rates of absorption of all rapid-acting insulin analogues and clinical efficacy in terms of glycemic control were similar.[76] Glulisine showed a faster onset of action in some studies with aspart and lispro, yet this advantage lasted less than 1 hour. Insulins may be subject to precipitation while in storage, resulting in infusion set occlusion. Aspart demonstrated the greatest chemical and physical stability in the insulin pump with lower rates of overall occlusion (aspart 9.2%, lispro 15.7%, glulisine 40.9%; $p < 0.01$) compared with glulisine and lispro. Thus, insulin aspart is the most compatible of the three rapid-acting insulins for pump use.

All fast-acting analogues are FDA approved for use in insulin pumps. Patients with severe insulin resistance who require high-volume basal and bolus flow rates, resulting in more than 150 U of daily insulin, might be candidates for concentrated U-500 regular insulin.[77] Pump reservoirs are designed to carry between 200 and 300 U of insulin. If a patient uses 200 U of insulin per day, the reservoir and infusion sets would have to be changed every 24 to 36 hours rather than every 3 days, adding to the overall expense for pump supplies. U-500 insulin can be beneficial for insulin-resistant patients. Because U-500 has a much slower onset of action than a rapid-acting insulin analogue, patients using concentrated insulin should delay eating for between 45 and 60 minutes after starting their dual-wave bolus. Because U-500 insulin is five times as potent as standard U-100 insulin, patients can reduce their basal and bolus rates by 80%. For example, a basal rate of 3.0 U per hour can be reduced to 0.6 U per hour on U-500. Meal boluses totaling 50 U can be changed to a dual-wave bolus of 5 U immediately and 5 U over a 3-hour period. Families of patients using U-500 insulin should be trained in the administration of emergency glucagon for rare cases of insulin-induced hypoglycemia.

7. *What instructions should be given regarding "pump emergency protocols"?*
Patients using insulin pumps must be able to anticipate, screen for, and manage short-term complications such as hyperglycemia, DKA, and hypoglycemia. Although these tasks are often taught by certified pump educators and CDEs, physicians should periodically assess patients' understanding of "emergency pump protocols."

If Jen awakens with a fasting blood glucose level of 280 mg per dL, she may administer a correction bolus to target the glucose level to 150 mg per dL. In Jen's case, her target blood glucose of 150 is 130 mg per dL below her current level. Knowing that her ISF is 1:30, Jen determines that she must provide an immediate bolus of 4.3 U for the correction. One hour after administering the bolus, another blood glucose level should be obtained. If the blood glucose level is decreasing, she can assume that the infusion set line is patent and the pump mechanics are in order. However, if the 1-hour post-correction blood glucose level is going *higher* despite the use of the supplemental bolus, she must proceed to troubleshoot the pump, infusion set, and the infusion site.

Hyperglycemia may result from a mismatch between the dose of insulin provided and the quantity of food consumed, a loss of insulin potency (incorrect shipping and packaging of mail-ordered insulin may result in reduced potency), an underlying infection resulting in an acute insulin-resistant state, an insulin-flow obstruction through the infusion set, or a pump mechanical malfunction. If a pump is subject to a static discharge, similar to a finger-tip shock one experiences in winter while walking on carpet, the pump parameters may be erased from the pump's internal memory. Most pumps will deliver an auditory or vibrating alarm if insulin delivery is interrupted. Insulin cannot be delivered if the infusion catheter is kinked within the insertion site. The pump will sense when abnormal pressure is required to pump insulin against an obstruction and subsequently emit an alarm.

When patients experience unexpected hyperglycemia, they should *always fix the diabetes first* by giving a subcutaneous correction dose of insulin via a syringe or pen device, targeting a 150 mg per dL blood glucose level. The infusion set and reservoir should be changed and an alternative infusion site chosen. Once the new infusion set has been inserted, the patient should carefully monitor blood glucose levels over the next 2- to 3-hour period, making certain that the hyperglycemia is not worsening (which could be indicative of a systemic infection) or that hypoglycemia has developed from using an excessive correction bolus.

Patients should always be provided with a copy of their prescribed parameters in case the pump needs emergency reprogramming. A delay in reprogramming the pump may result in hyperglycemia and DKA. Patients can get assistance on reprogramming their pumps from the manufacturers' websites (Table 13-6).

8. *Can Jen safely manage DKA while wearing an insulin pump?*

Because insulin pumps use rapid-acting insulin analogues, an interruption in drug delivery will quickly result in hyperglycemia. Any patient in whom hyperglycemia develops (blood glucose greater than 240 mg per dL) in association with nausea, vomiting, abdominal pain, and an altered level of consciousness should be evaluated for ketosis. Urine ketone test kits are readily available, and some home blood glucose monitors (Precision Xtra, Abbott) can be used to screen for the presence of ketone bodies. Table 13-8 lists the management strategies for DKA in pump patients.

9. *How often should Jen change the infusion set and pump reservoir?*

To prevent irritation and infection at the infusion-set insertion site while maintaining adequate insulin flow into the subcutaneous insulin depot site, the infusion sets and reservoirs should be changed every 2 to 3 days. Sites may need to be changed sooner if discomfort or irritability develops at the insertion site. A steady increase in glucose levels may be indicative of impaired insulin absorption from the infusion-site subcutaneous depot. After inserting a new infusion set into the skin, the patient should provide an immediate 1- to 2-U bolus of insulin to "prime the site" and establish a depot from which the insulin may be continuously absorbed. Some patients may prefer administering the priming bolus as dual wave, whereby half is administered immediately and the remaining insulin is infused over 30 to 60 minutes. The priming bolus will not reduce the patient's blood glucose level. Infusion sets should be changed only during the waking hours, because an improperly inserted set can result in significant hyperglycemia, which may go undetected while the patient sleeps. Two hours after the new infusion set is inserted, a blood glucose level should be determined to make certain that the patient's glycemic control is within the prescribed target range. Otherwise, a correction bolus may be administered.

Pump batteries should be replaced every 30 days. A bar on the pump screen flashes when the battery is low.

TABLE 13-8. Managing Diabetic Ketoacidosis in Patients Using Insulin Pumps

If nausea or vomiting is present, immediately check your blood glucose and ketones. If your blood glucose is above 250 mg/dL and/or ketones are present:

- Call your health-care provider
- Take an injection of a rapid-acting insulin analogue with a syringe or pen device (not through the pump). The amount should be the same as if you were taking a correction bolus
- Change entire infusion set system (new reservoir, infusion set, and cannula). Troubleshoot the pump. If help is needed, call the 24-h Product Help Line (the phone number is on the back of your pump)
- Drink liquids with no calories every 30 min (e.g., 8 oz diet ginger ale, broth, water)
- Check your blood glucose and urine ketones in 1 h. Blood ketones can be detected via the Precision QID home blood glucose meter (Abbott) (http://www.diabeteshealthconnection. com/products/monitors/precision/precisionxtra.aspx)
- Continue to take insulin as discussed with health-care professional
- Call your health-care professional immediately if your blood glucose and ketones are not decreasing or you are unable to drink fluids
- If your blood glucose is <200 mg/dL and ketones are present, drink liquids containing calories (e.g., juice or caffeine-free, non-diet soda). Also, additional insulin is usually required. Contact your health-care professional for specific guidelines for insulin doses when ketones are present

10. *What precautions should Jen take when she travels with the pump?*

    Patients on insulin pumps who travel should always have the following emergency supplies in their possession, *not in their checked baggage:*

    - Backup blood glucose meter, lancets, lancet device, and strips
    - Glucose tablets to manage hypoglycemia
    - A list of the pump parameters
    - Extra pump and blood glucose meter batteries
    - Extra infusion sets and reservoirs (if necessary, the infusion sets can be placed through the skin manually, without the use of a self-insertion device)
    - Extra vial of insulin
    - Pen injector of rapid-acting insulin analogue plus extra needles
    - Food and water, in case access is limited
    - If going to a foreign country, be sure to carry information on who to contact in case of a pump malfunction. The U.S. pump manufacturers can assist patients with this information

    Remember that insulin preparations available outside of the United States are not identical to what is marketed in this country. Plan accordingly when preparing to travel with any insulin-delivery devices

    Most pumpers, when traveling, do not adjust the insulin pump clock unless traveling across more than five time zones. Once patients arrive at their destination, routine bolus doses of insulin may be used. For the first day of long distance travel, running slightly higher than normal blood glucose readings would be preferable than risking a severe hypoglycemic event. Ideally, patients who travel frequently should use continuous glucose sensors.

    Patients should also be reminded to reset the internal clock of their insulin pumps twice each year at the beginning and end of daylight savings time. Most companies will send a blast e-mail to pump users suggesting that their clocks be changed 2 days prior to the scheduled event.

    Patients do not require a written note from their physician to pass through an airport security screening checkpoint with their insulin pumps. Pumpers are encouraged to disconnect their pumps (unless wearing an omnipod or other wireless device) and place them in their carry on bags while passing through the TSA checkpoint. Pumps will alarm if worn on clothing unless one walks through the metal detector slowly at a 45-degree angle. Unfortunately, this choreography will undoubtedly draw attention to your unique attempt to pass through the checkpoint with your pump undetected. Waiting for you on the other side of the scanner will be either a male or female member of the homeland security task force ready to place you in a rear naked choke hold and wipe your hands for some type of explosive material. All they will find is insulin residue. A better way to "fly" by the security checkpoint for frequent travelers is to join the TSA Pre Check program. This expedited screening procedure (available at www.globalentry.gov/tsa/html) allows qualified passengers to pass through expedited screening lanes at designated U.S. airports. Passengers can keep their shoes on, leave computers in their bags, keep their belts and pumps on, and do not have to remove jackets. TSA officers do not swipe the hands of all pumpers who pass through these precheck security checkpoints, although some passengers may still be subject to random searches.

11. *How should Jen manage "sick days" while on the pump?*

    Sick days are easily managed with pump therapy (Table 13-9).

    TBRs may need to be set for mild persistent hyperglycemia that may occur in response to a viral infection or the temporary use of corticosteroids (see Fig. 13-11). Patients should be instructed that mealtime boluses are not mandatory and should be programmed when a meal is consumed. If a patient is unable to eat, the basal insulin flow can be sufficient to control glycemia. Supplemental insulin may be used every 4 to 6 hours to control acute hyperglycemia.

TABLE 13-9. Sick-Day Protocol for Pump Users

- Monitor your blood glucose every 2 h while you are awake and at least once overnight
- Depending on the results of blood glucose and ketone testing, you may need to make periodic insulin adjustments while you are sick
- You will still require insulin, even when you are unable to eat
- If your blood glucose is above 250 mg/dL, follow the hyperglycemia protocol to avoid the potential of DKA from illness or infection
- Remember to call your health-care provider if your blood glucose is above 250 mg/dL and ketones are present

12. *What is the proper protocol for treating hypoglycemia?*
    Mild symptomatic hypoglycemia is managed by patients using the "rule of 15" (Fig. 13-12). Pump patients and their families should always be trained in using a glucagon emergency kit for reversing severe hypoglycemia.

Fine-tuning Pump Therapy

Patients should be reevaluated within 1 to 2 weeks of pump initiation to begin their parameter adjustments. Basal and bolus doses are adjusted according to the patient's blood glucose measurements taken before meals, 2 hours after meals, at bedtime, at midnight, and at 3:00 AM (Table 13-10).

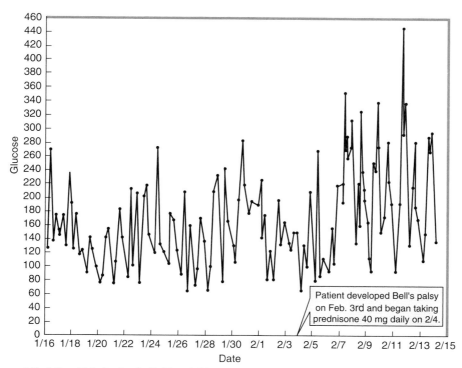

Figure 13-11 • **This is the Self–Blood Glucose Meter Download Graft of a 43-Year-Old Patient with T1DM Who Developed Bell's Palsy on February 3.** Following the initiation of prednisone the following day, the glycemic control deteriorated. Prednisone affects primarily PPG values, which would require an insulin pump patient to utilize a two- to threefold increase in the amount of extended bolus delivered over a 3-hour period beginning 1 to 2 days after prednisone is initiated. (Case supplied by Jeff Unger, MD)

If blood glucose is 60 mg/dL or below:

- Eat or drink **15 g** of carbohydrate*
- Recheck your blood glucose in **15** minutes. If the reading is not above 60 mg/dL, repeat treatment with another **15 g** of carbohydrate
- Test again in **15** minutes
- If blood glucose is not >60 mg/dL, repeat treatment with another **15 g** of carbohydrate, then call your health-care provider

*The following contain **15** grams of carbohydrate and are appropriate for the treatment of hypoglycemia:

- Glucose tablets (3, 5-gram tablets)
- 4 oz. (110 g) of juice or soda (not diet)
- 1 tablespoon of table sugar or honey
- 1 small box of raisins

Here is another useful formula that can help patients emerge safely from hypoglycemia without spiking into a glycemic state:

> (100 − blood glucose) × 0.2 = grams of carbohydrates necessary for blood glucose correction.

Thus, if the blood glucose is 50 mg/dL, the patient would consume 100 − 50 = 50; 50 × 0.2 = 10 g of carbohydrates.

Note: Pumpers should keep a glucagon emergency kit at home for rare occurrences of severe hypoglycemia. If a patient becomes unarousable, a 1-mg dose of glucagon is injected intramuscularly by a family member. This should result in a rapid rise in the blood glucose level.

Figure 13-12 • Managing Hypoglycemia. "The Rule of 15" and emerging safely from hypoglycemia.

The basal rate should be increased or decreased by 0.1 U per hour to keep the preprandial and overnight blood glucose levels within a 30-mg glucose excursion from baseline. If the glucose level increases more than 30 mg per dL from the 3:00 AM measurement to the prebreakfast measurement, a second basal rate (~1.5 times that of the initial basal rate) is added for 4 to 6 hours, beginning 2 to 3 hours before the usual breakfast time. Daytime basal rates are adjusted only if significant glucose excursions occur more than 4 hours after the mealtime bolus. To guide daytime basal-rate adjustments, the patient should be instructed to delay or skip a meal while monitoring blood glucose levels every 2 hours in the fasting state. This should be done periodically to ascertain that basal rates are not set too high or too low.

Bolus doses are adjusted according to blood glucose measurements taken 2 hours after meals. Patients are provided specific guidelines for adjusting insulin boluses or the I/C to maintain reasonable glucose excursions. If the blood glucose level 2 hours after eating is 50 mg or less higher than the premeal glucose level, the I/C was correctly determined. However, if the 2-hour postprandial level is greater than 50 mg per dL, a higher I/C for a given meal should be used the next time the patient eats that same meal. One common source of frustration among patients who attempt, yet fail to count carbohydrates correctly, is that this method of premeal insulin determination is best used when blood glucose levels are within the targeted range of 70 to 170 mg per dL. Carbohydrate counting when a patient's blood glucose values are consistently more than 300 mg per dL, for example, will only result in persistent hyperglycemia. Patients can use both carbohydrate counting and their ISFs to determine their premeal insulin dose; a calculation that is performed automatically by the Bolus Wizard feature on several pumps.

Using electronic home blood glucose download data is very helpful in determining the efficacy of the patient's bolus regimen. If at least 50% of the patient's postmeal glucose levels (taken 2 hours after eating) for each meal is within the 70 to 170 mg per dL range, the patient boluses are adequate. If more than 3% of the patient's postprandial levels is less than 70 mg per dL, the patient should be advised to reduce the total bolus for that particular meal by 10% to 20% to avoid hypoglycemia.[78]

TABLE 13-10. Adjusting Pump Parameters

Basal and bolus doses should be adjusted for and based on blood glucose levels at:
- Preprandial
- 1- to 2-h postprandial
- At bedtime
- At 3:00 AM (monitor for nocturnal hypoglycemia occurring between 2:00 and 4:00 AM)
- Dawn phenomenon (hyperglycemia occurring on waking)

Overnight blood glucose
- Goal of 100 mg/dL (±30 mg/dL)
- If blood glucose >100 mg/dL at 3:00 AM, program a second bolus at 1.5 × the basal dose. This second bolus dose should begin between 3:00 and 4:00 AM for 4–6 h
- Adjust basal rate during day to compensate for skipped or delayed meals
- Teach patient to check blood glucose in a daytime fasting state every 2 h

Bolus dose should be based on the carbohydrate-to-insulin ratio and adjusted for:
- 1- to 2-h postprandial blood glucose
- Changes in carbohydrate to insulin ratios adjusted every 2 d to maintain 1- to 2-h postprandial blood glucose <180 mg/dL
- Carbohydrate-to-insulin ratio for each meal can be estimated (after the bolus dose is well matched to a stable meal plan)
- Optimal ratio ranges from 1 U/5 g CHO to 1 U/25 g CHO (most patients require 1 U/10 g CHO)

CHO, cholesterol.

Patients who show persistent elevations in PPG levels should increase their premeal insulin bolus or consider working harder on correctly counting carbohydrates.

Paired (structured) glucose testing should be emphasized periodically to determine if 2-hour PPG levels for any given meal are between 0 and 50 mg per dL from baseline. If the "delta" consistently exceeds 50 mg per dL, the mealtime bolus or lag time (delay between the time of bolusing and onset of eating) will need to be increased (Table 13-11). Any 2-hour PPG level that is lower than baseline (i.e., a "negative delta") should prompt the pumper to monitor closely for hypoglycemia.[41] Remember, any insulin bolus will have a duration of 4 hours. If at 2 hours the glucose level is lower than at baseline and insulin is still "on board" waiting to be absorbed from the subcutaneous depot, glucose levels will likely be dropping. The insulin pump can be suspended or placed on a "temporary basal rate" until glucose levels stabilize. Table 13-12 provides an explanation for deltas outside of the physiologic range. Pump patients should be encouraged to perform structured testing prior to each meal and 2 hours postprandial each month in order to fine-tune their baseline bolus requirements.

Some blood glucose meters, such as the iBG Star, can be downloaded directly into an iPhone. An app appears on the smartphone screen, which may be used to review and e-mail the data to the patient's provider. Clinicians may suggest basal or bolus dosing adjustments based on the e-mails they receive directly from the patient's iPhone app. Additional information regarding the iBG Star may be found at: www.ibgstar.us.

TABLE 13-11. Structured Glucose Testing Method to Fine-tune Mealtime Boluses

Date	Premeal Glucose	2-h Postmeal Glucose	Delta (Difference between Pre- and Postmeal Glucose)	Possible Reasons Delta Could be > or < 50 mg/dL

On a monthly basis, patient is advised to record blood glucose values via a handwritten log before and 2 h after each meal. The blood glucose value 2 h after eating should be 0–50 mg/dL from baseline. Patients should determine possible reasons why their blood glucose values may be outside of the targeted delta range by using Table 13-12.

TABLE 13-12. Interpretation of 2-h Postmeal Glucose Excursions (Delta Values)

Delta Value at 2-h Postmeal Consumption	Interpretation of Delta Value
0–50 mg/dL	• Correct amount of insulin was provided to cover the carbohydrates consumed for this meal • Insulin correction factor calculation was correctly applied if the premeal glucose value was >200 mg/dL • Insulin bolus was administered appropriately with a 10–15 min lag time if the premeal glucose value was >80 mg/dL. If the premeal glucose was <80 mg/dL, the premeal bolus should be administered at the time the meal is consumed
>50 mg/dL	• Insulin to carbohydrate calculation mismatch • No insulin bolus lag time. Bolus given at time of meal rather than 10–15 min prior to eating • Snack consumption between end of meal and 2 h blood glucose test • Use of caffeine in AM that can increase hepatic glucose production • Improper type of pump bolus given (extended wave only rather than dual wave; immediate bolus only rather than use of a dual-wave bolus)
>100 mg/dL	• Forgot to bolus insulin • Too many carbs consumed • Failure to correct premeal hyperglycemia, resulting in postmeal insulin resistance. (ISF can minimize this postprandial excursion.)
>200 mg/dL	• Forgot to bolus insulin • Watch for DKA • Is your insulin pump functioning properly? Troubleshoot pump now • Sick day • Use of corticosteroids • Severe insulin:carb mismatch for pizza or Chinese food consumption
<Negative delta at 2 h (−25)	• Too much insulin used in relation to carbohydrates consumed • Postmeal activity increased glucose utilization in muscles • Drinking alcohol reduces hepatic glucose production increasing the risk of postmeal hypoglycemia • Insulin stacking (Insulin was used without taking into consideration the "amount of insulin on board" from a prior bolus • Note: Any negative delta at 2 h should prompt repeat testing at 3 h to make certain that glucose values are not dropping <70 mg/dL, which will result in hypoglycemia

Patients with an A1C level greater than 8.5% should focus their pump adjustments on improving their fasting blood glucose levels. As A1C levels become normalized (A1C less than 8.5%), adjustments in boluses will further improve the A1C levels:

- Change I/C for certain meals
- Change ISF
- Determine and use one's personal lag time
- Carry extended bolus over a 2- to 3-hour period
- Provide 25% of total bolus immediately with the onset of the meal and 75% over the following 2- to 3-hour period
- Consider using pramlintide (or liraglutide-off label) to improve glycemic variability (see Chapter 11).

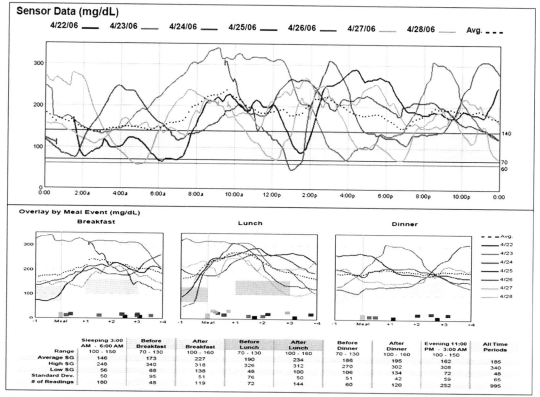

	Sleeping 3:00 AM - 6:00 AM	Before Breakfast	After Breakfast	Before Lunch	After Lunch	Before Dinner	After Dinner	Evening 11:00 PM - 3:00 AM	All Time Periods
Range	100 - 150	70 - 130	100 - 160	70 - 130	100 - 160	70 - 130	100 - 160	100 - 150	
Average SG	146	173	227	190	234	186	195	162	185
High SG	248	340	318	326	312	270	302	308	340
Low SG	56	88	138	48	100	106	134	72	48
Standard Dev.	50	95	51	76	50	51	42	59	65
# of Readings	180	48	119	72	144	60	120	252	995

Figure 13-13 • One of the Many Reports Available on CareLink. This report provides a day-to-day (modal day) comparison of CGMS data displayed in a series of overlaid 24-hour data plots (upper graph). The solid line represents the patient's targeted glucose values. Trending above the target indicates trending in the range of hyperglycemia, whereas glucose values that lie below the target suggest that the patient has become hypoglycemic during that period of time. The lower graph shows the sensor overlay by mealtime allowing the patient and clinician the opportunity to identify mealtime trends in glycemic control, thereby providing the "team" with suggestions by which insulin to carb ratios, insulin lag times, or total insulin dosing may be modified. Additional information regarding CareLink may be found at https://carelink.minimed.com.

▌ Downloading Pumps

Insulin pump manufacturers have marketed a number of management software programs designed to assist patients and physicians integrate data downloaded from pumps, CGMS, blood glucose meters, and logbooks. The data that are displayed in simplified charts, graphs, and tables may be useful in adjusting intensive insulin pump therapy. One Internet-based integrated system, Care-Link, was shown to reduce the aggregate A1C by 0.3% in 94 children with T1DM over 3 years when compared with age-matched controls who had no access to data management system.[79]

CareLink is also useful in providing insight into the effects of specific foods, exercise, stress, and acute illness on blood glucose trends. An example of the integrated data system is shown in Figure 13-13.

Other pump manufactures have equally effective data management systems available to both patients and providers who prescribe pump therapy. Table 13-13 lists the currently available software systems.

TABLE 13-13. Insulin Pump Software Management Systems

Roche	Medtronic
	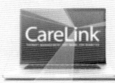
Accu-Check 360 Diabetes Management System	CareLink
http://www.accu-chekinsulinpumps.com/ipus/products/informationmanagement/index.html	http://www.medtronicdiabetes.net/products/carelinkpersonalsoftware
PC Only	PC and Mac
Downloads Roche insulin pumps and Accu-Check meter family	Downloads Medtronic insulin pumps and sensors, as well as multiple blood glucose meters
Animas	Omnipod (Insulet)
	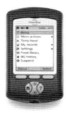
exManager Max	
	Pathfinder Data Management Software
http://www.animas.com/animas-insulin-pumps/ezmanager-max-software	http://www.myomnipod.com/customer-care/download-software/
PC and Mac	PC
Downloads Animas pumps and One Touch blood glucose meters	Downloads Freestyle Navigator CGMS, Dexcom CGMS, Omnipod insulin pump, and Freestyle blood glucose meters

■ Long-term Follow-up of Insulin Pump Patients

Once the patient is stabilized on the pump parameters, patients may be reevaluated every 3 to 5 months, with attention paid to the following issues:

1. Home blood glucose monitoring electronic logs should be carefully inspected to determine if fine-tuning of the basal and boluses is necessary.
2. Review the protocol for managing hypoglycemia (Fig. 13-12), hyperglycemia (using supplemental insulin), prevention, and initial treatment of DKA, sick-day management (Table 13-9), and the emergency protocol for pump malfunction (Fig. 13-14).
3. Review the pump parameters to make certain that the physician-directed basal rates have not been changed by the patient. Patients should understand that they are in charge of their mealtime and supplemental boluses. However, the medical team should direct any alterations in basal rates.
4. Evaluate the areas surrounding the infusion sites to make certain that abscesses and scar tissue are not forming. Areas of inflammation may be indicative of a localized insulin allergy, which may require switching to a different short-acting insulin analogue.

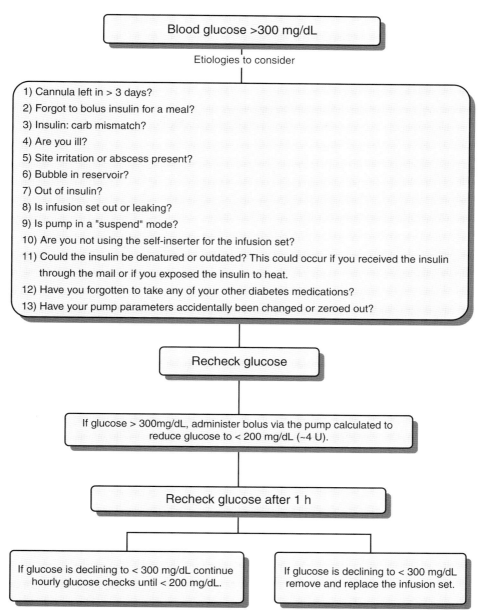

Figure 13-14 • **Troubleshooting and Managing Acute Hyperglycemia While on Insulin Pump Therapy.**

5. Insulin stacking should be discussed, especially for patients experiencing more than 5% hypoglycemia on their electronic logs.
6. A1C levels should be monitored three to four times a year.
7. Remember that approximately 50% of the patient's total daily insulin dose should be provided as bolus insulin, and 50%, as basal insulin. If the patient is providing multiple correction and supplemental boluses, the ratio of basal to bolus insulin will be far less than 1:1. The basal rates will have to be analyzed and readjusted.

Table 13-14 discusses questions that should be explored for pump patients having difficulty achieving a targeted A1C of less than 7%.

TABLE 13-14. Questions to Ask Pump Patients When Their Follow-up A1C Levels Are >7%

1. Is the patient monitoring his or her blood glucose levels 4–6 times/d?

2. Is the basal insulin rate set properly? Can the patient skip a meal without experiencing hypoglycemia or hyperglycemia?

3. Does the patient count carbohydrates accurately and give proper boluses? Is the patient using the dual-wave (or extended) boluses or are only immediate (normal boluses) being used to dose the insulin?

4. Does the patient use the proper correction bolus factor to treat elevated blood glucose levels?

5. Does the patient treat low blood glucose levels with the appropriate amount of carbohydrates?

6. Has the personal lag time for insulin been determined?

7. Is the patient forgetting to administer bolus insulin for some meals?

8. Is the patient "guessing" what his or her preprandial glucose level is rather than actually performing a test before "guessing" how much insulin to administer for the meal?

9. Has the patient experienced any significant weight gain? If so, his or her insulin requirements will increase.

10. Is the patient taking any medications that may cause insulin resistance, abnormal blood glucose values, or A1C levels that do not appear to be reflective of the patient's overall glycemic control (see Chapter 7)?

11. Is the patient pregnant?

12. Does the patient have insulin requirements that appear to increase during menstruation?

13. Is the patient inserting the infusion set by hand or using the autoinserter?

14. Is the patient wearing the pump? (Some may refuse to wear the pump for employment reasons or they may stop using the pump while on vacation and never restart the pump.)

15. Make certain that another diagnosis is NOT being overlooked, such as hemochromatosis, Cushing's disease, sleep apnea, monogenetic diabetes, eating disorders, bipolar depression, or substance abuse.

16. Could the patient be using heat denatured or expired insulin?

Exercising with an Insulin Pump

Exercise is beneficial for patients with diabetes. The use of an insulin pump can facilitate the administration of insulin to maintain normoglycemia and avoid dangerous hypoglycemia after exercise. Exercise can result in initial hyperglycemia, followed by postexercise hypoglycemia. As exercise begins, free fatty acids are released from the adipose tissue as an initial source of energy. Within 10 minutes of beginning exercise, the liver accelerates the production and release of glucose, which provides skeletal muscles with a sustainable source of energy. If glucose levels increase in an insulinopenic patient who is already hyperglycemic (blood glucose level >240 mg per dL), exercise-induced ketosis may occur. Some individuals may need to give a small insulin bolus at the onset of exercise if their blood glucose level is more than 240 mg per dL.

An insulin pump can be worn during most exercise and sports activities. Precautions must be addressed in patients involved in contact sports. Patients need to be taught to make safe basal-rate alterations in preparation for exercise and how to prevent inadvertent disruption/dislocation of catheter or pump during intense exercise or sports activities.

Adjustments in basal insulin delivery while exercising should be individualized. The basic rule of thumb is that a well-conditioned athlete who is participating in the same activity for which he has been training rarely needs to alter the rate of insulin delivery or suspend the pump while exercising. However, a poorly conditioned individual who is embarking on a moderate or more intensive exercise regimen will need to reduce or suspend the insulin delivery while active. Patients should always check the blood glucose levels before beginning exercise and every 30 minutes during exercise to determine how a given activity might affect their glycemic control. The blood glucose should also be monitored immediately after exercising as well as 4 hours after completing the activity in case a delayed hypoglycemic response to the exercise develops. Blood glucose levels should be maintained in the target range of 120 to 180 mg per dL during the exercise program.

When exercising in the basal state (before breakfast or more than 4 hours after the previous meal), the basal infusion rate is initially reduced by 50%. Subsequently, the adjusted temporary basal infusion rate is adjusted according to self-monitoring blood glucose (SMBG). For example, if a patient with a usual basal rate of 1.6 U per hour jogs or cycles for 1 hour in the early morning before breakfast, this rate is reduced to 0.8 U per hour. After individual SMBG measurements, this temporary basal infusion rate can be further adjusted. Some athletes choose to decrease the infusion rate for 30 to 60 minutes during the postexercise period because of increased insulin sensitivity. In addition, the subsequent mealtime bolus is often reduced by 30% to 50%. When the insulin pump is continued during any exercise, the patient should monitor for hyperglycemia due to malfunction or dislodging of the infusion catheter. To limit weight gain, many exercising patients choose insulin adjustment rather than supplemental food intake.

With prolonged endurance exercise (e.g., hiking, walking, running, cycling), a "steady state" develops, and patients maintain plasma glucose levels within a predictable range while balancing carbohydrate intake and exercise. They may balance a low-dose temporary basal infusion rate with intermittent food to offset caloric expenditure. In this situation, the TBR is set at 0.1 to 0.2 U per hour. With experience, many patients maintain glucose levels between 100 and 140 mg per dL during several hours of activity.

A general guideline for carbohydrate consumption with exercise is 15 to 30 g every 30 to 60 minutes. Less insulin and fewer calories are required with improved fitness level and favorable environmental conditions. When the individual is exercising during weather extremes, adjustments in both basal insulin and caloric intake are often necessary. Exercising at a lower fitness level in cold weather may require more calories, whereas exercising in a hot environment may lead to hypoglycemia due to poor appetite and reduced caloric intake, suggesting a lower insulin requirement.

Antecedent hypoglycemia can blunt the metabolic counter-regulatory responses to recurrent episodes of rapidly falling blood glucose levels in patients with insulin requiring diabetes.[14] Patients with T1DM have shown a blunted neuroendocrine (catecholamine and glucagon), autonomic nervous system (muscle sympathetic activity), and metabolic (lipolysis and glucose kinetics) during exercise which occurs within hours of experiencing a mild hypoglycemic event.[80] Exercise-induced hypoglycemia is likely to induce "feed-forward cycles" of malglycemia, which may occur during sleep and are likely to be repeated the following day.

Patients who use insulin and exercise regularly should consider using continuous glucose sensors that monitor and alert the user to rapid change of interstitial glucose levels as shown in Figure 13-15. Table 13-15 summarizes recommendations for exercising with insulin pumps.

"Patch Pumps" and Futuristic Insulin Delivery Devices for Patients with T2DM

Several novel insulin pumps are being tested for use in patients with T2DM. Among them is the Valeritas h-Patch, the first disposable "patch pump" designed and FDA. The V-Go provides delivery of insulin both in preset basal rates and on-demand bolusing as shown in Table 13-16.

The V-Go is purely mechanical, does not require a battery-driven pump or external controller, and can be operated through clothing. Although the pump is user-friendly, only a single

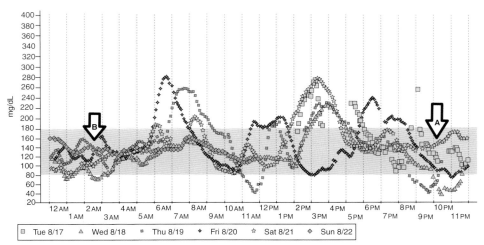

Figure 13-15 • **Exercise-Induced Hypoglycemia.** A 52-year-old patient with T1DM who uses an insulin pump and a continuous glucose sensor. The patient has very good glycemic control throughout the day. Six days each week, he performs 45 to 60 minutes of high-intensity cardiovascular conditioning at the gym from 6:00 to 7:00 PM and experiences postexercise hypoglycemia from 9:00 to 11:00 PM after 50% of his workouts are completed (*arrow* A). On one occasion during this 7-day interval, the patient also experienced an episode of nocturnal hypoglycemia from 2:10 to 2:45 AM (*arrow*, B). In response to this pattern of recurrent hypoglycemia, the patient was advised to reduce his insulin pump basal rate by 0.1 U per hour beginning 1 hour prior to exercise continuing until midnight. He was also given a secondary basal rate pattern to be used on days when he did not exercise, during which time the basal rate was maintained at 0.6 U per hour from 5:00 PM through 12:00 AM as he had been established previously. (Case supplied by Jeff Unger, MD)

predetermined basal flow of insulin may be deployed by each device. The primary drawback of V-Go pumping is that most patients will not receive optimal physiologic insulin delivery. Dual-wave mealtime bolusing is not possible with this pump. Likely candidates for V-Go pumps would be patients with T2DM who require basal insulin to augment the use of either oral agents or GLP-1 agonists.

 TABLE 13-15. **Recommendations for Exercising While Pumping Insulin**

- Check blood glucose at the time of exercise. The target blood glucose level for beginning exercise is 120–180 mg/dL. If the blood glucose is >240 mg/dL, check for urine ketones. If positive (+), delay or postpone exercise until ketones clear and blood glucose levels return to the target range. If ketones are negative (–), consider giving a small bolus of insulin before beginning exercise.

- If blood glucose levels are <120 mg/dL before exercise, consume 15 g of carbohydrates and begin a TBR, as described later.

- Check blood glucose 30–45 min after beginning to exercise in order to adjust insulin delivery for trending toward extreme hyperglycemia or hypoglycemia.

- Check blood glucose 2–4 h after completion of exercise to monitor for hypoglycemia.

- In general, physical conditioning over time reduces glycemic variability associated with exercise. Untrained athletes may experience more glucose fluctuations and become hypoglycemic after concluding exercise.

- If exercise times are consistent, basal rates may be lowered beginning at the onset of anticipated exercise and continued for 2–4 h after exercise is completed.

- Patients may choose to set a TBR while exercising. Reduce the prescribed basal rate by 50%–75% while exercising, and continue this TBR for 1–2 h after finishing the training.

- When possible, consider exercising while using a continuous glucose sensor.

TABLE 13-16. V-Go Pump Parameters

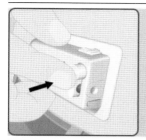 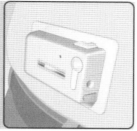

V-Go Pump	Maximum 24 h Basal Insulin Delivery (U-100 Insulin-Lispro, Aspart or Glulisine)	Preset Basal Delivery Rate (U/h)	Prandial Bolus Capabilities
V-Go 20	20 U	0.83	2-U increments up to 36 U/24 h
V-Go 30	30 U	1.25	2-U increments up to 36 U/24 h
V-Go 40	40 U	1.67	2-U increments up to 36 U/24 h

From http://www.valeritas.com. Accessed March 22, 2011., with permission.

The Calibra Finesse disposable pump (Fig. 13-16) provides only prandial insulin to patients with either T1DM or T2DM.[81] The device, which contains no electronics, is inserted subcutaneously once every 3 days. The pump reservoir contains 200 U of rapid-acting insulin analogue from which the bolus may be released by pressing two small buttons on each side of the device. Each press will release 1 or 2 U of insulin. Perspective patients include those who tend to forget their syringes, vials, or pen devices at home, individuals who attend business meetings and prefer discrete bolusing, or people who travel. Patch pumps allow patients to have access to a continuous supply of insulin and

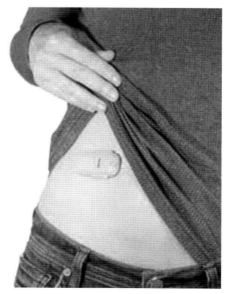

Figure 13-16 • **Calibra Finesse Disposable Pump. (Available at www.myfinesse.com)**

allow greater flexibility in daily activities. An extra pump may be carried by the patient and imme-diately inserted subcutaneously if the primary pump runs out of insulin.

The MedSolve Technologies Freehand pump is designed for use in patients with both T1DM and T2DM. This tubeless unit is considerably smaller than currently available devices, with a remote controller, allowing multiple basal rates as well as delivering small bolus increments. The pump is designed to be replaced every 3 months.[82] Other very small pumps in development include a novel device from Cellnovo, a Welsh company using microfluidics for drug delivery; a patch pump from Starbridge Systems; the NiliMEDIX single-use disposable pump, which may incorporate a CGM sen-sor; and the STMicroelectronics and Debiotech insulin nanopump that integrates a patch system with a separate electronic controller. This pump is smaller than traditional pumps, yet has a large insulin reservoir.

Another approach to basal insulin delivery being developed by Altea Therapeutics is the Pass-Port transdermal insulin patch.[83] Unlike other insulin pumps, the PassPort delivers insulin via trans-dermal absorption of the drug rather than by subcutaneous injection. Use of the transdermal patch may encourage early adoption of basal insulin therapy for patients with T2DM who prefer pump-ing over subcutaneous injections. These pumps may be useful in the future as well as for patients who wish to pump basal insulin and control prandial excursions with inhaled insulin. If a patient becomes hypoglycemic, the patch can be removed and blood glucose levels will rise. This company is also developing a transdermal exenatide preparation, and devices are being developed for delivery of glucagon-like peptide-1 and pramlintide as well as insulin.

New Integrated Pump Systems for Patients with T1DM or T2DM

Roche Diabetes Care is working on several types of insulin pumps that they hope to market in 2012. The "SOLO system" is a wireless semi-disposable patch micropump (Fig. 13-17). A 90-day reusable

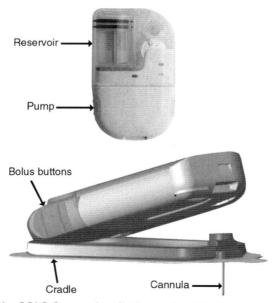

Figure 13-17 • Roche SOLO System Insulin Pump. The SOLO micropump consists of wireless remote controller, and a cradle with a built-in cannula. The 200 U insulin reservoir, which attaches to the disposable pump, is replaced every 2 days. The cradle is replaced every 90 days. (Roche Diabetes Care. Used with permission)

pump base stores all pump parameters so that boluses may be delivered with or without a remote activator. A SOLO pump base contains the electronics, memory, pump motor, bolus activator, and safety alarms. Although the pump base is designed to stay on the skin for 3 months, the disposable 200 U insulin reservoir is detachable and replaced every 2 to 3 days.[84]

The Accu-Chek Spirit Combo insulin pump interfaces with the Aviva blood glucose meter via *Bluetooth* wireless technology to assist the user in determining one's insulin dose based on carbohydrate intake and a blood glucose entry. By setting "time blocks" that correlate with specific activity levels one normally experiences throughout the day, bolus "advice" is provided and reviewed by the patient prior to delivery. Bolus advice may also be determined based on one's acceptable blood glucose target range during each time block, one's insulin to carbohydrate ratio, and the ISF to correct any aberrant readings prior to bolusing. The Aviva blood glucose meter also stores up to 1,000 data points that may be reviewed and downloaded with compatible software.

Steady progress has been made toward the development of the "artificial pancreas" fully automated, external, closed-loop system for insulin delivery (Fig. 13-18). Under experimental conditions, closed-loop glucose control using continuous glucose sensing, insulin pumps, and pump-controlled algorithms has demonstrated superiority over open-loop control in being able to achieve greater time within a designated glycemic target range with less treatment emergent hypoglycemia.[85]

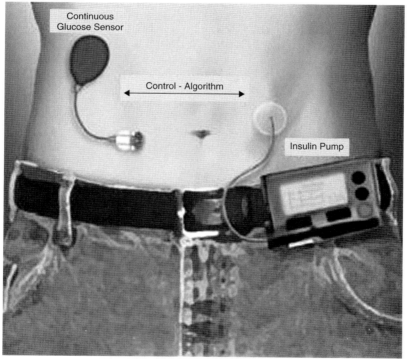

Figure 13-18 • **A Prototype of the Artificial Pancreas Closed-Loop Fully Automated Insulin Delivery Device.** The closed-loop system consists of an insulin pump, continuous glucose sensor and mathematically determined insulin delivery algorithms designed to minimize glycemic variability during exercise, rest, sleep, and the postprandial state.

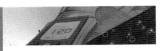

SUMMARY

Intensive diabetes management can be achieved with the use of insulin pump therapy. Compared with MDIs, CSII has better insulin pharmacokinetics, less variability in insulin absorption, and decreased risk of hypoglycemia. Patients using insulin pumps enjoy greater lifestyle flexibility and often become more proactive in their approach to diabetes self-management. Although more expensive than MDIs, pump therapy offers patients a much more physiologic approach to controlling their diabetes. Careful evaluation of pump candidates, patient education, and timely follow-up visits are vital to the success of pump therapy.

As we enter the dawn of a new age of diabetes management with mechanical sensors and pumps working in unison, improvement in glycemic control for patients with diabetes seems to be heading in a positive direction. Until a closed-loop feedback system between the pump and sensor is developed and marketed, basal bolus insulin therapy using an insulin pump remains state of the art. In the future, more patients with T2DM will be using patch pump or transdermal insulin delivery technology. With hundreds of thousands of satisfied and highly motivated American insulin pump users among our diabetes population, family physicians are very likely to see these patients in their practices. As a group, insulin pump patients experience better glycemic control and fewer long-term complications than patients using MDI. They are a pleasure to manage in clinical practice.

Appendix 13-1

Personalized Insulin Pump Parameter Form
Insulin Pump Setting Form

Name: _____   ID: _____

Date: _____   Age: _____

Insulin: Lispro   Aspart   Glulisine   U-500

Parameter: Setting:

Calculated TDD of Insulin (0.7 U per 24 hours × wt in kg) _____

Total calculated **bolus** insulin per 24 h (50% of TDD)

(Suggested initial bolus calculation: 0.1 U per kg per meal)

(Suggested initial bolus adjustment based on meal size, not carb content

- Large-size meal + dessert Add 3 U to immediate bolus
- Moderate-size meal Add 2 U to immediate bolus
- Slightly more than usual meal Add 1 to 2 U to immediate bolus
- Less than usual meal Subtract 1 to 2 U from immediate bolus

Total calculated **basal** insulin per 24 h (50% of TDD)

Insulin/Carb Ratio (500/TDD): _____

Insulin Sensitivity Factor (1,800/TDD): _____

1 U lowers BG _____ mg per dL

Target BG (Default value: 150 mg per dL)

Time 1 _____

Time 2 _____

Time 3 _____

Lag Time (15 minutes unless blood glucose is less than 80 mg per dL)
Or
Personal Lag Time

To determine personal lag time:

- Begin with a normal blood glucose value between 100 and 120 mg per dL
- Bolus insulin

Check blood glucose levels every 15 minutes until the starting blood glucose is reduced by 15 mg per dL. The time required for reduction from the baseline reading – 15 mg per dL = personal lag time

Change out insulin reservoir and infusion sets: every 2 days
                                                        every 3 days

Basal rate maximum setting/h =
Suggested boluses: Rate

Breakfast

Lunch

Dinner

Maximum bolus:

Rate

Extended   Dual Wave

Extended   **Time (over what time)**

Monitoring blood glucose levels should be performed (check all that apply):

- Before meals
- After meals (1, 2, 3 h)
- At bedtime
- At 3:00 AM
- Before/During/After exercise
- Before driving
- At 1 h after giving a supplemental (correction) insulin dose
- Structured glucose testing as follows:

Note: Bring your home blood glucose meter and structured glucose testing logs with you on each follow-up visit.

Appendix 13-2

2011 Medicare Laboratory Guidelines to Qualify for an External Insulin Pump

(A patient may qualify for an insulin pump under Medicare guidelines if they meet one of the following criteria):

- Positive Islet cell autoantibodies.
- A C-peptide value that can be not greater than 110% of the lowest value in the reference range. For example, if the lowest reference value is 0.8 ng per mL, the qualifying result can be equal to, but not greater than 0.88 ng per mL. The C-peptide result is valid *only* if accompanied by a *fasting* blood glucose drawn at the same time with a result that is ≤225 mg per dL.
- A patient with renal insufficiency may qualify for a pump under the following conditions:

  1. Serum creatinine is obtained.
  2. The C-peptide value is ≤200% of the lowest limit in the reference range for the patient to qualify. Thus, if the creatinine is 1.6 mg per dL, the lowest C-peptide reference value is 0.8 ng per mL, a C-peptide result ≤1.6 ng per mL would qualify the patient for a pump. The fasting blood glucose value of less than 225 mg per dL must be submitted with the C-peptide report.

REFERENCES

1. Weissbert-Benchell J, Antisdel-Lomaglio J, Seshadri R. Insulin pump therapy: a metaanalysis. *Diabetes Care*. 2003;26:1079–1087.
2. Graff MR, Rubin RR, Walker EA. How diabetes specialists treat their own diabetes: findings from a study of AADE and ADA membership. *Diabetes Educ*. 2000;26:460–467.
3. Boland EA, Greg M, Oesterle A, et al. Continuous subcutaneous insulin infusion: a new way to lower risk of severe hypoglycemia, improve metabolic control, and enhance coping in adolescents with type 1 diabetes. *Diabetes Care*. 1999;22:1779–1784.
4. Weinzimer S, Ahern J, Boland E, et al. Continuous subcutaneous insulin infusion is safe and effective in very young children with type 1 diabetes: program and abstracts of the 63rd Scientific Sessions of the American Diabetes Association; June 13–17, 2003. New Orleans, Louisiana: Abstract 1744-P.
5. Saudek C. Johns Hopkins Point-of-Care Information Technology Center. http://www.hopkins-diabetesguide.org/management/type_1_diabetes/full_insulin_pump_management.html?contentInstanceId =528245&siteId=496641 N10115. Accessed March 17, 2011.
6. Millennium Research Group. *US Markets for Drug Delivery 2005*. Toronto: Millenium Research Group; 2004.
7. Pickup JC, Keen H, Parsons JA, et al. The use of continuous subcutaneous insulin infusion to achieve normoglycaemia in diabetic patients [abstract]. *Diabetologia*. 1977;13:425A.
8. Bode BW, Tamborlane WV, Davidson PC. Insulin pump therapy in the 21st century: strategies for successful use in adults, adolescents, and children with diabetes. *Postgrad Med*. 2002;111. Online: URL: http://www.postgradmed.com/issues/2002/05_02/bode3.htm. Accessed November 13, 2005.
9. The Diabetes Control and Complications Trial Research Group. The effect of intensive treatment of diabetes on the development and progression of long-term complications in insulin-dependent diabetes mellitus. *N Engl J Med*. 1993;329:977–986.
10. Davis SN, Horton ES, Battelino T, et al. STAR 3 randomized controlled trial to compare sensoraugmented insulin pump therapy with multiple daily injections in the treatment of type 1 diabetes: research design, methods, and baseline characteristics of enrolled subjects. *Diabetes Technol Ther*. 2010;12:249–255.
11. Bergenstal RM, Tamborlane WV, Ahmann A, et al. Sensor-augmented pump therapy for A1C reduction (STAR 3) study: results from the 6-month continuation phase. *Diabetes Care*. 2011;34:2403–2405.
12. Choudhary P, Shin J, Wang Y, et al. Insulin pump therapy with automated insulin suspension in response to hypoglycemia: reduction in nocturnal hypoglycemia in those at greatest risk. *Diabetes Care*. 2011;34:2023–2025.
13. Nielsen JK, Djurhuus CB, Gravholt, et al. Continuous glucose monitoring in interstitial subcutaneous adipose tissue and skeletal muscle reflects excursions in cerebral cortex. *Diabetes* 2005;54:1635–1639.
14. Unger J, Parkin C. Recognition, prevention and proactive management of hypoglycemia in patients with type 1 diabetes. *Postgrad Med*. 2011;123(4):71–80.
15. Deiss D, Bolinder J, Riveline JP, et al. Improved glycemic control in poorly controlled patients with type 1 diabetes using real-time continuous glucose monitoring. *Diabetes Care*. 2006;29:2730–2732.
16. Zick R, Petersen B, Richter M, et al. SAFIR Study Group. Comparison of continuous blood glucose measurement with conventional documentation of hypoglycemia in patients with type 2 diabetes on multiple daily insulin injection therapy. *Diabetes Technol Ther*. 2007;9:483–449.
17. Castle JR, Pitts A, Hanavan K, et al. The accuracy benefit of multiple amperometric glucose sensors in people with type 1 diabetes. *Diabetes Care*. 2012;35(4):706–710.
18. Stratton IM, Adler AI, Neil HA, et al. Association of glycaemia with macrovascular and microvascular complications of type 2 diabetes (UKPDS 35): prospective observational study. *BMJ* 2000;321:405–412.
19. The Writing Team for the DCCT/EDIC Research Group. Effect of intensive therapy on the microvascular complications of type 1 diabetes mellitus. *JAMA* 2002;287:2563–2569.
20. Cryer PE. Hypoglycaemia: the limiting factor in the glycaemic management of type I and type II diabetes. *Diabetologia*. 2002;45:937–948.
21. Bode BW, Steed RD, Davidson PC. Reduction in severe hypoglycemia with long-term continuous subcutaneous insulin infusion in type I diabetes. *Diabetes Care*. 1996;19:324–327.
22. Nielsen S, Kain D, Szudzik E, et al. Use of continuous subcutaneous insulin infusion pump in patients with type 2 diabetes mellitus. *Diabetes Educ*. 2005;31:843–848.
23. Melki V, Renard E, Lassmann-Vague V, et al. Improvement of HbA1c and blood glucose stability in IDDM patients treated with lispro insulin analog in external pumps. *Diabetes Care*. 1998;21:977–982.

24. Downie E, Craig ME, Hing S, et al. Continued reduction in the prevalence of retinopathy in adolescents with type 1 diabetes: role of insulin therapy and glycemic control. *Diabetes Care.* 2011;34:2368–2373.

25. Hirsch IB, Brownlee M. Beyond hemoglobin A1c: need for additional markers of risk for diabetic microvascular complications. *JAMA.* 2010;303(22):2291–2292.

26. Unger J. A primary care approach to continuous subcutaneous insulin infusion. *Clin Diabetes.* 1999;7:113–120.

27. Camilleri M. Diabetic gastroparesis. *N Engl J Med.* 2007;356:820–829.

28. Fraser RJ, Horowitz M, Maddox AF, et al. Hyperglycaemia slows gastric emptying in type 1 (insulin-dependent) diabetes mellitus. *Diabetologia.* 1990;33:675–680.

29. Couturier O, Bodet-Milin C, Querellou S, et al. Gastric scintigraphy with a liquid-solid radiolabelled meal: performances of solid and liquid parameters. *Nucl Med Commun.* 2004;25:1143–1150.

30. Sharma D, Morrison G, Joseph F, et al. The role of continuous subcutaneous insulin infusion therapy in patients with diabetic gastroparesis. *Diabetologia.* 2011;54(11):2768–2770.

31. Aragona M, Giannarelli R, Coppelli A. Improvement in retinopathy in type 1 diabetic patients treated with continuous subcutaneous insulin infusion: program and abstracts of the 63rd Scientific Sessions of the American Diabetes Association; June 13–17, 2003, New Orleans, Louisiana, Abstract 435-P.

32. Wainstein J, Metzger M, Boaz M, et al. Insulin pump therapy vs. multiple daily injections in obese type 2 diabetic patients. *Diabet Med.* 2005;22:1037–1046.

33. Pickup J, Mattock M, Kerry S. Glycaemic control with continuous subcutaneous insulin infusion compared with intensive insulin injections in patients with type 1 diabetes: metaanalysis of randomized controlled trials. *Br Med J.* 2002;324:705–710.

34. Retnakaran R, Hochman J, DeVries JH, et al. Continuous subcutaneous insulin infusion versus multiple daily injections: the impact of baseline A1C. *Diabetes Care.* 1994;27:2590–2596.

35. Doyle EA, Weinzimer SA, Steffen AT, et al. A randomized, prospective trial comparing the efficacy of continuous subcutaneous insulin infusion with multiple daily injections using insulin glargine. *Diabetes Care.* 2004;27:1554–1558.

36. Bloomgarden Z. Aspects of insulin treatment. *Diabetes Care.* 2010;33(1):e1–e6.

37. Chantelau E, Spraul M, Muhlhauser I, et al. Long-term safety, efficacy and side effects of continuous subcutaneous insulin infusion treatment for type 1 (insulin-dependent) diabetes mellitus: a one centre experience. *Diabetologia.* 1989;32:421–426.

38. O'Connell SM, Cooper MN, Bulsara MK, et al. Reducing rates of severe hypoglycemia in a population-based cohort of children and adolescents with type 1 diabetes over the decade 2000–2009. *Diabetes Care.* 2011;34:2379–2380.

39. Shade DS, Valentine V. To pump or not to pump. *Diabetes Care.* 2002;25:2100–2102.

40. Rodbard HW, Schnell O, Unger J, et al. Use of an automated decision support tool optimizes clinicians ability to interpret and appropriately respond to structured self-monitoring of blood glucose data. *Diabetes Care.* 2012. doi: 10.2337/dc11-1351.

41. Unger J. Uncovering undetected hypoglycemic events. *Diabetes Metab Syndr Obes.* 2012;5(1):57–74.

42. Bode BW, Gross T, Steed D, et al. A recent assessment of continuation rates for continuous subcutaneous insulin infusion (CSII) [abstract 393]. *Diabetes.* 1998;21(suppl 1):393.

43. Gabbe SG, Holing E, Temple P, et al. Benefits, risks, costs, and patient satisfaction associated with insulin pump therapy for the pregnancy complicated by type 1 diabetes mellitus. *Am J Obstet Gynecol.* 2000;182:1283–1291.

44. Kanakis SJ, Watts C, Leichter SB. The business of insulin pumps in diabetes care: clinical and economic considerations. *Clin Diabetes.* 2002;20:214–216.

45. Medicare national coverage determinations manual. Chapter 1, Part 4 (Sections 200–310.1). Rev. 135, 09-22-11. http://www.cms.gov/manuals/downloads/ncd103c1_Part4.pdf. P. 126-127. Accessed November 21, 2011.

46. U.S. Food and Drug Administration, General Hospital and Personal Use Medical Devices Panel Insulin Infusion Pumps Panel Information, 2010.

47. Guilhem I, Leguerrier AM, Lecordier F, et al. Technical risks with subcutaneous insulin infusion. *Diabetes Metab.* 2006;32:279–284.

48. Abraham MR, al-Sharafi BA, Saavedra GA, et al. Lispro in the treatment of insulin allergy. *Diabetes Care.* 1999;22:1916–1917.

49. Ottensen JL, Nilsson P, Jami J, et al. The potential immunogenicity of human insulin and insulin analogues evaluated in transgenic mouse model. *Diabetologia.* 1994;37:1178–1185.

50. Patterson R, Lucena G, Metz R, et al. Reaginic antibody against insulin: demonstration of antigenic distinction between native and extracted insulin. *J Immunol*. 1969;103:1061–1071.
51. Oakley WG, Jones VE, Cunliffe AC. Insulin resistance. *Br Med J*. 1967;2:134–138.
52. Kahn CR, Rosenthal AS. Immunologic reactions to insulin: insulin allergy, insulin resistance, and the autoimmune insulin syndrome. *Diabetes Care*. 1979;2:283–295.
53. Schernthaner G, Borkenstein M, Fink M, et al. Immunogenicity of human insulin (Novo) or pork mono-component insulin in HLA-DR-typed insulin-dependent diabetic individuals. *Diabetes Care*. 1983;6 (suppl 1):43–48.
54. Fineberg SE, Kawabata TT, Finco-Kent D, et al. Immunological responses to exogenous insulin. *Endocr Rev*. 2007;28(6):625–652.
55. Dahl-Jorgensen K, Torjesen P, Hanssen KF, et al. Increase in insulin antibodies during continuous subcutaneous insulin infusion and multiple-injection therapy in contrast to conventional treatment. *Diabetes*. 1987;36:1–5.
56. Bolli GB, Kerr D, Thomas R, et al. Comparison of a multiple daily insulin injection (basal once daily glargine plus mealtime lispro) and continuous subcutaneous insulin infusion (lispro) in type 1 diabetes: a randomized open parallel multicenter study. *Diabetes Care*. 2009;32(7):1170–1176.
57. Misso ML, Egberts KJ, Page M, et al. Continuous subcutaneous insulin infusion (CSII) versus multiple insulin injections for type 1 diabetes mellitus. *Cochrane Database Syst Rev*. 2010;1:CD005103.
58. Grunberger G, Bailey TS, Cohen TM, et al. Statement by the American Association of Clinical Endocrinologists consensus panel on insulin pump management. *Endocr Pract*. 2010;16(5):747–762.
59. Monami M, Lamanna C, Marchionni N, et al. Continuous subcutaneous insulin infusion versus multiple daily injections in type 2 diabetes: a meta-analysis. *Exp Clin Endocrinol Diabetes*. 2009;117:220–222.
60. Unger J, Marcus A. Insulin pump therapy: what you need to know. *Emerg Med*. 2002;34:P24–P33.
61. Unger J. Preconception management of women with type 1 diabetes. *Female Patient* (OB/GYN edition). 2001;26:45–51.
62. Simmons D, Thompson CF, Conroy C, et al. Use of insulin pumps in pregnancies complicated by type 2 diabetes and gestational diabetes in a multiethnic community. *Diabetes Care*. 2001;24:2078–2082.
63. Lac G, Chamoux A. Elevated salivary cortisol levels as a result of sleep deprivation in a shift worker. *Occup Med*. 2003;53:143–145.
64. Unger J. Intensive management of type 1 diabetes. *Emerg Med*. 2001;33:30–42.
65. Bailon RM, Partlow BJ, Miller-Cage V, et al. Continuous subcutaneous insulin infusion (insulin pump) therapy can be safely used in the hospital in select patients. *Endocr Pract*. 2009;15:24–29.
66. Alemzadeh R, Ellis JN, Holzum MK, et al. Comparison of continuous subcutaneous insulin infusion (CSII) with flexible multiple daily insulin (FMDI) regimen using insulin glargine in pediatric type 1 diabetes mellitus: program and abstracts of the 63rd Scientific Sessions of the American Diabetes Association, June 13–17, 2003. New Orleans, Louisiana. Abstract 434-P.
67. Wilson D, Buckingham B, Kunselman E, et al. A two center randomized controlled trial of insulin pump therapy in young children with diabetes: program and abstracts of the 63rd Scientific Sessions of the American Diabetes Association, June 13–17, 2003. New Orleans, Louisiana. Abstract 1745-P.
68. Bryden KS, Neil A, Mayou RA, et al. Eating habits, body weight, and insulin misuse: a longitudinal study of teenagers and young adults with type 1 diabetes. *Diabetes Care*. 1999;22:1956–1960.
69. Jeitler K, Horvath K, Berghold A, et al. Continuous subcutaneous insulin infusion versus multiple daily insulin injections in patients with diabetes mellitus: systematic review and meta-analysis. *Diabetologia*. 2008;51(6):941–951.
70. Linkeschova R, Raoul M, Bott U, et al. Less severe hypoglycaemia, better metabolic control, and improved quality of life in Type 1 diabetes mellitus with continuous subcutaneous insulin infusion (CSII) therapy; an observational study of 100 consecutive patients followed for a mean of 2 years. *Diabetic Med*. 2002;19:746–751.
71. Roze S, Valentine WJ, Zakrzewska KE, et al. Health-economic comparison of continuous subcutaneous insulin infusion with multiple daily injection for the treatment of Type 1 diabetes in the UK. *Diabetic Med*. 2005;22(9):1239–1245.
72. Bode BW. Use of rapid-acting insulin analogues in the treatment of patients with type 1 and type 2 diabetes mellitus: insulin pump therapy versus multiple daily injections. *Clin Ther*. 2007;29(suppl D): S135–S144.
73. Hammond P, Liebl A, Grunderc S. International survey of insulin pump users: impact of continuous subcutaneous insulin infusion therapy on glucose control and quality of life. *Prim Care Diabetes*. 2007;1(3):143–146.

74. Lenhard M, Maser R. Success is relative: CSII in challenged patients: program and abstracts of the 63rd Scientific Sessions of the American Diabetes Association; June 13–17, 2003. New Orleans, Louisiana. Abstract 2129-PO.

75. Hirsch IB. Intensive treatment of type 1 diabetes. *Med Clin North Am*. 1998;82:689–719.

76. Bode B. Comparison of pharmacokinetic properties, physiochemical stability and pump compatibility of three rapid-acting insulin analogs: aspart, lispro and glulisine. *Endocr Pract*. 2011;17:271–280.

77. Knee TS, Seidensticker DF, Walton JL, et al. A novel use of U-500 insulin for continuous subcutaneous insulin infusion in patients with insulin resistance: a case series. *Endocr Pract*. 2003;9:181–186.

78. Brewer KW, Chase HP, Owen S, et al. Slicing the pie. Correlating HbA1C values with average blood glucose values in a pie chart form. *Diabetes Care*. 1998;21(2):209–212.

79. Corriveau EA, Durso PJ, Kaufman ED, et al. Effect of Carelink, an internet-based insulin pump monitoring system, on glycemic control in rural and urban children with type 1 diabetes mellitus. *Pediatr Diabetes*. 2008;9(4 Pt 2):360–366.

80. Briscoe VJ, Tate DB, Devisa SN. Type 1 diabetes: exercise and hypoglycemia. *Appl Physiol Nutr Metab*. 2007;32:(3):576–582.

81. http://www.myfinesse.com/.Accessed March 22, 2011.

82. Anhalt H, Bohannon NJV. Insulin patch pumps: their development and future in closed-loop systems. *Diabetes Technol Ther*. 2010;12(suppl 1):S51–S58.

83. http://www.alteatherapeutics.com/mediacoverage/OnDrugDelivery_Final.pdf- Accessed March 23, 2011.

84. http://www.roche.com/investors/ir_update/inv-update-2010-04-13.htm Accessed March 23, 2011.

85. Bruttomesso D, Farret A, Costa S, et al. Closed-loop artificial pancreas using subcutaneous glucose sensing and insulin delivery and a model predictive control algorithm: preliminary studies in Padova and Montpellier. *J Diabetes Sci Technol*. 2009;3:1014–1021.

14

Addressing Cultural Competency in Diabetes Care

These men ask for just the same thing,
fairness, and fairness only. This, so far as in
my power, they, and all others, shall have.
—*Abraham Lincoln, 16th U.S. president*

Introduction Primary care providers see patients of all ages, ethnicities, sexual orientations, educational levels, psychological profiles, and religious beliefs. This chapter examines how being culturally competent can optimize care management for virtually all patients afflicted with diabetes.

Cultural competency is defined as having "awareness of and sensitivity to cultural differences; knowledge of cultural values, beliefs, and behaviors; and skill in working with culturally diverse populations."[1] The first step in developing cultural competency is understanding the distinction between *race* and *culture*. Race refers to specific populations defined by unique physical characteristics, whereas culture refers to the shared beliefs, values, customs and behaviors of specific populations.

Although race and culture are often interrelated, there is a tendency to stereotype patients' cultural influences based solely upon their race. This can result in misunderstanding and miscommunication because patients of different races may, in fact, share the same culture. For example, Cuban Americans represent several races—Africans, Latinos and whites—yet, they are all influenced by the shared values and customs associated with Cuban culture.

The characteristics that best define a culturally competent provider include (1) one whose practice is based upon value diversity, (2) one who has the capacity and willingness for cultural diversity self-assessment, (3) one who possesses a knowledge base that includes the fundamental philosophical, religious, and family values related to the cultural groups to which treatment is rendered, and (4) one who adapts one's professional service delivery to reflect the needs of the cultures that are being treated.

Valuing diversity implies that one has accepted and developed a respect toward cultural and ethnic differences. Not all ethnic groups respond equally to evidence-based treatment protocols. Asian Americans, for example, are highly insulin resistant despite having a physical appearance that suggests ideal metabolic functioning.

Traditions that have been passed on through generations may strongly influence a patient's approval of therapeutic options. Adherence to prescribed therapies is greatly influenced by family dynamics, religious beliefs, immigrant status, and literacy comprehension rates. During the Islamic calendar's holy month of Ramadan, Muslims fast from dawn to sunset, a gesture that is thought to figuratively burn away all sins. Yet this can be a challenge for Muslims with diabetes: a large epidemiologic study conducted in 13 Islamic countries on 12,243 individuals with diabetes who fasted during Ramadan showed a high rate of acute complications (DKA, hypoglycemia, dehydration and thrombosis).[2] Table 14-1 presents recommendations for managing glycemic control in Muslim patients during fasts.

Cultural self-assessment implies that a conscious effort be made by the practitioner to customize interviewing and physical examining techniques consistent with the patient's ethnic, cultural, and religious values. The most important actions that must be adopted during cultural diversity training are usually taken for granted. For instance, comfortable physical distance during social interactions varies by culture. Sitting too far away from a gay couple could infer an anxious attitude on the part of the examiner. Elderly Native American patients will typically discourse in a slow speech pattern that may also make the examiner feel uncomfortable and hurried. Yet attempting to speed up the conversation would be a sign of disrespect.

Even shaking hands with a patient upon entering the room may influence how the clinician is perceived from a cultural perspective. In some cultures, an excessively firm grip on a patient's hand

TABLE 14-1. Suggested Guidelines for Managing Diabetes during Ramadan and Public Fasting Days on the Jewish Calendar

- Frequent blood glucose self-monitoring is required of all patients using insulin.

- The common practice of ingesting large amounts of foods rich in carbohydrate and fat, especially at the sunset meal, should be avoided. Because of the delay in digestion and absorption, ingestion of foods containing "complex" carbohydrates may be advisable at the predawn meal, while foods with more simple carbohydrates may be more appropriate at the sunset meal.

- Normal levels of physical activity may be maintained. However, excessive physical activity may lead to higher risk of hypoglycemia and should be avoided, particularly during the few hours before the sunset meal.

- Patients must immediately end the fast if they become hypoglycemic (blood glucose, 60 mg/dL) or if the blood glucose level reaches <70 mg/dL within the first few hours of initiating the fast especially if insulin or a sulfonylurea is being used.

- No fasts should be undertaken on "sick days."

- Use of a medical alert bracelet is strongly encouraged.

- Patients with wide glycemic variability should not fast.

- Patients with T1DM who insist on fasting should be placed on an insulin pump and a continuous glucose sensor, which will alarm in response to either a rapid decrease in blood glucose or an actual hypoglycemic event.

- In patients with T2DM who are well controlled with diet alone, the risk associated with fasting is quite low. However, there is still a potential risk for occurrence of postprandial hyperglycemia after the predawn and sunset meals if patients overindulge in eating. Distributing calories over two to three smaller meals during the non-fasting interval may help prevent excessive postprandial hyperglycemia.

- Elderly patients should consume extra fluids during non-fasting times to minimize the risk of dehydration and thrombosis.

Adapted from Al-Arouj M, Bouguerra R, Buse J, et al. Recommendations for management of diabetes during ramadan. *Diabetes Care.* 2005;28(9):2305–2311.

is perceived as an attempt to demonstrate intellectual and personal superiority over that individual, whereas use of a lighter grip suggests equality.

Cultural self-assessment takes time and practice. Patient clinicians will learn how effective use and interpretation of "body language" may be used to their advantage to improve patients' diabetes care.

Many factors may influence cross-cultural (clinician vs. patient) interactions. For example, biases based on historical cultural experiences can explain some patients' reluctance to comply with chronic care interventions. Some Native American tribal members may blame the "white man" for bringing diabetes to their people, while anyone who remembers the "Tuskegee Study of Untreated Syphilis in the Negro Male" can see that ethnicity can affect standards of care. This study, conducted by the Public Health Service in 1932, attempted to record the natural history of syphilis in hopes of justifying a treatment programs for blacks. The study initially involved 600 black men—399 with syphilis and 201 who served as "healthy controls." The study was conducted *without* the benefit of patients' informed consent. Researchers told the men they were being treated for "bad blood," a local term used to describe several ailments, including syphilis, anemia, and fatigue. However, patients never received treatment for syphilis. This study, which was originally projected to last 6 months, was continued for over 40 years. When penicillin became the drug of choice for treating syphilis in 1947, researchers did not provide this treatment option to the Tuskegee subjects. In 1974, a $10 million out-of-court settlement was reached. As part of the settlement, the U.S. government promised to give lifetime medical benefits and burial services to all living participants.[3] The Tuskegee Study led to important federal regulations related to human clinical trials. All patients who participate in a clinical trial are now required to sign informed consent. Institutional Review Boards (IRBs) provide oversight and protection for all subjects who participate as volunteers in human clinical trials.

The integration of ethnic and cultural dynamics into one's practice will relax patient barriers toward diabetes self-management. Culturally competent practices are able to provide unique services to patients suffering from a globally epidemic disorder. Medical practices that service diverse populations will certainly grow as a result of their attempts to become culturally competent.

Estimates of complementary and alternative medicine (CAM) use in individuals with diabetes are comparable to those with other common chronic medical disorders.[4] In one study, 57% of individuals with diabetes who used CAM discussed it with their regular physician and 43% were actually referred to CAM users by a physician.[4] This is reassuring because it means that patients with diabetes are not abandoning conventional treatments, which have been rigorously tested, for unconventional treatments, which lack properly designed efficacy trials. Enterprising PCPs will acknowledge CAM use by their patients and allow them to incorporate modalities that may augment traditional therapeutic options.

Culturally competent practices should strive to develop tools that enhance education of divergent patient populations. Group diabetes classes targeting specific ethnic or religious populations within a given community may be developed. (See Chapter 1 for tips on establishing group diabetes visits.). Certified Diabetic Educators may be selected to assist with the group sessions. High-risk patients who attend the group sessions may even be screened for diabetes complications that are highly prevalent within that selected patient population. The possibilities for enhancing one's practice by targeting cultural competency are electrifying and well within the realm of primary care.

■ Barriers to Health Care

Many minority populations face cultural obstacles to the acquisition of health care. Although some assume that the American system of health care is universally accepted and accessible, for a variety of reasons, ethnic minorities receive suboptimal care in the United States. Barriers to care include patients' and providers' cultural beliefs and misalignment between the American health-care system and culturally based health assumptions.

• Delays in Seeking Health Care

Delays in seeking care in a timely manner are an essential barrier and may be culturally based. Some cultures believe that diabetes indicates a failure to live properly, represents a lack of spiritual strength, or is a punishment for immoral behavior.[1] Patients who resist seeking health care because they associate illness with a morally inferior lifestyle deny themselves timely access to care.

• Cultural Beliefs versus American Health-care Attitudes

Violation of cultural ideals by American health-care attitudes is another barrier against early diabetes diagnosis and intensive therapeutic intervention. Sound diabetes management is based upon integrating healthy lifestyle choices with appropriate and timely pharmacologic therapies. In the ideal world, patients should eat well balanced meals, exercise for 30 minutes 5 days a week, lose 7 to 10 lb when advised to do so by their physician and get 6 to 8 hours of uninterrupted sleep each night. Doctors expect that all of their patients should become phenotypic clones of the late Jack LaLanne after one to two consultations. If everyone in the world possessed Jack LaLanne's genetic good fortune, there would probably be no need for physicians!

Cultural diversity demands that clinicians carefully assess each patient to determine their individual glycemic and metabolic baseline and targeted goals. An Asian American patient, for example, may have a BMI of only 24 kg per m^2, yet be diagnosed with diabetes and hypertriglyceridemia. This hesitant patient may even argue his or her case against having diabetes by saying, "I thought only heavy people have diabetes and I'm not even overweight!"

The clinician will need to be forthright in explaining the ethnic differences in BMIs between Asians and non-Asian Americans. Non-white Hispanics may view slight obesity as a sign of being healthy rather than carrying risk for diabetes or cardiovascular disease (CVD).[1] Although much evidence links obesity and T2DM, patients who consider weight control measures to be contrary to their cultural ideals may devalue the advice of their physician. PCPs must exercise care in offering health-care advice to their patients to avoid conflicts between their patients' cultural beliefs and any preexisting notions of the superiority of the traditional American approach to medical care.

▌ Race and Racial Disparities

• Diabetes Prevalence

Diabetes touches Americans from all walks of lives. The *defenseless* pancreatic β-cell is an equally opportunistic target of apoptosis and disease progression regardless of age, race, gender, family history, or lifestyle choices. That being said, certain ethnic populations are disproportionately affected by diabetes. The prevalence of diabetes is two to six times higher among Hispanic Americans, African Americans, Native Americans, and Asian Americans than among white Americans. The National Institutes of Health reports that Native Americans are 2.2 times more likely to have diabetes than are non-Hispanic whites.[5] Even among Native Americans, diabetes prevalence rates vary, ranging from 6% in Alaskan Natives to 29.3% in the Pima Indians living in southern Arizona.[5]

From 1997 to 2009 the age-adjusted incidence of diagnosed diabetes was 8.5/1,000 among whites, 11.7/1,000 among blacks, and 13.1/1,000 among Hispanics in patients aged 18 to 79 as shown in Figure 14-1. The prevalence of diabetes by race from 1980 to 2009 is shown in Figure 14-2.

Trends in immigration suggest that the number of Latino, African, and Asian Americans will rise. Currently, Latino Americans make up 12.5% of the population, followed by African Americans at 12.3%, and Asian Americans at 3.6%. By 2050, 30% of the U.S. adult population will have diabetes. Thus, the number of adults aged 20 and older with diabetes will have increased 165% from 11 million (prevalence of 4%) in 2000 to 29 million in 2050. The fastest growing ethnic group with diagnosed diabetes is expected to be black males (+363% from 2000 to 2050), with black females (+217%), white males (+148%), and white females (+107%) following.[6]

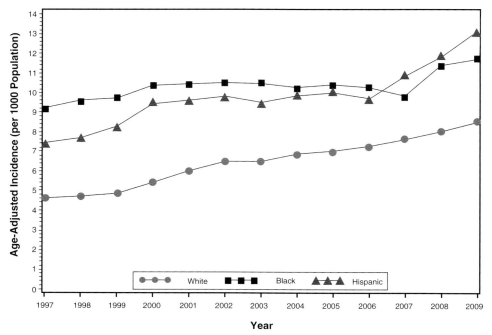

Figure 14-1 • **Age-Adjusted Incidence of Diagnosed Diabetes per 1,000 Population Aged 18 to 79 Years by Race/Ethnicity in the United States 1997 to 2009.**
Reference: Centers for Disease Control and Prevention. Data and Trends. http://www.cdc.gov/diabetes/statistics/incidence/fig6.htm. Accessed January 8, 2012.

• Metabolic Parameters

Successful management of diabetes requires implementation of the most appropriate lifestyle and pharmacologic interventions that will allow each patient to achieve his or her customized glycemic, blood pressure, and cholesterol targets. Epidemiologic data suggest that metabolic parameters are achieved more often among white patients with diabetes than blacks and non white Hispanics.[7]

Working with patient data from a large managed care population, Brown and colleagues found that mean A1C was significantly higher among Latinos (8.1%, $p < 0.0001$), Asians/Pacific Islanders (8.1%, $p < 0.0001$), and African Americans (7.9%, $P = 0.0009$) than among white Americans (7.7%). Mean LDL was higher among African Americans than among white Americans (118 vs. 111 mg per dL, $p < 0.0001$), and African Americans were also more likely to have inadequate blood pressure control (greater than 140/90 mm Hg) than were white Americans (55.5% vs. 44.1%, $p < 0.0001$).

• Physiologic Disparities

Although practice guidelines for the diagnosis and management of diabetes provide a valuable resource for physicians, they often fail to emphasize key physiologic differences among the various ethnic populations that can impact care. For example, first-generation Asian Americans tend to have lower body weight and BMI measurements, yet they have a greater prevalence of T2DM than the general population. Compared with whites, Asian Americans are more likely to be overweight but less likely to be obese after applying the modified Asian criteria (Table 14-2). Yet, considered as an ethnic population, Asian Americans are approximately 30% more likely to have T2DM than their white counterparts.[8] PCPs who fail to screen for diabetes in Asian American patients having a BMI of ≥23 kg per m[2] could miss the diagnosis in this high-risk population.

Even at BMI ranges thought to be acceptable, the risk of diabetes may be markedly underestimated in non-white ethnic groups, several of which appear to be particularly sensitive to weight gain in

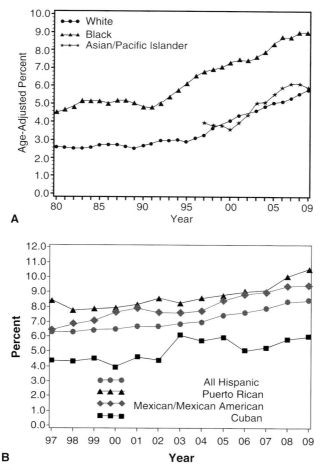

Figure 14-2 • A. Prevalence of Diabetes Among Whites, Blacks, and Asian/Pacific Islanders from 1980 to 2009. B. Prevalence of Diabetes Among Non white Hispanic Populations from 1997 to 2009.
Reference: Centers for Disease Control and Prevention. Data and Trends. http://apps.nccd.cdc.gov/DDT-STRS/default.aspx. Accessed January 9, 2012.)

terms of diabetes risk. As shown in Figure 14-3, for the equivalent incidence of diabetes at BMI of 30 kg per m^2 for white subjects, the BMI cutoff values are 24 for South Asians, 25 for Chinese, and 26 for black subjects.[9] A population shift from the normal to the obese BMI range could theoretically result in a 12-fold increase in the incidence of diabetes among the Asian population groups compared with a four- to sixfold increase in diabetes in other ethnic groups.

 TABLE 14-2. National Heart, Lung, and Blood Institute and World Health Organization Guidelines for Defining Obesity

BMI (kg/m²)	Obesity Category	Asian Standard (kg/m²)
<18.5	Underweight	<18.5
18.5–24.9	Normal weight	18.5–22.9
25 to ≤30	Overweight	23 to ≤27.5
≥30	Obese	>27.5

From World Health Organization Expert Consultation. Appropriate body-mass index for Asian populations and its implications for policy and intervention strategies. *Lancet.* 2004;363:157–163.
NHLBI Obesity Education Initiative: http://www.nhlbi.nih.gov/guidelines/obesity/prctgd_c.pdf. Assessed January 9, 2012.

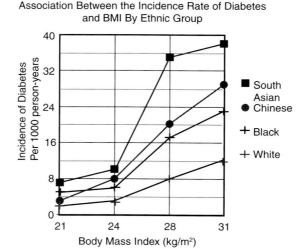

Association Between the Incidence Rate of Diabetes and BMI By Ethnic Group

Figure 14-3 • For the equivalent incidence rate of diabetes at BMI of 30 kg per m² for white subjects, the BMI cutoff values are 24 for South Asians, 25 for Chinese, and 26 for black subjects. (Adapted from Chiu M, Austin PC, Manuel DG, et al. Deriving ethnic-specific BMI cutoff points for assessing diabetes risk. *Diabetes Care*. 2011;34:1741–1748.)

Several hypotheses have been suggested to explain why Asian Americans may have a higher risk of diabetes than other ethnic groups. Asians may be more susceptible to inheritance of the "thrifty gene" because their ancestors were more likely to be exposed to extended periods of starvation. The thrifty gene was advantageous during feast or famine cycles as it enabled individuals to store calories more efficiently as food became scarce. Today, where high-fat and high-calorie foods are readily accessible, the thrifty gene may make weight control difficult under non-starvation conditions.[10]

Genetic susceptibility to insulin resistance as well as higher central adiposity at similar BMI levels also favors increased risk of developing T2DM in Asians. Adaptation of the sedentary Western lifestyle has undoubtedly promoted a trend toward diabetes on a global scale. Each 2-hour per day increment of time spent watching television is associated with a 14% increase in diabetes risk, whereas each 1-hour per day of brisk walking reduces the risk of diabetes by 34%.[11] In all ethnic populations, the diabetes epidemic may be contained simply by having at-risk patients incorporate weight management and moderately intense exercise into their daily routines. Primary prevention of T2DM should become a global primary care initiative.

Quality Improvement in Medical Care Delivery May Not Lead to More Equitable Care for Patients With Diabetes

In the ideal world, physicians attempt to improve the quality, expand access, and eliminate disparities in their health-care delivery. Yet, the improvements observed in health-care quality over the past decade have not translated into more equitable care, because high-risk diabetes population groups are less likely to have access to specialized diabetes care providers.[12] NHANES data from 1999 to 2006 suggest that rates of blood pressure control were significantly lower and mean systolic blood pressure was significantly higher for black and non-white Hispanic adults than for white adults with hypertension. Among adults with diabetes, rates of glycemic control were lower and A1C levels were higher for black and non-white Hispanics. Glycemic control was worse for less educated adults. Interestingly, near-universal Medicare coverage for patients after age 65 *improved* disease control for greater numbers of minorities and less educated adults. This suggests that the underinsured or intermittently insured patients may benefit from acquiring access to some form of health-care coverage.[12,13]

Patient-centered Diabetes Care-based Cultural and Religious Diversity

The foundation of effective chronic disease management relies upon effective communication between patients and their providers. Cultural competency becomes the ally of the clinician, who may increase the health literacy of his or her diverse patient population. Culturally competent clinicians develop flexibility toward their personal attitudes and beliefs, which helps direct their patients toward achieving their targeted metabolic goals. Providers should address both the strengths and weaknesses of each patient's self-management skill set. Interventions that incorporate ethnic and cultural ideologies are likely to result in successful outcomes.

• Native Americans

Historically, diabetes prevalence rates were very low among Native Americans prior to 1940. The epidemic of T2DM within the Native American population, which began in the 1960s, corresponds with the westernization of many of these tribal members. Daily caloric consumption increased and energy expenditure declined.

In the 1950s, the Cornell University Medical Team provided care and conducted physical examinations for the majority of the members of the Many Farms Navajo community in North Eastern Arizona and found few cases of T2DM. When comparison data were collected once again in 1988, the 168,000 inhabitants at this site were found to be 10 times more likely to have developed diabetes than were members of their previous generation. Key changes in the community included a reliance on the federally subsidized commodities food program that distributed excess farm produce, consisting primarily of refined flour, cheese, lard, and refined sugar. The recent conceptualization of fry bread as a traditional Native American food is largely a result of the commodities food distribution program established by the Agricultural Act of 1949.[14] These factors, coupled with a dramatic reduction in physical activity resulting from altered traditional work patterns and greater access to fast foods, have resulted in an epidemic of diabetes in this and other Native American communities.[15] Thus, the purchase and donation of surplus commodities by the U.S. government to the Agricultural Department are believed to have triggered the explosive epidemic of diabetes within the Native American population. Prior to 1950, Native Americans were busy farming their own lands and caring for their own needs. Because the Federal Government continues to provide high-fat food to tribes at no cost, the recipients of the free commodities have determined that farming their own lands is no longer cost-effective. Thus, the Federal Government has eliminated all incentives for primary prevention of T2DM by giving this high-risk population free food that is high in fat and carbohydrates! Native Americans stop farming because they cannot compete with the Federal Government. There is little incentive to work within some tribal communities because they are receiving financial support and free medical care from the government. Meanwhile, the aggregate weight of the population increases and boredom begins to set in. People with extra time on their hands may indulge in alcohol intake, which increases their blood pressure and weight even further. Is the white man to blame for increasing the prevalence of diabetes within the Native American population? One could clearly identify why Native Americans might mistrust the "white man."

The impact of diabetes within the Native American populace is staggering. Native Americans are nearly three times more likely to be diagnosed with diabetes than non-Hispanic whites of similar ages. Up to 70% of Native Americans ages 45 to 74 have diabetes. The incidence of T2DM in Native American youths ages 15 to 19 has increased 54% since 1996.[16]

Native Americans have a higher prevalence of many of the complications associated with diabetes. The high prevalence of T2DM, combined with a poorer prognosis, contributes to a disproportionately high and increasing diabetes mortality rate among Native American populations. In New Mexico, diabetes-related mortality increased by 564% and 1,110% for Native American men and women, respectively, from 1958 to 1994.[17,18] Using the 2005 MarketScan health expenditure for an adult with average risk ($3,050), a U.S. adult with diabetes was estimated to cost approximately

TABLE 14-3. Considerations for Patients of Different Cultural Backgrounds

Ethnic Population	Cultural Modifications Targeting Patient Interviews	Cultural Modifications Targeting Physical Examinations	Belief Systems Related to Diabetes	Cultural Issues that May Conflict with Allopathic Patient Management
Native Americans	Use indirect communication. Rather than respond by saying, "You should" one should say, "Someone with a similar problem as yours would consider this type of treatment…" Listening is valued over talking. Slow down when speaking. Long periods of silence between speakers is common. Do not interrupt, especially if the speaker is elderly. Eye contact is not direct or only briefly direct. Gaze may be directed over the shoulder.	Modesty and privacy are valued. Permission should be obtained before examination of each area. Care should be taken to keep the body covered. In some reservations clothes are removed only if absolutely necessary.	Belief that diabetes results from consuming too much sugar or too much food in general. Having diabetes indicates a failure to live properly due to a lack of spiritual strength. Patients feel shamed by the diagnosis and are reluctant to tell friends or family. Suggest, "Eat less sugar. Become more active."	Monitor for use of herbs, some of which can cause hypoglycemia such as nopal (prickly pear cactus) and hintonia (copalquin). Hintonia can also cause liver failure. Sharing of medicine between family members is common. Patients may discontinue medications when they "feel better." "Cost of medications may be a factor in urban or rural areas, where IHS benefits are not available Patients are taught traditionally to withstand pain for survival. They are generally undertreated for acute and chronic pain. Some IHS facilities are short on staff, lack efficiency, and do not practice patient-centered care. The time spent waiting to see a midlevel practitioner adds to the frustration that patients feel regarding diabetes self-management.
Asian Americans	Direct interrogation of physicians by patients is a sign of disrespect Disagreeing with a PCP is disrespectful Speak in short, simple sentences Ask close-ended questions ("yes" and "no").	"Low touch society." Explain what will transpire during a physical exam.	Family obligations trump personal health needs. Explain that "body is out of balance," which is affecting the patient's ability to function normally Advise family to use foods that "can restore balance."	Monitor for traditional herbal remedies. Non adherence common due to use of TCM herbs.

| African Americans | Eye contact important during the history and any discussion point. When entering the exam room, do not stand while interviewing patient. Maintain eye level interview to minimize appearance of cultural superiority and affect trust. Proactively question about erectile dysfunction in men or sexual dysfunction in women. | Prostate exam in males age 40 and up Higher risk of chronic kidney disease and cancers. Screen when appropriate. Screen for glaucoma, especially in patients with a positive family history | Some research has shown that African Americans have a strong sense of living in the present, willingly accept obesity as the norm, and express the view that T2DM is hereditary and therefore cannot be prevented. Elderly patients may be less trusting of physicians. Patients remember the Tuskegee experiment. Trust must be earned. Belief that religion may have an impact on disease could delay intensification of treatment. | Religious teachings suggest that patient developed diabetes due to living a "prior" life of sin. If patient believes in reincarnation, the thought of having diabetes may therefore be embarrassing. The patient will opt against using insulin or checking blood glucose levels in public. Avoid speaking to patients in public about their diabetes. | If patient becomes non adherent in regards to medical regimen or home blood glucose monitoring ask patient about financial burden of medications. Consider co-pay cards when appropriate. |

(Continued)

Table 14-3. Considerations for Patients of Different Cultural Backgrounds *(Continued)*

Ethnic Population	Cultural Modifications Targeting Patient Interviews	Cultural Modifications Targeting Physical Examinations	Belief Systems Related to Diabetes	Cultural Issues that May Conflict with Allopathic Patient Management
Latino American	Indirect eye contact preferred and is a show of "respect" toward the clinician Start interview with "small talk" rather than rapidly interrogating the patient Use "proper names" such as Senor or Senora rather than the patient's first name. Sit or stand in close proximity to the patient to show respect	Explain link between "stress" and disease. Explain that improved blood glucose control will likely improve symptomatology (blurred vision, fatigue, erectile dysfunction, parenthesis, nocturia, and reduce dry skin). Do NOT attempt to scare patients into using medications by mentioning that failure to treat diabetes aggressively is likely to result in long-term complications When shaking hands with patients, avoid a firm grip as this would imply that the clinician is attempting to "overpower" them. Simply put your hand forward and have the patient apply the pressure.	Anger or strong emotions may predispose one's body to develop diabetes but is not the specific trigger for inducing acute or chronic hyperglycemia	Herbal remedies often used, but not often disclosed to clinician for fear of being "scolded." Patients may adopt a fatalist attitude toward diabetes, believing their future is "in God's hands." This may increase likelihood of non adherence.
Observant Jews	Direct communication acceptable and respected	Modesty and privacy must be respected especially when examining members of the opposite sex. Asking permission when examining patients is suggested. Chaperone, or patient's husband should be present when examining a female patient.	Patients respect and accept the treatment protocols prescribed by physicians.	Patients believe that their bodies are shrines on loan from God. They must do whatever possible to protect their bodies and keep themselves as healthy as possible.

	Avoid scheduling appointments on Friday afternoon, which may interfere with the celebration of the Sabbath. Observant Jews may only walk on the Sabbath and may not accept any other mode of transportation.			For patients with no contraindications to prolonged fasting, alterations in insulin and oral agent regimens may be necessary for Jewish holidays, such as Yom Kippur. Using an ultra long basal insulin, such as degludec or IDegAsp might be useful. Insulin pumping may be continued while fasting using the patient's standard basal rate profile.
LGBT patients	Avoid sitting farther from the patient than necessary Develop a comfort level using terms such as "husband" "spouse" "wife" "partner"	High risk of alcohol abuse (binge drinking), cigarette smoking, polycystic ovary syndrome, depression, suicide ideation, obesity, HIV, and insulin resistance. Don't forget pap smears and cancer screening.	Management of diabetes may take a back seat other psychosocial issues.	Patients who are being treated for HIV often have significant insulin resistance. Binge drinking, common in Lesbian patients with T1DM, can develop severe hypoglycemia.

References
1. Ahn AC, Ngo-Metzger Q, Legedza AT, et al. Complementary and alternative medical therapy use among Chinese and Vietnamese Americans: prevalence, associated factors, and effects of patient-clinician communication. *Am J Public Health.* 2006;96(4):647–653.
2. ETHNOGERIATRIC CURRICULUM MODULE. Stanford University. http://www.stanford.edu/group/ethnoger/americanindian.html. Accessed February 6, 2011.
3. American Jewish Diabetes noes Association. http://www.jewishdiabetes.org/alon/kippur_english.pdf. Accessed February 8, 2011.
4. Gavin JR, Wright EE. Building cultural competency for improved diabetes care: African Americans and diabetes. *J Fam Pract.* 2007;56(9):S22–S28.
5. Caballero EA, Tenzer P. Building cultural competency for improved diabetes care: Latino Americans and diabetes. *J Fam Pract.* 2007;56(9):S29–S38.
6. Garnero TL. Providing culturally sensitive diabetes care and education for the Lesbian, Gay, Bisexual, and Transgender (LGBT) community. *Diabetes Spectrum.* 2010;23(3):178–182.

$12,800 during 2005 and an American Indian adult with diabetes approximately $19,260.[19] Diabetes management alone comprises over 40% of the total federal Indian Health Service (IHS) budget of $1.46 billion.[16] The morbidity burden among Native Americans with diabetes far exceeds that of commercially insured U.S. adults with diabetes. Considering the disproportionate burden of T2DM within this ethnic group, primary care interventions should mandate screening high-risk individuals for prediabetes. Those patients identified as having impaired fasting glucose or impaired glucose tolerance should be introduced to a comprehensive program designed to restore normal β-cell function through weight loss, increased physical activity, and intensive pharmacotherapy if one's A1C exceeds 6.0%. Patients should be advised to discontinue their use of alcohol and nicotine. Obese patients should also be screened for the presence of obstructive sleep apnea (see Chapter 8).

The IHS provides health services to more than 300,000 American Indians and Alaska Natives throughout the United States with diabetes.[20] The 2010 IHS annual budget of more than $4.05 billion equates to approximately $2,700 per individual (compared with $6900 per capita personal health-care expenditures for the total U.S. population.[21] In 1997, Congress passed legislation to create Special Diabetes Program for Indians (SDPI) to provide additional IHS funding for diabetes prevention and treatment programs, funding nearly 400 diabetes programs in American Indian and Alaska Native communities in 2007.[20] Since the enactment of SDPI, intermediate clinical outcomes (e.g., blood glucose, blood pressure, and cholesterol levels) among American Indians and Alaska Natives with diabetes have improved, and the rate of diabetes-related end-stage renal disease has decreased.[19]

Many Native American tribes (e.g., Ojibwa, Cree, Dakota, Navajo, Kiowa, Ute), believe that diabetes is, in fact, a new disease introduced by the "white man." Tribal belief is that diabetes results from a state of imbalance caused by consuming too much sugar, overeating, drinking alcohol, and behaving immorally. Because one should strive to follow a righteous and spiritual life, being diagnosed with diabetes may imply a personal failure to achieve a productive and virtuous life. Those afflicted with diabetes may feel ashamed by a diagnosis that they may be reluctant to share openly with family or friends.[22]

The severity of a chronic illness is judged by the amount of pain, disability, and discomfort it causes. Those who suffer most tend to seek comfort from a spiritual leader's ritual healing interventions and the use of herbal remedies. Once ritual healings restore balance to one's mind, body, and spirit a patient will theoretically commit to living a life of humility and harmony. Patients should begin to incorporate healthier lifestyle choices into their daily living with respect to food, physical activity, prayer, sleep, and social relationships.

Herbs widely used in the Southwest and Mexico include those with known hypoglycemic activity, such as nopal (prickly pear cactus), hintonia (copalquin), garlic, and onion (Table 14-4). Unfortunately, some of these agents also have toxic effects. Hintonia, for example, contains pyrrolizidine alkaloids that can cause severe liver damage (Table 14-5).[1]

Foods are an essential to many religious and social ceremonies. Among most Native American groups, participating in ceremonial feasts is a key component of maintaining tribal identity. For example, the Navajo categorize food as being either "strong" or "fillers." Strong foods (corn products, mutton, stew, fry bread, beef, coffee) provide satiety, strength for heavy work, and protection against illness. Strong foods are served at social and religious functions and donated to kin in times of need. Fillers include commodities such as cheese, refined flour, and canned meat. Studies have described many reasons for non adherence to dietary recommendations among Native Americans. Members of the Cherokee tribe reported difficulty in using the carbohydrate exchange system as well as a reluctance to incorporate healthier foods and cooking practices in their daily lives.[23] For the Navajo and Ute tribes, the suggestion to withhold certain foods, limit their consumption, or not participate in religious feasts is unconscionable. Thus, simply suggesting that Native Americans adopt a totally Western style diet, limit carbohydrates and saturated fats, or increase fiber intake becomes a cultural nightmare, one that is likely to result in distrust toward the prescriber and non adherence by the patient. CDEs specially trained to assist with dietary modification for this special population should be consulted within the IHS system whenever possible.

Introducing cultural competency to clinicians managing Native Americans through the IHS or privately contracted organizations has encountered bureaucratic roadblocks. Some agencies lack professional presence or may be staffed by transient newly trained residents paying back student

TABLE 14-4. Commonly Used Natural Medications for Treating Diabetes

Drug Class	Natural Remedy	Existing Scientific Evidence Supporting Products
Hypoglycemic agents	Banaba (Lagerstroemia speciosa)[a] Bitter melon (Momordica charantia) Fenugreek (Trigonella foenum-graecum) Gymnema (Gymnema sylvestre)	T2DM patients who took Banaba extract for 2 wk had an average 10% lowered BG than placebo Gymnema 200–400 mg daily may allow some patients to reduce doses of oral agents and insulin. In small trials has been shown to increase C-peptide levels for up to 20 mo. However, reliable scientific evidence is lacking.
Insulin sensitizers	Agaricus mushroom (Agaricus blazei) American ginseng (Panax quinquefolius) Banaba (Lagerstroemia speciosa) Cassia cinnamon (Cinnamomum aromaticum) Chromium Magnesium Panax ginseng Prickly pear cactus (Opuntia ficus-indica) Soy (Glycine max) Vanadium	Some studies demonstrate improvement in A1C when certain brands of cinnamon are consumed. However, Other trials have shown no change in glycemic control with cinnamon. Chromium picolinate is only useful in patients with a documented chromium deficiency. However, chromium deficiency is difficult to document clinically. American ginseng 3 g taken 2 h before meals reduces postprandial blood glucose excursions. More studies are needed before this can be recommended. One prickly pear cactus species, Opuntia streptacantha, can reduce blood glucose levels by 17%–46%. Mechanism is unclear. Reliable evidence for use is lacking.
Carbohydrate absorption inhibitors	Bean pod (Phaseolus vulgaris) Blond psyllium (Plantago ovata) Fenugreek (Trigonella foenum-graecum)	White mulberry leaf extract inhibits α-glucosidase enzymes in the gut preventing absorption of carbohydrates. Mulberry leaf powder 1 g taken three times daily for 4 wk reduced fasting blood glucose by 27% in patients with T2DM, but longer studies have not been completed. Blond psyllium seed (soluble fiber) in several small-scale studies have demonstrated a reduction in postprandial glucose by 14%–20%. LDL-cholesterol is also improved. Guar gum, a soluble fiber from the guar plant, has also been shown to reduce fasting and postprandial glucose levels in both T1DM and T2DM patients.

(Continued)

TABLE 14-4. Commonly Used Natural Medications for Treating Diabetes *(Continued)*

Drug Class	Natural Remedy	Existing Scientific Evidence Supporting Products
	Glucomannan (*Amorphophallus konjac*) Guar gum (*Cyamopsis tetragonoloba*) Oat bran (*Avena sativa*) Prickly pear cactus (*Opuntia ficus-indica*) Soy (*Glycine max*) White mulberry (*Morus alba*)	Oat bran taken on daily basis can reduce blood glucose levels. Soy, taken at 30 g/d reduces insulin resistance, lowers fasting blood glucose and lowers A1C. Glucomannan, an insoluble polysaccharide, delays glucose absorption. Taken daily at doses of 3.6–7.2 g for 90 d, fasting glucose levels can be reduced by 29%. Lipid profiles also improve.
Drugs for diabetes-related complications	α-lipoic acid Chia (*Salvia hispanica*) Coenzyme Q10 Selenium Stevia (*Stevia rebaudiana*) Power 1 walnut Santi Bovine Penis Erecting Capsule Zhong Hua Niu Bian	α-lipoic acid is an antioxidant that may lessen the symptoms of diabetic peripheral neuropathy. The dose is 600–1,200 mg/d. Effects may be noticed in 3–5 wk Coenzyme Q10 is an antioxidant. May minimize myalgias in "statin intolerant" patients. Chia extract in pill form is not beneficial to improving metabolic parameters.

References
1. Natural medicines clinical database. http://naturaldatabase.therapeuticresearch.com/ce/ceCourse.aspx?s=ND&cs=&pc=10%2D107&cec=1&pm=5. Accessed February 12, 2011.
2. Chan TYK. Outbreaks of severe hypoglycaemia due to illegal sexual enhancement products containing undeclared glibenclamide. *Pharmacoepidemiology and Drug Safety.* 2009;18(12):1250–1251.

TABLE 14-5. Potential Harmful Effects of Herbal Remedies Commonly Used for the Management of Diabetes

Herbal Remedy	Potential Adverse Effect of Herbal Remedy
Bitter melon	When used in combination with prescribed oral antihypoglycemic agents may result in hypoglycemia.
Fenugreek	Inhibits platelet aggregation. Caution should be taken when used with aspirin, warfarin, or any other prescription blood thinners. May cause excessive bleeding during surgery and interact with some anesthetic agents. Peanut sensitive patients must avoid using this herb due to potential for anaphylaxis.
Gymnema	Hypoglycemia may occur when herb is used in combination with insulin or an oral antidiabetic agent.
Cassia cinnamon	Potential for hepatotoxicity.
Chromium	May worsen chronic kidney disease.
Vanadium	Renal toxicity and excessive bleeding during surgery. This herbal remedy should be completely avoided in patients with diabetes.
Psyllium, glucomannan, guar gum, and oat bran	Delays absorption of oral prescription medications. Prescription drugs should be taken either 1 h before or 4 h after using these herbal supplements.
Stevia	FDA is investigation potential toxic adverse events linked to this herbal remedy. This popular agent should not be used in managing diabetes until safety issues are further clarified.
Selenium	May actually increase one's risk of developing diabetes!
Ginseng	May potentiate the anticoagulation effect of warfarin resulting in significant bleeding. Has been associated with spontaneous induction of mania in several patients.
Power 1 walnut, Santi Bovine Penis Erecting Capsule, Zhong Hua Niu Bian	When used with a sulfonylurea and a PDE-5 inhibitor will likely result in severe, prolonged and life-threatening hypoglycemia.
Gingko leaf	Has been associated with spontaneous bleeding. When used in combination with aspirin, anti-inflammatory drugs or warfarin, can induce hemorrhaging.
St. John's wort	Phototoxicity and serotonin syndrome has been reported (even when used as monotherapy). Can alter the pharmacokinetics of multiple prescription drugs including amitriptyline, nortriptyline, digoxin, simvastatin, and theophylline. Can cause menstrual irregularities in patients using oral contraceptives.

References
1. Natural medicines clinical database. http://naturaldatabase.therapeuticresearch.com/ce/ceCourse.aspx?s=ND&cs=&pc=10%2D107&cec=1&pm=5. Accessed February 12, 2011.
2. Chan TYK. Outbreaks of severe hypoglycaemia due to illegal sexual enhancement products containing undeclared glibenclamide. *Pharmacoepidemiol Drug Safety.*2009;18(12):1250–1251.
3. Wood AJJ. Herbal remedies. *N Engl J Med.*2002;347:2046–2065.

loans. IHS services are not located in large urban centers. Therefore, Native Americans who seek medical care outside of their local clinics and hospitals are likely to encounter clinicians who have limited or no experience with their culture. Due to budget constraints within the IHS, rationing of care within the system results in gaps and delays in treatment. The end result within IHS creates a program in which diagnoses and treatment interventions are delayed, exacerbating the severity of a patient's underlying disease state. The inefficiency of the IHS implies that Native Americans may live with more disabling chronic diseases, which will become more costly to manage over time. The U.S. Government Accountability Office (GAO) visited 13 IHS-funded facilities in 2005 and discovered that wait times at 4 IHS-funded facilities ranged from 2 to 6 months for women's health care, and general physicals. Some patients had to travel over 90 miles one way to obtain care. After waiting all day to see a midlevel practitioner, many patients delay travel until their condition is truly emergent.

Like other patients, Native Americans must feel a sense of comfort and trust with their primary care provider. Some patients believe that physicians may be using them for "experimentation" with their own practices. Trust can develop when care providers are bicultural. In addition, continuity of care can enhance patient–provider relationships. A single clinician (such as a family physician) who provides all services to a patient and his or her Family (including dietary counseling, foot care, lifestyle intervention, diabetes self-management, pre-conception planning, and intensive diabetes management) and is consistent with messaging will increase confidence and satisfaction of care for Native Americans.[1]

The keys for successful management of Native Americans with diabetes are noted in Table 14-6.

Because the prevalence of T2DM in Native Americans is projected to increase, there is an urgent need for the development and dissemination of more interventions that are both culturally appropriate and clinically comprehensive, including emphasis on self-management of diabetes care, to prevent and/or delay complications of diabetes in this high-risk population.

• Asian Americans

Asian Americans are a diverse and rapidly growing segment of the American population. Between 1990 and 2000, the Asian American population grew by 48%, far above the national growth rate of 13%. The "metabolically obese" phenotype (normal body weight with increased abdominal obesity) is common in Asian populations, adding to the risk of genetically prone individuals to rapidly progress toward clinical diabetes and end-stage complications. The prevalence of diabetes within the adult (aged 20 or older) Asian American population is 8.4%.[24] In an international survey, 55% of Asian and 40% of white patients with T2DM had increased albuminuria, suggesting that Asian patients exhibit high risk for renal complications.[25] Asian Americans have an increased risk of gestational diabetes that contributes to the increasing diabetes epidemic in the United States.[26]

TABLE 14-6. Considerations for Native American Patients with Diabetes

- Do not rush the slow speech of elder Native Americans. To do so is a sign of disrespect. Direct eye contact should be avoided.

- Lifestyle interventions such as "eating less" intake and increasing one's activity level might restore the balance that is disrupted. Medications can also be used to help restore a normal glucose level within the body.

- Carefully monitor patients' use of herbal medicines. Some may result in toxicity and drug interactions.

- Clearly identify individual metabolic targets for each patient (A1C, blood pressure, lipids).

- Make certain that patients understand that successful metabolic management requires that patients are adherent to their treatment regimen. Native Americans tend to discontinue medications when the begin to "feel better."

- Take advantage of the Certified Diabetes Educators that are available through the IHS.

Community-based prospective surveys, including those conducted in Asia, reported independent associations of fasting and 2-hour postprandial glucose levels with cancer risk.[26]

Within the Asian American population, 49 diverse groups, speaking more than 100 languages and dialects, have been identified. These include: Chinese, East Indians, Filipinos, Vietnamese, Koreans, Japanese, Indians and Pacific Islanders. From 2000 to 2010, the Asian American population in the United States increased 45% from 11.9 million to 17.3 million.[27,28]

Philosophical differences related to wellness, health, and disease state exist between Asian and traditional American values. Within the Asian American community, environmental factors, food choices, emotional stability, and family values impact the development and progression of disease. A key aspect of the Asian American assessment of one's health is based upon maintaining balance between life's opposite forces, a philosophical concept referred to as yin and yang. Yin and yang are not opposing forces, but complementary opposites that interact within a greater whole. Everything must have both yin and yang. Light cannot exist without darkness and vice versa. Balancing life's physical and emotional demands forms the basis of the Traditional Chinese Medicine (TCM) philosophy.

Within the Asian American community, increased irritability has been frequently cited as a "symptom of diabetes."[29] Patients with poorly controlled diabetes "get angry easily" and throw "temper tantrums" when they become hyperglycemic. Emotional variability held particular resonance for Chinese immigrants because social ease, avoidance of overt expression of strong negative emotions, and accommodation of family members' expressed and unexpressed needs were culturally valued. Emotional fluctuations were most often attributed to the disease rather than to the person. Wife: "Before he was diagnosed, he wasn't like this. He was REALLY GOOD. After he was diagnosed, when he became upset, he would yell at his mother or whomever." Within the Asian American community, family members may tend to focus more on the social aspects of glucose regulation rather than the physiologic symptoms of hyperglycemia (nocturia, fatigue, weight loss).[29]

Food choices, treatments, and complications may also be viewed as being "hot" or "cold." A patient with diabetes is experiencing a metabolic disparity that is best managed through the use of traditional foods, herbal remedies, acupuncture, Asian physical therapies, and conventional medication. Minimizing the importance of any of these interventions is likely to result in less favorable glycemic control.

TCM proposes that an elaborate internal system helps the human body maintain equilibrium and well-being. Taoist philosophy is deeply rooted in contemporary China and is an unavoidable part of modern Chinese life. TCM follows the principle of Taoist philosophical and religious traditions: all human beings are governed by the laws of the universe (harmonious and ordered) and all life is interconnected; illness results when disruption to the natural order occurs or as a direct result of changes in one's environment.

Chinese medicine was developed to strategically restore the imbalances of one's mind, body, and spirit in response to disease. Liu Wangu, a Chinese physician from the 10th century theorized that diseases are caused by heat in the body and should be counteracted by herbs with a cold nature. This theory is still advocated today. In modern China, the pathogenesis of diabetes is described as a deficiency of yin manifested externally as excessive heat.

Patients with diabetes have organs that are "overworked" and produce heat. Insulin resistance causes the pancreas to become "hot" in an attempt to overproduce insulin and restore euglycemia. The stomach is also considered "hot" because gastric emptying is more rapid. Thus, one may have more "yang" or heat and become dehydrated. To counter this, TCM practitioners prescribe foods that restore the body's natural balance. Dietary plans suggesting food restrictions that Westerners may consider important for glycemic control will not be accepted in many Asian communities. "Pleasurable foods" are appreciated as being crucial to mental health and balance. If patients are restricted by their diet, they are likely to believe that life has "lost its meaning."

Restricting food during illness is counterintuitive for many Chinese Americans.[30] Rather, special foods and disease-specific medicinal foods should be provided for patients as both a means of supporting health and demonstrating family solicitousness.

Many Asian American patients will attempt to supplement or replace their prescription medications with traditional herbs to neutralize "side effects" of prescription medications. Some express guilt for using Western medications that family members and friends claim could disrupt the normal balance of their internal organs. A patient who insists on using TCM remedies should be educated as to the natural progression of the diabetes disease process. In addition, patients should be reminded that TCM herbal remedies can result in adverse events such as drug interactions, confusion, elevated liver function studies, and fatigue.[31] Unlike prescription medicine, few randomized controlled clinical trials have been published proving superior efficacy or providing dosing algorithms for TCM herbal remedies.

Teaching Asian Americans and their families about diabetes self-management requires sensitivity to the social relevance of common symptoms, particularly pain, irritability, and emotional lability. Open expression of strong emotions, particularly negative emotions, may be considered culturally inappropriate and negatively affect family harmony.[32] Indirect, muted, and contained expressions of emotions may be both valued and directly challenged by patients' perceived lack of self- control when symptomatic.

For many elderly patients, remaining stoic while experiencing significant pain is perceived as a badge of courage and honor. The challenge for clinicians is to directly question patients regarding specific symptomatology rather than assume that all is well when asking, "How have you been feeling since our last visit?"

Dietary restrictions on carbohydrates can be particularly challenging to a population that has historic, symbolic, and ritualized inclusion of rice in their daily diets. Recommended reductions in rice may be highly distressing and may challenge core beliefs about health maintenance. Rice is a symbolically vital food for many Asian people. Attempting to reduce the intake of this staple commodity or alter the type of rice consumed is likely to fail. Rice is viewed not only as necessary for survival, but also as a symbolically comforting food. Stepwise approximations to an ideal diet may ease the transition and allow patients and families to explore healthy alternatives to highly processed white rice or rice noodles. Teaching patients about how rice affects blood glucose may dispel cultural myths. Consultation with dietitians who are familiar with Asian food preferences and can offer culturally acceptable food substitutions is warranted.

Table 14-7 summarizes the key factors for successful diabetes management and cultural competency toward Asian Americans within a primary care practice.

TABLE 14-7. Considerations for Asian American Patients with Diabetes

- Ask open ended questions in an attempt to determine if patients are experiencing any uncomfortable diabetes symptomatology or medication adverse effects. Cultural belief systems within the Asian community holds that patients who ask questions of physicians are being "disrespectful."

- Professional interpreters may provide less biased feedback from patients than family members.

- Family obligations within the Asian culture takes priority over one's personal health. Thus, if there are two patients with diabetes in a home (husband and wife), the wife may devote all of her effort toward managing the husband and minimize the importance of her own diabetes self-management. Her diabetes will worsen as his improves.

- When medications are needed for metabolic control, clinicians should refer to the drugs as a means by which "balance may be restored in the body" rather than a way to get the blood pressure and glucose controlled.

- Allow patients to continue using TCM to seek balance in their lives. However, monitor the types of herbal medicines used and make certain that the prescribed medications are continued. Some herbal medicines may interact with prescribed medications to induce hypoglycemia.

- Additional resources for managing Asian Americans with diabetes at the Asian American Diabetes Initiative (AADI), Joslin Diabetes Center: http://aadi.joslin.harvard.edu

• African Americans

Approximately 13% of the African American population in the United States aged 20 and older has T2DM and about one third of these individuals are undiagnosed.[33] Although findings from the Diabetes Prevention Program indicate that no apparent ethnic disparity was evident in the risk of developing T2DM, African Americans are 1.8 times more likely than non-Latino white Americans of similar age to have T2DM.[33,34]

Studies have demonstrated significant ethnic disparities in quality of care and disease-state outcomes among white and African American patients with diabetes despite recent impressive clinical, and scientific innovations.[35,36] Although HEDIS scores improved on 9 measures monitored for over 1.8 million Medicare beneficiaries from 1997 to 2003, significant racial disparities were noted for patients with diabetes and heart disease. Important differences were noted in the control of LDL cholesterol and A1C for whites versus African Americans.[35]

The economic burden of diabetes care is significant among African Americans who are prone to ketosis and require insulin for survival. A study of 56 African American patients admitted to the hospital for diabetic ketoacidosis (DKA) demonstrated that half discontinued their insulin therapy for economic reasons. 14% stopped insulin because they were provided with no sick day education and therefore assumed that nausea, vomiting, and anorexia implied insulin was not necessary.[37] Thus, 75% of admissions for acute DKA can be avoided with improved access to care and proper patient education regarding appropriate insulin use. Education and access to care should be viewed as critical targeted goals for improving both short- and long-term glycemic outcomes for African Americans.

Outcomes for any patient with diabetes can be improved with timely screening and early intervention. Several chronic diseases, such as diabetes and hypertension, lack prodromal symptoms. Patients may be unwilling to seek medical care until the appearance of symptoms that interfere with their quality of life. Diabetes is often not detected within the African American community until complications are already apparent.[38]

Community-based screening programs have been developed that have been enormously successful at preempting diabetes within African Americans. One of the most unique concepts for African American diabetes screening is the Black Barbershop Health Outreach Program, which screened men right in their barbershops. Initiated in 2007 by Bill Releford, DPM and partially funded by the CDC, the Black Barbershop Health Outreach Program had three primary objectives:

1. SCREEN: Cardiovascular disease (diabetes and hypertension)
2. EDUCATE: Preventive education about diet and exercise as well as education about the signs and symptoms of common chronic diseases.
3. REFER: Through the "Real Black Book/Medical Resource Guide," men will be referred to local health-care providers that offer free or low-cost health services.

Why screen black men for diabetes, hypertension, and cardiovascular disease in barbershops? For decades, the barbershop has served as a centralized gathering place where many African American men feel comfortable discussing the important issues that impact their lives such as politics, social trends, family, and finances. Some men hang out at their local barbershop with no intention of getting a haircut. They simply want to spend some time with the guys in a stress-free environment. Dr. Releford and his team of local volunteers decided to use the peer pressure of local neighborhood black barbershops to their advantage. In 2007, 80 black barbershops and 2,500 patients participated in the screening process. By 2011, over 23 U.S. cities screened 15,000 patients for diabetes, hypertension, and cardiovascular disease. Dr. Releford and his team of volunteers hope to screen 250,000 patients in 2012.

The protocol used to "encourage" participation within the barbershops is based upon both "peer pressure" and positive reinforcement. The team shows up on their scheduled date with their blood glucose and A1C screening testing station, blood pressure meters, and simple instruments that allow them to monitor for diabetic sensory neuropathy in the feet. A patient who screens positive for diabetes or hypertension is provided with a "pass" to a free clinic where he is evaluated, treated, and educated about his chronic disease. Each patient who presents to the free clinic is also rewarded with a coupon for a free haircut, thereby allowing him to return to his home barbershop and spread the word about the simplicity and importance of the screening process. Most importantly, patients encourage their peers to undergo screening for possible chronic diseases. Often, receiving a gentle push from a buddy within the comforts of one's own neighborhood barbershop tends to have a greater impact on opportune testing than when diabetes screening is suggested by family members or church goers. More information on the Black Barbershop Outreach Program is available at: http://blackbarbershop.org.

African Americans have distinctive opinions as to the origin of their diabetes. Rural southern African Americans may believe that the condition "sugar" or "sweet blood" is caused by an imbalance due to eating too much sugar and starchy foods. Constant stress and worry simply magnifies their hyperglycemia. Patients will often ask if "stress impacts their diabetes control." Common treatments for any abnormal glucose level within the African American community may include prayer, trusting in God, and the use of herbal remedies (lemon juice, garlic, juniper berries).[1]

During an initial assessment of a new patient with diabetes, the clinician is advised to enter the room and immediately sit positioning himself or herself at a level equal to or lower than the patient. Patient and practitioner should always be at comparable eye levels when communicating even if both parties are of the same ethnic background. For example, an African American female who graduated cum laude from her medical school class is likely to achieve a more favorable degree of successful communication with an African American Harvard University professor if both are seated and talking at eye level, rather than having the clinician standing above the patient while taking a history. Direct eye contact should be maintained during the history intake and whenever a treatment regimen is discussed.

Showing respect is particularly important with elderly African Americans, who may have negative views toward non-African American physicians due to the unethical syphilis research projects performed as part of the Tuskegee experiments.[39] Trust, once earned, is likely to be tenured.

Faith plays an important role in the lives of many African Americans with chronic diseases. Many African Americans believe spiritual faith has more curative potential than allopathic therapies. Patients may request that intensification of diabetes therapy be delayed for "a few months" yet provide only vague reasons for wanting to buy time. Although clinicians may express frustration over what they perceive as deferred action or "non compliance" on behalf of their patient, this "delay of game" is most often used to establish prayer groups within churches. Patients simply hope to use the power of prayer to eliminate, slow, or reverse their progressive disease. In their own way, they are doing what they can personally to take control of their own diabetes management. Unless one is gravely ill, allowing a patient 2 months by the clock to experiment with prayer is certainly reasonable. Matters of faith are never to be regarded lightly, regardless of cultural setting. Churches would be happy to partner with health-care providers to screen their own congregants for chronic diseases. Patients should be encouraged to continue their religious interventions with the hope that their doctor's treatment decisions may be augmented by their prayers.

Faith-based primary prevention of diabetes has been tested in one clinical trial.[40] Thirty-seven participants at five different churches participated in 6- or 12-week diabetes prevention program protocols with follow-ups at 6 and 12 months. The primary outcomes were changes in fasting glucose and weight. Two churches participated in a 6-week church-based diabetes prevention program and three churches participated in a 16-week church-based diabetes prevention program, with follow-up at 6 and 12 months. Overall, the fasting glucose decreased from 108.1 to 101.7 mg per dL post intervention ($P = 0.037$), and this reduction persisted at the 12-month follow-up without any planned maintenance following the intervention. Weight decreased 1.7 kg post intervention with 0.9 kg regained at 12 months. Body mass index (BMI) decreased from 33.2 to 32.6 kg per m^2 post intervention with a final mean BMI of 32.9 kg per m^2 at the 12-month check ($p < 0.05$). Thus, translation of the diabetes prevention program can be achieved in at-risk African Americans if clinicians build successful community-based relationships with members of local churches.

In cases where religious affiliation and/or inclination is not known, a physician might ask an open-ended question, such as "Where do you find support during times of stress or illness?" The response needs to be honored, supported, encouraged, and integrated into the care management plan.

A thorough history is paramount in discovering patients' beliefs about T2DM, their basic knowledge of the disease, how they monitor the disease, and the treatment options they are using. This information will help identify knowledge deficits and personal beliefs that can guide patient education efforts. In gathering this information, patients should not feel as though they are being interrogated. Obtaining a family history is also critical. African Americans are more likely than whites to be diagnosed with chronic kidney disease,[41] and the risk of diabetes-related complications appears to be higher among family members within the African American community. African Americans are twice as likely to develop and die from cancer as other race and ethnic groups.[42] Discussing the importance of screening, early diagnosis, and slowing disease progression can enhance a patient's willingness to participate in diabetes self-management and incorporate appropriate lifestyle interventions into their daily routines.

Another way of showing concern and establishing trust is to proactively discuss issues that, although important to patients, may be uncomfortable for them to discuss with a provider. For example, erectile dysfunction and stroke are two common concerns of male patients with T2DM. By initiating conversation about these very personal concerns, a high degree of trust can often be established, thereby helping build a long-term, patient–provider relationship that is essential for successful diabetes management.

Table 14-8 summarizes strategies for successful management of African American patients with diabetes.

• Latino (Hispanic) Americans

The incidence of T2DM has reached epidemic proportions in the Latino (or Hispanic) American community. Approximately 14% of Latino Americans have T2DM in comparison with 7% of non-Hispanic white Americans.[43] The Latino community also demonstrates poorer disease control, higher rates of complications (retinopathy, nephropathy, peripheral vascular disease and amputations), as well as an increase in all-cause mortality.[43] Latino children born today have a 50% likelihood of developing T2DM during their lifetime.[44]

Latino Americans are a heterogeneous group, which includes people from Mexico, Puerto Rico, Cuba, Central and South America, and individuals of Spanish descent, among others. Although Latino Americans share a common language, their history, dialects, cultural beliefs, traditions, and family values vary widely. Philosophical differences with regard to diabetes management among

TABLE 14-8. Considerations for African American Patients with Diabetes

- Interview and speak to patients while maintaining eye contact and equal eye level.
- Allow the patient to integrate his or her fate with allopathic medicine treatment programs.
- Consider allying your practice with local community churches to establish screening programs for diabetes, hypertension, and cardiovascular disease.
- Become proactive when discussing possible complications such as erectile dysfunction and painful neuropathy.
- Always obtain a family history as complications from diabetes tend to have a genetic predilection within African Americans.
- Inquire about the burden of drug costs. High costs of medications favor non-adherence and inappropriate cessation of insulin.
- The traditional image of insulin involves injection with a long needle, large syringe, and a cold vial of milky colored medicine. Use of an insulin pen may allay patient's fears as many have never realized that the drug could be administered with such a novel device. Remind the patient that beside being virtually painless, he or she will probably be the first person in his or her neighborhood using this form of "injection technology." This will make the patient feel very special!

Latino American subgroups are dependent upon age, generation, gender, economic and immigration status, and availability of homeopathic care.

Latino Americans vary in their degree of acculturation and in the values and beliefs to which they subscribe. New immigrants and those residing in communities with strong ties to the home culture are more likely to hold to traditional values. Second- and third-generation immigrants and those with more time spent in the American education system may favor the values of the dominant American culture. Physicians can assess their patients' degree of acculturation by inquiring about their background, asking whether they were born in the United States or are recent immigrants, their language preference, the type of community in which they reside and the level of education they have received in the United States.

Latino American attitudes toward medicine and treatment may also differ from the Western medical model. Latino culture places a high value on herbal remedies and other natural treatments. A small study of 22 individuals with T2DM living in El Paso County, Texas, revealed that Latino American patients frequently mix herbal and Western treatments but often do not disclose this information to their physicians for fear of being "scolded." Physicians who are able to establish an open and nonjudgmental dialogue with their patients about medical beliefs will help to foster trust and mutual understanding.[45]

Although Latinos tend to have a good, basic conceptual framework as to the true pathogenesis of diabetes, cultural issues play a strong role in disease progression. For example, many Latinos believe that the emotional life is intertwined with the physical. Thus, emotions can affect one's overall health.[46] Anger, fright, or a life-changing emotional experience may predispose one's body to developing diabetes but is not the direct trigger that induces chronic hyperglycemia.[45] Mexican American and Puerto Rican patients may believe that diabetes results from both excessive consumption of sugar and as God's will or punishment. These populations report symptoms indicative of hyperglycemia including weakness, headache, anxiety, leg pain, forgetfulness, and anger.[1] In one study of elderly Puerto Ricans with diabetes, over half used herbs and prayer to manage diabetes, reporting that these modalities provided them with peace and improvement in their glycemic control.[47]

The prevalence of overweight and obesity among Latino Americans has been estimated to be 73%.[48] In the Latino culture, a degree of excess weight may be tolerated or even celebrated, effectively lessening social pressure to lose weight. Especially among children, being slightly overweight or plump is equated with health and good parental care; whereas, being thin may be associated with being undernourished or even neglected.

The traditional Latino cuisine is rich in legumes, rice, and fresh fruits, high in fiber and low in fat. However, as Latinos become acculturated into American society, the content of their diet becomes lower in nutrients and higher in fat. They may exchange traditional corn tortillas for refined flour tortillas, which are easier to use. Those living in economically disadvantaged areas may have difficulty finding affordable fresh fruits and vegetables. Convenience foods, which are typically higher in fat, may be preferred because they are easy to prepare and are generally affordable. These dietary changes, along with the increasingly sedentary lifestyle that characterizes American life, undoubtedly contribute to the epidemic of obesity and its associated health problems, such as T2DM.

Expecting patients to replace their diet with unfamiliar, "healthier" foods is asking them to make a further sacrifice, giving up one of the few remaining ties to their homeland. This type of intervention is not likely to be effective. Dietary changes that are easy to incorporate into the traditional diet, such as pouring off excess grease after cooking meat or substituting healthier oils for lard, are more culturally acceptable options and, therefore, are more likely to be successful. Referring patients to a certified diabetes educator with cultural diversity skills would be of obvious benefit for many Latino American patients with diabetes.

Despite the integration of lifestyle changes and pharmacotherapy into the lives of patients with diabetes, many Latino Americans maintain a fatalistic attitude. Believing that diabetes is a "curse" that will not likely be reversed or delayed, little can be done to prevent the inevitable onslaught of complications. Thus, for some patients, simply being diagnosed with diabetes implies that loss of sight or a limb is just weeks away. A discussion regarding possible insulin initiation may be considered the "nail in the coffin" for not only the patient, but his or her family. All Latino patients know of someone with diabetes who was admitted to the hospital yet never made it home to spend another night with friends or relatives. Thus, the hospital is viewed as the last stop for nearly all people with diabetes, and for this reason, they may think it is best to avoid intensifying one's therapy or even seeing a doctor for the disorder in the first place! Along similar lines, some Latino Americans may be more focused on the "here and now" and, thus, may "leave the future in God's hands."[44]

Some clinicians may attempt to panic patients into a state of improved compliance by suggesting that they are "very likely to go blind or lose a foot to diabetes unless they start insulin!" Obviously, this approach will do nothing except shorten the doctor's work day. A more effective approach would be to assure patients with poorly controlled diabetes that they are more likely to feel better (less fatigued, improved vision, less frequent urination, improved sexual function) if their blood glucose levels are better controlled. Patients can be assured that with so many different types of interventions available, we will pick the one most likely to ease the patient's symptoms and allow for successful achievement of their metabolic goals. Additional medications may be added sequentially according to the customized targets of the patient. Although the clinician is interested in immediate improvement in symptomatology, the ultimate goal is to minimize one's risk of developing long-term complications. For this goal to be achieved, the doctor, patient, and family will need to work together as a single unit.

The initiation of insulin is often anxiety provoking for both the patient and the family. Clinicians must address insulin initiation openly with their patients so that fears and misconceptions can be addressed. A common misconception is the belief that the need for insulin indicates a patient's personal failure to manage his or her disease, and that if insulin is needed, the patient must be very ill. By initiating a discussion with patients early about the progressive nature of diabetes, and by explaining that escalating doses of oral medications and the use of insulin as replacement therapy should be expected, physicians can begin to allay some of their patients' fears long before the need for insulin becomes apparent.

With the approval of GLP-1 analogues, clinicians have another therapeutic intervention that can be initiated at any point in time once a patient has been diagnosed with T2DM. Patients must be told that despite being injected, GLP-1 analogues promote the release of insulin from one's own pancreas in a glucose-dependent manner. Thus, hypoglycemia is unlikely to occur. Use of GLP-1 analogues will improve A1C, fasting and postprandial glucose levels, and often result in weight loss.[49]

Some patients have even greater fears about insulin. The survey of Latino Americans with T2DM in El Paso County, Texas, (discussed earlier) found that some participants believed insulin caused blindness, and several patients related stories about relatives who became blind shortly after beginning insulin therapy. Others were concerned that continued insulin use would lead to dependence.[45]

Latino patients often have difficulty understanding and adhering to prescribed treatment plans if a language barrier is present. Use of interpreters from within the family may be useful. Professional translators will eliminate interpretation bias expressed by family members during the interview process. When possible, instructions should be expressed in written form in the patient's native language.

Communication with Latino patients may be enhanced in several ways. First, when greeting patients of Latino ethnicity, the forceful grip on the handshake between the clinician and the patient should be reduced so as to imply that both parties are on equal ground. The handshake in the 1800s was traditionally meant to show that each party was "unarmed." In medicine, a strong grip by the clinician could demonstrate superior education, knowledge base, and even economic superiority between the two individuals.

Elderly patients should always be respectfully addressed by using "Senor" or "Senora" rather than their first names. Whenever possible, a physical examination should be performed during which time the clinician touches the patient's body with his or her hands. Patients view the examination as being part of the healing process.

Table 14-9 summarizes the strategies for successful management of Latino American patients with diabetes.

TABLE 14-9. Considerations for Latino American Patients with Diabetes

- Elderly patients should be referred to as "Senor" and "Senora."
- Attempt to touch each patient at each exam.
- Patient's indirect eye contact should be interpreted as a sign of respect for the clinician.
- Lightening the greeting handshake will imply equal superiority between the clinician and the patient.
- Emotions can affect health, according to most patients. Patients with comorbid psychological disorders should have the emotional component stabilized prior to attempting improving glycemic control.
- Mexican Americans are 23% more likely to lack appropriate medical insurance coverage than non-white Hispanics.
- Use insulin pens whenever possible for patients requiring insulin.

(Brown AF, Gerzoff RB, Karter AJ, et al. Health behaviors and quality of care among Latinos with diabetes in managed care. *Am J Public Health.* 2003;93:1694–1698).

• Observant Jews

The prevalence of diabetes within the Jewish community is difficult to ascertain, but data from Israeli studies may give some insight. A retrospective population-based cross-sectional study of patients in two large Israeli health maintenance organizations demonstrated that the prevalence of diabetes increased from 20.2/1,000 in 1995 to 63.7/1,000 in 2007.[50] The metabolic control of patients with diabetes in this population appeared to be improving. The proportion of patients having A1C ≤ 7% increased from 10% to 53% over 12 years, while the percentage of individuals reporting A1C greater than 9% declined from 40% to 13%.

When compared with Arab individuals of similar sex and age, the development of T2DM in Jews is delayed an average of 11 years (mean corresponding age of onset = 68 years).[51] This implies that culturally sensitive interventions aimed at maintaining normal body weight and active lifestyle may delay the progression toward clinical diabetes in those patients who screen positive for prediabetes.

Jews are at higher risk for developing certain diabetes-related complications than other ethnic sub groups. In Israel, advanced age-related macular degeneration is less common in the Arab population than in the Jewish population.[52] Differences in complication rates and end-stage disease progression exist even among various sects within the Jewish population. For example, the Sephardic Jews (immigrants from North Africa and the Middle East) with T1DM are more likely to develop proliferative retinopathy than are the Ashkenazi Jews (immigrants from Europe and North and South America).[53] Although Asian-Indian Jews have a higher prevalence of kidney disease, intracultural ethnicity does not affect the frequency of cardiovascular disease.[54]

Jews believe in one universal God. They must obey the Ten Commandments and the Torah given to Moses on Mount Sinai, while practicing charity and tolerance toward fellow human beings. The Jewish Sabbath is a "day of rest" that begins before nightfall on Friday and ends on Saturday evening. Observant Jews will not write, travel, work, or switch on electrical appliances on the Sabbath. Instead, the holiest day of the week is dedicated to Torah study. Religious services are held in the synagogue on Friday evenings and Saturday mornings led by the rabbi, who is the religious leader of the community.

Judaism views medical treatment as a necessity, even as an obligation. One's body is considered a blessed sanctuary that is to be honored and preserved to the best of one's ability. To help maintain one's body, God has created physicians, many of whom have traditionally been accorded high status over the past centuries. In fact, many leading rabbis and scholars from the Talmudic period through the Middle Ages and beyond were also physicians. Rabbi Maimonides, one of the greatest

Torah scholars and physicians in 1135, viewed the responsibility of physicians as returning to the patient "anything he has lost." Interestingly, in some Middle Age societies, medicine was one of the few professions open to Jews.

Jewish philosophy clearly dictates proper decorum for accepting or declining medical intervention for any disease including diabetes. Jews should refuse any medical treatment that is likely to be unsafe, is considered "experimental," is likely to cause harm or injury to the person, or shorten one's lifespan by even a single day. Moreover, any activity that endangers one's health, such as smoking or substance abuse, is clearly unjustified. Interventions that have a 50% or greater chance of prolonging life should be accepted. Thus, currently marketed diabetes interventions, including insulin, would all be considered reasonable therapies for any Jewish patient with diabetes.

During each calendar year, observant Jews participate in 6 public fasting days during which time eating and drinking should be avoided for up to 25 hours. Fasting is also traditionally required for the bride and groom on the day of their wedding ceremony. This will expose patients with diabetes to hypoglycemia, erratic glycemic control, dehydration, and place them at higher risk of thrombosis. Some patients may insist on discontinuing insulin or their oral agents during fast days. A patient with T1DM who discontinues insulin for 24 hours may develop DKA. Therefore, primary care physicians must proactively address appropriate diabetes management during fast days as suggested in Table 14-10. If necessary, patients and physicians may also seek counsel of a qualified rabbi to serve as a mediator.

When possible, patients with T2DM should be placed on medications that are less likely to induce hypoglycemic events such as metformin, DPP-4 inhibitors, and GLP-1 agonists. Sulfonylureas and mixed insulin analogues should be avoided on public fast days as these interventions have a high risk of inducing hypoglycemia, especially when doses remain unadjusted for minimal food consumption.

Although most Jews have historically expressed little doubt about the benefits of exercise, the majority of one's physical activity is performed on the Sabbath as one walks to the Temple. This poses an increased threat of exercise induced hypoglycemia for patients who inject insulin 1 to 2 hours prior to beginning a 30- to 90-minute walk. Jewish law (Halacha) also forbids individuals from carrying any objects other than the clothes they are wearing on the Sabbath. However, Rabbinical intervention is critical to explain the loophole in Jewish law that demands that patients must continue to use medications and monitor their glucose levels in order to minimize any medical risks associated with fasting. The use of continuous glucose sensors, blood glucose monitors, insulin pump therapy, multiple daily injections, and other medications used to maintain metabolic control must be continued on the Sabbath and during public fast days. To ignore Halacha against the advice of one's Rabbi or physician implies that one has committed a grave sin.

The Jewish Diabetes Association provides an outstanding source of education for patients who would like recipes and information related to low-carbohydrate, low-fat kosher cooking. The JDA web site may be found at: www.jewishdiabetes.org.

Physicians should not hesitate to encourage their Jewish patients to adopt exercise as a means of supporting a healthy lifestyle. In most communities exercise is traditionally segregated among the sexes. Women and men may be encouraged to form individual walking "clubs" within their neighborhoods. Some Orthodox Jewish rabbis have actually become black belts in martial arts and teach these same skills to members of their congregations.[55]

Clinicians should be mindful of scheduling observant Jews on Friday afternoons. Because Jews are unable to travel on the Sabbath, all business, personal, and social events must be concluded by sundown each Friday night allowing the individual to get home in time to begin the Sabbath tradition.

Disparities in diabetes care, especially among low socioeconomic patients and those belonging to ethnic minorities are well documented. A population-based study in England showed that diabetic women of white British ethnicity and those of higher socioeconomic status were more likely to receive perception counseling.[56]

TABLE 14-10. Suggested Management of Insulin Regimen for Orthodox Jews on Religious Fast Days

Type of Insulin Regimen	Suggested Adjustments
Insulin pump	No change in basal insulin rate. Check blood glucose levels every 4 h. Give compensatory bolus every 4 h to keep blood glucose level 150–200 mg/dL. If blood glucose falls below 100 mg/dL consider using a temporary basal rate for 1-2 h to raise blood glucose into target range of 150–220 mg/dL.
Basal insulin	No change in dose required. Suggest use of insulin degludec when this product becomes available. This insulin may be dosed flexibly at any time of day without compromising glycemic control. Degludec has a duration of action of 40–42 h (1).
Basal bolus insulin	No change in basal insulin. Check blood glucose every 4–6 h. Give 2–3 U of fast-acting insulin every 4–6 h if blood glucose level is >200 mg/dL. Target blood glucose is 150–200 mg/dL. May consider changing the basal insulin component to degludec for reasons stated above. Confirmed episodes of nocturnal hypoglycemia appear to be less frequent with insulin degludec than with insulin glargine (2). For patients with T1DM, insulin degludec appears to induce a greater counter-regulatory hormone response to hypoglycemia than does insulin glargine (4).
Mixed insulin analogues	Fasting not recommended. Monitor blood glucose level at 8:00 AM, noon, 4:00 PM, 8:00 PM, bedtime and 3:00 AM. If blood glucose is <80 mg/dL consider breaking fast and consuming carbohydrates (see Table 14-1). Switch to insulin degludec. Less nocturnal hypoglycemic events reported with IDegAsp than with Biphasic Insulin Aspart 30 (3).

References
1. Meneghini L, Atkin SL, Bain S, et al. Flexible once-daily dosing of insulin degludec does not compromise glycemic control of safety compared to insulin glargine givein once daily at the same time each day in people with type 2 diabetes. American Diabetes Association. *71st Scientific Sessions*. 35-LP poster. San Diego, CA. June 24–28, 2011.
2. Garber AJ, King AB, Francisco AMO, et al. Insulin degludec improves long-term glycemic control with less nocturnal hypoglycemia compared with insulin glargine: 1-year results from a randomized basal-bolus trial in people with type 2 diabetes. American Diabetes Association. *71st Scientific Sessions*. 74-OR. San Diego, CA. June 24–28, 2011.
3. Vaag A, Leiter L, Franek E, et al. Use of a new basal insulin with a bolus boost (IDegAso) in Type 2 Diabetes: comparison with Biphasic Insulin Aspart 30. American Diabetes Association. *71st Scientific Sessions*. Poster 1141. San Diego, CA June 24-28, 2011.
4. Pieber T, Korsatko S, Kohler G, et al. Response to induce hypoglycemia in type 1 diabetes: insulin degludec elicits an enhanced counter-regulatory hormone response compared with insulin glargine. American Diabetes Association. *71st Scientific Sessions*. Poster 498. San Diego, CA. June 24–28, 2011.
Note that higher insulin doses may increase hunger and likelihood of hypoglycemia. This should be explained to each patient who is insulin requiring.

Women with suboptimal control of T1DM should receive preconception counseling. Patients may be provided with oral contraceptives if case appropriate, which may be used until targeted glycemic control is achieved. Condoms are generally regarded as being unallowable by observant Jews.

Finally, advanced directives should not be forced upon any Jewish patient. Jews believe that one's life should be extended allowing the soul to have complete access to God's human sanctuary for as long as possible. As physicians our role is to preserve life. The patient's role is to live life to its fullest extent.

Table 14-11 summarizes the strategies for successful management of observant Jews with diabetes.

TABLE 14-11. Considerations for Observant Jews with Diabetes

- Avoid scheduling appointments on Friday afternoons to allow patients the opportunity to have adequate time to return home in time for celebration of the holy Sabbath.

- Refer patients to the Jewish Diabetes Association web site for information related to kosher recipes, and guidance on management of glycemic control for special festive holidays.

- Patients with excellent glycemic control may safely fast provided they obtain medical clearance from their physician. Patients with T1DM should be maintained on continuous subcutaneous insulin infusion (pump therapy) while fasting. The use of continuous glucose sensors is strongly encouraged. The rules for breaking the fast are found in Table 14-7.

- Encourage high-risk patients to carry their blood glucose meters and glucose tablets with them on the Sabbath. In order to identify and reverse hypoglycemia, patients with poor glycemic control should avoid fasting.

- Advanced directives are culturally unacceptable to observant Jews.

• Lesbian, Gay, Bisexual, and Transgender Americans

The prevalence of diabetes within the United States Lesbian, Gay, Bisexual, and Transgender (LGBT) community is estimated to be 1.3 million, far surpassing the population of both T1DM and gestational diabetes. The delivery of diabetes care and education to members of the LGBT community presents a unique set of challenges that are frequently ignored at national and regional primary care meetings.

The LGBT population has distinctive health matters placing them at high risk for developing diabetes and increasing their likelihood of developing complications while limiting their access to health care. The metabolic, psychological, and behavioral risk factors that impact diabetes care within the LGBT community are listed in Table 14-12.

The foundation of quality care is the assessment. If critical information is missed and appropriate questions are not raised, the diabetes care plan will be drafted with the assumption that the individual is a member of the heterosexual community. This could trigger distrust by the patient toward the clinician and concern that disclosure of one's sexual orientation would become imbedded in the EMR, resulting in health-care discrimination.[57] Nevertheless, the National Standards for Diabetes Self-Management Education require an individualized assessment inclusive of cultural information, family support, and general psychosocial problems that may pose barriers to planning care effectively.[58] Denoting one's sexual preference is therefore essential in providing optimal and customized care for all primary care patients.

When managing LGBT patients, clinicians should avoid making any demeaning or judgmental comments. Unsolicited referrals to mental health resources, and engagement in verbal hostility is inappropriate. Direct eye contact should be maintained and the clinician should not be sitting farther from the patient than necessary.

Cultural competency in managing LGBT individuals begins with accepting responsibility for personal beliefs and biases, and becoming sensitive to the norms that shape these patients' lives. This includes showing respect for family structures and roles within the LGBT culture. Competency assumes the ability and willingness to effectively serve the public health needs of LGBT individuals and their community. Primary care physicians who practice at university health-care centers are well trained to effectively manage the LGBT population. Community physicians may advance their roles as cultural advocates for the LGBT community by providing patient history intake forms, which include the term "domestic partnership" in the relationship status bar. Beside listing genders as being "male and female," one could include "transgender (male-to-female and female-to-male)" options. Including sexual orientation as a standard demographic variable in patient history intake

TABLE 14-12. Metabolic, Psychological and Behavioral Risk Factors That Impact Diabetes Care within the LGBT Community

- Cigarette smoking prevalence rate ranges from 38% to 69% in adolescents and 11%–50% in adults. Smoking increases risk of insulin resistance, stroke, cardiovascular disease, neuropathy, chronic kidney disease and retinopathy.

- Polycystic ovary syndrome prevalence is highest among lesbians (38% vs. 14% among heterosexual women). Women with PCOS constitute the largest group of women at risk for developing CVD and diabetes.

- Patients with PCOS often have infertility, hypertension, sleep apnea and depression all of which may increase insulin resistance. Depression reduces adherence to prescribed treatment regimens.

- Rates in delaying or not filling prescription medicines are highest for LGB African-Americans.

- Overweight and obesity rates are higher among lesbians than among heterosexual women.

- Progression from prediabetes to clinical T2DM risk is increased in overweight transgender women who are on hormone therapy.

- Diabetes rates among men receiving HIV treatment are four times that of HIV-negative men (not that HIV only affects gays). Diabetes rates are highest among LGB African-American adults. Treatments for HIV often result in severe insulin resistance.

- Uninsured rates and difficulty obtaining medical care occur most frequently for lesbians, bisexual women, and LGB Latino adults. Access to health care affects the detection of diabetes.

- Depression and suicide attempts are highest among LGB individuals.

- Suicide attempts among LGBT youth are between 20% and 42%; gay men are six times more likely and lesbians are twice as likely as their heterosexual counterparts to attempt suicide. This may explain why some type 1 (albeit closeted LGBT) youths withhold insulin, not as a "diabulemic" maneuver, but possibly as a suicidal gesture.

- Psychological distress is most likely experienced by LGB Asian or Pacific Islander adults.

- Illicit substance use is a serious health problem for the LGBT community. These patients should be screened for bipolar depression.

- Binge and heavy drinking is significantly more likely to occur in lesbians than in heterosexual women. Alcohol intoxication can result in severe hypoglycemia.

- Papanicolaou tests and breast exams are less likely to occur in lesbian populations. Cancer rates are increased in all patients with diabetes, especially those who are overweight.

- Homeless adolescents include up to 40% LGBT individuals.

- Outright hostility from health care providers is a common LGBT experience. Up to 39% of transgender people face harassment when seeking routine health care. This barrier in health care services could delay screening, management and treatment of diabetes and diabetes related complications.

From Garnero TL. Providing culturally sensitive diabetes care and education for the Lesbian, Gay, Bisexual, and Transgender (LGBT) community. *Diabetes Spectrum.* 2010;23(3):178–182.

forms or in direct questioning demonstrates one's interest and desire to work with this unique population.

Posted non-discrimination policies and medical brochures that address the health needs of LGBT patients would be welcomed by many individuals. Most importantly, clinicians must demonstrate a degree of comfort when managing these patients by using words such as "spouse" or "partner" in addition to "husband" and "wife." Without clear and visible signals from health care facilities and verbal interactions with health care professionals that demonstrate acceptance, many LGBT people will not feel safe "outing" themselves.

TABLE 14-13. Considerations for Lesbian, Gay, Bisexual and Transgender Patients with Diabetes

- Prepare to investigate and workup the many co-existing disorders associated with LGBT patients (PCOS, sleep apnea, obesity, depression, cancer risk, vaccination requirements, etc.).
- Demographic office forms should include LGBT specific headings.
- Examiner should be nonjudgemental and focus on managing the patient's metabolic disorder.
- Sitting further away from the patient than necessary suggest that the physician is uncomfortable with the status of the encounter.
- The Gay and Lesbian Medical Association Web site is an excellent resource for physicians who would like additional information on cultural competency related to the LGBT population in their community.
- Encourage vaccinations for Hepatitis A and B.
- HPV vaccination for men and women up to 26 years of age.

Clinicians must be prepared to manage non–diabetes-related patient queries related to sexually transmitted diseases, breast cancer, mental health, hepatitis vaccinations, and hormonal therapy. Further information related to management of LGBT patients may be found on the Gay and Lesbian Medical Association website: www.glma.org.

Table 14-13 summarizes the strategies for successful management of LGBT patients with diabetes.

• Illiteracy

Limited literacy in adults contributes to racial disparities in health. According to the Institute of Medicine, 90 million people in the United States lack the literacy proficiency needed to effectively understand and act on health information.[59]

Low literacy is common among patients with diabetes. A study of patients with diabetes at two urban public hospitals found that 55% of patients had inadequate literacy.[60] Of those patients with inadequate literacy, 50% did not know the symptoms of hypoglycemia, 62% did not know how to treat hypoglycemic episodes, and 42% did not know the normal blood glucose range, despite the fact that 73% of the patients had attended multiple diabetes education classes. Another study, involving over 400 patients with T2DM, found that poor literacy was associated with worse glycemic control and higher rates of retinopathy.[61]

While there is a strong correlation between verbal literacy and quantitative skills, there are many patients who have adequate verbal literacy but are still unable to use math skills appropriately.[62] This has important implications for patients who are asked to perform daily critical tasks such as carb count, insulin dosing calculations and adjustments, or determining the amount of "insulin on board" to minimize the risk of iatrogenic hypoglycemia due to stacking. Those patients who have been challenged their entire life with the acquisition of basic math skills, may become overwhelmed at the prospect of insulin self-titration protocols.

Numeracy refers to one's ability to demonstrate proficiency with numbers and basic mathematical concepts. Numeracy is particularly important for patients with diabetes because many self-management tasks, such as carbohydrate counting, interpreting blood glucose monitoring results, paired (structured) glucose testing, and correction dose insulin calculations rely on mathematics. Patients who are "innumerate" are prone to episodes of hypoglycemia and wide glycemic variability.[62] Unlike illiteracy, mathematical incompetence may be observed in prominent and well-educated patients.[63] Some patients may even boast about their lack of mathematical prowess by proclaiming that they "inherited their dysfunctional math skills from their 'children'!" Nevertheless, innumerate and illiterate patients should be identified and referred to skilled Certified Diabetic Educators who may introduce them to specialized programs designed to improve their self-management and metabolic control.[62]

TABLE 14-14. Action Plan to Enhance Diabetes Self-management for Patients Suspected of Having Either Low Literacy Skills or Innumeracy

1. Provide educational material that is written at the fourth to sixth grade level. The Diabetes literacy and numeracy toolkit (DLNT) from the Vanderbilt Diabetes Research and Training Center can be downloaded from this Web site. http://www.mc.vanderbilt.edu/diabetes/drtc/preventionandcontrol/registration.php?accesscode=3462DD5B&username=&position=&location=&email=&downloadreason=&actionTtype=download&catid=3

2. Limit the number of topics covered in one teaching session.

3. Use the "teach back" method of education, which encourages the patient to teach information back to the instructor making certain that the primary goals of education have been properly interpreted.

4. Encourage and support patients who have difficulty understanding basic concepts. Do not embarrass or humiliate patients. Remind patients that diabetes is a very challenging chronic disorder and that eventually the educational objectives for them will be met. If a patient requests to stop his or her treatments or education, remind him or her "failure is not an option on my watch. Now, let's start again…".

One may quickly assess literacy by asking a patient to read a pill bottle and explain how that medication is to be taken. Patients exhibiting clinical evidence of either low literacy skills or innumeracy may be managed using the action plans noted in Table 14-14.

Low literacy and diabetes numeracy presents potentially modifiable barrier to successful diabetes self-management. Educational programs and adaptive tools designed to facilitate effective patient–clinician communication have been published and have proven to be successful at improving glycemic control.[62] Clinicians who detect low literacy or diabetes numeracy, should consider referring these patients to Certified Diabetes Educators who can provide comprehensive training to these individuals.

TABLE 14-15. Phases of Cultural Assessment

Phase	Intervention
General assessment	Obtain an overview of patient's physical, behavioral, and medical requirements. Determine ethnicity, degree of affiliation within the ethnic group, religion, patterns of decision-making, and preferred communication style.
Elicit situation-specific cultural information	Identify patient's reasons for seeking care, belief's about disease state, prior treatments, and anticipated outcomes.
Determine influential cultural factors that will likely influence interventions	Identify patient's current and preferred diet, specifics related to food preparation and meaning of food in patient's life.
Incorporate family assistance	Encourage the assistance of family members to target treatment goals.

A cultural assessment is a focused and systematic appraisal of beliefs, values, and practices conducted to determine the context and substance of client needs and then to best adapt (or construct) and evaluate health interventions. Unlike physical assessments, cultural assessments are necessary for each of the three phases of professional practice: problem identification, intervention, and evaluation. Cultural assessments are not exhaustive of all aspects of culture, but rather are focused on those elements relevant to the presenting problem, necessary intervention, and participatory evaluation. From Tripp-Reimer T, Choi E, Kelley LS, et al. Cultural barriers to care: inverting the problem. *Diabetes Spectrum*. 2001;14(1):13–22.

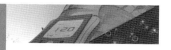

SUMMARY

Diabetes is a disease with a variety of presentations, treatment options, and complications. By better understanding our patients as individuals, within the context of their cultural beliefs, PCPs can better individualize each patient's overall care and, specifically, his or her diabetes care.

Culturally competent providers have the ability to provide medical care to patients with diverse values, beliefs, and behaviors while customizing management to comply with one's social, cultural, ethical, religious, and linguistic requests. The ultimate goal of primary care physicians should be to deliver the highest quality of care to each patient regardless of race, ethnicity, religious or cultural background, or proficiency of the English language.

A cultural assessment (Table 14-15) should be performed on all patients having challenging ethnic ideologies. The assessment is a focused and systematic appraisal of beliefs, values, and practices conducted to determine the context and substance of patient needs prior to initiation of targeted interventions. Cultural assessments should focus on elements relevant to the patient's presenting complaint, prescribed interventions, and family participation.

Expert primary care diabetes management requires that clinicians implement appropriate therapeutic interventions while considering the cultural implications of each patient. Practicing cultural competency allows clinicians to look beyond "evidence-based medicine," randomized clinical trials, meta-analysis observational studies, and head-to-head drug wars sponsored by pharmaceutical companies.

Although achieving cultural competency may be time-consuming and challenging, the potential for enhancing metabolic targets and long-term outcomes is apparent. Cultural competency reminds us that individualized care trumps an expert opinion position statement on hyperglycemic management.

In our offices, the best medicine remains individualized care, based around the needs of the patient and his or her family. I believe my own Uncle Charlie may have been the original purveyor of cultural competency. As a general practitioner in the 1960s, Uncle Charlie was one of the most popular clinicians in Chicago. Unfortunately, after graduating from medical school in 1942, Uncle Charlie never opened a medical textbook, read a medical journal, or attended a medical meeting.

There were two reasons for Uncle Charlie's tremendous success as a physician: (1) he never hurt anyone because he rarely used any medication other than sulfa, penicillin, or aspirin; and (2) he was a world-class listener. He was in no hurry to whisk his patients in and out of a "treatment room." Patients would wait for an hour just to have their concerns heard. Sometimes Uncle Charlie didn't speak their language, but he listened, smiled, touched the patients' hands, and told them all that they would be fine. Uncle Charlie's cultural sensitivity came from within his eyes and from his touch. From his slow pace on a hectic day he would give everyone their time and space. To me, this is what we must do with all our patients—rich or poor, happy or depressed, gay or straight.

We are clinicians who must provide our patients with an appearance and understanding of cultural individuality and individual pride. This is how we can improve the care of diabetes in the United States: listen, touch, understand, confide, educate, and praise.

REFERENCES

1. Tripp-Reimer T, Choi E, Skemp Kelley L, et al. Cultural barriers to care: inverting the problem. *Diabetes Spectrum*. 2001;14:13–22.
2. Salti I, Benard E, Detournay B, et al. The EPIDIAR Study Group. A population-based study of diabetes and its characteristics during the fasting month of Ramadan in 13 countries: results of the Epidemiology of Diabetes and Ramadan 1422/2001 (EPIDIAR) study. *Diabetes Care*. 2004;27:2306–2311.
3. Centers for Disease Control and Prevention. U.S. Public Health Service Syphilis Study at Tuskegee. http://www.cdc.gov/tuskegee/timeline.htm. Accessed January 25, 2012.
4. Egede LE, Xiaobou Y, Zheng D, et al. The prevalence and pattern of complementary and alternative medicine use in individuals with diabetes. *Diabetes Care*. 2002;25(2):324–329.
5. National Institutes of Health. The diabetes epidemic among American Indians and Native Alaskans. http://ndep.nih.gov/diabetes/pubs/FS_AmIndian.pdf. Accessed February 4, 2011.
6. Venkat Narayan KM, Boyle JP, Thompson TJ, et al. Lifetime risk for diabetes mellitus in the United States. *JAMA*. 2003;290:1884–1890.
7. Brown AF, Gregg EW, Stevens, MR, et al. Variation in percent mean A1C level for patients of white American, African American, Latino American, and Asian American/Pacific Islander ethnicity. *Diabetes Care*. 2005;28:2864–2870.
8. Lee JWR, Brancati FL, Yeh H-C. Trends in the prevalence of type 2 diabetes in asians versus whites: results from the United States National Health Interview Survey, 1997–2008. *Diabetes Care*. 2011;34(2):353–357.
9. Chiu M, Austin PC, Manuel DG, et al. Deriving ethnic-specific BMI cutoff points for assessing diabetes risk. *Diabetes Care*. 2011;34:1741–1748.
10. Goh KP, Sum CF. Connecting the dots: molecular and epigenetic mechanisms in type 2 diabetes. *Curr Diabetes Rev*. 2010;6 (4):255–265.
11. Hu FB, Li TY, Colditz GA, et al. Television watching and other sedentary behaviors in relation to risk of obesity and type 2 diabetes mellitus in women. *JAMA*. 2003;289:1785–1791.
12. McWilliams JM, Meara E, Zaslavsky AM, et al. Differences in control of cardiovascular disease and diabetes by race, ethnicity, and education: U.S. Trends from 1999 to 2006 and effects of Medicare coverage. *Ann Internal Med*. 2009;150(8):505–515.
13. McWilliams JM, Meara E, Zaslavsky AM, Ayanian JZ. Health of previously uninsured adults after acquiring Medicare coverage. *JAMA*. 2007;298:2886–2894.
14. http://www.nationalaglawcenter.org/assets/farmbills/1949.pdf. Accessed January 25, 2012.
15. Hall TR, Hickey ME, Young TB. Many Farms revisited: evidence of increasing weight and non-insulin dependent diabetes in a Navajo community. In: Joe JR, Young RS, eds. *Diabetes as a Disease of Civilization: The Impact of Culture Change on Indigenous Peoples*. New York, NY: Mouton de Gruyter; 1993:129–146.
16. U.S. Commission on Civil Rights. Broken promises: evaluating the Native American health care system, 1994. http://academic.udayton.edu/health/03access/indian01.pdf. Accessed January 25, 2012.
17. Carter JS, Wiggins CL, Becker TM, et al: Diabetes mortality among New Mexico's American Indian, Hispanic, and non-Hispanic white populations, 1958–1987. *Diabetes Care*. 1993;16:306–309.
18. Gilliland FD, Owen C, Gilliland SS, et al. Temporal trends in diabetes mortality among American Indians and Hispanics in New Mexico: birth cohort and period effects. *Am J Epidemiol*. 1997;145:422–431.
19. O'Connell J, Yi R, Wilson C, et al. Racial disparities in health status: a comparison of the morbidity among American Indian and U.S. Adults with diabetes. *Diabetes Care*. 2010;33(7):1463–1470.
20. Indian Health Service. *Special Diabetes Program for Indians, 2007 Report to Congress: On the Path to a Healthier Future*. Bethesda, MD: Indian Health Service; 2009.
21. IHS Fact Sheet. 2011 Profile. Available online: http://www.ihs.gov/PublicAffairs/IHSBrochure/Profile2010.asp. Accessed January 10, 2012.
22. Tom-Orme L. Traditional beliefs and attitudes about diabetes among Navajos and Utes. In: Joe JR, Young RS, eds. *Diabetes as a Disease of Civilization: The Impact of Culture Change on Indigenous Peoples*. New York, NY: Mouton de Gruyter; 1993:272–291.
23. Broussard BA, Baas MA, Jackson MY. Reasons for diabetes diet noncompliance among Cherokee Indians. *J Nutr Educ*. 1982;14:56–67.
24. American Diabetes Association. Diabetes Basics. http://www.diabetes.org/diabetes-basics/diabetes-statistics/. Accessed January 11, 2012.
25. Parving HH, Lewis JB, Ravid M, et al. Prevalence and risk factors for microalbuminuria in a referred cohort of type II diabetic patients: a global perspective. *Kidney Int*. 2006;69(11):2057–2063.

26. Chan JCN, Malik V, Jia W, et al. Diabetes in Asia: epidemiology, risk factors and pathophysiology. *JAMA*. 2009;301(20):2129–2140.

27. Barnes JE, Bennett CE. The Asian Population: Census 2000 Brief, February 2002, http://www.census.gov/prod/2002pubs/c2kbr01-16.pdf. Accessed February 2, 2012.

28. U.S. Census Bureau News CB11-FF.06, http://www.census.gov/newsroom/releases/pdf/cb11ff-06_asian.pdf. Accessed February 2, 2012.

29. Chesla CA, Chun KM, Kwan CML. Cultural and family challenges to managing type 2 diabetes in immigrant Chinese Americans. *Diabetes Care*. 2009;32(10):1812–1816.

30. Chesla CA, Chun KA. Accommodating type 2 diabetes in the Chinese American family. *Qual Health Res*. 2005;15:240–255.

31. Sampson W. Studying herbal remedies. *N Engl J Med*. 2005;353:337–339.

32. Sue DW, Sue D. *Counseling the Culturally Diverse: Theory and Practice*. 4th ed. New York, NY: John Wiley; 2003.

33. National Diabetes Education Program. National Institutes of Health. The diabetes epidemic among African Americans. Updated 2005. http://ndep.nih.gov/diabetes/pubs/FS_AfricanAm.pdf. Accessed February 11, 2011.

34. Diabetes Prevention Program Research Group. Reduction in the incidence of type 2 diabetes with lifestyle intervention or metformin. *N Engl J Med*. 2002;346:393–403.

35. Trivedi AN, Zaslavsky AM, Schneider EC, et al. Trends in the quality of care and racial disparities in medicare managed care. *N Engl J Med*. 2005;353:692–700.

36. Ibrahim NH, Wang C, Ishani A, et al. Screening for chronic kidney disease complications in U.S. adults: Racial implications of a single GFR Threshold. *Clin J Am Soc Nephrol*. 2008;3:1792–1799.

37. Musey VC, Lee JK, Crawford R, et al. Diabetes in urban African-Americans. I. Cessation of insulin therapy is the major precipitating cause of diabetic ketoacidosis. *Diabetes Care*. 1995;18:483–489.

38. Boult L, Boult C. Underuse of physician services by older Asian-Americans. *J Am Geriatr Soc*. 1995;43:408–411.

39. Fourtner AW, Fourtner CR, Herreid CF. "Bad Blood:" A case study of the Tuskegee syphilis experiment. *J Coll Sci Teaching*. 1994;23:277–285.

40. Boltri JM, Davis-Smith M, Okosun IS, et al. Translation of the National Institutes of Health Diabetes Prevention Program in African American churches. *J Natl Med Assoc*. 2011;103(3):194–202.

41. United States Renal Data System. USRDS 2000 Annual Data Report, Bethesda, MD: National Institutes of Health, National Institute of Diabetes and Digestive and Kidney Diseases; 2000.

42. Giovannucci E, Harlan DM, Archer MC, et al. Diabetes and cancer. *Diabetes Care*. 2010;33:1674–1685.

43. Bonds DE, Zaccaro DJ, Karter AJ, et al. Ethnic and racial differences in diabetes care: The Insulin Resistance Atherosclerosis Study. *Diabetes Care*. 2003;26:1040–1046.

44. Caballero EA, Tenzer P. Building cultural competency for improved diabetes care: Latino Americans and diabetes. *J Fam Pract*. 2007;56(9):S29–S38.

45. Poss JE, Jezewski MA, Gonzalez Stuart A. Home remedies for type 2 diabetes used by Mexican Americans in El Paso, Texas. *Clin Nurs Res*. 2003;12:304–323.

46. Weller SC, Baer RD, Pachter LM, et al. Latino beliefs about diabetes. *Diabetes Care*. 1999;22:722–728.

47. Rios H. *Hispanic Diabetic Elders: Self-Care Behaviors and Explanatory Models*. Iowa City, IO: The University of Iowa Press; 1992.

48. Foreyt JP. Cultural competence in the prevention and treatment of obesity: Latino Americans. *Permanente J*. 2003;7:42–45.

49. Unger J, Parkin C. Type 2 diabetes: an expanded view of pathophysiology and therapy. *Postgr Med*. 2010;122 (3):145–157.

50. Goldfract M, Levin D, Peled O, et al. Twelve-year follow-up of a population-based primary care diabetes program in Israel. *Int J Qual Health Care*. 2011;23(6):674–681.

51. Kalter-Leibovici O, Chetrit A, Lubin F, et al. Adult-onset diabetes among Arabs and Jews in Israel: a population-based study. *Diabet Med*. 2011;Nov 3. doi: 10.1111/j.1464-5491.2011.03516.x.

52. Asleh SA, Chowers I. Ethnic background as a risk factor for advanced age-related macular degeneration in Israel. *Isr Med Assoc J*. 2007;9(9):656–658.

53. Kalter-Leibovici O, Leibovici L, Loya N, et al. The development and progression of diabetic retinopathy in type I diabetic patients: a cohort study. *Diabet Med*. 1997;14(10):858–866.

54. Wolak T, Anfanger S, Wolak A. Target organ damage in hypertensive patients of different ethnic groups. *Int J Cardiol*. 2007;20;116(2):219–224.

55. Jewish Federation of Delaware. http://www.shalomdelaware.org/page.aspx?id=211321. Accessed January 22, 2012.
56. Tripathi A, Rankin J, Aarvold J, et al. Preconception counseling in women with diabetes: a population-based study in the north of England. *Diabetes Care*. 2010;33:586–588.
57. Garnero TL. Providing culturally sensitive diabetes care and education for the Lesbian, Gay, Bisexual, and Transgender (LGBT) community. Diabetes Spectrum 2010;23(3):178–182.
58. Funnell MM, Brown TL, Childs BP, et al. National standards for diabetes self-management education. *Diabetes Care*. 2010;33(suppl 1):S89–S96.
59. Institute of Medicine. *Health Literacy: A Prescription to End Confusion*. Washington, DC: National Academies Press; 2004.
60. Williams MV, Baker DW, Parker RM, et al. Relationship of functional health literacy to patients' knowledge of their chronic disease: a study of patients with hypertension and diabetes. *Arch Intern Med*. 1998;158:166–172.
61. Schillinger D, Grumbach K, Piette J, et al. Association of health literacy with diabetes outcomes. *JAMA*. 2002;288:475–482.
62. Osborn CY, Cavanaugh K, Wallston KA, et al. Diabetes numeracy: an overlooked factor in understanding disparities in glycemic control. *Diabetes Care*. 2009;32(9):1614–1619.
63. Paulos JA. *Innumeracy: Mathematical Illiteracy and Its Consequences*. 1st ed. New York, NY: Hill & Wang; 1988.

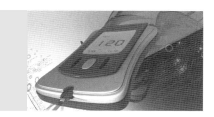

Index

Note: Page numbers followed by f indicate figures; those followed by t indicate tables.

583